HANDBOOK OF ASSESSMENT
AND TREATMENT PLANNING
FOR PSYCHOLOGICAL DISORDERS

HANDBOOK OF ASSESSMENT AND TREATMENT PLANNING FOR PSYCHOLOGICAL DISORDERS

Martin M. Antony
David H. Barlow

Editors

OKANAGAN UNIVERSITY COLLEGE
LIBRARY
BRITISH COLUMBIA

THE GUILFORD PRESS
New York   London

©2002 The Guilford Press
A Division of Guilford Publications, Inc.
72 Spring Street, New York, NY 10012
www.guilford.com

All rights reserved

Paperback edition 2004

No part of this book may be reproduced, translated, stored in a
retrieval system, or transmitted, in any form or by any means,
electronic, mechanical, photocopying, microfilming, recording,
or otherwise, without written permission from the Publisher.

Printed in the United States of America

This book is printed on acid-free paper.

Last digit is print number: 9 8 7 6 5 4 3 2

Library of Congress Cataloging-in-Publication Data

Handbook of assessment and treatment planning for psychological disorders / Martin M.
Antony, David H. Barlow, editors.
    p. cm.
  Includes bibliographical references and index.
  ISBN 1-57230-703-X (hardcover)   1-59385-013-1 (paper)
    1. Mental illness—Diagnosis—Handbooks, manuals, etc. 2. Mental
illness—Treatment—Handbooks, manuals, etc. I. Antony, Martin M. II. Barlow, David H.

RC469 .H356 2002
616.89—dc21   2001040518

To Cindy, Sita, and Kalinda, for their continuing positive assessments of me
—M. M. A.

To Beverly, Deneige, and Jeremy, for love, loyalty, and patience
—D. H. B.

About the Editors

Martin M. Antony, PhD, is Associate Professor in the Department of Psychiatry and Behavioural Neurosciences at McMaster University, as well as Chief Psychologist and Director of the Anxiety Treatment and Research Centre at St. Joseph's Hospital in Hamilton, Ontario. Formerly, he was Assistant Professor in the Department of Psychiatry at the University of Toronto, and was a staff psychologist in the Anxiety Disorders Clinic at the Clarke Institute of Psychiatry (now part of the Centre for Addiction and Mental Health).

Dr. Antony has published eight books, the most recent of which include *The Shyness and Social Anxiety Workbook: Proven Techniques for Overcoming Your Fears* (New Harbinger, 2000), *Phobic Disorders and Panic in Adults: A Guide to Assessment and Treatment* (American Psychological Association, 2000), *When Perfect Isn't Good Enough: Strategies for Coping with Perfectionism* (New Harbinger, 1998), all with Richard P. Swinson, and *Practitioner's Guide to Empirically-Based Measures of Anxiety* (Kluwer Academic/Plenum, 2001), with Susan M. Orsillo and Lizabeth Roemer. He has also published more than 50 research papers and book chapters in the areas of cognitive-behavioral therapy, panic disorder, social phobia, specific phobia, and obsessive–compulsive disorder.

Dr. Antony has received early career awards from the Society of Clinical Psychology (American Psychological Association, Division 12), the Canadian Psychological Association, and the Anxiety Disorders Association of America. He is currently President of the Anxiety Disorders Special Interest Group of the Association for Advancement of Behavior Therapy (AABT) and is Program Chair for the 2001 AABT meeting. Dr. Antony was an advisor to the DSM-IV Text Revision Work Group (Anxiety Disorders) and was involved in producing Ontario practice guidelines for the management of anxiety disorders in primary care. He is Scientific Advisory Editor for *Cognitive and Behavioral Practice,* and is on the editorial boards of *Behavior Therapy, Behaviour Research and Therapy, Clinical Psychology: Science and Practice,* and *Journal of Psychopathology and Behavioral Assessment.* Dr. Antony is actively involved in clinical research in the area of anxiety disorders. He also teaches and maintains a clinical practice.

David H. Barlow, PhD, is Professor of Psychology, Research Professor of Psychiatry, Director of Clinical Training Programs, and Director of the Center for Anxiety and Related Disorders at Boston University. He was formerly Professor of Psychiatry at the University of Mississippi Medical Center and Professor of Psychiatry and Psychology at Brown University, and founded clinical psychology internships in both settings. He was also Distinguished Professor in the Department of Psychology and Director of the Phobia and Anxiety Disorders Clinic at the University at Albany, State University of New York.

Dr. Barlow has published over 400 articles and chapters and over 20 books, mostly in the area of anxiety disorders, sexual problems, and clinical research methodology. His books include *Single Case Experimental Designs: Strategies for Studying Behavioral Change,* Second Edition (Pergamon Press, 1984), with Michel Hersen; *Anxiety and Its Disorders: The Nature and Treatment of Anxiety and Panic,* Second Edition (Guilford Press, 2002); *Clinical Handbook of Psychological Disorders,* Third Edition (Guilford Press, 2001); *Abnormal Psychology: An Integrative Approach,* Second Edition (Brooks/Cole, 1999), with V. Mark Durand; and *The Scientist Practitioner: Research and Accountability in the Age of Managed Care,* Second Edition (Allyn & Bacon, 1999), with Steven C. Hayes and Rosemary O. Nelson-Gray.

Dr. Barlow is the recipient of the 2000 American Psychological Association (APA) Distinguished Scientific Award for the Applications of Psychology, the first annual Science Dissemination Award from the Society for a Science of Clinical Psychology of the APA, as well as the 2000 Distinguished Scientific Contribution Award from the Society of Clinical Psychology of the APA. He also received an award in appreciation of outstanding achievements from the General Hospital of the Chinese People's Liberation Army, Beijing, China, with an appointment as Honorary Visiting Professor of Clinical Psychology. Dr. Barlow is past president of both the Division of Clinical Psychology of the APA and the Association for Advancement of Behavior Therapy and past editor of *Behavior Therapy* and *Journal of Applied Behavior Analysis.* He currently is Editor of *Clinical Psychology: Science and Practice.* A member of the DSM-IV Task Force of the American Psychiatric Association, Dr. Barlow was chair of the APA Task Force on Psychological Intervention Guidelines and cochair of the Work Group for revising the anxiety disorder categories. He is also a Diplomate in Clinical Psychology of the American Board of Professional Psychology and maintains a private practice.

Contributors

Brian V. Abbott, MS, Department of Psychology, Texas A&M University, College Station, Texas

Martin M. Antony, PhD, Anxiety Treatment and Research Centre, St. Joseph's Healthcare, Hamilton, and Department of Psychiatry and Behavioural Neurosciences, McMaster University, Hamilton, Ontario, Canada

Sandra L. Baker, PhD, Center for Anxiety and Related Disorders, Department of Psychology, Boston University, Boston, Massachusetts

David H. Barlow, PhD, Center for Anxiety and Related Disorders, Department of Psychology, Boston University, Boston, Massachusetts

Timothy A. Brown, PsyD, Center for Anxiety and Related Disorders, Department of Psychology, Boston University, Boston, Massachusetts

Lynn F. Bufka, PhD, Center for Anxiety and Related Disorders, Department of Psychology, Boston University, Boston, Massachusetts

Laura A. Campbell, MA, Center for Anxiety and Related Disorders, Department of Psychology, Boston University, Boston, Massachusetts

Linda W. Craighead, PhD, Department of Psychology, University of Colorado, Boulder, Colorado

Jeanne I. Crawford, PhD, MPH, Access Measurement Systems, Ashland, Massachusetts

Keith S. Dobson, PhD, Department of Psychology, University of Calgary, Calgary, Alberta, Canada

David J. A. Dozois, PhD, Department of Psychology, University of Western Ontario, London, Ontario, Canada

Jill T. Levitt, MA, Center for Anxiety and Related Disorders, Department of Psychology, Boston University, Boston, Massachusetts

Brett T. Litz, PhD, Boston University School of Medicine and Boston Veterans Affairs Medical Center, Boston, Massachusetts

Randi E. McCabe, PhD, Anxiety Treatment and Research Centre, St. Joseph's Healthcare, Hamilton, and Department of Psychiatry and Behavioural Neurosciences, McMaster University, Hamilton, Ontario, Canada

Lisa M. McTeague, BA, Center for the Study of Emotion and Attention, University of Florida, Gainesville, Florida

Mark W. Miller, PhD, Boston University School of Medicine and Boston Veterans Affairs Medical Center, Boston, Massachusetts

Charles M. Morin, PhD, School of Psychology, Université Laval, Québec, Canada

Kim T. Mueser, PhD, New Hampshire–Dartmouth Psychiatric Research Center and Department of Psychiatry, Dartmouth Medical School, Concord, New Hampshire

James G. Murphy, MS, Department of Psychology, Auburn University, Auburn, Alabama

Marcus D. Patterson, MA, Department of Psychology, Boston University, Boston, Massachusetts

Sarah I. Pratt, PhD, New Hampshire–Dartmouth Psychiatric Research Center and Department of Psychiatry, Dartmouth Medical School, Concord, New Hampshire

Anna M. Ruef, PhD, Boston University School of Medicine and Boston Veterans Affairs Medical Center, Boston, Massachusetts

Josée Savard, PhD, School of Psychology and Cancer Research Center, Université Laval, Québec, Canada

Douglas K. Snyder, PhD, Department of Psychology, Texas A&M University, College Station, Texas

Ingrid Söchting, PhD, Richmond Mental Health Outpatient Program, Richmond Hospital, Richmond, British Columbia, Canada

Laura J. Summerfeldt, PhD, Department of Psychology, Trent University, Peterborough, Ontario, Canada; Anxiety Treatment and Research Centre, St. Joseph's Healthcare, Hamilton, and Department of Psychiatry and Behavioural Neurosciences, McMaster University, Hamilton, Ontario, Canada

Steven Taylor, PhD, Department of Psychiatry, University of British Columbia, Vancouver, British Columbia, Canada

Dana S. Thordarson, PhD, Department of Psychiatry, University of British Columbia, Vancouver, British Columbia, Canada

Jalie A. Tucker, PhD, MPH, Department of Health Behavior, University of Alabama at Birmingham School of Public Health, Birmingham, Alabama

Rudy E. Vuchinich, PhD, Department of Psychology, University of Alabama at Birmingham, Birmingham, Alabama

Thomas A. Widiger, PhD, Department of Psychology, University of Kentucky, Lexington, Kentucky

Markus Wiegel, MA, Center for Anxiety and Related Disorders, Department of Psychology, Boston University, Boston, Massachusetts

John P. Wincze, PhD, Department of Psychology, Brown University, Providence, Rhode Island; Center for Anxiety and Related Disorders, Department of Psychology, Boston University, Boston, Massachusetts

Preface

With the increased role of managed care in recent years, clinicians have been under pressure to provide services in fewer sessions and to demonstrate the effectiveness of their interventions. In the context of psychological treatments, there has been a movement to develop criteria for identifying empirically valid (or evidence-based) treatments and to use those criteria to select interventions for particular conditions (Chambless & Ollendick, 2001; Weisz, Hawley, Pilkonis, Woody, & Follette, 2000). Increasingly, clinicians are recognizing that not all treatments are equally effective for all psychological problems. Many are seeking specialized training to provide empirically supported treatments (e.g., cognitive-behavioral therapy for anxiety disorders, interpersonal psychotherapy for depression, dialectical behavior therapy for borderline personality disorder).

At the same time, there has been increased recognition that treatments shown to be useful in research settings may not always be as effective when used in typical clinical settings (Seligman, 1996), where patients often have somewhat different presentations than individuals admitted to clinical research trials. In other words, findings from treatment efficacy studies do not always produce exactly the same outcomes when the same strategies are used in the community. Although there is increased awareness of the importance of training in empirically supported treatments, there is also recognition that these treatments need to be researched in the clinical settings where they are most likely to be used (i.e., effectiveness studies).

The recent shift in emphasis to empirically supported treatments has important implications for assessment, an essential component of almost every clinician's training and practice. Only through the process of assessment can a practitioner thoroughly identify the parameters of a patient's problem, choose an effective course of treatment, and measure the outcome of treatment. Just as it is important to select treatments that are supported through controlled research, it is equally important that clinicians use assessment techniques with proven reliability and validity for answering the most important assessment questions. However, it is also important that assessment strategies be brief, practical, and psychometrically sound for the population and setting where they are to be used.

The purpose of this book is to provide clinicians, researchers, and students from a wide range of disciplines with detailed guidelines for assessing individuals suffering from psychological disorders. In addition, chapters discuss how assessment results can be used to select effective interventions and how a clinician can use standard assessment tools to measure the outcome of treatment.

This book is different from other books on assessment in a number of ways. First, traditional psychological assessment texts often emphasize general assessment strategies designed to measure broad aspects of personality, cognitive functioning, and psychopathology. Although these traditional, nonspecific strategies for assessment may be appropriate in settings where nonspecific treatments are likely to be delivered, they often do not provide the information needed to deliver standardized, evidence-based treatments for particular psychological disorders. Instead, selection of an appropriate treatment protocol typically requires that the clinician generate an appropriate diagnosis and select appropriate treatment strategies based on a thorough assessment of relevant symptoms. This book is one of the only assessment texts that is organized with respect to problem areas, rather than assessment modalities. It provides clinicians and researchers with suggestions regarding which instruments should be used when assessing individuals with particular psychological disorders.

This book also differs from other books with respect to breadth of coverage. Although there are other books on the assessment of particular conditions (e.g., addictions, posttraumatic stress disorder), this is one of the few books that thoroughly covers the topic of assessment for a full range of clinical conditions. In addition, this book takes the topic of assessment to the next level, by including detailed suggestions regarding how assessment data can be used to plan an effective course of treatment and how specific assessment tools can be used to measure outcome. Each chapter also includes information about assessing psychological problems in primary care and managed care settings.

The first part of this book contains two chapters that discuss screening methods for various psychological problems. The first chapter, by Summerfeldt and Antony, discusses the use of structured and semistructured interviews to identify particular syndromes. This chapter describes the most popular interviews and reviews the psychometric properties and key features of each. Chapter 2, by Bufka, Crawford, and Levitt, reviews brief assessments that can be used to identify people suffering from specific disorders who present to managed care or primary care settings.

The second part, making up the bulk of the book, contains chapters that each provide detailed information on the assessment of a particular psychological disorder. This section includes chapters on panic disorder and agoraphobia (Baker, Patterson, and Barlow), specific and social phobia (McCabe and Antony), generalized anxiety disorder (Campbell and Brown), obsessive–compulsive disorder (Taylor, Thordarson, and Söchting), trauma (Litz, Miller, Ruef, and McTeague), depression (Dozois and Dobson), obesity and eating disorders (Craighead), couple distress (Snyder and Abbott), schizophrenia (Pratt and Mueser), substance use disorders (Tucker, Vuchinich, and Murphy), personality disorders (Widiger), sexual dysfunction (Wiegel, Wincze, and Barlow), and insomnia (Savard and Morin).

Topics covered in each chapter include (1) an overview of the empirical literature on the most popular tools for screening and for assessing the key features of the disorder, (2) practical suggestions for multimodal assessment of individuals suffering from the disorder, (3) assessment in primary care and managed care settings, (4) using the information collected during the assessment to aid in treatment planning, and (5) strategies for assessing treatment outcome. Many of the chapters include detailed tables comparing and contrasting relevant measures. Most chapters also include a detailed case example, illustrating typical assessment procedures.

We would like to thank the authors of each chapter for their outstanding contributions. In addition, a special thanks to the staff at The Guilford Press for their hard work and support for this project. Finally, we would like to thank Jennifer Mills for providing comments and assisting with the editorial process for certain sections.

Martin M. Antony
David H. Barlow

REFERENCES

Chambless, D. L., & Ollendick, T. H. (2001). Empirically supported psychological interventions: Controversies and evidence. *Annual Review of Psychology, 52,* 685–716.

Seligman, M. E. P. (1996). Science as an ally of practice. *American Psychologist, 51,* 1072–1079.

Weisz, J. R., Hawley, K. M., Pilkonis, P. A., Woody, S. R., & Follette, W. C. (2000). Stressing the (other) three Rs in the search for empirically supported treatments: Review procedures, research quality, relevance to practice and the public interest. *Clinical Psychology: Science and Practice, 7,* 243–258.

Contents

Contents

PART I

SCREENING FOR
PSYCHOLOGICAL DISORDERS

1

Structured and Semistructured Diagnostic Interviews

Laura J. Summerfeldt
Martin M. Antony

The last three decades of the 20th century witnessed a cascade of interest in the development and use of standardized structured and semistructured interviews for the diagnosis of mental disorders. This activity was the culmination of several decades of growing dissatisfaction with the outcomes of traditional unstructured interviews. By the 1970s it was recognized that by using such methods, clinicians commonly arrived at dissimilar diagnoses and rates of diagnostic agreement were no better than could be expected by chance (see Beck, Ward, Mendelson, Mock, & Erbaugh, 1962; Spitzer & Fleiss, 1974). Clearly, this state of affairs hampered advancement of knowledge about psychopathology. Improving the reliability of psychiatric diagnoses became a research priority.

Structured and semistructured interviews are specifically designed to minimize the sources of variability that render diagnoses unreliable. In traditional unstructured interviews, the clinician is entirely responsible for determining what questions to ask and how the resulting information is to be used in arriving at a diagnosis. Substantial inconsistency in outcomes is often the result, even when explicit diagnostic criteria are available for reference. Structured interviews address such issues by standardizing the content, format, and order of questions to be asked and by providing algorithms for arriving at diagnostic conclusions from the information obtained that are in accordance with the diagnostic framework that is being employed.

The use of structured and semistructured interviews is now the standard in research settings. These strategies, administered in various ways, are also becoming the hallmark of empirically driven clinical practice. For example, as outlined in subsequent chapters, many empirically oriented clinicians administer select sections of these interviews to confirm suspected diagnoses or to rule out alternative diagnoses, particularly if time is not available to administer the full instrument. This chapter discusses essential issues in the evaluation and use of structured diagnostic interviews, and reviews several instruments that are currently in widespread use.

ESSENTIAL ISSUES

Criteria for Selecting an Interview

Several factors need to be considered when choosing a structured or a semistructured interview. These are related not only to factors characteristic of the interview itself—such as its demonstrated psychometric qualities, degree of structure (i.e., highly structured vs. semistructured, allowing for additional inquiry) and breadth of diagnostic coverage—but also to the context in which the interview is to be used. Some of the potential considerations, many of them consistently identified in reviews of this literature (e.g., Blanchard & Brown, 1998), are presented in Table 1.1. These pertain to the content, format, and coverage of the diagnostic interview; the level of expertise required for its administration; and the psychometric characteristics and the availability of support and guidelines for its use.

No one instrument best fits the requirements of all clinicians and researchers: When selecting an interview, health care workers must consider their specific needs, priorities, and resources. For example, it might be tempting to consider broad diagnostic coverage, excellent reliability, and validity to be essential criteria in all instances; however, each of these has the potential for drawbacks, and they can sometimes be mutually exclusive. Broad diagnostic coverage (i.e., number of disorders assessed for) often comes at the cost of in-depth information about specific diagnoses—this is the classic "bandwidth versus fidelity" dilemma (Widiger & Frances, 1987). Reliability, or the reproducibility of results, is enhanced by increasing the degree of structure of the interview (i.e., minimizing the flexibility permitted in inquiry and format of administration). However, this inflexibility has the potential to undermine the validity of the diagnosis. Customized questions posed by an experienced clinician may clarify responses that would otherwise lead to erroneous diagnostic conclusions. Such issues warrant consideration.

Understanding Psychometric Characteristics of Diagnostic Interviews

Psychometric qualities are a foremost consideration in judging the worth of any measurement instrument and are equally important to consider when critically evaluating the diagnoses generated by structured and semistructured interviews.

Reliability

The reliability of a diagnostic interview refers to its replicability, or the stability of its diagnostic outcomes. As already discussed, the historically poor reliability of psychiatric diagnoses was a principal basis for the development of structured interview techniques, and this issue continues to be of foremost importance. Inconsistency in diagnoses can arise from multiple sources (see Ward, Beck, Mendelson, Mock, & Erbaugh, 1962, for a seminal discussion), and two of these are particularly worth noting. *Information variance* derives from different amounts and types of information being used by different clinicians to arrive at the diagnosis. *Criterion variance* arises from the same information being assembled in different ways by different clinicians to arrive at a diagnosis and from the use of different standards for deciding when diagnostic criteria are met. Another source of diagnostic inconsistency is patient variance, or variations within the respondent that result in inconsistent reporting or clinical presentation.

Two strategies are principally used to test the reliability of diagnostic interviews. *Interrater* (or *joint*) *reliability* is the most common reliability measure used in this area; here, two or more independent evaluators usually rate identical interview material, which was obtained through either direct observation or videotape of a single assessment; in this case,

TABLE 1.1. Potential Considerations in Selection of a Diagnostic Interview

Coverage and content

- Does the interview cover the time period of interest (e.g., lifetime occurrence, current episode, worst episode)?
- Can the interview assess the course of the disorders of interest?
- Can the interview be used longitudinally to assess change in target symptoms or syndromes?
- Does the interview allow for diagnosis according to the relevant diagnostic system(s) (e.g., DSM-IV, ICD-10)?
- Does the interview cover the disorders of interest?
- Does the interview provide a sufficiently detailed assessment (i.e., Is diagnostic information above and beyond that necessary to meet criteria assessed? Are other variables of interest assessed, such as longitudinal course, demographics, and risk factors)?
- Are chronological markers obtained for comparison with course of disorders (e.g., age when first left home, age of first child)?
- How are symptoms and symptom severity rated (e.g., categorical ratings of present vs. absent, clinical vs. subclinical, or dimensional ratings of continuous degrees)?
- Does the interview assess causes of symptoms for the purpose of differential diagnosis or etiological analysis (e.g., potential organic correlates)?

Target population

- Is the interview developed for, validated with, or applicable to the population of interest (e.g., community respondents, primary care patients, psychiatric patients, specific diagnostic groups)?
- What translations are available, and what validation has been made with the translated version of interest?

Psychometric features

- Is the interview sufficiently reliable for the diagnoses and populations of interest?
- What types of reliability have been established (e.g., interrater, test–retest)?
- Are validity data available for the diagnoses and populations of interest?
- Do validity data support the sensitivity of the measure for subthreshold conditions, if this is a focus of investigation (e.g., in family studies)?
- What types of validation methods have been used for the interview (e.g., comparisons with expert clinical diagnosis, other well-established structured interviews)?

Practical issues

- How long does the interview take to administer, particularly in the population of interest? Estimates often differ significantly for clinical vs. nonclinical respondents.
- Does the interview include a screening module to expedite the assessment?
- Can disorders of lesser relevance be easily omitted?
- Is augmentation with other sources of information (e.g., informants, chart data) required or recommended?
- How feasible is the training required for the interview's use (e.g., self-administered vs. course-based)?

Administration requirements

- Who can administer the interview (e.g., lay interviewers, mental health professionals)?
- What are the system requirements for any computer programs required for scoring or administration (e.g., on site vs. off site)?

Backup

- Are standardized guidelines for administration and scoring available (e.g., user's manual, algorithms/scoring systems for ascertaining diagnoses)?
- Are adequate training materials available?
- Is continued support available for clarification of questions arising from training or the interview's use?

there is only one set of responses to be interpreted and rated. In contrast, *test–retest reliability* involves the administration of a diagnostic interview on two independent occasions, usually separated by a maximum of 2 weeks and often conducted by different evaluators. This, the less commonly used of the two, is a more stringent test of reliability, as variability is potentially introduced due to inconsistencies in styles of inquiry or in respondents self-reports. For example, whereas some respondents may attempt to be overly self-consistent, others may be primed by the initial interview and report novel information at retest. There is also a growing body of evidence that discrepant reporting at retest is due to systematic *attenuation*—that is, respondents' increased tendency to say "no" to items endorsed in the initial interview, perhaps due to their learning more about the nature and purpose of the interview as they gain experience (Lucas et al., 1999).

Interpretation of reports of test–retest reliability is sometimes made difficult due to variations in the methods employed. For example, if supplemental questions are permitted in the follow-up interview to resolve diagnostic ambiguities (e.g., Helzer et al., 1985), the question arises as to whether data should be considered evidence of test–retest reliability rather than a form of validity, as discussed later in this chapter. Interpretability of results is also made challenging by a lack of consistency in the usage of the terms. For example, reliability studies may be described as having a test–retest design only if readministration at retest is conducted by the same rater (see Segal & Falk, 1998) or even when different raters are used (see Rogers, 1995).

Whether test–retest or joint interview designs are employed, the statistic most commonly used to report the degree of reliability observed is Cohen's kappa. Different kappa statistics can be used in different circumstances, such as when several diagnostic categories are possible and when multiple raters' assessments are being compared. The kappa index is superior to a measure such as percentage of agreement because it corrects for chance levels of agreement; this correction can lead to highly variable kappa values due to differing base rates, however. Essentially, the lower the base rate (or higher if base rate is greater than 50%), the lower the kappa, posing a problem for researchers interested in phenomena where the base rates are generally low, such as psychiatric diagnoses. For this reason, another statistic, Yule's Y, is sometimes used because of its greater stability with low to medium base rates (Spitznagel & Helzer, 1985). Intraclass correlation coefficients (ICCs) are also sometimes reported as an index of diagnostic reliability; these are calculated based on variance in ratings accounted for by differences among clinicians and are best used with large samples.

Kappa coefficients range in value from –1.00 (perfect disagreement) to 1.00 (perfect agreement); a kappa of 0 indicates agreement no better or worse than chance. Conventional standards for interpreting kappa values suggest that values greater than .75 indicate good reliability, those between .50 and .75 indicate fair reliability, and those below .50 denote poor reliability (Spitzer, Fleiss, & Endicott, 1978). However, there is some disagreement regarding these benchmarks. Landis and Koch (1977) proposed that kappas within the range of .21 to .40 suggest fair agreement. In summary, there are no definitive guidelines for the interpretation of the kappa statistic; however, researchers usually consider kappas of .40 to .50 as the lower limits of acceptability for structured interviews.

The reliability of a diagnostic interview is determined by many factors. These include the clarity and nature of the questions asked and how well they are understood by the respondent, the degree and consistency of training and experience of interviewers, the conditions in which the interview is conducted, the type of reliability assessed (e.g., test–retest, interrater), the range and complexity of disorders under investigation, and the base rate (or prevalence) of the diagnosis in the target population. In light of this, researchers and clinicians should keep in mind that reliability is not an integral feature of a measurement instrument: it is a product of the context in which it was produced. Thus, reliability estimates are truly meaningful only to other applications of the interview that have comparable circumstances (e.g., administration format, training of interviewers, population). Each study should attempt to establish some form of reliability within its particular constraints. The same caveat applies to the issue of validity.

Validity

The validity of a diagnostic interview is closely bound to the validity of the diagnostic framework it operationalizes. If the way a disorder is conceptualized by, for example, the fourth edition of the *Diagnostic and Statistical Manual of Mental Disorders* (DSM-IV; American Psychiatric Association, 1994) is problematic, a structured interview that loyally adheres to this framework will be invalid, no matter how psychometrically sound it is. Simple convergence between the two, in the words of Rogers (1995), is "hardly more than a tautological exercise" (p. 4). Thus, the matter of "validity" encompasses much larger issues than simple psychometrics and pertains to the very conventions adopted in framing and defining mental disorders (see Widiger & Clark, 2000, for a recent discussion).

Much early work focused on the validity of alternate diagnostic frameworks and criteria (e.g., Feighner or Research Diagnostic Criteria [RDC] vs. DSM; see Feighner et al., 1972; Spitzer, Endicott, & Robins, 1978), or how well they captured the core characteristics of mental disorders. This research focus, though not its underlying premises, has been rendered somewhat obsolete by the widespread adoption of DSM as the predominant psychiatric nosology. Most contemporary research on the validity of structured interviews revolves around the issue of how well they approximate the DSM standard.

Even presupposing the validity of the diagnostic framework used, determining the validity of a diagnostic instrument or how accurately it assesses the conditions it purports to assess poses a considerable challenge for researchers. Primarily, this is because there is no infallible criterion index (i.e., "gold standard") with which interview-generated diagnoses can be compared. Conventional strategy for investigating the validity of a measurement instrument consists of comparing its outcomes to those of another source, known to be a valid index of the concept in question. In the case of diagnostic interviews, other sources of information about diagnoses might include expert diagnosis and/or clinical interview, chart review, or other diagnostic interviews or indexes. Therein lies the problem. Other diagnostic instruments may themselves suffer from psychometric weaknesses, and reliance on clinical diagnosis as an ultimate criterion seems misguided, begging the question of why structured interviews began to be used in the first place. Indeed, Robins, Helzer, Croughan, and Ratcliff (1981) referred to such procedures as "bootstrapping," or using one imprecise method to improve the classificatory accuracy of another.

In light of these issues, Spitzer (1983) proposed the LEAD standard—Longitudinal observation by Experts using All available Data—as an optimal method to establish the procedural validity of a diagnostic instrument. Procedural validity in this case refers to the congruence between diagnoses generated by structured interview versus expert clinicians. The LEAD standard, also known as a *best estimate* diagnosis, incorporates data collected longitudinally from interviews, chart review, and other informants. Expert clinicians then use all available data to come to a consensus diagnosis, which serves as the criterion measure. Unfortunately, this rigorous method is time-consuming and expensive to apply, and has not been widely adopted in validation research to date (see Booth, Kirchner, Hamilton, Harrell, & Smith, 1998, for a recent exception).

There are three principal categories of procedures for determining a test's validity: content-related, construct-related, and criterion-related. In contemporary research on diagnostic interviews, the chief focus has been on the latter, with several forms of particular relevance. Although rarely seen outside of the diagnostic assessment literature, the term *procedural validity* is generally used to denote the degree of congruence between diagnoses generated by structured interview versus expert clinicians. *Concurrent validity* refers to the degree of correlation between scores on the interview in question and scores on another established instrument administered simultaneously. *Predictive validity* denotes the degree to which ratings on the interview are associated with a specified criterion over a time interval (e.g., diagnostic status of the individual or intervening course of the disorder, at follow-up). There is some inconsistency in the use of this terminology, however. It is at times difficult to determine the comparability of validation results because researchers have reported them using different terms. On a more basic level, it has been suggested that the very term "validity" is often erroneously used in this literature (Malgady, Rogler, & Tryon, 1992), in part because of reference to data better regarded as evidence of a diagnostic interview's reliability.

Statistics commonly reported in the context of validity research include the following: (1) *specificity*, or the percentage of noncases of a disorder that has been identified correctly (i.e., poor specificity results in overdetection); (2) *sensitivity*, or the percentage of true cases of a disorder that has been identified correctly (i.e., poor sensitivity results in underdetection); specificity and sensitivity figures are proportional to the total number of noncases and cases, respectively, identified by the instrument; (3) *positive* and *negative predictive values*, or the probability that individuals positive or negative for a diagnosis, according to the instrument being validated, are similarly identified according to the criterion; and (4) *hit rate*, or the number of correct classifications relative to the total number of classifications made. The kappa statistic is commonly reported as a general index of agreement.

In summary, an understanding of the ways in which reliability and validity are defined and evaluated in the literature on psychiatric diagnosis is essential when appraising the relative merits of the many standardized interviews currently available.

REVIEW OF DIAGNOSTIC INTERVIEWS

This section reviews standardized structured and semistructured interviews currently in widespread use. All the instruments reviewed are designed for adult populations and for the principal assessment of symptom syndromes (i.e., those found on Axis I of DSM-IV). Interviews directed solely at specific diagnoses (e.g., mood and anxiety disorders) are discussed elsewhere in this volume and are not included here. Five major instruments are discussed in detail, followed by lesser coverage of three interviews of interest but less widespread application. Table 1.2 presents general characteristics for the former in a highly summarized form. In all cases, contact information is provided for readers who are interested in obtaining or learning more about these interviews.

Anxiety Disorders Interview Schedule for DSM-IV (ADIS-IV)

Context and Description

The ADIS-IV is a clinician-administered, semistructured, diagnostic interview that was developed to establish differential diagnosis among the anxiety disorders, according to DSM-IV criteria. Sections are also included for the diagnosis of mood disorders, somatoform disorders, and substance use disorders, because of their high rates of comorbidity with anxiety disorders. This instrument is one of the most frequently used diagnostic measures among researchers of anxiety disorders. The ADIS-IV provides considerably more detail about

TABLE 1.2. Comparison of Features of Principal Axis I Diagnostic Interviews

Variables	ADIS	DIS	PRIME-MD	SADS	SCID
Relative breadth of diagnostic coverage?	Average	Average	Narrow	Average	Superior
Time in minutes to administer (nonpsychiatric samples)?	45–60	90–120	10–20	60	60
Target population designed for?	Medical and psychiatric patients, community	Community respondents	Primary care patients	Medical and psychiatric patients, community	Medical and psychiatric patients, community
Etiology queried at length?	Yes	Yes	No	No	No
Present diagnosis ascertained?	Yes	Yes	Yes	Yes	Yes
Lifetime diagnosis ascertained?	Yes	Yes	No	Yes	Yes
Recommended rater qualifications?	Trained mental health professionals	Lay interviewers with intensive training	Trained health professionals	Trained mental health professionals	Trained mental health professionals
Dimensional severity ratings possible?	Yes	No	No	Yes[a]	Somewhat[b]
Degree of structure?	Semistructured	Fully structured	Semistructured	Semistructured	Semistructured
Consistent with DSM-IV criteria?	Yes	Yes	Somewhat[c]	No[d]	Yes
Suitable as primary diagnostic measure in psychiatric setting?	Yes	No	No	Yes	Yes

Note. ADIS, Anxiety Disorders Interview Schedule; DIS, Diagnostic Interview Schedule; PRIME-MD, Primary Care Evaluation of Mental Disorders; SADS, Schedule for Affective Disorders and Schizophrenia; SCID, Structured Clinical Interview for Axis I Disorders.

[a]For most current nonpsychotic symptoms only.

[b]Three-point scale: "1," absent; "2," subthreshold; "3," present.

[c]See text regarding its partial exclusion of distress and impairment criteria.

[d]Based on RDC criteria; see text regarding modified versions.

anxiety-related problems than any other popular semistructured interview. This instrument is designed to be used in both clinical and research settings.

Two versions of the adult ADIS-IV are available, both published by the Psychological Corporation/Graywind Publications. The standard version (Brown, Di Nardo, & Barlow, 1994) provides information about current diagnoses only. The lifetime version (ADIS-IV-L; Di Nardo, Brown, & Barlow, 1994) provides diagnostic information for past and current problems. A clinician's manual and a training video are also available from the publisher.

Coverage. The ADIS-IV begins with questions about demographic information, a description of the presenting problem, and information about recent life stresses. This introductory section is followed by sections for assessing the presence of Axis I disorders, beginning with the anxiety disorders (i.e., panic disorder, agoraphobia, social phobia, generalized anxiety disorder [GAD], obsessive–compulsive disorder [OCD], specific phobia, posttraumatic stress disorder [PTSD]/acute stress disorder). The anxiety disorders section is followed by sections for mood disorders (i.e., major depressive disorder, dysthymic disorder, mania/cyclothymia), somatoform disorders (i.e., hypochondriasis, somatization disorder), mixed anxiety-depression (included in Appendix B in DSM-IV, among the criteria sets and axes provided for further study), alcohol abuse/dependence, and substance abuse/dependence. The instrument also includes screening questions for psychotic disorders, conversion symptoms, and familial psychiatric history.

Detailed questions are also included to assess medical history and history of treatment for psychological problems. The Hamilton Anxiety Rating Scale (HARS; Hamilton, 1959) and the Hamilton Rating Scale for Depression (HRSD; Hamilton, 1960) are reprinted in a format that allows both scales to be administered simultaneously. These scales assess the severity of a broad range of symptoms that are often associated with anxiety and depression, and they generate separate anxiety and depression severity scores. Finally, the ADIS-IV also includes questions for coding diagnostic information for DSM-IV Axes III, IV, and V, in addition to Axis I conditions.

Alternate Forms and Translations. A version of the ADIS-IV for children was developed by Silverman and Albano (1996). This version consists of separate child and parent interviews; a manual for clinicians is also available. Like the adult versions of the ADIS-IV, the child versions are published by the Psychological Corporation/Graywind Publications. The child and adult versions of the ADIS-IV have been translated into several languages, including Dutch, French, German, Portuguese, and Spanish.

Format. Each ADIS-IV section includes questions to assess all DSM-IV criteria for the disorder. The section begins with an initial inquiry that typically contains a dichotomous question that can be answered with either "yes" or "no." A positive response to the initial inquiry is followed by more detailed questions about the problem, including questions about each of the DSM-IV criteria. A negative response to the initial inquiry leads the clinician to skip to the next section. For many of the key features of each disorder (e.g., intensity of fear, frequency of avoidance, level of distress and interference), severity is rated on a 9-point scale, ranging from 0 (no fear, avoidance, etc.) to 8 (maximum fear, avoidance, etc.). Each section ends with questions about the etiology and age of onset for the disorder.

As an example, the initial inquiry for the section on panic disorder contains the question "Do you currently have times when you feel a sudden rush of intense fear or discomfort?" followed by questions about the types of situations that trigger the rushes, whether the rushes ever occur out of the blue, the time taken for the rush to reach a peak, and how long the rush lasts at its peak. For individuals who report uncued rushes of fear, the inquiry is continued with detailed questions about the current episode. The ADIS-IV-L also includes sections to assess past episodes. If there is no history of uncued panic attacks, the clinician is instructed to skip to the next section (i.e., agoraphobia).

Psychometric Properties

Reliability. Studies on the ADIS-IV (Brown, Di Nardo, Lehman, & Campbell, 2001) and its predecessors (e.g., Di Nardo, Moras, Barlow, Rapee, & Brown, 1993; Di Nardo, O'Brien, Barlow, Waddell, & Blanchard, 1983) have supported the reliability of this interview. Brown et al. (2001) investigated the reliability of the DSM-IV anxiety and mood disorders based on 362 outpatients who underwent two independent interviews with the ADIS-IV-L. For almost all diagnostic categories, reliability was good to excellent, with most kappas between .60 and .86. Dysthymic disorder was the only condition with poor reliability, with kappas as low as .22.

The most common sources of unreliability varied across disorders. For social phobia, specific phobia, and obsessive–compulsive disorder (but not other disorders), a common reason for diagnostic disagreements involved one clinician assigning the condition at a clinical level and the other clinician assigning the diagnosis at a subclinical level. Differences in patient reports across the two interviews was also a common reason for diagnostic disagreements.

For certain disorders (e.g., social phobia, OCD, PTSD), fewer than 20% of disagreements involved difficulty distinguishing between two disorders, whereas for other problems (e.g., GAD and depression) this was frequently a source of disagreement. For example, patients who received a diagnosis of GAD from one interviewer often received other diagnoses such as major depression, dysthymic disorder, and anxiety disorder not otherwise specified from the other interviewer.

Brown et al. (2001) also evaluated the interrater reliability of the continuous ratings provided in the ADIS-IV (e.g., clinical severity ratings, number of panic attacks, avoidance ratings, severity of depression symptoms). Acceptable levels of reliability were found for most dimensional ratings.

Validity. There are no published studies on the validity of the ADIS-IV. However, many studies have used this instrument to examine features of particular anxiety disorders, and they indirectly support the construct validity of the instrument, as well as the validity of DSM-IV categories. For example, in a panic attack induction study using carbon dioxide inhalation and hyperventilation challenges, Rapee, Brown, Antony, and Barlow (1992) used the ADIS-R (the predecessor of the ADIS-IV) to assign a DSM-III-R diagnosis to outpatients (American Psychiatric Association, 1987). Consistent with previous studies using other diagnostic measures, individuals diagnosed with panic disorder were found to have the strongest response to these challenges, compared to individuals with other conditions.

Summary of Special Issues and Implications for Clinical Application

The ADIS-IV has several features that are worth noting. First, its semistructured format allows the clinician to ask additional questions to clarify the patient's responses and to subsidize the information obtained in the standard interview. The authors of the ADIS-IV recommend that the clinician be familiar not only with the ADIS-IV but also with DSM-IV. Clinical judgment is often needed to generate appropriate follow-up questions. In addition, it may be necessary to differentiate particular conditions from other disorders that are not assessed by the ADIS-IV (e.g., obsessive–compulsive personality disorder, avoidant personality disorder, and body dysmorphic disorder).

Compared to other popular semistructured interviews, such as the Structured Clinical Interview for DSM-IV (SCID-IV), the ADIS-IV has several advantages. The ADIS-IV provides more detailed information about the conditions it assesses, including dimensional ratings for symptoms, inquiries about a larger number of symptom subtypes, and questions about etiology. The ADIS-IV is also one of the only semistructured diagnostic interviews to be available in separate current and lifetime versions. The ADIS-IV has several disadvantages over other structured and semistructured interviews, however. First, the ADIS-IV is relatively time-consuming to administer, with the lifetime version typically taking between

2 and 4 hours in clinical samples. Second, compared to the SCID-IV, the ADIS-IV assesses a more narrow range of disorders.

Contact Information

The ADIS-IV interview and manual are available from Psychological Corporation, Harcourt Brace & Company, 555 Academic Court, San Antonio, TX 78204-2498 (phone: 800-211-8378; Canadian office: 800-387-7278; website: www.psychcorp.com).

Diagnostic Interview Schedule (DIS)

Context and Description

The DIS is a fully structured interview developed to enable both professional and lay interviewers to assess an extensive range of psychiatric diagnoses and their associated features (e.g., duration, age of onset, treatment received). Its most recent version, revised for DSM-IV, is the Diagnostic Interview Schedule, Version IV (DIS-IV; Robins, Cottler, Bucholz, & Compton, 1995). The DIS is the most structured of the interviews reviewed in this chapter, reflecting its origins. It was developed, starting in 1978, at the request of the National Institute of Mental Health, to be used in its large-scale multicenter epidemiological research—the Epidemiologic Catchment Area (ECA) Program. Practical issues dictated the structured format of the DIS. Budgetary considerations compelled the ECA Program to rely on lay interviewers; thus minimization of interviewer judgment—via simplification and standardization of diagnostic questions—was a paramount consideration in its development. A full account of the evolution of the DIS can be found in Eaton and Kessler's (1985) book detailing the methods and rationale of the ECA Program. Although previous versions of the DIS served several diagnostic frameworks, the DIS-IV content and wording focus exclusively on DSM-IV criteria; diagnoses according to alternate systems may at best be approximated; computer scoring is available only for the DIS-IV.

The DIS was also the prototype for the Composite International Diagnostic Interview (CIDI), which expanded on the DIS to permit (1) epidemiological research across a range of cultures and (2) diagnoses according to both the DSM system and the *International Classification of Diseases* (ICD) of the World Health Organization (Robins et al., 1988). The most recent revision of the CIDI, designed to be consistent with DSM-IV and the 10th revision of the ICD (ICD-10), is CIDI version 2.1 (World Health Organization, 1993). The format and coverage of the CIDI 2.1 is relatively comparable to that of the DIS-IV; as such, it will not be discussed in detail here. Andrews and Peters (1998) provide a comprehensive review of the psychometric and practical features of the most recent version of the CIDI, and a review of the last version of the CIDI can also be found in *The Thirteenth Mental Measurements Yearbook* (Impara & Plake, 1998).

Coverage. The DIS-IV comprises 19 diagnostic modules and covers more than 30 major DSM-IV Axis I diagnoses from such categories as mood disorders, anxiety disorders, substance-use disorders, and psychotic disorders, along with one Axis II condition: antisocial personality disorder. DSM-IV Axis I conditions not covered by the DIS-IV include most somatoform disorders (other than somatoform pain disorder), dissociative disorders, most sexual disorders, and delusional disorders. The DIS-IV expanded on previous versions by (1) including four diagnoses found in the DSM-IV Axis I category of disorders first diagnosed in infancy, childhood, and adolescence, including attention-deficit/hyperactivity disorder, separation anxiety disorder, oppositional defiant disorder, and conduct disorder; and

(2) permitting subtyping of several disorders, in line with DSM-IV, including pain disorders, specific phobias, and depressive episodes.

The modular design of the DIS permits investigators to customize the interview by including only those sections relevant to their interests. Each diagnostic section is independent, except in cases where one diagnosis preempts another; sections that can be safely dropped without compromising retained sections are clearly indicated by a mnemonic coding system that is provided in the margins of the measure itself. In addition, the DIS-IV provides termination points, or "exits," to indicate where to drop questioning for particular disorders once it is clear that too few symptoms are present to meet diagnostic criteria. Because these exits are optional, they can be ignored by investigators interested in full-symptom profiles, even in subsyndromal cases.

Alternate Forms and Translations. The fully structured format of the DIS eases its transfer to a computer-administered format, and several self-administered computerized variations of an earlier version of the DIS exist (see Blouin, Perez, & Blouin, 1988). Although these computerized alternatives have the potential advantage of reducing variability that may have been introduced by different raters, they share the common limitation of not covering all DIS diagnoses. A computer-administered version of the DIS-IV, the CDIS-IV, is currently available and can be interviewer- or self-administered with each diagnostic module administered in full, as a screen, or omitted. As yet, no published accounts exist to compare the CDIS-IV with the standard DIS-IV. (See Erdman et al., 1992, for a discussion of pertinent issues with an earlier version.)

An abbreviated paper-and-pencil self-report version of the DIS-III-R was also developed (DIS Self-Administered [DISSA]; Kovess & Fournier, 1990). Importantly, the DISSA restricted its coverage to three conditions thought to be most prevalent in community samples: depressive disorders, anxiety disorders, and alcohol dependence.

The DIS has been translated into Chinese and Spanish, with the Spanish version in particular receiving extensive cross-cultural validation work (see Rogers, 1995, pp. 77–79, for a review). The CIDI 2.1 has been translated into more than 20 languages, among them Arabic, Cantonese, Czech, Dutch, French, German, Greek, Hebrew, Hindi, Italian, Japanese, Korean, Lithuanian, Mandarin, Nepali, Norwegian, Persian, Polish, Portuguese, Russian, Spanish, and Turkish.

Format. All aspects of the format of the DIS reflect the goal of eliminating the need for clinical judgment in the measure's administration. Because the DIS was originally designed for epidemiological research in normative samples, no inquiry is made about a chief complaint or presenting problem; rather, questions proceed through symptoms in a standardized order. The diagnostic sections consist of required core questions about specific symptoms, formatted according to a flowchart. Questions are read verbatim; the interviewer is not free to initiate unstructured, "customized," or reworded questions, and a lack of understanding is to be addressed by repeating the question in the wording provided.

The interview begins with a demographic section. This section expands on standard demographic information (e.g., respondent's education, parenthood status, etc.) in two ways: (1) by asking about chronological markers that might link life events causally with the symptoms reported (e.g., questions about current marital status include ages at which the respondent married, divorced, or was widowed); and (2) by assessing demographic risk factors that are not commonly incorporated into diagnostic interviews, such as history of childhood separation from parents and indices of social status in childhood. Risk factors in other forms are also identified in a section on health behavior and social indicators. Questions included in this section consider such variables as history of problematic or illegal activities (e.g., spousal abuse, use of weapons, and promiscuity), lifetime relationship patterns (e.g., cohabitations), and ages and patterns of such health-related behaviors as tobacco, drug, and alcohol use. The interview then proceeds to the diagnostic modules.

All questions are written to evoke closed-ended answers, with replies coded with a forced-choice "yes"/"no" format. When a respondent answers in the affirmative a question about whether a symptom has ever been experienced, the interviewer then proceeds to a series of standardized contingent questions provided by the measure's Probe Flow Chart. These probe questions, applied to each endorsed symptom, are designed to permit lay interviewers to identify whether a symptom has clinical significance and to rule out any symptoms that can be fully explained by physical conditions or by the taking of drugs, medication, or alcohol. In short, they are designed to ascertain whether each symptom should be counted as a significant psychiatric symptom. As illustration, probes to ascertain clinical significance include questions about whether professional help was sought for the symptom or whether medication was prescribed for it more than once. Probe questions to ascertain whether a symptom should be considered exclusively psychiatric include whether it was the result of an injury or illness and what diagnosis, if any, was made by a physician. This second category of probe questions, designed to ensure that nonpsychiatric symptoms are not counted as criteria for Axis I disorders, has considerable complexity. For example, the interviewer must determine for each symptom not only if the symptom was ever accounted for by organic etiologies but whether this was the case for every occurrence of the symptom. Not surprisingly, these types of differential inquiries can make the DIS quite unwieldy to administer—the original DIS had over 800 contingent probe questions—and administration time for the most recent version (DIS-IV) is estimated by its authors to be 90 to 120 minutes for community-based participants.

Based on answers to the core and subsequent probe questions, each symptom is assigned one of five possible codes: 1 = did not occur; 2 = lack of clinical significance; 3 = medication, drugs, or alcohol; 4 = physical illness or injury (or physical illness plus substance use); or 5 = possible psychiatric syndrome. Thus, unlike most other diagnostic interviews, appraisals of likely etiology are incorporated into assessments of each individual symptom. If a threshold number of symptoms is endorsed (i.e., rated 5) for a specific disorder, the interviewer returns to ask additional questions about the episode or syndrome, including questions regarding its frequency of occurrence and respondent's age at first and last occurrence. Several new features of this part of the interview were introduced with the DIS-IV, including (1) a determination of continuity of symptoms, (2) chronological order of appearance of disorders, and (3) whether the complete syndrome (in addition to its constituent symptoms) appeared in the last year. Data collected in the interview are scored by a computer program, which also assigns diagnoses.

Psychometric Properties

At this time, most available information about the reliability and validity of the DIS derives from studies of earlier versions, and several revisions were made for the DIS-IV. However, consistency in the measure's essential format and much of its content suggest that much of this information remains pertinent. It is important to note that researchers interested in detailed psychometric information for specific populations or disorders are provided with a unique resource by the measure's developers, who, for a small fee, offer a compilation of published articles dating back to 1981.

Reliability. Investigations of the reliability of the DIS have yielded mixed results. The most commonly cited source for reliability data was provided by a series of studies by

Robins et al. (1981; Robins, Helzer, Ratcliff, & Seyfried, 1982), which used a test–retest design to determine the comparability of diagnoses produced by DIS interviews conducted by lay versus professional (i.e., psychiatrist) interviewers. Here, kappas for all DSM-III lifetime disorders, with the exception of panic disorder (.40), were .50 or greater, and the investigators noted that the least reliable diagnoses were for disorders that were in remission or of marginal severity. However, these figures were obtained with a sample that consisted primarily of current or former psychiatric patients, which suggests that the findings might not be generalizable to the more heterogeneous community population for which the DIS was designed. Moreover, subsequent major studies of the reliability of the DIS, employing comparable designs in clinical samples, reported more modest levels of interrater agreement. Helzer et al. (1985; Helzer, Spitznagel, & McEvoy, 1987), for example, using a sample of 370 patients preselected on 11 diagnoses, reported average kappas for lifetime diagnoses of .43 and .37, for test–retests at 6-week and 12-month intervals, respectively. When large nonclinical samples are used, comparable reliability coefficients have been obtained. In a study of 486 undergraduate students using a 9-month test–retest design with lay interviewers only, Vandiver and Sher (1991) reported median kappas of .46 for current diagnoses and .43 for lifetime diagnoses. These investigators also attributed much of the observed unreliability to subthreshold cases.

Study has also been made of the reliability of specific symptom ratings made with the DIS; this issue is important to researchers interested in changes within syndromes (e.g., due to longitudinal course or treatment response). Reported data have been generally promising. For example, Wittchen et al. (1989) found very high levels of agreement regarding the onset and duration of critical symptoms, with most intraclass coefficients greater than .70.

Validity. The literature on the validity of the DIS is at times difficult to interpret and has been critiqued for confusing validity with reliability (see Malgady et al., 1992). Primary studies of the validity of the DIS have traditionally focused on its concurrent/procedural validity or the equivalence of DIS diagnoses with those generated by clinical interview. As already discussed, this is a questionable practice, as it presupposes that psychiatrists' diagnoses represent a truly accurate criterion for validity. Results from this body of research have been variable and controversial. Several early studies reported generally poor concordance. Robins et al. (1982) found a mean agreement of 55% between lay-administered DIS diagnoses and medical chart diagnoses. Using ECA data, Anthony et al. (1985), compared lay-administered DIS diagnoses to DSM-III diagnoses by psychiatrists in a sample of over 800 community residents and found generally poor interrater agreements—kappas ranged from –.02 (panic disorder) to .35 (alcohol use disorder), with an average of .15. However, other investigations in community samples have reported slightly less discouraging figures. Helzer et al. (1985), for example, reported agreement between psychiatrist-administered DIS interviews and clinical diagnoses ranging from .12 to .63, with an average kappa of .40. Therefore, it is not unlikely that threats to the validity of the DIS arise in part from the use of lay interviewers. Indeed, Helzer et al. (1985) observed that nonprofessional interviewers tended to overdiagnose major depression,[1] although underdetection of this diagnosis by the DIS has also been recently noted, relative to clinician diagnosis using the Schedules for Clinical Assessment in Neuropsychiatry (SCAN) (Eaton, Neufeld, Chen, & Cai, 2000). Other problematic categories for the DIS have historically included panic disorder,

---

[1]Evidence for the sensitivity of the DIS, however, can be found in a recent report on the Baltimore ECA Program follow-up study (Eaton et al., 1997). It was found that of the 4.3% of the sample who developed major depression during the follow-up period (median interval of 12.6 years), all had been identified by the original lay-administered DIS as displaying "prodromal" depressive features.

social phobia, and schizophrenia (see Anthony et al., 1985; Cooney, Kadden, & Litt, 1990; Erdman et al., 1987), with the greatest difficulty commonly posed by subthreshold and re-mitted cases (see also Neufeld, Swartz, Bienvenu, Eaton, & Cai, 1999). In general, the speci-ficity of the DIS appears to be stronger than its sensitivity (see Eaton et al., 2000; Murphy, Monson, Laird, Sobol, & Leighton, 2000). Although such findings have led some to con-clude that the DIS's validity does not warrant its use in epidemiological research (e.g., Fol-stein et al., 1985), a more widely held opinion is that while adequate for this application, DIS data should not be considered the sole source of diagnostic information in clinical set-tings (Erdman et al., 1987; Segal & Falk, 1998).

Clearly, investigation of the validity of the DIS for DSM-IV is needed, and some focus areas have been suggested by existing published work. It is worth noting that several revi-sions made for the DIS-IV are pertinent to the areas of concern mentioned. For example, the aforementioned overdiagnosis of major depression may be partly addressed by the new in-clusion of vignettes for this and several other syndromes; such vignettes are used to enhance the respondent's ability to identify symptoms as a cluster. The earlier strategy of relying solely on sequential reporting of discrete symptoms may have inflated estimates due to in-clusion of features common to many physical conditions (e.g., fatigue and appetite loss). Special attention was also paid in the revision to reducing false negatives (i.e., increasing sensitivity) in the ascertainment of panic disorder—identified as problematic for the DIS (Wittchen, 1994)—by its increased emphasis on somatic symptoms, even if fear or anxiety are not endorsed.

Summary of Special Issues and Implications for Clinical Application

The DIS is a well-designed structured interview that has no equal for large-scale epidemio-logical research. The DIS is the only broad-based diagnostic interview specifically designed for use by nonprofessionals, and thus it has both methodological and economic advantages. However, given some of the variable psychometric data reported in the literature, it is key that potential users observe the training recommendations provided by the developers for lay interviewers. Optimal training consists of completion of a 5-day training course, which includes lectures, workbook exercises, small-group practice, and supervised administration with volunteer subjects. Prepared materials for teaching interviewers, such as mock inter-views and homework, are also available; these may be particularly useful for refreshing training as studies progress.

Several unique features of the DIS-IV may be of particular value for certain research questions. These include its coverage of both current and lifetime conditions, its enhanced coverage of demographic and risk factors, its ascertainment of chronology of symptoms and syndromes, and its potential for etiological analysis (i.e., of organic bases of symptoms). Detection of the latter entails complex inquiry and judgment on the part of the interviewer, however. Indeed, Rogers (1995) has suggested that the etiologic component of the DIS is "overly elaborate and unduly refined" (p. 83), given the elusiveness of such conclusive an-swers even when much more sophisticated methods (i.e., laboratory procedures) are used.

Researchers working with some populations should note that the DIS-IV may be vul-nerable to response styles and deliberate faking. Although no published study has been made of this, it is a possibility due to the high face validity of the measure's content and the disallowance of additional inquiry when such strategies are suspected (see Rogers, 1995). Less calculated but similarly confounding response tendencies have been noted in some populations: Eaton et al. (2000) observed consistent underreporting of depressive symp-toms attributed to life crises or medical illness in older respondents and male respondents. Indeed, researchers interested in mood disorders should be generally cautious about using this measure, as these authors and others (Murphy et al., 2000) have concluded that it underestimates the prevalence of major depression in community samples.

The DIS-IV is not suitable as the primary diagnostic method in clinical settings. This arises principally from the history of poor agreement between DIS-based and clinical diagnoses, suggesting the need for augmentation with other sources of data or, preferentially, the use of alternate semistructured interviews (e.g., SCID) that permit more customized inquiry (Blanchard & Brown, 1998). Other practical issues pertinent to clinical settings are worth noting. The standard administration time for the DIS-IV of 90 to 120 minutes is significantly increased for severely ill patients or those with multiple comorbidities, and its detailed etiologic and chronologic inquiry may render the DIS-IV unwieldy in such cases. Although the DIS manual provides instructions for several strategies that can be used to shorten the interview, as discussed earlier in this section, these often come with a loss of potentially valuable information.

Contact Information

For information on DIS materials and training, contact Dr. Lee Robins, Department of Psychiatry, Washington University School of Medicine, 4940 Children's Place, St. Louis, MO 63110-1093 (phone: 314-362-2469). Information on CIDI 2.1 can be obtained from the World Health Organization website: www.who.int.

Primary Care Evaluation of Mental Disorders (PRIME-MD)

Context and Description

The PRIME-MD is a brief clinician-administered, semistructured interview. It was first developed—in the PRIME-MD 1000 study—to permit quick but standardized identification by primary care physicians of DSM-III-R mental disorders most commonly seen in primary care settings (Spitzer et al., 1994), and has been updated for DSM-IV (Spitzer et al., 1995). It is designed for use either as a screening device with all new or established patients or as a diagnostic clarification tool for clients in whom psychiatric difficulties are suspected but not yet identified.

The PRIME-MD has two components:

1. The Patient Questionnaire (PQ), a one-page self-report questionnaire, completed by the patient prior to seeing the physician, containing 25 "yes"/"no" questions about psychiatric symptoms and 1 question about general health.
2. The Clinician Evaluation Guide (CEG), a nine-page interview consisting of five diagnostic modules, used by the interviewer to follow up on items endorsed by the patient on the PQ. The CEG also contains a diagnostic summary sheet.

Coverage.   The PRIME-MD for DSM-IV covers, in part, five current DSM-IV Axis I categories: mood (major depressive [current, recurrent, or partial remission], minor depressive and bipolar disorders, and dysthymia), anxiety (panic disorder, GAD, and anxiety disorder not otherwise specified), somatoform ("multisomataform" or undifferentiated somatoform disorder and somatoform disorder not otherwise specified), eating (bulimia nervosa [purging and nonpurging types] and binge eating disorder), and alcohol-related (alcohol abuse or dependence) disorders. Of these 16 specific conditions, 8 correspond to DSM-IV diagnoses; 3 are "rule-outs" (R/O) (i.e., 1 R/O bipolar disorder, 2 R/O depressive disorder or anxiety disorder) due to general medical condition, medication, or other drug;

and 5 are subthreshold, being characterized by fewer symptoms than are required for specific diagnoses. The self-report PQ screen contains from one to four questions that tap the key symptoms of each of these five categories. Somatic complaints comprise the bulk of the scale's items (15 of 25), and in some cases these may prompt the physician to enter a diagnostic module (e.g., insomnia may trigger questions about depression).

Alternate Forms and Translations. In light of concerns about the time needed for physicians to complete the PRIME-MD for patients who screened positive on the initial questionnaire, an entirely self-administered version of the full measure has been developed (Spitzer, Kroenke, & Williams, 1999). The Patient Health Questionnaire (PHQ), which combines the PQ and the CEQ, covers eight of the original DSM-IV diagnoses found in the PRIME-MD (albeit with some simplification, such as the merging of several depressive disorders into a single category). This version only requires the clinician to confirm self-identified diagnoses and to apply diagnostic algorithms. The PRIME-MD can also be administered by computer, using either desktop or telephone (i.e., interactive voice response [IVR]). The PRIME-MD has been translated into several languages, including Chinese, French, German, and Spanish.

Format. The two components of the PRIME-MD are administered sequentially, with items endorsed by the patient on the PQ triggering the interviewer to enter specific diagnostic modules of the CEG. Within each of the five modules, the interviewer proceeds through questions in sequence and prompts (i.e., "go to") are provided for shifts to ensuing questions. In most cases, these questions are simplified versions of the corresponding DSM-IV criteria. For example, the question "Have you had problems with little interest or pleasure in doing things?" is used to tap DSM-IV major depressive episode criterion symptom of markedly diminished interest or pleasure in all or almost all activities. Because of this, the authors encourage interviewers to supplement the questions with their own requests for further information. Answers are rated as either "yes" or "no." In the mood and anxiety modules, after inquiring about the entire syndrome, the interviewer must determine whether a physical disorder, medication, or other drug could be biologically causing the symptoms. If this is thought to be the case, the diagnosis of "rule out due to physical disorder, medication, or other drug" would be made for the specific disorder.

Psychometric Properties

Reliability. Few true reliability data exist for the PRIME-MD. Existing information consists primarily of comparisons of its diagnoses with those made using different methods. As such, these data are best considered a form of criterion validity and are reported in the following paragraphs. Note, however, that as Skodol and Bender (2000) have indicated, given the similarity of the comparison criteria used in these studies, they might be safely viewed as evidence of joint reliability.

Validity. Evidence for the convergent validity of the PRIME-MD for DSM-III-R was provided by the PRIME-MD 1000 study, where for 431 patients, the measure was compared to telephone interviews with mental health professionals using relevant questions from the SCID for DSM-III-R. Here, the sensitivity of the PRIME-MD for detecting any diagnosis was good (.83), with figures for specific diagnoses ranging from .22 for minor depressive disorder to .81 for probable alcohol abuse or dependence. Specificity was excellent for diagnostic modules, ranging from .92 for any mood disorder to .99 for any eating disorder. Overall diagnostic accuracy was very good to excellent, ranging from .84 for any mood disorder to .96 for any eating disorder, though the validity of the somatoform module was not investigated.

More recent data are available for the two new alternate forms of the measure developed for DSM-IV. In a validation study of the PHQ, the self-report version for DSM-IV (Spitzer et al., 1999), 3,000 patients from a range of primary care settings completed the PHQ, 585 of whom then underwent a blind telephone diagnostic assessment with a mental health professional. Kappas for categories of disorder ranged from .58 for any mood disorder to .61 for any eating disorder, with an overall agreement regarding the presence of any diagnosis of .65 and overall accuracy of .85, sensitivity of .75, and specificity of .90. These figures, though the kappas fall only within the "fair" range, suggest that the PHQ provides information comparable to that of the PRIME-MD. As well, there is evidence for the criterion validity of the computer-administered version for DSM-IV: in a study with 200 outpatients from multiple primary care and specialty clinics, Kobak et al. (1997) compared outcomes of interactive voice response (IVR) PRIME-MDs with telephone interviews (SCID for DSM-IV) with a trained clinician and found comparable prevalence rates for specific disorders and fair overall agreement for the presence of any diagnosis (kappa = .67).

Evidence for the construct validity of the PRIME-MD also derives from findings that its positive diagnoses are highly associated with specific indices of functional impairment. Such findings have been reported using the PRIME-MD for DSM-III-R (Nease, Volk, & Cass, 1999; Spitzer et al., 1995; see also Linzer et al., 1996) and the PHQ (Spitzer et al., 1999).

Findings with specific populations similarly support its validity and clinical utility. Positive diagnoses on its mood module have been found to predict prior history of depression and pain in patients undergoing radiation therapy (Leopold et al., 1998) and high utilization of services in primary care patients (Lefevre et al., 1999). Diagnoses on the mood and anxiety modules have also been found to be associated with patient dissatisfaction following a visit to a general medical clinic regarding physical complaints and with physicians' ratings of the perceived difficulty of this encounter (Kroenke, Jackson, & Chamberlin, 1997).

In short, evidence for the validity of the PRIME-MD is quickly accumulating and points to its utility with a range of primary care patients and special populations. Particular study needs to be made of the validity of the somatoform module, however, given its implications for approaches to patient difficulties in primary care settings.

Summary of Special Issues and Implications for Clinical Application

Both the PRIME-MD and PHQ provide primary care physicians with much-needed, extremely time-efficient, standardized tools for identifying the mental disorders most commonly seen in their settings. In the PRIME-MD 1000 study, the average time required for completion of the CEG was 11.4 minutes for patients with PRIME-MD diagnoses and 5.6 minutes for those without (Spitzer et al., 1994). The PHQ, the newer self-report DSM-IV version, further reduces this time commitment, typically to less than 3 minutes.

The price paid for the efficiency of the PRIME-MD is breadth and detail. Its limited diagnostic coverage is one aspect of this; another is that diagnosis with the PRIME-MD does not absolutely correspond to DSM diagnosis. For example, an important feature of DSM-IV is the inclusion, for most disorders, of an explicit functional impairment and subjective distress criterion. That is, the diagnosis cannot be given unless the syndrome causes clinically significant subjective distress and/or functional impairment. The PRIME-MD does not include this criterion in its sections for major depressive and somatoform disorders, suggesting that the measure could lead to overdiagnosis of these conditions. Similarly, the PRIME-MD directs the interviewer to proceed through all questions for major depression, irrespective of whether key criterion symptoms have been met.

Test–retest and interrater reliabilities for the measure are needed, particularly in light of features of the contexts in which it is used. Although the measure's developers encourage interviewers to supplement questions with further inquiry, time constraints in primary care settings likely preclude this. Systematic investigation of whether inconsistencies in this practice result in poor reliabilities would be of value, particularly for subsets of patients where rates of PRIME-MD diagnosis for multiple disorders have been found to be high (see, e.g., Linzer et al., 1996).

Users should note that although the PRIME-MD includes bipolar disorder in its list of rule-out diagnoses, requisite symptoms for this syndrome are not included in the standard questions and the one question devoted to it—"Did the doctor ever say you were manic-depressive or give you lithium?"—may be inadequate to detect bipolar disorders, particularly if past episodes were of hypomania.

In summary, the PRIME-MD is an adequate measure when used for the purposes for which it was designed. However, it is limited by its basic coverage of only a few of the mental disorders seen in psychiatric settings and by its only rough equivalence to DSM-IV criteria for those disorders it does cover. This is even more true of the PHQ. Clearly, neither one should be seen as a substitute for a more thorough diagnostic interview for Axis I disorders, particularly for complex cases where differential diagnosis may be of importance. More detailed information on the PRIME-MD and its use in primary care settings is included in a recent review chapter by Hahn, Kroenke, Williams, and Spitzer (2000).

Contact Information

The PRIME-MD is under copyright to Pfizer, Inc. Free copies of PRIME-MD and PHQ materials can be obtained from Dr. Robert L. Spitzer, Biometrics Research Department, New York State Psychiatric Institute, Unit 60, 1051 Riverside Drive, New York, NY 10032 (phone: 212-543-5524).

Schedule for Affective Disorders and Schizophrenia (SADS)

Context and Description

The SADS (Endicott & Spitzer, 1978) is a clinician-administered, semistructured interview that was developed to permit diagnosis of a range of psychiatric diagnoses according to the research diagnostic criteria (RDC) of Spitzer, Endicott, and Robins (1978). The history and rationale of this diagnostic system have been described in detail by these authors (see also Zwick, 1983). A precursor of DSM-III, RDC was proposed in an effort to address diagnostic error (i.e., arising from information and criterion variance) at a time when such error was a widely recognized impediment to psychiatric research. The developers of the SADS were particularly interested in this issue as it pertained to the description and diagnosis of depressive disorders, and the measure was first used in a large, NIMH-sponsored collaborative study of the psychobiology of depression. Subsequently, the SADS has undergone several expansions, though its permutations remain wedded to the RDC diagnostic system and continue to offer unparalleled coverage of issues germane to research on depression.

The SADS is available in several versions, each designed to meet a different need. The versions differ primarily in terms of the time period that is the focus of assessment:

1. The regular version (SADS) has two parts: Part I covers symptoms of current (i.e., within the past year) mental disorders, and Part II covers past history (i.e., beyond the past year before assessment) of mental disorders.
2. The lifetime version (SADS-L) is similar to Part II of the SADS, except that the time period is not restricted to the past and includes any current symptoms.
3. The change version (SADS-C).

The SADS and SADS-L are the most widely used, and it is important to note that their different temporal focus has implications for depth of coverage. Although the SADS-L permits lifetime (i.e., past and present) diagnostic coverage, information about current episodes is considerably less detailed than that provided by the SADS. As Arbisi (1995) has noted, the SADS-L is therefore more suitable for use in nonpsychiatric samples or when the interviewee is currently symptom free, or where such detail is deemed unnecessary. Also available are the following:

4. The SADS-LB, which is similar to the SADS-L but contains additional items related to bipolar illness.
5. The SADS-I (interval) version, similar to the SADS-C but with a lifetime emphasis.
6. The family history version, the FH-RDC, designed to elicit diagnostic data from family members about their relatives.
7. The SADS-LA, similar to the SADS-L, but with expanded coverage of anxiety disorders.

Importantly, the SADS-LA is alone among these in incorporating not only RDC criteria but also those from DSM-III and DSM-III-R (Fyer, Endicott, Mannuzza, & Klein, 1985), and, most recently, DSM-IV (SADS-LA-IV; Fyer, Endicott, Mannuza, & Klein, 1995).

Coverage. In general, the SADS has less breadth of coverage than other general diagnostic interviews currently available, although there are differences among its various versions. The original versions (SADS and SADS-L) enable coverage of 23 major diagnostic categories according to the RDC, a few of which also have multiple subtypes. Disorders covered include schizophrenia spectrum disorders, mood disorders (major depressive, manic–depressive [i.e., bipolar], and minor depressive disorders), anxiety disorders (panic, obsessive–compulsive, phobic, and generalized anxiety disorders), alcohol and drug use disorders, three personality disorders (cyclothymic, labile, and antisocial disorders), two categories of "unspecified functional psychosis," and other psychiatric disorders. The SADS also yields scores for eight dimensional "summary scales" that were derived through factor analysis: depressive mood and ideation, endogenous features, depressive-associated features, suicidal ideation and behavior, anxiety, manic syndrome, delusions-hallucinations, and formal thought disorder (Endicott & Spitzer, 1978). The design of the SADS permits investigators to skip sections that are considered to be less relevant and/or as indicated by nonendorsement of screening questions.

Historically, investigators have been in the practice of modifying the SADS according to their needs. These modifications may occur (1) at the item level (i.e., incorporating additional items within existing categories to allow DSM diagnoses), and/or (2) at the level of diagnostic category (i.e., adding sections to allow for identification of diagnoses not covered by the SADS). For example, one of the most recent additions to the SADS family—the aforementioned SADS-LA-IV (Fyer et al., 1995)—has modifications at both the item and category levels. The former were made to permit diagnoses according to both RDC and to all versions of DSM after and including DSM-III. The latter include expanded and updated (i.e., DSM-IV-congruent) coverage of anxiety disorders (including posttraumatic stress disorder and panic disorder subtypes) and antisocial personality disorder, and the addition of such diagnostic categories as separation anxiety disorder in childhood, hypochondriasis, and somatization and tic disorders.

Alternate Forms and Translations. Neither the SADS nor its more recent modified versions are available in a computerized format, primarily because of the flexibility and clinical judgment necessary in its administration. The SADS has been translated into 10 languages, and information about these translations is available from Jean Endicott (see contact information at the end of this section). Translations have also been made of subsequent modified versions (e.g., SADS-LA; see Leboyer et al., 1991).

Format. The versions of the SADS differ somewhat in their overall layout and format. The SADS begins with a brief scorable overview of the interviewee's background and demographics (i.e., education, peer relations, marital status, work history, hospitalizations) and open-ended questions about the course of any past illnesses. The interviewer then proceeds to the main diagnostic body of the SADS.

In Part I, individual symptoms for each of the covered disorders are rated (1) for the worst period of the current episode and (2) for the current time period (i.e., the week before the interview). This unique and valuable feature of the SADS minimizes day-to-day fluctuations in symptoms that might obscure ascertainment of the disorder's severity (Endicott & Spitzer, 1978; Rogers, 1995). Another noteworthy feature of Part I is its reliance on dimensional ratings of severity of symptoms. For both of the time periods rated (i.e., at worst and in past week), most individual symptoms are rated on multipoint scales. Except in the case of psychotic symptoms, typically rated on a 3-point scale, a 6-point scale is usually employed, having such values as, 1 = not at all; 3 = moderate, a frequent symptom or symptoms of low to medium intensity; and 6 = extreme, unremitting symptoms of high intensity. A rating of 0 is used if no information is available or if the item is not applicable. Clinically significant symptoms are identified with cut points on these scales. Furthermore, each of these numeric ratings is accompanied by a descriptive severity anchor for the symptom in question. For example, anchors for ratings for the manic syndrome criterion of increased energy include 3 = "little change in activity level but less fatigued than usual," and 6 = "usually active all day long with little or no fatigue."

Part II of the SADS, as well as the SADS-L, is organized by specific syndrome. Within each section, questions are provided regarding: (1) screening criteria, (2) individual symptoms of the condition, (3) degree of severity/impairment (i.e., evidence of clinical intervention or change in functioning), and (4) associated features. Importantly, this component of the SADS employs only dichotomous scoring for specific symptoms ("no," "yes," or "no information") as respondents' recall for precise details of past episodes is considered unreliable. After all symptoms are rated, the interviewer consults the RDC to arrive at diagnoses according to the clinically significant symptom ratings.

The SADS, particularly its Part I, is a truly semistructured interview. Several levels of inquiry may be used for each symptom: standard questions; optional probes, in order to clarify or challenge ambiguous responses; and nonstandardized "custom" questions, formulated by the interviewer and used, as needed, to further clarify responses and facilitate the rating process. In addition, for many diagnostic sections of the SADS, key branching questions serve as screens; their nonendorsement allows the interviewer to skip sections of the interview, though investigators often choose to ignore such "skip out" opportunities, depending on their specific interests and purposes (Rogers, 1995; Segal, 1997). Use of all these levels of inquiry is strongly encouraged by the measure's developers, as is the use of gentle challenges and/or reference to all available sources of information (e.g., patient charts, reports from relatives) when necessary.

Questions regarding associated features, included in many of the diagnostic sections, provide such clinically significant information as mode of onset, duration, life context and relationship to psychosocial stressors, physical illness, drugs or medications, and treatment history for the syndrome in question.

Psychometric Properties

In part because of the number of modifications of the SADS, coverage of all information regarding its reliability and validity is beyond the scope of this review. Conoley and Impara (1995, pp. 908–917) include a discussion of its applications with specific populations and provide a list of over 400 test references.

Reliability. A detailed summary of studies of reliability of the SADS may be found in Rogers (1995), where it is noted that "more than other diagnostic interviews, the SADS has benefited from careful attention to the various elements of reliability" (p. 88). In general, studies using a range of designs have demonstrated good to excellent reliabilities, and this is consistent with the findings of the comprehensive studies originally conducted by the measure's developers. Researchers have sought to determine reliability of all levels of SADS output: diagnosis, summary scale scores, and symptom ratings.

Reliability of diagnoses was evaluated by Spitzer, Endicott, and Robins (1978) using a test–retest design in two inpatient samples. Concordance rates were high for current (median kappa = .91) and lifetime (median kappa = .93) RDC diagnoses, although a greater range was found for the latter. Also using a test–retest design, Andreasen et al. (1981) found equally impressive reliabilities for lifetime RDC diagnoses in a nonpatient sample, with results based on both immediate (average ICC = .87) and 6-month (average ICC = .72) test–retest intervals. In a study using an extended interrater design that involved challenging videotaped interviews and 36 independent raters, Andreasen et al. (1982) also found high rates of agreement (average ICC = .75). More recently, Leboyer et al. (1991) used a combined interrater and test–retest design to study a translated version of the SADS-L in psychiatric patients and their relatives; they reported concordance to be good for current DSM-III-R diagnoses (all kappa > .80), though less so for lifetime diagnoses (average kappa = .52). In these and other studies, hypomania has emerged as among the least reliable of SADS-generated diagnoses.

Reliability of the SADS at the level of summary scales has also been well demonstrated. Endicott and Spitzer (1978) reported the results of the two original studies. One used an interrater design with joint interviews of psychiatric inpatients and found very high agreement (average ICC = .96) for all summary scales, as well as evidence for the good internal consistency of all but the anxiety and formal thought disorder scales. The second study used a test–retest design with an inpatient sample and produced agreement rates for summary scales that were slightly lower than those from the joint evaluations but still sizeable (median ICC = .83) for all but formal thought disorder.

Evidence of the reliability of specific symptoms (i.e., SADS items) is without equal among diagnostic interviews. In the samples described previously, Endicott and Spitzer (1978) found the 120 items of the current section of the SADS to display substantial reliability for both joint and test–retest interviews (i.e., the majority of ICCs ≥ .60). Subsequent investigations of these items or subsets thereof have reported comparable and often more robust reliabilities (e.g., Andreasen et al., 1982; Keller et al., 1981; McDonald-Scott & Endicott, 1984).

In summary, compelling evidence exists for the reliability of the SADS at all levels of assessment.

Validity. More than other structured interviews, evidence for the criterion-related validity of the SADS derives from studies not only of its concordance with other methods of diagnosis (i.e., concurrent validity) but of its ability to predict meaningful patterns in the syndromes it assesses. Many studies have used versions of the SADS to examine genetic and familial correlates of mental disorders. Indeed, Maziade et al. (1992), in their review of existing genetic-linkage studies for bipolar disorders, found that the majority of those using structured diagnostic interviews used some version of the SADS. SADS-generated diagnoses have also been used to successfully detect familial patterns of schizophrenia and related disorders (Kendler, Gruenberg, & Kinney, 1994; Stompe, Ortwein-Swoboda, Strobl, & Friedmann, 2000) and obsessive–compulsive and related disorders (Bienvenu et al., 2000). In addition, the instrument's diagnoses and summary scale scores have been found to predict course, clinical features, and/or outcome in schizophrenia (Loebel et al., 1992; Stompe et al., 2000), major depression (Coryell et al., 1994), and bipolar disorder (Vieta et al., 2000). It also bears mentioning that convergent validity is of particular relevance in the case of the SADS, based as it is on a diagnostic system other than that of DSM. Concordance between specific SADS-generated RDC and DSM-based diagnoses is detailed in the reference list provided by Conoley and Impara (1995).

Summary of Special Issues and Implications for Clinical Application

The SADS offers unparalleled coverage of subtypes and gradations of severity of mood disorders, and an extensive literature exists on its applications in research. Its use of multipoint ratings permits a more fine-grained picture of current status than is found in many diagnostic instruments. This depth of coverage has several strengths, among them (1) increasing the reliability values that can be expected at both the symptom and diagnosis level; and (2) enabling greater sensitivity to change in symptoms, even when they appear at subthreshold levels. In particular, researchers interested in the assessment of lifetime mood disorders should note the SADS's record of reliably establishing prior episodes and the evidence that has accrued for its predictive validity regarding future course of the disorder. The cost of this depth of coverage is breadth: the SADS includes fewer diagnoses than other general interviews. Although this deficit has been addressed in part by more recent revisions, even for those that have undergone standardization (i.e., SADS-LA and SADS-LA-IV) less multisite study has been made of their psychometric characteristics.

For many researchers, a pivotal issue to be considered in the use of the SADS is its linkage to RDC. For many of the disorders covered by the interview, particularly in the categories of mood and schizophrenia, the criteria used correspond quite closely to those of DSM-IV. In other cases, however, clinicians and researchers interested in DSM-based diagnostic classification must augment pertinent sections with items congruent with DSM-IV. This is particularly true for the anxiety and somatoform disorder categories. Deficiencies in the SADS with regard to the former category and to a lesser extent to the latter have been addressed by the development of the SADS-LA and later the SADS-LA-IV, both of which offer complete coverage of DSM anxiety disorders. The antisocial personality disorder sections in the SADS Part II and SADS-L also bear particular mention. Criteria for this disorder have undergone several changes throughout the revisions of DSM that are not reflected in the RDC; researchers and clinicians interested in this diagnosis must either augment the SADS with extensive DSM-IV-based questions (see Carroll, Ball, & Rounsaville, 1993) or use the SADS-LA-IV, which has updated items in this section to correspond to DSM-IV. This all said, it must be noted that reliance on a diagnostic system other than DSM should not necessarily be seen as an intrinsic flaw, as discussed earlier in this chapter. As Skodol and Bender (2000) have noted, many of the principles that inform current understanding of major depression—including its clinical features (e.g., course, prognosis), etiology, and treatment—have derived from studies that have relied not on DSM-IV, but on the RDC.

The level of clinical expertise needed for administration of the SADS has long been noted by reviewers. Clinical judgment, interviewing skills, and familiarity with diagnostic criteria and issues germane to differential diagnosis are all crucial for its competent administration (Rogers, 1995; Segal, 1997; Skodol & Bender, 2000). Indeed, the measure's developers recommend that it be given only by professionals who have graduate degrees and clinical backgrounds, such as psychiatrists, clinical psychologists, and psychiatric social workers. Furthermore, special training in SADS interviewing is requisite; this is an intensive and potentially lengthy (i.e., several-week) process, with such recommended elements as (1) reading the most recent SADS manual and articles on both the SADS and the RDC, (2) practice rating of both written case vignettes and videotaped SADS interviews, (3) establishing interrater agreement among trainee and experienced clinician ratings of practice cases, and (4) administration of real SADS interviews under the direct supervision of experienced SADS interviewers. In short, the SADS is not suitable in contexts where (1) lay interviewers or junior clinicians are used, (2) access to clinicians with SADS experience is limited, or (3) the necessary training program is precluded by time constraints.

Administration of the SADS can be similarly time-consuming. Although the SADS can be administered to healthy respondents in 1 hour or less, employment of multiple gradations of rating for each symptom in Part I means that the interview commonly requires 2 to 4 hours for psychiatric patients. This may be of particular concern to researchers in settings that serve clinical populations where multiple comorbidities may be anticipated.

Contact Information

Copies of the SADS and related materials are available from Dr. Jean Endicott, Department of Research Assessment and Training, New York State Psychiatric Institute, Unit 123, 1051 Riverside Drive, New York, NY 10032 (phone: 212-543-5536).

Structured Clinical Interview for DSM-IV Axis I Disorders (SCID)

Context and Description

The SCID is a clinician-administered, semistructured interview developed to permit diagnosis of a broad range of psychiatric disorders according to DSM-IV. Of the interviews reviewed in this chapter, the SCID is probably the most widely used in North American research; in a review of its predecessor, the SCID for DSM-III-R, Williams et al. (1992) noted that "[this is] attested to by more than 100 published studies that have used the instrument to select or describe their study samples" (p. 630). This popularity has continued with the measure's latest revision. The instrument was initially designed to address the perceived need for an interview to closely operationalize diagnostic criteria for DSM-III, and has subsequently undergone several revisions and expansions. Its mandate of remaining closely tied to DSM criteria has persevered, however. The history and rationale of its development have been described in detail elsewhere (see Segal, Hersen, & van Hasselt, 1994; Spitzer, Williams, Gibbon, & First, 1992).

In light of criticisms that earlier versions had sacrificed useful diagnostic information in order to render them less cumbersome for clinicians, the SCID for DSM-IV Axis I disorders was made available in two versions designed to meet different needs: the SCID-CV (clinician version) (First, Spitzer, Gibbon, & Williams, 1997), and SCID-I (research version)

(First, Spitzer, Gibbon, & Williams, 1996). In addition, a separate and complementary interview for Axis II personality disorders is available (SCID-II).

The clinician version (SCID-CV), the briefest of these versions, serves to provide standardized assessment in clinical settings but includes full diagnostic coverage of only those DSM-IV disorders commonly seen in clinical practice. In contrast, the research version (SCID-I) is intended for use in research settings and is much longer than the clinician version. It permits ascertainment of information that is potentially of interest only to researchers, including more disorders and their subtypes, severity and course specifiers, and provisions for coding the details of past mood episodes. The SCID-I is itself available in three standard versions.

1. SCID-I/P—the broadest of these versions—is designed for subjects already identified as psychiatric patients.
2. The SCID-I/P with Psychotic Screen, an abridged version of the SCID-I/P, is designed for patients also in psychiatric settings but where psychotic disorders are expected to be rare or where a screen for psychotic disorders would suffice. Here, screening questions about psychotic symptoms replace the lengthy and complex psychotic disorders module of the SCID-I/P.
3. The SCID-I/NP (nonpatient version), for use with subjects who are not identified as psychiatric patients (e.g., in community surveys, family studies, research in primary care, or general medical settings). This last version makes no assumption of a chief complaint and uses other questions to inquire about a history of psychopathology.

Coverage. As already indicated, the various versions of the SCID differ primarily in their breadth of coverage of Axis I disorders. The full version (SCID-I/P) enables the broadest range of diagnostic coverage of all the widely used diagnostic interviews, with the main body comprising nine diagnostic modules: Mood Episodes, Psychotic Symptoms, Psychotic Disorders Differential, Mood Disorders Differential, Substance Use Disorders, Anxiety Disorders, Somatoform Disorders, Eating Disorders, and Adjustment Disorders. In addition, an optional module is provided to enable diagnosis of disorders potentially of research interest, including some currently appendixed in DSM-IV (e.g., minor depressive disorder). A total of 51 DSM-IV Axis I disorders are covered by the SCID-I/P. The modular design of the SCID permits investigators to customize the interview by including only those modules that are relevant to their needs—a practice encouraged by the interview's developers.

Alternate Forms and Translations. Computerized versions of the SCID are available as (1) clinician-administered programs for diagnosis of DSM-IV (both Axis I and Axis II) disorders, in which the program acts as an "interview-driver"; (2) patient self-report screening questionnaires for Axis I disorders; and (3) comprehensive patient self-reports for both Axis I and Axis II disorders. Although the SCID may be administered by telephone, findings with the DSM-III-R version suggest that this may result in poor congruence with in-person findings, particularly for current diagnoses (Cacciola, Alterman, Rutherford, McKay, & May, 1999).

Format. The SCID begins with an open-ended overview that provides demographic information (e.g., marital status), work history, chief complaint, history of present and past periods of psychopathology, treatment history, and assessment of current functioning. This preliminary section elicits responses in the subject's own words and has several benefits. First, it encourages rapport building prior to the more structured symptom-focused format of the main body of the SCID. Second, the information elicited provides context (i.e., life events, psychosocial stressors) that are potentially useful in interpreting responses to subsequent diagnostic questions. This overview concludes with an optional screener, containing 12 questions that can be used to decide whether subsequent diagnostic sections may be skipped. The interviewer then proceeds to the main body of the SCID, composed of the diagnostic modules.

The diagnostic sections consist of required probe questions and suggested follow-up questions. Next to each probe the SCID presents the corresponding DSM-IV diagnostic criteria for each disorder, which are to be rated in a three-column format as follows: (1) absent or false, (2) subthreshold (i.e., present but of subthreshold duration or severity and therefore not counted), or (3) true (i.e., present and of clinically significant duration or severity). A fourth rating option—?—is used when there is insufficient information (e.g., the interviewee cannot recall or is uncertain). Ratings are made on the basis of the probe question and any follow-up questions deemed necessary. Although probe questions, to be asked verbatim, may produce an unelaborated "yes" or "no" answer, this answer is often inadequate to determine whether the corresponding criteria have been met and additional clarifying questions are necessary. For example, First et al. (1996) recommend that an affirmative answer to the delusion of reference question—"Has it ever seemed like people were talking about you or taking special interest in you?"—should be followed up by a request for specific examples that establish the psychotic nature of the belief as the standard question, alone, has a high false positive rate. This is an important feature of the SCID, as recorded ratings are of diagnostic criteria, not of the interviewee's answers to the questions. Another key feature is the regular use of "skip-out" directions, which direct the interviewer to skip subsequent questions when a subject does not meet a critical criterion required for a particular disorder (e.g., the 2-week duration criterion for depressed mood or loss of interest in a major depressive episode). In other words, inquiry into additional symptoms of a condition is not then standardly made. As a consequence of these and other features, the SCID requires considerable clinical judgment on the part of the interviewer.

Psychometric Properties

At this time, most available information about the reliability and validity of the SCID derives from studies of its earlier DSM-III-R version. Nonetheless, the minimal changes entailed in its revisions for DSM-IV suggest that this information remains pertinent.

Reliability. A complete summary of reliability studies for the SCID for DSM-III-R may be found in Segal et al. (1994). By far the most comprehensive examination of the reliability of the full version SCID for DSM-III-R was undertaken in a multisite study conducted by its developers (Williams et al., 1992). This study used a rigorous test–retest design, in which randomly matched pairs of mental health professionals trained in using the SCID independently evaluated and rated the same individual within a 2-week period. The sample included 390 patient and 202 nonpatient subjects. In general, overall reliability for current disorders was fair to good in the patient sample (overall weighted kappa = .61) but poor in the nonpatient sample (overall weighted kappa = .37). There was considerable variability in kappas for specific disorders in the patient sample, ranging from a low of .40 for dysthymia to a high of .86 for bulimia nervosa. Reliabilities for some common disorders were good (>.75) for bipolar disorder, drug abuse/dependence, alcohol abuse/dependence and fair (between .50 and .75) for major depression, schizophrenia, panic disorder, and generalized anxiety disorder. Although the investigators concluded that the measure's reliability was "roughly similar, across categories, to that obtained with other major diagnostic instruments" (Williams et al., 1992, p. 636), their and others' findings in studies on a smaller scale have pointed to areas of lesser strength. Particularly noteworthy is an often cited finding by Skre, Onstad, Torgersen, and Kringlen (1991) of poor reliabilities (< .41) for the diagnoses of somatoform, obsessive–compulsive, and agoraphobia (without history of panic) disorders in a Norwegian sample; this finding warrants cautious interpretation, however, given their low base rates for these disorders. In general, acceptable joint reliabilities (kappa > .70) have been reported in most studies for disorders commonly seen in clinical settings, such as major depressive disorder and the anxiety disorders, including generalized anxiety disorder and panic disorder and its subtypes. Patient characteristics may also have an impact on SCID reliabilities. A study of lifetime comorbidity of Axis I disorders in substance abusers found poorer test–retest reliabilities for the SCID for DSM-III-R than those generally reported (Ross, Swinson, Doumani, & Larkin, 1995).

It is important to note that the SCID's semistructured format and its dependence on clinical judgment, ability to elicit augmenting information, and diagnostic experience of the interviewer go a long way to explain the variability in kappas reported in the literature. As already noted, this approach, though having its strengths, renders the instrument vulnerable to the effects of all of the threats to reliability reviewed earlier in this chapter. For example, the impact of information and criterion variance can be seen in the findings of the Ross et al. (1995) study, where the authors concluded that disagreements about levels and significance of organicity accounted for many diagnostic inconsistencies. Indeed, kappas reported in large-scale studies may not be representative of those to be expected in regular practice settings. Interviewers in these studies are highly trained, and much attention is paid to standardization of administration. In short, reliability of the instrument depends on the skills and training of the person administering it.

Validity. Few studies have been made of the criterion validity of the SCID, primarily because its content closely corresponds to DSM criteria; this is particularly true of the DSM-IV version. Evidence for criterion-related validity of the DSM-III-R version is restricted to studies of specific conditions, particularly panic disorder (e.g., Noyes et al., 1990). In general, as summarized in Rogers (1995), such studies showed high correspondence of SCID findings with such variables as clinical features, course and treatment outcome, and dimensional ratings of symptoms with other standardized measures.

Clearly, additional investigation of the validity of the SCID for DSM-IV is needed, with some focus areas suggested by existing published work. Several studies have found poor general agreement between SCID and standard clinical and/or chart diagnoses (e.g., Parks, Kmetz, & Hillard, 1995; Shear et al., 2000; Steiner, Tebes, Sledge, & Walker, 1995). The SCID's sensitivity in special populations particularly warrants further study: in Parks et al.'s (1995) sample of mentally ill homeless subjects, for example, the negative predictive power (i.e., accurately identifying a negative history) was found to be low.

Summary of Special Issues and Implications for Clinical Application

The SCID is a user-friendly instrument with an unmatched breadth of diagnostic coverage that adheres closely to DSM criteria.

Its semistructured format—although allowing for customization of the measure and additional inquiry when deemed necessary by the interviewer—leaves it open to threats to reliability. Diagnostic experience and/or training in SCID administration is essential, and it has been recommended that the SCID be administered by someone "with enough clinical experience and knowledge of psychopathology and psychiatric diagnosis to conduct a diagnostic interview without an interview guide" (Skodol & Bender, 2000, p. 51). A detailed user's guide and available support materials (e.g., 11-hour training video) will help, but caution should be exercised in sites where lay interviewers are used.

Researchers working with some populations should note that the SCID may be vulnerable to response styles and deliberate faking, likely in part due to the high face validity of its content questions. Rogers (1995) reported that in an unpublished study with schizophrenic patients, he and his colleagues found that individuals suspected of fabricating symptoms produced profiles indistinguishable from those of honest patients on disorder-relevant items on the SCID-P for DSM-III-R.

Depending on the research interests of its users, some deficiencies in the SCID may necessitate augmentation with other measures or adjustments to the standard procedure. For example, several DSM-IV syndromes of potential interest to researchers are not covered by the SCID—among them disorders usually first diagnosed during childhood and adolescence (e.g., tic-related disorders) and sexual, sleep, and cognitive disorders. There are also several conditions for which the standard SCID asks only about current episode (i.e., in the last month) rather than lifetime prevalence: dysthymic disorder, generalized anxiety disorder, all somatoform disorders, and adjustment disorder. In addition, the SCID's close adherence to the DSM framework means that questions beyond those needed for DSM criteria are not provided. The authors encourage researchers interested in specific disorders to add supplemental material such as dimensional severity ratings. Finally, the decision-tree format, employing skip-outs, although making administration more efficient, means that information about subthreshold conditions is standardly lost. Researchers interested in phenomenology or symptomatology of specific conditions may wish to disregard skip-out rules and inquire about the full complement of symptoms of target conditions whether or not probe criteria are met.

Contact Information

The research version of the SCID, as well as a user's manual, can be obtained from SCID Central, Biometrics Research Department, New York State Psychiatric Institute, Unit 60, 1051 Riverside Drive, New York, NY 10032 (phone: 212-543-5524). The clinician's version, manual, and score sheets are available from American Psychiatric Press, Inc., 1400 K Street, NW, Washington, DC 20005 (phone: 800-368-5777; fax: 202-789-2648; website: www.appi.org). The computerized version is available from Multi-Health Systems Inc., 908 Niagara Falls Boulevard, North Tonawanda, NY 14120-2060 (phone: 800-456-3003; Canadian office: 800-268-6011; website: www.mhs.com).

The Mini-International Neuropsychiatric Interview (MINI)

The MINI, version 5.0 (Sheehan et al., 1999) is a clinician-administered structured diagnostic interview developed to permit diagnoses according to both DSM-IV and ICD-10 criteria. Disorders covered include most anxiety disorders and eating disorders, most mood disorders, alcohol and drug abuse and dependence, and psychotic disorders. Many of these are ascertained as current disorders only. Despite this breadth of coverage, the MINI is extremely short, with an administration time of approximately 15 minutes, and was designed to meet the perceived need for an abbreviated but valid structured psychiatric interview for specific research and clinical contexts, including multicenter clinical trials and epidemiological studies, and outcome tracking in nonresearch clinical settings. The development and applications of the MINI and related interviews, including a version with expanded diagnostic coverage—the MINI-Plus—are discussed in a recent article by the measure's developers (Sheehan et al., 1998), which also reports efforts to establish the convergent validity of the MINI using several indices, including expert clinical diagnosis, as well as such established diagnostic instruments as the SCID and the CIDI. Prior efforts, using DSM-III-R criteria, found good interrater and test–retest reliability, as well as sensitivity and specificity for almost all diagnoses (Lecrubier et al., 1997). The MINI has been translated into over 30 languages.

Contact Information

Permission for use of the MINI can be obtained from Dr. David Sheehan, Department of Psychiatry, University of South Florida, 3513 East Fletcher Avenue, Tampa, FL 33613 (phone: 813-974-4544; fax 813-974-4575). It may also be downloaded from www.medical-outcomes.com.

Schedules for Clinical Assessment in Neuropsychiatry (SCAN)

The SCAN comprises a set of instruments designed to assess and measure experiences and behavior that are common among adults presenting with major psychiatric disorders and to permit cross-cultural comparisons of diagnoses. It is unique among the instruments reviewed in this chapter in its primary emphasis not on diagnosis of specific categories of disorder but on describing and ascertaining key signs and symptoms of psychopathology.

The SCAN, currently in version 2.1 (World Health Organization, 1998) has four components: (1) a clinician-administered semistructured clinical interview; this is version 10.2 of the Present State Examination (PSE), out of which the SCAN evolved (see Wing, 1998); (2) a glossary of detailed differential definitions to be used in rating experiences endorsed in the interview by respondents; (3) the Item Group Checklist, used for rating information obtained from sources other than the respondent (e.g., case records and informants) to either supplement PSE information or provide a rough substitute when the PSE cannot be fully completed; and (4) the optional Clinical History Schedule, used to supplement the PSE information with data relevant to the broader developmental, clinical, or social history (e.g., childhood and education, intellectual level, physical illnesses, social roles). Extensive discussion of both the rationale behind, and the nature of, the SCAN 2.1 can be found in its reference manual (Wing, Sartorius, & Üstün, 1998).

The PSE, which forms the core of the SCAN, has two parts comprising 25 sections; it covers a broad range of psychopathology. The first part includes nonpsychotic symptoms and disorders, as well as limited coverage of physical features (e.g., weight, bodily functions). The second part covers psychotic and cognitive conditions and abnormalities of behavior, speech, and affect. In line with the aforementioned descriptive focus of the SCAN, symptoms are organized by symptom types rather than diagnosis, thus reflecting the idea that each symptom should be assessed individually rather than according to prior nosologically based expectations of how it should cluster with others.

In using the SCAN 2.1, the interviewer must select a time period to be used to classify the phenomena being assessed. These include (1) "present state," or the month before examination; or (2) "lifetime before" or any time previously; and, less commonly, (3) "representative episode," chosen because it is highly characteristic of the respondent's experience. A computer program is available to process data and generate ICD-10 and DSM-IV diagnoses. The SCAN 2.1 has been widely translated, including into all major languages and several of less widespread usage such as Kannada and Yoruba.

The SCAN may be a particularly valuable tool for researchers interested in the phenomenology of psychopathology and for those engaged in cross-cultural research. It is primarily designed for administration by experienced clinicians, although there is some evidence for its feasibility with carefully trained lay interviewers (Brugha, Nienhuis, Bagchi,

Smith, & Metzler, 1999). In its development, the SCAN was extensively field-tested (see Wing et al., 1990), and analyses of these data suggest that it possesses acceptable psychometric features, including generally high interrater and test–retest reliabilities for diagnoses and symptom types (see Wing, Sartorius, & Der, 1998). Not surprisingly, some researchers have found lower interrater diagnostic agreement for the SCAN than for more structured interviews. In their comparison of SCAN- and CIDI-generated mood and anxiety disorder diagnoses, Andrews, Peters, Guzman, and Bird (1995) suggested that the level of clinical judgment involved in administering the SCAN resulted in more moderate, though still acceptable, levels of interrater agreement. The flexibility in inquiry permitted by the SCAN, however, also has advantages: Eaton et al. (2000) found that it was less vulnerable to underreporting of mood symptoms than was the rigidly structured DIS.

Contact Information

Up-to-date information on the SCAN 2.1 and its components, and instructions on how to obtain them, as well as a list of SCAN training and references centers is available on the World Health Organization website (www.who.ch/msa/scan).

Symptom-Driven Diagnostic System for Primary Care (SDDS-PC)

The SDSS-PC is a brief, highly structured, physician-administered diagnostic interview designed to facilitate recognition of common psychiatric disorders in primary care settings. The measure was initially designed in accordance with DSM-III-R criteria (Broadhead et al., 1995; Weissman et al., 1995) and subsequently was revised for DSM-IV and for computer administration (Weissman et al., 1998). Diagnostic coverage includes major depression, alcohol and drug dependence, generalized anxiety, panic, and obsessive–compulsive disorders; suicidal behavior is also ascertained. Its administration involves the completion of a self-administered symptom screen by patients, and a brief (i.e., less than 5-minute) diagnostic interview conducted by a nurse or staff member, which yields a one-page summary of positive symptoms and a provisional computer-generated diagnosis and suggested rule-outs to be reviewed by the physician, who then makes the final diagnosis.

Evidence exists for the clinical utility of the SDDS-PC. Physicians have reported enhanced detection of previously unknown or only suspected psychiatric conditions (Weissman et al., 1995). Evidence for its validity, though promising, is less compelling. In a sample of more than 1,000 patients, Weissman et al. (1998) found modest agreement between physicians' SDDS-PC-based diagnoses and those made a few days later by mental health professionals (kappas ranging from .28 to .43). The earlier version of the measure was also found to display marginal to weak concordance with the SCID-based diagnoses (i.e., kappas ≤ .50 for all disorders) (Weissman et al., 1995). However, such findings of validity should be weighted by the value of having these data available at all. Indeed, based on their examination of diagnostic errors with the SDDS-PC screening component, Leon et al. (1999) concluded that erring on the side of sensitivity (i.e., increasing false positives) is preferable at such an early stage of ascertainment, given the nominal burden of follow-up assessments for patients. In summary, within the logistical constraints imposed by primary care settings, the SDDS-PC may provide a useful and feasible initial diagnostic tool.

Contact Information

The SDDS-PC is copyrighted by Pharmacia & Upjohn, and at this time is not readily available for general distribution.

SUMMARY

A vast amount of research has accumulated over the last 30 years on the development and use of structured and semistructured diagnostic interviews. Researchers and clinicians are now faced with the challenging prospect of deciding among many potential instruments, each with its relative advantages and disadvantages. It has been our intent in this chapter to provide an overview of standardized diagnostic interviews that are currently in widespread use, along with the many considerations to be weighed in their selection. We hope that this review will aid researchers, and clinicians committed to empirically driven practice, in the task of selecting the structured or semistructured interview that best suits their unique needs.

ACKNOWLEDGMENT

Laura J. Summerfeldt would like to acknowledge the general support provided during the writing of this chapter by the Ontario Mental Health Foundation, in the form of a New Investigator Fellowship.

REFERENCES

American Psychiatric Association. (1987). *Diagnostic and statistical manual of mental disorders* (3rd ed., rev.). Washington, DC: Author.

American Psychiatric Association. (1994). *Diagnostic and statistical manual of mental disorders* (4th ed.). Washington, DC: Author.

Andreasen, N. C., Grove, W. M., Shapiro, R. W., Keller, M. B., Hirschfeld, R. M. A., & McDonald-Scott, P. (1981). Reliability of lifetime diagnosis. *Archives of General Psychiatry, 39,* 400–405.

Andreasen, N. C., McDonald-Scott, P., Grove, W. M., Keller, M. B., Shapiro, R. W., & Hirshfeld, R. M. A. (1982). Assessment of reliability in multicenter collaborative research with a videotape approach. *American Journal of Psychiatry, 139,* 876–882.

Andrews, G., & Peters, L. (1998). The psychometric properties of the Composite International Diagnostic Interview. *Social Psychiatry and Psychiatric Epidemiology, 33,* 80–88.

Andrews, G., Peters, L., Guzman, A., & Bird, K. (1995). A comparison of two structured diagnostic interviews: CIDI and SCAN. *Australian and New Zealand Journal of Psychiatry, 29,* 124–132.

Anthony, J. C., Folstein, M., Romanoski, A. J., Von Korff, M. R., Nestadt, G. R., Chahal, R., Merchant, A., Brown, H., Shapiro, S., Kramer, M., & Gruenberg, E. M. (1985). Comparison of the lay Diagnostic Interview Schedule and a standardized psychiatric diagnosis: Experience in eastern Baltimore. *Archives of General Psychiatry, 42,* 667–675.

Arbisi, P. A. (1995). Review of the Schedule for Affective Disorders and Schizophrenia, third edition. In J. C. Conoley & J. C. Impara (Eds.), *The twelfth mental measurements yearbook* (pp. 917–918). Lincoln, NE: Buros Institute of Mental Measurements.

Beck, A. T., Ward, C. H., Mendelson, M., Mock, J. E., & Erbaugh, J. K. (1962). Reliability of psychiatric diagnoses: 2. A study of consistency of clinical judgments and ratings. *American Journal of Psychiatry, 119,* 351–357.

Bienvenu, O. J., Samuels, J. F., Riddle, M. A., Hoehn-Saric, R., Liang, K., Cullen, B. A. M., Grados, M. A., & Nestadt, G. (2000). The relationship of obsessive–compulsive disorder to possible spectrum disorders: Results from a family study. *Biological Psychiatry, 48,* 287–293.

Blanchard, J. J., & Brown, S. A. (1998). Structured diagnostic interview schedules. In C. R. Reynolds (Ed.), *Comprehensive clinical psychology: Vol. 3. Assessment* (pp. 97–130). London: Elsevier Science.

Blouin, A. G., Perez, E. L., & Blouin, J. H. (1988). Computerized administration of the Diagnostic Interview Schedule. *Psychiatry Research, 23,* 335–344.

Booth, B. M., Kirchner, J. E., Hamilton, G., Harrell, R., & Smith, G. R. (1998). Diagnosing depression in the medically ill: Validity of a lay-administered structured diagnostic interview. *Journal of Psychiatric Research, 32,* 353–360.

Broadhead, W. E., Leon, A. C., Weissman, M. M., Barrett, J. E., Blacklow, R. S., Gilbert, T. T., Keller, M. B., Olfson, M., & Higgins, E. S. (1995). Development and validation of the SDDS-PC screen for multiple mental disorders in primary care. *Archives of Family Medicine, 4,* 211–219.

Brown, T. A., Di Nardo, P. A., & Barlow, D. H. (1994). *Anxiety Disorders Interview Schedule for DSM-IV (ADIS-IV).* San Antonio, TX: Psychological Corporation.

Brown, T. A., Di Nardo, P. A., Lehman, C. L., & Campbell, L. A. (2001). Reliability of DSM-IV anxiety and mood disorders: Implications for the classification of emotional disorders. *Journal of Abnormal Psychology, 110,* 49–58.

Brugha, T. S., Nienhuis, F., Bagchi, D., Smith, J., & Metzler, H. (1999). The survey form of SCAN: The feasibility of using experienced lay survey interviewers to administer a semi-structured systematic clinical assessment of psychiatric and non-psychotic disorders. *Psychological Medicine, 29,* 703–711.

Cacciola, J. S., Alterman, A. I., Rutherford, M. J., McKay, J. R., & May, D. J. (1999). Comparability of telephone and in-person structured clinical interview for DSM-III-R (SCID) diagnoses. *Assessment, 6,* 235–242.

Carroll, K. M., Ball, S. A., & Rounsaville, B. J. (1993). A comparison of alternate systems for diagnosing antisocial personality disorder in cocaine abusers. *Journal of Nervous and Mental Disease, 181,* 436–443.

Conoley, J. C., & Impara, J. C. (Eds.). (1995). *The twelfth mental measurements yearbook.* Lincoln, NE: Buros Institute of Mental Measurements.

Cooney, N. L., Kadden, R. M., & Litt, M. D. (1990). A comparison of methods for assessing sociopathy in male and female alcoholics. *Journal of Studies on Alcohol, 51,* 42–48.

Coryell, W., Winckur, G., Maser, J. D., Akiskal, H. S., Keller, M. B., & Endicott, J. (1994). Recurrently situational (reactive) depression: A study of course, phenomenology and familial psychopathology. *Journal of Affective Disorders, 31,* 203–210.

Di Nardo, P. A., Brown, T. A., & Barlow, D. H. (1994). *Anxiety Disorders Interview Schedule for DSM-IV: Lifetime Version.* San Antonio, TX: Psychological Corporation.

Di Nardo, P. A., Moras, K., Barlow, D. H., Rapee, R. M., & Brown, T. A. (1993). Reliability of DSM-III-R anxiety disorder categories: Using the Anxiety Disorders Interview Schedule—Revised (ADIS-R). *Archives of General Psychiatry, 50,* 251–256.

Di Nardo, P. A., O'Brien, G. T., Barlow, D. H., Waddell, M. T., & Blanchard, E. B. (1983). Reliability of DSM-III anxiety disorder categories using a new structured interview. *Archives of General Psychiatry, 40,* 1070–1074.

Eaton, W. W., Anthony, J. C., Gallo, J., Cai, G., Tien, A., Romanoski, A., Lyketsos, C., & Chen, L. (1997). Natural history of Diagnostic Interview Schedule/DSM-IV major depression: The Baltimore epidemiologic catchment area follow-up. *Archives of General Psychiatry, 54,* 993–999.

Eaton, W., & Kessler, L. (Eds.). (1985). *Epidemiologic field methods in psychiatry: The NIMH epidemiologic catchment area program.* New York: Academic Press.

Eaton, W. W., Neufeld, K., Chen, L., & Cai, G. (2000). A comparison of self-report and clinical diagnostic interviews for depression. *Archives of General Psychiatry, 57,* 217–222.

Endicott, J., & Spitzer, R. L. (1978). A diagnostic interview: The Schedule for Affective Disorders and Schizophrenia. *Archives of General Psychiatry, 35,* 837–844.

Erdman, H. P., Klein, M. H., Greist, J. H., Bass, S. M., Bires, J. K., & Machtinger, P. E. (1987). A comparison of the Diagnostic Interview Schedule and clinical diagnosis. *American Journal of Psychiatry, 144,* 1477–1480.

Erdman, H. P., Klein, M. H., Greist, J. H., Skare, S. S., Husted, J. J., Robins, L. N., Helzer, J. E., Goldring, E., Hamburger, M., & Miller, J. P. (1992). A comparison of two computer-administered versions of the NIMH Diagnostic Interview Schedule. *Journal of Psychiatric Research, 26,* 85–95.

Feighner, J. P., Robings, E., Guze, S. B., Woodruff, R. A., Winokur, G., & Munoz, R. (1972). Diagnostic criteria for use in psychiatric research. *Archives of General Psychiatry, 26,* 57–63.

First, M. B., Spitzer, R. L., Gibbon, M., & Williams, J. B. W. (1996). *Structured Clinical Interview for Axis I DSM-IV Disorders Research Version—Patient Edition (SCID-I/P, ver. 2.0).* New York: New York State Psychiatric Institute, Biometrics Research Department.

First, M. B., Spitzer, R. L., Gibbon, M., & Williams, J. B. W. (1997). *Structured Clinical Interview for*

DSM-IV Axis I Disorders (SCID-I)—Clinician Version. Washington, DC: American Psychiatric Press.

Folstein, M. F., Romanoski, A. J., Nestadt, G., Chahal, R., Merchant, A., Shapiro, S., Kramer, M., Anthony, J., Gruenberg, E. M., & McHugh, P. R. (1985). Brief report on the clinical reappraisal of the Diagnostic Interview Schedule carried out at the Johns Hopkins site of the Epidemiological Catchment Area Program of the NIMH. *Psychological Medicine, 15,* 809–814.

Fyer, A. J., Endicott, J., Mannuzza, S., & Klein, D. F. (1985). *Schedule for Affective Disorders and Schizophrenia—Lifetime Version, modified for the study of anxiety disorders (SADS-LA).* Unpublished measure, Anxiety Genetics Unit, New York State Psychiatric Institute, New York, NY.

Fyer, A. J., Endicott, J., Mannuzza, S., & Klein, D. F. (1995). *Schedule for Affective Disorders and Schizophrenia—Lifetime Version, modified for the study of anxiety disorders, updated for DSM-IV (SADS-LA-IV).* Unpublished measure, Anxiety Genetics Unit, New York State Psychiatric Institute, New York, NY.

Hahn, S. R., Kroenke, K., Williams, J. B. W., & Spitzer, R. L. (2000). Evaluation of mental disorders with the PRIME-MD. In M. E. Mariush (Ed.), *Handbook of psychological assessment in primary care settings* (pp. 191–254). London: Erlbaum.

Hamilton, M. (1959). The assessment of anxiety states by rating. *British Journal of Medical Psychology, 32,* 50–55.

Hamilton, M. (1960). A rating scale for depression. *Journal of Neurology, Neurosurgery, and Psychiatry, 23,* 56–62.

Helzer, J. E., Robins, L. N., McEvoy, L. T., Sptznagel, E. L., Stolzman, R. K., Farmer, A., & Brockington, I. F. (1985). A comparison of clinical and diagnostic interview schedule diagnoses: Physician reexamination of lay-interviewed cases in the general population. *Archives of General Psychiatry, 42,* 657–666.

Helzer, J. E., Spitznagel, E. L., & McEvoy, L. (1987). The predictive validity of lay Diagnostic Interview Schedule diagnoses in the general population: A comparison with physician examiners. *Archives of General Psychiatry, 44,* 1069–1077.

Impara, J. C., & Plake, B. S. (Eds.). (1998). *The thirteenth mental measurements yearbook.* Lincoln, NE: Buros Institute of Mental Measurement.

Keller, M. B., Lavori, P. W., McDonald-Scott, P., Scheftner, W. A., Andreasen, N. C., Shapiro, R. W., & Croughan, J. (1981). Reliability of lifetime diagnoses and symptoms in patients with a current psychiatric disorder. *Journal of Psychiatric Research, 16,* 229–240.

Kendler, K. S., Gruenberg, A. M., & Kinney, D. K. (1994). Independent diagnoses of adoptees and relatives as defined by DSM-III in the provincial and national samples of the Danish Adoption Study of Schizophrenia. *Archives of General Psychiatry, 51,* 456–468.

Kobak, K. A., Taylor, L. H., Dottl, S. L., Greist, J. H., Jefferson, J. W., Burroughs, D., Mantle, J. M., Katzelnick, D. J., Norton, R., Henk, H. J., & Serlin, R. C. (1997). A computer-administered telephone interview to identify mental disorders. *Journal of the American Medical Association, 278,* 905–910.

Kovess, V., & Fournier, L. (1990). The DISSA: An abridged self-administered version of the DIS. Approach by episode. *Social Psychiatry and Psychiatric Epidemiology, 25,* 179–186.

Kroenke, K., Jackson, J. L., & Chamberlin, J. (1997). Depressive and anxiety disorders in patients presenting with physical complaints: Clinical predictors and outcome. *Amercian Journal of Medicine, 103,* 339–347.

Landis, J. R., & Koch, G. G. (1977). The measurement of observer agreement for categorical data. *Biometrics, 33,* 159–174.

Leboyer, M., Maier, W., Teherani, M., Lichtermann, D., D'Amato, T., Franke, P., Lepine, J. P., Minges, J., & McGuffin, P. (1991). The reliability of the SADS-LA in a family study setting. *European Archives of Psychiatry and Clinical Neuroscience, 241,* 165–169.

Lecrubier, Y., Sheehan, D. V., Weiller, E., Amorim, P., Bonora, I., Sheehan, K. H., Janavs, J., & Dunbar, G. C. (1997). The Mini International Neuropsychiatric Interview (MINI): A short diagnostic structured interview—Reliability and validity according to the CIDI. *European Psychiatry, 12,* 224–231.

Lefevre, F., Reifler, D., Lee, P., Sbenghe, M., Nwadiaro, N., Verma, S., & Yarnold, P. R. (1999). Screening for undetected mental disorders in high utilizers of primary care services. *Journal of General Internal Medicine, 14,* 425–431.

Leon, A. C., Portera, L., Olfson, M., Kathol, R., Farber, L., Lowell, K. N., & Sheehan, D. V. (1999). Diagnostic errors of primary care screens for depression and panic disorder. *International Journal of Psychiatry and Medicine, 29,* 1–11.

Leopold, K. A., Ahles, T. A., Walch, S., Amdur, R. J., Mott, L. A., Wiegand-Packard, L., & Oxman, T. E. (1998). Prevalence of mood disorders and utility of the PRIME-MD in patients undergoing radiation therapy. *International Journal of Radiation, Oncology, Biology, and Physics, 42,* 1105–1112.

Linzer, M., Spitzer, R., Kroenke, K., Williams, J. B., Hahn, S., Brody, D., & de Gruy F. (1996). Gender, quality of life, and mental disorders in primary care: Results from the PRIME-MD 1000 study. *American Journal of Medicine, 101,* 526–533.

Loebel, A. D., Lieberman, J. A., Alvir, J. M., Mayerhoff, D. I., Geisler, S. H., & Szymanski, S. R. (1992). Duration of psychosis and outcome in first-episode schizophrenia. *American Journal of Psychiatry, 149,* 1183–1188.

Lucas, C. P., Fisher, P., Piacentini, J., Zhang, H., Jensen, P. S., Shaffer, D., Dulcan, M., Schwab-Stone, M., Regier, D., & Canino, G. (1999). Features of interview questions associated with attenuation of symptom reports. *Journal of Abnormal Child Psychology, 2,* 429–437.

Malgady, R. G., Rogler, L. H., & Tryon, W. W. (1992). Issues of validity in the Diagnostic Interview Schedule. *Journal of Psychiatric Research, 26,* 59–67.

Maziade, M., Roy, M. A., Fournier, J. P., Cliché, D., Merette, C., Caron, C., Garneau, Y., Montgrain, N., Shriqui, C., & Dion C. (1992). Reliability of best-estimate diagnosis in genetic linkage studies of major psychoses: Results from the Quebec pedigree studies. *American Journal of Psychiatry, 149,* 1674–1686.

McDonald-Scott, P., & Endicott, J. (1984). Informed versus blind: The reliability of cross-sectional ratings of psychopathology. *Psychiatry Research, 12,* 207–217.

Murphy, J. M., Monson, R. R., Laird, N. M., Sobol, A. M., & Leighton, A. H. (2000). A comparison of diagnostic interviews for depression in the Stirling County Study: Challenges for psychiatric epidemiology. *Archives of General Psychiatry, 57,* 230–236.

Nease, D. E., Volk, R. J., & Cass, A. R. (1999). Investigation of a severity-based classification of mood and anxiety symptoms in primary care patients. *Journal of the American Board of Family Practitioners, 12,* 21–23.

Neufeld, K. J., Swartz, K. L., Bienvenu, O. J., Eaton, W. W., & Cai, G. (1999). Incidence of DIS/DSM-IV social phobia in adults. *Acta Psychiatrica Scandinavica, 100,* 186–192.

Noyes, R., Reich, J., Christiansen, J., Suelzer, M., Pfohl, B., & Coryell, W. A. (1990). Outcome of panic disorder: Relationship to diagnostic subtypes and comorbidity. *Archives of General Psychiatry, 47,* 809–818.

Parks, J. J., Kmetz, G., & Hillard, J. R. (1995). Underdiagnosis using SCIDR in the homeless mentally ill. *Psychiatric Quarterly, 66,* 1–8.

Rapee, R. M., Brown, T. A., Antony, M. M., & Barlow, D. H. (1992). Response to hyperventilation and inhalation of 5.5% carbon dioxide–enriched air across the DSM-III-R anxiety disorders. *Journal of Abnormal Psychology, 101,* 538–552.

Robins, L. N., Cottler, L., Bucholz, K., & Compton, W. (1995). *The Diagnostic Interview Schedule, Version IV.* St. Louis, MO: Washington University Medical School.

Robins, L. N., Helzer, J. E., Croughan, J., & Ratcliff, K. S. (1981). National Institute of Mental Health Diagnostic Interview Schedule: Its history, characteristics, and validity. *Archives of General Psychiatry, 38,* 381–389.

Robins, L. N., Helzer, J. E., Ratcliff, K. S., & Seyfried, W. (1982). Validity of the diagnostic interview schedule, version II: DSM-III diagnoses. *Psychological Medicine, 12,* 855–870.

Robins, L. N., Wing, J., Wittchen, H. U., Helzer, J. E., Babor, T. F., Burke, J., Farmer, A., Jablenski, A., Pickens, R., Regier, D. A., Sartorius, N., & Towle, L. H. (1988). The Composite International Diagnostic Interview: An epidemiological instrument suitable for use in conjunction with different diagnostic systems and in different cultures. *Archives of General Psychiatry, 45,* 1069–1077.

Rogers, R. (1995). *Diagnostic and structured interviewing: A handbook for psychologists*. Odessa, FL: Psychological Assessment Resources.

Ross, H. E., Swinson, R., Doumani, S., & Larkin, E. J. (1995). Diagnosing comorbidity in substance abusers: A comparison of the test–retest reliability of two interviews. *American Journal of Drug and Alcohol Abuse, 21,* 167–185.

Segal, D. L. (1997). Structured interviewing and DSM classification. In S. M. Turner & M. Hersen (Eds.), *Adult psychopathology and diagnosis* (3rd ed., pp. 24–57). New York: Wiley.

Segal, D. L., & Falk, S. B. (1997). Structured interviews and rating scales. In A. S. Bellack & M. Hersen (Eds.), *Behavioral assessment: A practical handbook* (4th ed., pp. 158–178). Boston: Allyn & Bacon.

Segal, D. L., Hersen, M., & van Hasselt, V. B. (1994). Reliability of the Structured Clinical Interview for DSM-III-R: An evaluative review. *Comprehensive Psychiatry, 35,* 316–327.

Shear, M. K., Greeno, C., Kang, J., Ludewig, D., Frank, E., Swartz, H. A., & Hanekamp, M. (2000). Diagnosis of nonpsychotic patients in community clinics. *American Journal of Psychiatry, 157,* 581–587.

Sheehan, D. V., Janavs, R., Baker, R., Harnett-Sheehan, K., Knapp, E., & Sheehan, M. (1999). *Mini International Neuropsychiatric Interview*. Tampa: University of South Florida Press.

Sheehan, D. V., Lecrubier, Y., Sheehan, K. H., Amorim, P., Janavs, J., Weiller, E., Hergueta, T., Baker, R., & Dunbar, G. C. (1998). The Mini-International Neuropsychiatric Interview (M.I.N.I.): The development and validation of a structured diagnostic psychiatric interview for DSM-IV and ICD-10. *Journal of Clinical Psychiatry, 59* (Suppl. 20), 22–33.

Silverman, W. K., & Albano, A. M. (1996). *Anxiety Disorders Interview Schedule for Children*. San Antonio, TX: Psychological Corporation.

Skodol, A. E., & Bender, D. S. (2000). Diagnostic interviews for adults. In American Psychiatric Association Taskforce for the Handbook (Ed.), *Handbook of psychiatric measures* (pp. 45–70). Washington, DC: American Psychiatric Association Press.

Skre, I., Onstad, S., Torgersen, S., & Kringlen, E. (1991). High interrater reliability for the Structured Clinical Interview for DSM-III-R Axis I (SCID-I). *Acta Psychiatrica Scandinavica, 84,* 167–173.

Spitzer, R. L. (1983). Psychiatric diagnosis: Are clinicians still necessary? *Comprehensive Psychiatry, 24,* 399–411.

Spitzer, R. L., Endicott, J., & Robins, E. (1978). Research diagnostic criteria. *Archives of General Psychiatry, 35,* 773–782.

Spitzer, R. L., & Fleiss, J. L. (1974). A re-analysis of the reliability of psychiatric diagnosis. *British Journal of Psychiatry, 125,* 341–347.

Spitzer, R. L., Fleiss, J. L., & Endicott, J. (1978). Problems of classification: Reliability and validity. In M. A. Lipton, A. DiMascio, & K. Killam (Eds.), *Psychopharmacology: A generation of progress* (pp. 857–869). New York: Raven Press.

Spitzer, R. L., Kroenke, K., Linzer, M., Hahn, S. R., Williams, J. B., deGruy, F. V., Brody, D., & Davies, M. (1995). Health-related quality of life in primary care patients with mental disorder: Results from the PRIME-MD study. *Journal of the American Medical Association, 274,* 1511–1517.

Spitzer, R. L., Kroenke, K., & Williams, J. B. (1999). Validation and utility of a self-report version of PRIME-MD: The PHQ primary care study. Primary Care Evaluation of Mental Disorders. Patient Health Questionnaire. *Journal of the American Medical Association, 282,* 1737–1744.

Spitzer, R. L., Williams, J. B. W., Gibbon, M., & First, M. B. (1992). The Structured Clinical Interview for DSM-III-R (SCID): History, rationale, and description. *Archives of General Psychiatry, 49,* 624–629.

Spitzer, R. L., Williams, J. B. W., Kroenke, K., Linzer, M., deGruy, F. V., Hahn, S. R., Brody, D., & Johnson, J. G. (1994). Utility of a new procedure for diagnosing mental disorders in primary care: The PRIME-MD 1000 study. *Journal of the American Medical Association, 272,* 1749–1756.

Spitznagel, E. L., & Helzer, J. E. (1985). A proposed solution to the base rate problem in the kappa statistic. *Archives of General Psychiatry, 42,* 725–728.

Steiner, J. L., Tebes, J. K., Sledge, W. H., & Walker, M. L. (1995). A comparison of the structured clinical interview for DSM-III-R and clinical diagnoses. *Journal of Nervous and Mental Disease, 183,* 365–369.

Stompe, T., Ortwein-Swoboda, G., Strobl, R., & Friedmann, A. (2000). The age of onset of schizophrenia and the theory of anticipation. *Psychiatry Research, 93,* 125–134.

Vandiver, T., & Sher, K. (1991). Temporal stability of the Diagnostic Interview Schedule. *Psychological Assessment, 3,* 277–281.

Vieta, E., Colom, F., Martinez-Aran, A., Benabarre, A., Reinares, M., & Gasto, C. (2000). Bipolar II disorder and comorbidity. *Comprehensive Psychiatry, 41,* 339–343.

Ward, C. H., Beck, A. T., Mendelson, M., Mock, J. E., & Erbaugh, J. K. (1962). The psychiatric nomenclature: Reasons for diagnostic disagreement. *Archives of General Psychiatry, 7,* 198–205.

Weissman, M. M., Broadhead, W. E., Olfson, M., Sheehan, D. V., Hoven, C., Conolly, P., Fireman, B. H., Farber, L., Blacklow, R. S., Higgins, E. S., & Leon, A. C. (1998). A diagnostic aid for detecting (DSM-IV) mental disorders in primary care. *General Hospital Psychiatry, 20,* 1–11.

Weissman, M. M., Olfson, M., Leon, A. C., Broadhead, W. E., Gilbert, T. T., Higgins, E. S., Barrett, J. E., Blacklow, R. S., Keller, M. B., & Hoven, C. (1995). Brief diagnostic interviews (SDDS-PC) for multiple mental disorders in primary care: A pilot study. *Archives of Family Medicine, 4,* 220–227.

Widiger, T. A., & Clark, L. A. (2000). Toward DSM-V and the classification of psychopathology. *Psychological Bulletin, 126,* 946–963.

Widiger, T. A., & Frances A. (1987). Definitions and diagnoses: A brief response to Morey and McNamara. *Journal of Abnormal Psychology, 96,* 286–287.

Williams, J. B. W., Gibbon, M., Frist, M. B., Spitzer, R. L., Davies, M., Borus, J., Howes, M. J., Kane, J., Pope, H. G., Rounsaville, B., & Wittchen, H. (1992). The Structured Clinical Interview for DSM-III-R (SCID): Multisite test–retest reliability. *Archives of General Psychiatry, 49,* 630–636.

Wing, J. K. (1998). The PSE tradition and its continuation in SCAN. In J. K. Wing, N. Sartorius, & T. B. Üstün (Eds.), *Diagnosis and clinical measurement in psychiatry: A reference manual for SCAN* (pp. 12–24). Cambridge, UK: Cambridge University Press.

Wing, J. K., Babor, T., Brugha, T., Burke, J., Cooper, J. E., Giel, R., Jablenski, A., Regier, D., & Sartorius, N. (1990). SCAN. Schedules for Clinical Assessment in Neuropsychiatry. *Archives of General Psychiatry, 47,* 589–593.

Wing, J. K., Sartorius, N., & Der, G. (1998). International field trials: SCAN-O. In J. K. Wing, N. Sartorius, & T. B. Üstün (Eds.), *Diagnosis and clinical measurement in psychiatry: A reference manual for SCAN* (pp. 86–109). Cambridge, UK: Cambridge University Press.

Wing, J. K., Sartorius, N., & Üstün, T. B. (Eds.). (1998). *Diagnosis and clinical measurement in psychiatry: A reference manual for SCAN.* Cambridge, UK: Cambridge University Press.

Wittchen, H. U. (1994). Reliability and validity studies of the WHO-Composite International Diagnostic Interview: A critical review. *Journal of Psychiatric Research, 28,* 57–84.

Wittchen, H. U., Burke, J. D., Semier, G., Pfister, H., Von Cranach, M., & Zaudig, M. (1989). Recall and dating of psychiatric symptoms: Test–retest reliability of time-related symptom questions in a standardized psychiatric interview. *Archives of General Psychiatry, 46,* 437–443.

World Health Organization. (1993). *International classification of diseases* (10th ed.). Geneva: World Health Organization.

World Health Organization. (1998). *Schedules for Clinical Assessment in Neuropsychiatry, Version 2.1.* Geneva: World Health Organization.

Zwick, D. I. (1983). Establishing national health goals and standards. *Public Health Reports, 98,* 416–425.

2

Brief Screening Assessments for Managed Care and Primary Care

Lynn F. Bufka
Jeanne I. Crawford
Jill T. Levitt

As managed care has continued to make inroads into health care in the United States, the use of the primary care physician (PCP) and associated medical staff, such as nurse practitioners and physician assistants, as the "gatekeepers" to the health care system has grown. Increasingly greater numbers of individuals see their PCPs for the majority of their health care needs or, at the very least, see their PCPs at the beginning of their search for appropriate treatment. At the same time, many patients who present for treatment in primary care and managed care settings have either co-occurring behavioral problems or primary mental health problems (e.g., Rinaldi, 1992). Indeed, according to the National Institute of Mental Health, more PCPs see patients for psychiatric problems than do mental health professionals (Narrow, Regier, Rae, Manderscheid, & Locke, 1993). Furthermore, much treatment for depression occurs in the primary care setting (Schurman, Kramer, & Mitchell, 1985).

In theory, as health care costs spiraled well above the cost of inflation, the use of the PCP as gatekeeper appeared to make good sense as a cost-cutting procedure. In practice, however, while the gatekeeper model has given responsibility for identifying mental health problems in many patients to the PCP, the data indicate that PCPs are doing an inadequate job of recognizing mental health problems and that existing mental illness remains undetected in many patients (Simon & Von Korff, 1996). One complication is that many symptoms of mental illness can present as physical symptoms, which further obscures their recognition. Numerous studies document problems in PCP recognition of mental disorders. For example, an elegant study conducted by Perez-Stable and colleagues showed that PCPs underdiagnosed depression in 35.7% of the clients, but also diagnosed depression in 36 (out of 256) patients who, according to independent assessment with the Diagnostic Interview Schedule, were *not* depressed (Perez-Stable, Miranda, Munoz, & Ying, 1990).

THE COST OF UNDERDIAGNOSIS

Underdiagnosis of emotional disorders is a major problem from several vantage points, including increased medical costs, work loss, and increased human suffering. In addition, undiagnosed and untreated mental health problems are known to complicate medical treatment. Financially, untreated mental illness is expensive. Studies have shown that patients who did not receive mental health services visited a medical doctor twice as often for unnecessary care than did patients who received appropriate mental health care (Lechnyr, 1992). In addition, in a review of medical utilization at the Columbia Medical Plan in Maryland, researchers found that patients with treated mental illness averaged 21% fewer nonpsychiatric visits than an untreated group of patients with mental illness. In fact, from 1974 to 1975, the untreated group had a 41% increase in the use of nonpsychiatric services, while the treated group had only an 11% increase (Hankin, Kessler, & Goldberg, 1983). It is clearly essential that payers, who are already assessing cost and utilization in the primary care setting, begin to look at outcomes of quality of life, depression disability days, and general issues of medical cost offset as related to both psychiatric problems and appropriate psychiatric treatment.

In addition to the financial cost of underdiagnosis in the primary care setting, there is a clear social cost. The consequences of untreated mental disorders can be serious on multiple levels. It is well documented that untreated depression leads to significant loss of work time and productivity, and it follows that other untreated mental illnesses may lead to similar losses. One analysis of the relationship between depression and work loss found that depressed workers had between 1.5 and 3.2 more short-term work disability days out of 30 than did nondepressed workers, with a salary productivity equivalent loss of $182 to $395 (Kessler et al., 1999). Untreated anxiety disorders show similar trends (Zimmerman et al., 1994). Also, anxiety (like depression) is associated with increased morbidity and mortality in adult populations (Wetherell & Arean, 1997).

Fortunately, a wealth of data demonstrates that the treatment of depression and other emotional disorders leads to decreased medical utilization and increased work functioning, as well as improved life functioning and remission of psychiatric symptoms. In an analysis of 58 controlled studies of the effect of mental health treatment on medical utilization, medical offset data suggest decreases in medical utilization of up to 182% (Mumford, Schlesinger, Glass, & Cuerdon, 1984). Mental health treatment also contributes to positive changes in work functioning. In a study conducted by the Rand Corporation, after successful treatment of depression, patients who had used a large quantity of medical services reduced the number of days of disability and increased employment (Broadhead, Blazer, George, & Tse, 1990).

Because primary care medical staff are often not able to accurately assess mental illness, what can be done to increase appropriate recognition of mental health issues in the primary care setting? One strategy that seems to hold great promise is the use of mental health screening tools. Because staff frequently do not have sufficient time to assess for all potential emotional problems, and because such staff rarely have specific training in mental health concerns, the prudent use of screening tools and brief assessments for mental illness can serve to maximize the appropriate identification of mental health problems. The dissemination of knowledge about easy-to-use tools that accurately assess psychiatric conditions commonly seen in the primary care setting is therefore critical.

The data that have been collected to date seem to indicate that the use of brief screening tools leads to more accurate diagnosis of mental illness in the primary care setting. For example, one study assessed 100 patients using the Zung Self-Rating Depression Scale. The intervention consisted of randomly informing (or not informing) the PCP of the patient's status on the self-rating scale. The study demonstrated that informing PCPs of a positive score on the Zung depression scale for previously undiagnosed patients led to greater recognition (56.2% vs. 34.6%) and treatment (56.2% vs. 42.3%) of depression (Magruder-Habib, Zung, & Feussner, 1990). In another study, use of the Beck Depression Inventory in the primary care setting indicated that only a subset of items from this scale were needed to accurately identify depression (Carmin & Klocek, 1998.) In addition, a study conducted in Sweden demonstrated that the brief Geriatric Depression Scale (GDS-20) is an effective screening tool that can be used to diagnose geriatric depression in the primary care setting (Noltorp, Gottfries, & Norgaard, 1998).

Research at the Kaiser Permanente Oakland Medical Center suggests that a fully integrated approach to medical and behavioral health care may be beneficial. This setting provides behavioral screening of all primary care patients who visit the clinic for regularly scheduled appointments. Patients are screened with brief screening tools for depression, anxiety, somatization, substance abuse, and social difficulties, and counselors are available on a drop-in basis. Data collected at the medical center indicate that patients who saw a counselor were more positive and satisfied with their health care than previously and felt less need to talk to their physician about personal or emotional needs (Miller & Farber, 1996). Thus, psychological screening instruments may prove useful for the patient, as well as for the practitioner.

QUESTIONS TO CONSIDER WHEN DECIDING WHICH INSTRUMENT TO USE

Before choosing a screening instrument to be used in the primary care setting, a variety of factors must be taken into account. Careful selection of screening tools or assessment approaches appropriate to the setting is essential. The regular use of some type of screening instrument is encouraged to ensure systematic evaluation of all patients and lessen the problem of undetected symptoms due to reliance on interviews by untrained staff. A wide variety of screening approaches exist, each with different attributes that make them appealing in different settings. Screening approaches include self-report surveys administered by paper and pencil, computerized questionnaires, and very brief interview screens administered by the PCP or trained staff members. Whichever approach is adopted, implementation of a standard, structured approach ensures that all patients are assessed for psychopathology. Earlier assessment will help identify those individuals who would benefit from more thorough psychological and psychiatric assessment.

Existing screening tools currently available to identify mental health problems range from older, well-established tools such as the Symptom Checklist-90—Revised (SCL-90-R; Derogatis, 1977, 1994) to newer tools such as the Mini-International Neuropsychiatric Interview (MINI; Sheehan et al., 1998). These measures, and others, will be described in greater detail later in this chapter. Some of the instruments are long, some are short, and most do a reasonably good job of recognizing psychological problems. However, they are not all equally user-friendly in the primary care setting, and the utility of the information given varies across instruments. Clearly, no one tool is best for all settings. The given approach must be functionally useful to the particular setting, and the benefits of implementing the approach must outweigh the burdens. Each setting will need to determine what is needed in a screening tool to make it useful to that primary care setting.

What Information Is Needed from the Assessment?

If the assessment tool is being used to assist the PCP in making a decision as to whether to refer the patient to a mental health practitioner, then a brief screening tool such as the 36-

Item Short-Form Health Survey (SF-36; Ware & Sherbourne, 1992) or even the 11-Item Short-Form Health Survey (SF-11; Ware & Sherbourne, 1992) may be sufficient. However, if the primary care physician is going to provide the mental health treatment, more detailed information may be needed from the assessment tool. Different assessment tools are designed to provide varying amounts of detail, ranging from simple information regarding the presence or absence of symptoms to complex diagnostic impressions. For example, the MINI is designed to provide *Diagnostic and Statistical Manual of Mental Disorders* (DSM-IV; American Psychiatric Association, 1994) diagnoses for 15 major categories and one Axis II diagnosis. Both the SCL-90-R and the Brief Treatment Outcome Package (TOP; Kraus, Jordan, Horan, & Crawford, in press) give a detailed profile of mental health status, unlike the SF-36, a questionnaire used in primary care settings that includes only five mental health questions and therefore provides a limited amount of behavioral health information. Before choosing an assessment tool, it is important to have a clear understanding of the needs of the particular primary care setting and how much diagnostic information is necessary.

Who Will Administer the Tool?

Assessment tools can be administered by the PCP or the support personnel, or it can be self-administered by the client. There are advantages and disadvantages to all of these options. Client self-report tools, like the TOP and the SCL-90-R, have the advantage of supplying the actual "voice" of the patient. Often the patient is uncomfortable talking about mental health issues in a "medical" setting and may be more comfortable responding to a questionnaire than directly to the physician. However, self-administered tools have a disadvantage for patients who are not prepared to focus on mental health problems in the primary care office. These instruments can be difficult to interpret when completed by patients who tend to minimize psychological factors and instead focus on somatic factors. Also, self-report measures cannot be used for clients who are unable to read, and they are difficult to use with severely disturbed patients. In contrast, physician-administered assessment systems such as the MINI or the clinician evaluation guide for the Primary Care Evaluation of Mental Disorders (PRIME-MD) (Spitzer et al., 1994) give the PCP the opportunity to interact with the patient but can take an inordinate amount of time to administer. In addition, patients are occasionally uncomfortable with the idea of talking directly with the PCP about mental health problems. Another option is for support personnel to administer or assist in the administration of the assessment. This option is contingent on personnel time, training, and sensitivity to patient issues.

How Long Does It Take?

There are three aspects of timing to consider: the length of time it takes to administer the assessment tool, the time it takes to score the tool, and the amount of time it takes to review the information and interpret the results.

Time of administration varies based on mode of administration and the length of the tool. The Brief TOP (self-administered) takes about 10 minutes for a patient to complete; the SCL-90-R (self-administered) takes about 15 minutes. The Behavior and Symptom Identification Scale (BASIS-32; Eisen, Dill, & Grob, 1994), the SF-36, and the Brief Symptom Inventory (BSI; Derogatis & Melisaratos, 1983) all take less time for self-completion. With experience, none of these five tools takes more than 2 or 3 minutes to review.

Most screening tools must be scored, thus ease of scoring is an important factor. Without some form of cutoff or clear diagnostic threshold, the collected information may be useless. The effort it takes to score the assessment tool must be factored into the cost/benefit of administration of the tool. Some tools, for example the BASIS-32, have software programs available for scoring, which make it possible to obtain rapid results. Other assessment tools are easily scored by the practitioner. Another scoring approach is a fax-back system, such as that used by the TOP: in this case, the assessment tool is faxed to a central scoring destination, and within 30 minutes a two-page report is returned. For screening and assessment tools to be of the most use, rapid scoring is essential. By using instruments that have quick administration and scoring, the clinician can potentially review the results of the assessment before the patient has left the office.

How Will the Data Be Used?

In many settings, the assessment tool will only be used as a screening tool—that is, it will indicate the likely presence of psychopathology and will be used only for clinical purposes. In this instance, relatively immediate results that are available for use soon after the tool is completed are ideal. In other settings, however the data will be used to help profile practice demographics and to track treatment outcomes. Some assessment tools are better suited for complex profiling than others. Tools such as the BASIS-32 that can be administered and scored by computer may be capable of exporting data into a spreadsheet for further analysis. Tools such as the TOP automatically provide monthly aggregate reports that detail overall patient demographics and symptom profiles.

Will Data Be Shared with Patients?

Mental health findings may often have to be demystified in the primary care setting. Frequently, patients present with somatic complaints—and they, and often their physicians, do not recognize possible connections between physical and mental health problems. The demystification process can be aided by actual reports that identify for the patient (and the physician) the exact nature of the mental health problems. For example, the report that is provided by the TOP provides information across multiple clinical domains, including anxiety, depression, and thought control. Because it is a self-report measure, the TOP is a reflection of the actual words of the patient. However, because the information is then analyzed within a mental health framework, both the physician and the patient are assisted in understanding the relationship between somatic concerns and mental health problems.

Does the Tool Make Sense to the Patient?

For a screening instrument to be useful in the primary care setting, it must make sense to the patient. The directions for completion and the purpose of the tool must be clear. This means that the tool should be worded in everyday language and should be written for the appropriate reading level of most patients. In addition, the instrument should be straightforward in nature and easy to fill out. For example, older patients may require a tool in larger print than younger patients, and patients taking certain psychotropic medicines may have difficulty filling in small circles. Finally, patients should be made aware of the purpose of the instrument, and the results should be integrated into their overall health care.

PSYCHOMETRICS AND TOOL DEVELOPMENT CONSIDERATIONS

In addition to the foregoing functional considerations, properties related to the psychometric soundness and development of the tool must also be evaluated. To evaluate an assessment approach in terms of psychometric soundness, several features should be considered. First, the approach must be reliable. That is, similar results should be obtained from one assessment to another assessment of the same patient, both over time (presuming no change in status has occurred due to symptom improvement) and with different evaluators. Second, the approach must be valid. In other words, the tool must assess what it purports to assess. Third, the approach needs to have been evaluated and determined to be appropriate for use with the given population or setting. Information on norms should be relevant to the given patient population in terms of gender, age, and ethnicity, at the very least.

Assessment instruments should also possess high levels of sensitivity and specificity. Sensitivity and specificity refer to how accurately an assessment approach identifies target "cases." The greater the sensitivity of the instrument, the greater the likelihood that an individual who actually has the particular problem that the approach is designed to identify will actually be identified by the assessment. Conversely, the greater the specificity of an assessment approach, the greater the likelihood that an individual who does not have the particular problem that the approach is designed to assess will not be identified by the assessment (Andrykowski, Cordova, Studts, & Miller, 1998). Clearly, tools with high specificity and sensitivity will identify the most individuals with the problem in question while yielding the fewest false positives. However, few screening tools are both highly sensitive and specific. Rather, it is useful to select a screening approach that is highly sensitive (that is, has a low false negative rate) and has moderate specificity. Such a tool will identify patients who might possibly meet diagnostic criteria but will still exclude a fair number of those who clearly do not have the problem in question (Baldessarini, Finkelstein, & Arana, 1983). One relevant study found that primary care patients who completed mental health screens that resulted in false positives for one diagnostic area still met diagnostic criteria for another disorder at a significantly higher proportion than those whose screens were true negatives (Leon et al., 1997). This again supports the idea that a screen that is highly sensitive with moderate specificity is appropriate for the primary care setting as the screening will, at the very least, identify those who need further assessment, even if the preliminary diagnosis is inaccurate.

Another important criterion in selecting an assessment approach is related to appropriate use in the given setting. That is, before choosing an assessment instrument for use in primary care, one should first consider the utility and feasibility of the approach for the specific setting. For instance, to ensure sound psychometric properties, an approach often must be conducted in a standardized fashion, but standardized administration is usually difficult in typical clinical settings. Therefore, selection of an assessment approach should take into consideration factors such as ease of administration, ability to train staff to appropriately administer the assessment, and the degree of variability of administration that will still yield accurate results. If the tool is easy to administer and interpret, more staff will willingly use it as part of their regular patient care. Once psychological screening is a routine part of patient care, staff will have greater information about all patients. And, as staff find routine psychological screening useful in their daily functioning, they will likely become more committed to widespread, accurate use of the screening measure.

The language of the assessment approach is also an important feature worthy of consideration. English is not the first language of many patients. Thus, for those who do not speak or read English, the assessment must be conducted in another language. Because a single assessment tool is usually preferable within a setting so that staff can easily compare patients and evaluate overall functioning of those who obtain care at the site, determining that psychometric properties are acceptable across languages is also important. However, because not all tools have acceptable translations, translators and interpreters might be employed instead, thus perhaps losing some reliability and validity but ensuring that all patients are screened. A second language consideration occurs when individuals with less than fluent mastery of English complete paper-and-pencil or computer-based measures in English. Little is currently known about how language fluency affects assessment accuracy, but it is likely to affect the validity of assessment results. A final language consideration is the level of literacy necessary for accurate completion of paper-and-pencil assessments. Some 20% of American adults cannot read at even a fifth-grade level (Literacy Volunteers of America, 2000), and therefore any assessment tool that requires reading must be written so that the majority of adults can understand the material.

The last important practical consideration is whether the assessment is culturally appropriate. Manifestations of psychopathology can vary across cultures, and various assessment strategies may be more or less culturally sensitive. In settings with highly diverse patient populations, this sensitivity is particularly important. Determining what adaptations to the assessment tool are acceptable so that meaningful scores will result is often necessary when selecting an instrument (Geisinger, 1998). Some tools have been evaluated cross-culturally and, thus, should be selected for use in settings with more diverse populations.

SCREENING AND ASSESSMENT INSTRUMENTS

Any assessment approach selected for wide-scale use in screening patients must meet several criteria. The importance of the criteria might vary by setting, but each should be considered when selecting an approach. In this section, specific assessment approaches are discussed in terms of psychometric soundness, sensitivity and specificity, and the utility and practical features associated with each approach. Information about all psychometric properties and clinical usefulness is not available for every measure, and not every measure has been thoroughly evaluated (for instance, relatively few measures have been tested cross-culturally). Furthermore, sensitivity and specificity are not known for all procedures. While a variety of assessment approaches exist, self-report tools are the principal focus of this chapter, as these require little specialized training on the part of the medical staff to administer and interpret. Primary care medical staff members typically have numerous duties to perform and must evaluate for many physical problems during patient appointments, so they have little time for added procedures. Following the discussion of a number of self-report screening tools, this chapter discusses three semistructured interviews designed for use in primary care settings.

Self-Report Measures

General Health Questionnaire (GHQ)

The GHQ (Goldberg, 1972) is a self-report questionnaire that is designed to detect nonpsychotic emotional disorders. It is not disorder-based but, rather, has a cutoff point that suggests the likely presence of a psychiatric disorder. The original instrument contains 60 items that refer to the severity of psychological symptoms during the past 4 weeks relative to the person's normal functioning. There is also a 30-item version of this questionnaire that has a corresponding cutoff point. The 60-item version takes 10 to 15 minutes to complete and has satisfactory sensitivity and specificity (Goldberg, 1989). Because the GHQ is a self-report measure, it is likely to miss those patients who underendorse symptoms. However, because it does not require a clinician-administered interview, it is more easily used than are structured diagnostic interviews. The GHQ has been used in a variety of studies, including those addressing community, social, and occupational research, as well as psychiatric morbidity associated with physical disorders (Shepherd, Cooper, Brown, & Kalton, 1981), suggesting that it is adequate across a variety of patient populations, although additional cross-cultural evaluation would be useful.

Symptom Checklist-90—Revised

The SCL-90-R (Derogatis, 1977, 1994) is a 90-item self-report questionnaire that was developed for the assessment of general psychopathology. Like the GHQ, SCL-90-R is not used as a diagnostic assessment tool, but can be used to screen for the presence of psychopathology. The SCL-90-R takes approximately 15–20 minutes to complete. The items in this questionnaire refer to the severity of psychological symptoms during the past week. Each item of the SCL-90-R is rated on a 5-point (0–4) scale of distress ranging from "not-at-all" to "extremely." Although the SCL-90-R is not disorder based, the symptoms cluster along nine symptom dimensions: anxiety, depression, hostility, interpersonal sensitivity, phobic anxiety, paranoid ideation, psychoticism, somatization, and obsessive–compulsive. Elevated scores on each of the subscales indicate possible psychopathology.

Interpretation of the SCL-90-R focuses on both the total score (with a higher score indicating more severe psychopathology) and the subscale scores, which can provide a profile of the patient's psychological functioning. In addition, three global indices can be calculated from the raw scores on the SCL-90-R: (1) the General Severity Index (GSI), a weighted frequency score based on the sum of the ratings the patient has assigned to each symptom; (2) the Positive Symptom Total (PST), a frequency count of the number of symptoms the patient has reported; and (3) the Positive Symptom Distress Index (PSDI), a score reflecting the intensity of distress, corrected for the number of symptoms endorsed. The reliability and validity of the SCL-90-R has been documented in several studies (e.g., Derogatis, Rickels, & Rock, 1976). It has been suggested that the SCL-90-R is best used as a global index of psychopathology or psychological distress, but that little reliance should be placed on the subscale profiles (Boulet & Boss, 1991), restricting its usefulness in the primary care setting. That is, the SCL-90-R has little utility as a diagnostic assessment, but it is helpful in assessing the general level of psychopathology. The SCL-90-R has been used widely in studies with diverse populations, has been translated into many languages (including German and Spanish), and has been found appropriate for use with numerous ethnic and cultural groups—including people from Cambodia (e.g., D'Avanzo & Barab, 1998), Germany (e.g., Maercker & Schuetzwohl, 1998), Arabic-speaking countries (e.g., Abdallah, 1998), Argentina (e.g., Bonicatto, Dew, Soria, & Seghezzo, 1997), Latino backgrounds (e.g., Peragallo, 1996), Korea (e.g., Noh & Avison, 1992), and French-Canadian backgrounds (e.g., Chartrand & Julien, 1994).

Brief Symptom Inventory

The BSI (Derogatis & Melisaratos, 1983) is a brief version of the SCL-90-R, and was developed as an adaptation of the longer scale. It is comprised of 53 items, each of which is rated on the same 5-point scale as the SCL-90-R. The BSI is a well-known and well-accepted instrument. It is easy to administer, takes little time to complete, and is relatively nonintrusive. As with the SCL-90-R, it is used as a general measure of psychopathology, rather than as a diagnostic tool. The BSI measures psychopathology along the same nine symptom dimensions and three global dimensions as in the SCL-90-R. Because it includes fewer items, however, the BSI takes only 10 minutes to complete. Scores on the BSI and the SCL-90-R are highly correlated, and both have been found to be reliable and valid psychometric instruments (Derogatis & Melisaratos, 1983).

Holden Psychological Screening Inventory (HPSI)

The HPSI (Holden, 1991) is a 36-item self-report questionnaire that is designed to identify individuals who might benefit from further assessment of psychological dysfunction. It is used as a screening instrument to measure general level of psychopathology, and it takes only 5 to 7 minutes to complete. The HPSI consists of three subscales: psychiatric symptomatology, social symptomatology, and depression. The subscale of psychiatric symptomatology reflects generalized psychopathology, including psychotic processes, anxiety, and somatic symptoms. The social symptomatology subscale includes such symptoms as interpersonal problems, inadequate socialization and problems with impulse control. The depression subscale includes feelings of pessimism, loss of confidence in abilities, self-deprecation, and introversion. Summing scores across the three subscales can also generate a total psychopathology score. The HPSI has shown excellent reliability and validity in a number of studies with both clinical as well as nonclinical populations (e.g., Holden, Mendonca, Mazmanian, & Reddon, 1992). Thus, in a primary care setting, where many patients do not have mental health problems, the HPSI can successfully identify those who do have such problems.

Multidimensional Health Profile, Part I: Psychosocial Functioning (MHP-P)

The MHP is a recently developed brief screening instrument that consists of two components—the MHP, Part I: Psychosocial Functioning (MHP-P; Ruehlman, Lanyon, & Karoly, 1999) and the MHP, Part II: Health Functioning. The MHP-P consists of 58 items assessing the following four areas: mental health, social resources, life stress, and coping skills. The mental health subscale screens for anxiety, depression, history of mental disorder, current global mental health, and life satisfaction. The social resources subscale assesses availability of social support, support satisfaction, use of social support, and negative social exchange. The life stress subscale includes questions regarding the number of stressful events experienced over the previous year, the perceived stressfulness of the events, and a single rating of the perceived impact of stress on one's life over the previous year (global stress). Finally, the coping skills subscale consists of emotion-focused coping skills, as well as problem-focused coping skills.

Although the MHP-P is not disorder-specific, and therefore cannot be used for diagnostic purposes, it does assess a wide range of psychosocial factors that are important in the primary care setting. Recent research supports the reliability and validity of this instrument using a nationally representative sample of English-speaking adults who were interviewed by telephone (Ruehlman, Lanyon, & Karoly, 1999). Because this scale was recently constructed, the data on reliability and validity that have been collected thus far are considered preliminary. Norms and raw score to T-score conversions have been developed for the MHP for six ages by gender groups. Interpretation of the scores is achieved by use of cutoff points. The authors of the scale have also suggested that future efforts will be directed toward the collection of much needed ethnic-group norms. Future research will also address the utility of this scale in primary care settings (Ruehlman et al., 1999).

Medical Outcomes Study 36-Item Short-Form Health Survey

The Medical Outcomes Study (MOS) was constructed to develop a series of outcomes instruments to assist in the collection of medical outcomes data for use in clinical practice, research, health policy evaluations, and general population surveys. A number of self-report instruments were created throughout this study, of which the most commonly used and most empirically sound is the SF-36 (Ware & Sherbourne, 1992). The SF-36 is a multi-item scale that measures each of eight health concepts: physical functioning (10 items); role limitations because of physical health problem (4 items); bodily pain (2 items); social functioning (2 items); general mental health (psychological distress and psychological well-being, 5 items); role limitations because of emotional problems (3 items); vitality (energy/fatigue, 4 items); and general health perceptions (5 items). One additional item asks respondents to rate the amount of change in their general health status over a 1-year period. All questions are scored using a Likert scale, and scores are summed to create eight indices of functioning and a general profile of physical and emotional health. These scales, and the items that they comprise, were selected to be consistent with the health status assessment literature.

The five-item general mental health subscale of the SF-36 is referred to as the Mental Health Inventory (MHI) and has been found to discriminate psychiatric patients from those with other medical conditions (Berwick et al., 1991). In addition, a number of studies have illustrated high reliability and convergent validity for the SF-36 (McHorney, Ware, & Raczek, 1993; Jenkinson, Layte, & Lawrence, 1997). The SF-36 differs from many of the other screening measures and assessment tools discussed in this chapter, as its main focus is on medical outcomes, rather than on psychological functioning or psychopathology. Like the other self-report instruments mentioned, the SF-36 gives no diagnosis-specific information. In the context of primary care, however, it may be helpful to use a measure that encompasses both physical and mental health assessment and that is used as an outcome tool, in addition to being an assessment instrument. The SF-36 has been translated for use in more than 40 countries; Chinese, Japanese, Spanish, and Vietnamese versions are in various stages of development and validation for use in the United States (Ware, 1999).

Psychiatric Diagnostic Screening Questionnaire (PDSQ)

Although several versions of the PDSQ are in circulation, the final version (Zimmerman & Mattia, 1999, 2001a, 2001b) is a 126-item self-administered questionnaire that screens for 13 DSM-IV disorders in five areas (eating, mood, anxiety, substance use, and somatoform disorders). It was designed to be brief enough to be completed by patients at a routine visit, yet comprehensive enough to cover the most common disorders for which patients seek treatment. The PDSQ takes approximately 10 to 15 minutes to complete and can be done in the waiting room, prior to an initial visit. The PDSQ consists of 13 subscales, each of which is related to a different DSM-IV diagnosis. For example, the depression subscale assesses each of the nine DSM-IV symptom criteria for major depressive disorder. For some of the disorders, the PDSQ's questions refer to the past 2 weeks. However, for phobias, substance use, generalized anxiety disorder, and somatoform disorders, the time frame of the questions is the past 6 months. Two of the 15 screening questions for posttraumatic stress disorder (PTSD) refer to a lifetime history of experiencing or witnessing a traumatic life event, and the remaining 13 questions inquire about PTSD symptoms within the past 2 weeks. The PDSQ subscales have been demonstrated to have good levels of internal consistency and test–retest reliability (Zimmerman & Mattia, 1999, 2001a, 2001b). In addition, the subscales have high levels of discriminant and convergent validity. The PDSQ is unique in that it is the first self-report questionnaire to screen for several different DSM-IV diagnoses; other self-report measures address the level of psychopathology but do not suggest the presence or absence of a number of specific diagnoses. Although many clinician-administered interviews assess for different diagnoses, the PDSQ is the only self-report measure to do so.

Behavior and Symptom Identification Scale

The BASIS-32 (Eisen et al., 1994) is a brief measure designed for use in assessing psychiatric symptoms and functional abilities. It has principally been used as a measure of treatment outcome. The measure does not provide diagnostic information but rather yields scores on five subscales: relation to self and others, daily living and role functioning, depression–anxiety, impulsive–addictive behaviors, and psychosis. The original instrument was developed for use as an interview in an inpatient setting but has subsequently been evaluated in outpatient settings and as a self-report measure (Hoffmann, Capelli, & Mastrianni, 1997; Klinkenberg, Cho, & Vieweg, 1998; Russo et al., 1997). Respondents provide ratings from 0 (none) to 4 (extreme) to indicate the degree of difficulty experienced for each item in the past week. Satisfactory concurrent and discriminant validity have been reported (Eisen et al., 1994) for the interview version and replicated for self-report administration (Russo et al., 1997). Internal consistency and reliability were also supported (Klinkenberg et al., 1998). The self-report version is an easily administered and scored tool, which suggests that it would be practical as a screening measure. Less information is available regarding the use of BASIS-32 with primary care populations, as most research has been conducted in mental health settings. The measure has been translated into several languages, including Cambodian, Chinese, French, Japanese, Korean, Spanish, Tagalog, and Vietnamese, and evaluation of these translations is occurring (Eisen & Culhane, 1999).

Treatment Outcome Package

The TOP (Kraus et al., in press) was developed to meet the growing need for clinically useful assessment and outcome tools designed specifically to assess important behavioral health clinical domains. The Brief TOP assesses clinical domains such as depression, anxiety, thought control, and paranoid ideation. The Brief TOP can be used in the primary care setting as a screening tool for psychiatric problems and takes between 5 and 10 minutes to complete. There is both an adult and a child version. The adult version is available in Spanish, as well as English.

The TOP uses fax-back technology: the patient completes a two-page questionnaire, the answer page is faxed to a central scoring facility, and a clinical report is returned to the primary care office within 30 minutes. The clinical report is based on the decision structure used by DSM-IV.

The Brief TOP was derived from the standard TOP, a longer tool that takes approximately 20 to 30 minutes to complete. The factor structure of the TOP has remained stable and consistent over three large, unique patient samples. The adult TOP yields 11 clinical scales: Depression, Violence, Interpersonal Functioning, Quality of Life, Mania, Psychosis, Sleep, Panic, Work Functioning, Sexual Functioning, and Suicidality. Concurrent validation studies have compared the adult TOP to the SF-36, BASIS-32, Minnesota Multiphasic Personality Inventory-2 (MMPI-2; Butcher, Dahlstrom, Grahm, Tellegen, & Kaemmer, 1989); BSI, and the Beck Depression Inventory (BDI; Beck, Ward, Mendelson, Mock, & Erbaugh, 1961). All studies suggest sufficient convergent and divergent validity for each of the summary scores (Kraus, Jordan, Horan, & Crawford, in press).

Table 2.1 summarizes these nine self-report measures available for use in primary care settings.

TABLE 2.1. Self-Report Measures for Use in Primary Care Settings

Title and citation	Acronym	Time length (minutes)	Content	Advantages	Possible disadvantages
General Health Questionnaire (Goldberg, 1972)	GHQ	15	Nonpsychotic emotional disorders; cutoff point suggests likely presence of a psychiatric disorder	Brief; useful across a variety of patient populations	Not recently researched; not disorder-specific; cannot be used for diagnostic purposes
Symptom Checklist-90—Revised (Derogatis, 1977, 1994)	SCL-90-R	15–20	Assessment of general psychopathology; 9 symptom dimensions	Reliability and validity well documented; translated into many languages; appropriate for use with various ethnic and cultural groups	Not disorder-specific
Brief Symptom Inventory (Derogatis & Melisaratos, 1983)	BSI	10	Brief version of the SCL-90; general measure of psychopathology	Brief; reliability and validity well documented	Not disorder-specific
Multidimensional Health Profile, Part I: Psychosocial Functioning (Ruehlman et al., 1999)	MHP-P	15	Assessment of mental health, social resources, life stress, and coping skills	Assesses wide range of psychosocial factors important in the primary care setting	New scale, reliability and validity data considered preliminary; not disorder-specific

(continued)

TABLE 2.1. (*continued*)

Title and citation	Acronym	Time length (minutes)	Content	Advantages	Possible disadvantages
Holden Psychological Screening Inventory (Holden, 1991)	HPSI	5–7	General measure of psycho-pathology; measures social and psychiatric symptoms	Brief; reliability and validity well documented, utilizing clinical and nonclinical populations; includes screening for psychotic symptoms	Not disorder-specific
Medical Outcomes Study (MOS) 36-Item Short-Form Health Survey (Ware & Sherbourne, 1992)	SF-36	5–10	Measures 8 health concepts, including physical functioning, social functioning, and general mental health	Useful in primary care due to focus on medical outcomes; translated for use in more than 40 countries	Not disorder-specific; psychological symptoms not emphasized
Psychiatric Diagnostic Screening Questionnaire (Zimmerman & Mattia, 1999, 2001a, 2001b)	PDSQ	10–15	Screens for 13 DSM-IV disorders 5 areas: eating, mood, anxiety, substance use, somatoform	Brief, yet fairly comprehensive; disorder-specific; items consistent with DSM-IV criteria	Specific to psychological diagnoses, no mention of general level of functioning or physical health/well-being
Behavior and Symptom Identification Scale (Eisen et al., 1994)	BASIS-32	10–20	Assesses psychiatric symptoms and functional abilities; measure of treatment outcome	Evaluated in outpatient settings; measure of psychotherapy treatment outcomes; available in many languages	Little research in primary care setting; cannot be used for diagnostic purposes
Brief Treatment Outcome Package (Kraus et al., in press)	Brief TOP	5–10	Assesses a variety of clinical domains; measure of treatment outcome	Useful in outpatient settings; measure of treatment outcomes; adult and child versions; available in Spanish; fax back technology	Limited in scope of diagnoses; few psychometrics reported on Brief TOP

Diagnostic Interviews

Primary Care Evaluation of Mental Disorders

The PRIME-MD (Spitzer et al., 1994) interview is based on the diagnostic criteria of DSM-IV and is used in primary care settings as a diagnostic instrument. It entails a two-stage evaluation process: a brief self-administered questionnaire, followed by a clinician-administered, structured diagnostic interview for individuals who indicate symptoms of psychiatric disorders. The first stage of the PRIME-MD, the Patient Questionnaire (PQ), is a one-page 26-item self-report questionnaire that includes "yes"/"no" questions about a wide range of symptoms. The PQ takes only a few minutes to complete. The symptoms from this questionnaire are categorized under five domains: depression, anxiety, alcohol, somatization, and eating disorders. If the patient endorses symptoms for any domain, the clinician then administers the appropriate module of the Clinician Evaluation Guide (CEG), a structured interview schedule that the physician uses to follow up on positive responses on the PQ.

The validity of the PRIME-MD was demonstrated in a multisite study in which the same patients were diagnosed by PCPs using the PRIME-MD and by experienced mental health professionals (Spitzer et al., 1994). The average amount of time spent by the physician administering the PRIME-MD was 8.4 minutes, with 95% of the cases requiring fewer than 20 minutes. A high level of agreement between PRIME-MD and independent mental health professionals for the presence of any diagnosis was found. The utility of the PRIME-MD also has been studied in a sample of American Indians at an urban Indian Health Service primary care clinic (Parker et al., 1997). In this study there was fair agreement between PRIME-MD diagnoses and the diagnoses of mental health professionals. In addition, the PRIME-MD was considered helpful in identifying the presence of psychopathology and in initiating treatment for those who had not previously been identified as requiring treatment for a psychiatric disorder. The PRIME-MD has also been evaluated for use with older (65+ years) populations and was found to increase rates of provider diagnosis and subsequent intervention (Valenstein et al., 1998). Although the PRIME-MD appears to have good sensitivity and specificity (Spitzer et al., 1994), it has not been widely adopted by PCPs (Joseph & Hermann, 1998). This is likely due to both the administration time and the training necessary to successfully administer this assessment.

A recent study examined the validity of a computer-administered version of the PRIME-MD, as well as a telephone-administered computer-assisted version that uses interactive voice response (IVR) technology and is referred to as the IVR PRIME-MD. Diagnoses obtained by these two methods were compared with diagnoses obtained by an expert clinician who conducted the Structured Clinical Interview for DSM-IV (SCID; First, Spitzer, Gibbon, & Williams, 1997), a widely used and well-validated instrument, by telephone (Kobak et al., 1997). Prevalence rates found by both computer interviews were similar to those obtained by the SCID-IV for the presence of any diagnosis, any affective disorder, and any anxiety disorder. Prevalence rates for specific diagnoses found by the computer interviews were also similar to those obtained by the SCID-IV, with the exception that the computer interviews determined that dysthymia and obsessive–compulsive disorder were more prevalent and the SCID-IV determined that panic disorder was more prevalent. Using the SCID-IV as the criterion, both computer-administered versions of the PRIME-MD had high sensitivity, high specificity, and positive predictive value for most diagnoses. In addition, no significant difference was found in how well patients liked each form of interview. This research supports the validity and utility of both forms of computerized diagnostic assessments.

Symptom-Driven Diagnostic System for Primary Care (SDDS-PC)

The SDDS-PC (Broadhead et al., 1995) is also based on the diagnostic criteria of DSM-IV, and can be used as a diagnostic instrument in primary care settings. It consists of a 16-item patient questionnaire, followed by a clinician-administered, structured diagnostic interview that is designed to assess alcohol abuse/dependence, panic disorder, generalized anxiety disorder, major depressive disorder, obsessive–compulsive disorder, and suicidal ideation. In general, with a large primary care sample, the SDDS-PC was found to have moderate to high reliability kappas and moderate validity for each disorder assessed (Leon, Olfson, Weissman, Portera, & Sheehan, 1996). The SDDS-PC has been compared with the SCID and has been found to have fair sensitivity and good specificity (Broadhead et al., 1995). However, because it takes approximately 35 minutes to administer in total, the SDDS-PC has not been widely adopted in primary care settings (Joseph & Hermann, 1998). In addition, the SDDS-PC was initially designed to be scored by computer, and that option is not available in all primary care settings. A computer-assisted telephone interview (CATI) of the SDDS-PC was developed and appears to be a viable first-stage screen in the assessment process (Leon et al., 1999).

Mini-International Neuropsychiatric Interview

The MINI (Sheehan et al., 1998) is an abbreviated structured psychiatric interview, developed jointly by psychiatrists and psychologists in the United States and Europe, for use with DSM-IV and the 10th edition of the *International Classification of Diseases* (ICD-10; World Health Organization, 1990) psychiatric disorders. It takes approximately 15 to 20 minutes to administer in total. The MINI was created to bridge the gap between very detailed, research-oriented interviews and short screening instruments designed for use in primary care settings. It is therefore shorter than typical research interviews but more comprehensive than typical screening instruments. The MINI consists of a one-page self-report questionnaire, including 25 questions that address symptoms of depression, anxiety, mania, suicidality, psychosis, eating disorders, alcohol and drug problems, and antisocial characteristics. In addition, a clinician-administered structured diagnostic interview is used to assess the major Axis I disorders in DSM-IV. This interview elicits most of the symptoms listed in the symptom criteria for DSM-IV for 15 major Axis I diagnostic categories and for antisocial personality disorder. The MINI is divided into modules, each of which corresponds to a diagnostic category. Its diagnostic algorithms are consistent with the DSM-IV diagnostic system.

The MINI was designed to be used by both licensed professionals and well-trained interviewers who do not have a background in psychiatry or psychology. In a large-scale study, the MINI was found to have good diagnostic concordance with the SCID (Sheehan et al., 1998); it produced the same diagnosis as the SCID in 85% to 95% of the cases. In addition to being a valid instrument, the MINI has been found to be a reliable measure of psychopathology. It has good sensitivity, specificity, and predictive value, with the level of each of these varying across diagnoses (Sheehan et al., 1998). The MINI is unique in that it has been translated into over 30 languages, and close attention has been paid to ensure adherence to the accuracy of questions across all languages. Like the PRIME-MD, the MINI now has a computerized version. It has also been included in an IVR/CATI that is integrated with a medical screening/triage interview for medical and primary care telephone screening. Studies are under way to assess the value of computerized versions of the MINI.

Table 2.2 summarizes the three diagnostic interview measures available for use in primary care settings.

TABLE 2.2. Clinician-Administered Diagnostic Interview Measures for Use in Primary Care Settings

Title and citation	Acronym	Time length (minutes)	Content	Advantages	Possible disadvantages
Primary Care Evaluation of Mental Disorders (Spitzer et al., 1994)	PRIME-MD	10–20 for the interview	Modules of interview include depression, anxiety, alcohol, somatization, and eating disorders	Questions consistent with DSM-IV diagnostic criteria; generates specific diagnoses; adequate reliability and validity	Inadequate provision of accurate diagnoses for many DSM-IV categories; time-consuming; extensive training necessary
Symptom-Driven Diagnostic System for Primary Care (Broadhead et al., 1995)	SDDS-PC	35 in total	Modules of interview include depression, anxiety, and alcohol disorders	Questions consistent with DSM-IV diagnostic criteria; generates specific diagnoses; adequate psychometrics	Time-consuming; training necessary; computer scoring not available in all primary care settings
Mini International Neuropsychiatric Interview (Sheehan et al, 1998)	MINI	15–20 in total	Assesses 15 major Axis I disorders and antisocial personality disorder	Questions consistent with DSM-IV and ICD-10 diagnostic criteria; comprehensive; generates specific diagnoses; strong psychometrics; translated into over 30 languages	Time-consuming; training necessary

ADDITIONAL AREAS FOR ASSESSMENT

Although research has largely focused on the assessment and treatment of depression and anxiety in the primary care setting, many other mental health problems and populations are amenable to primary care screening. This chapter has suggested tools designed primarily to assess overall psychopathology or common mental health concerns, such as depression, anxiety disorders and thought disturbances. However, it might prove beneficial in terms of enhanced treatment and cost savings in some primary care settings to assess for a wider variety of concerns, including issues related to anxiety before surgery, as well as smoking cessation. Additionally, many primary care settings serve populations ranging in age from the very young to the very old, possibly requiring age appropriate assessment tools. Here we briefly discuss research relevant to these issues.

Anxiety around surgery and invasive medical procedures is an area that is highly appropriate for primary care screening. Research has documented significant cost savings in the form of fewer days in the hospital, less use of pain medications, and fewer behavioral problems after psychological preparation for medical treatments (Groth-Marnat & Edkins, 1996). Psychological interventions prior to surgery are also useful, and many studies have found that patients who receive preoperative intervention stay in the hospital 1 to 2 days fewer than those who did not receive such intervention. In one study, Olbrisch (1981) found a reduction of 1.2 hospital days for adult surgical patients who received preoperative psychological interventions. In another study, preoperative biofeedback reduced hospital days by 72% and postoperative doctor visits by 63% (Anderson, 1987). Cost savings have also been documented for children who received preparations before medical procedures. In a study where children were shown a videotape to prepare them for hospitalization, the control children, who were not prepared for surgery, experienced hospitalization costs of about $200 more than those who saw the videotape (Pinto & Hollandsworth, 1989). Thus the time, money, and emotional well-being that can be saved by preparing patients for surgery and other medical procedures may greatly outweigh the actual cost of such preparations.

Another major area of cost in the primary care setting is that associated with cigarette smoking. The financial and emotional costs related to cigarette smoking are almost incalculable. One out of five Americans dies as a result of complications related to smoking, and direct annual costs for smoking related illnesses have been estimated to be about $47 billion per year (Groth-Marnat & Edkins, 1996). Although managed care generally does not pay for smoking cessation programs, and although there is a paucity of data looking at cost savings associated with smoking cessation programs, several studies have indicated that successful smoking cessation programs save money—not to mention lives. It was estimated that one smoking intervention program led to a $20,000 cost saving per year of life saved for patients who had a myocardial infarction (Groth-Marnat & Edkins, 1996). Thus, although there are few data on the contribution of behavioral health interventions such as psychological preparations for surgery or smoking cessation programs in the primary care setting, preliminary data suggest that such programs might have a positive impact on the emotional and physical lives of the patients and on the overall cost of medical care.

The question of just what to screen for in the primary care setting when working with patients who smoke is an important one. Most primary care providers inquire as to whether, and how much, a patient smokes and then encourage patients to quit. However, quitting smoking is extraordinarily difficult, even with available programs. A simple screening method to identify those smokers most likely to benefit from a behavioral intervention would be very useful in the primary care setting. At this point, encouraging data suggest that readiness to change (motivation), addiction level, and environmental barriers are areas that correlate with successful smoking cessation (Lichtenstein & Glasgow, 1997), but much more research is indicated before specific methodologies for such screening in the primary care setting can be recommended.

A final problem area often encountered in primary care settings is alcohol and other substance use. Substance use is another expensive problem at both the individual and societal level. In an adolescent population, alcohol abuse was found to undermine motivation, interfere with cognitive processes, contribute to debilitating mood disorders, and increase the risk of accidental injury or death (Hawkins, Catalano, & Miller, 1992). In addition, alcohol abuse in later life is associated with lung cancer, coronary heart disease, AIDS, violent crime, child abuse and neglect, and unemployment.

Alcohol use disorders affect from 3% to 20% of patients in the primary care setting (Johnson et al., 1995). However, PCPs often fail to recognize the existence of alcohol-related problems or other substance abuse. In fact, 45% of patients who requested treatment for addiction in a public health system reported that their physicians did not know about their substance abuse (Saitz, Mulvey, Plough, & Samet, 1997). Although the data on the efficacy of many alcohol and substance abuse treatment programs are mixed, and many managed care organizations are paying for only limited treatments, problem drinkers can benefit from physician intervention or referral to treatment programs at the time of a primary care visit (e.g., Fleming et al., 2000). In addition, many brief instruments that easily screen for alcoholism exist. These include the Quantity/Frequency Questions, Michigan Alcoholism Screening Test, the Alcohol Use Disorders Identification Test (AUDIT), the CAGE, and the TWEAK (the latter two are acronyms with each letter a prompt for the question to be asked) (see Cherpitel, 1997, for additional information on these measures).

Most assessment and screening instruments available for the primary care setting are designed to target the average adult population. However, both young and old patients may require assessment instruments tailored to the specific psychological issues relevant to the given age group. Pediatric and adolescent psychiatric disorders clearly warrant attention in terms of screening in the primary care setting. Childhood psychiatric disorders occur in 14% to 20% of American children and adolescents, and yet, similar to the problem for adults, only approximately one in five children with psychiatric disorders is identified (Cassidy & Jellinek, 1998; Costello et al., 1988). In addition, psychiatric disorders are underdiagnosed in adolescents in the primary care setting (Kramer & Garrada, 1998). Childhood psychiatric disorders are also associated with enhanced primary care attendance and expense (Garland, Bowman, & Mandalia, 1999). Thus, improvements in screening for child and adolescent psychiatric disorders in the primary care setting could result in significant improvements in mental and physical health of children, as well as in decreased spending on health care. Screening tools for children are typically designed to be completed by the parent or primary caregiver, rather than by the child. And there are relatively few, brief, general tools available for pediatric assessments, so much additional development is needed in this area.

In addition, primary care providers may need to devote specialized attention to assessments for geriatric populations. Overall, it appears that older patients are less likely to seek out mental health providers or accept referrals from their physicians so the PCP, by default, becomes the major provider of all services (Katz, 1998). The majority of research on psychological screening in the elderly focuses on the assessment of depression. However, one study that screened for a wide variety of disorders found that "substantial proportions of those who screened positive for each of the non-depressive disorders were screen-negative for depression" (Lish et al., 1995). In other words, screening for depression alone might preclude identification of numerous other psychological problems. Some screening tools have been evaluated for use with geriatric populations, but if a tool that has not been evaluated for such use is selected for a primary care setting, providers must be aware of possible mental health screening complications. Due to the greater likelihood of multiple medical problems and/or cognitive changes in the elderly, increases are often seen in such symptoms as fatigue, difficulty sleeping, and impairments in concentration. It is extremely important that PCPs who screen for psychological symptoms in the elderly are careful to differentiate between symptoms that stem from psychological versus physical disorders.

BARRIERS TO THE IMPLEMENTATION OF STANDARDIZED SCREENING FOR MENTAL HEALTH PROBLEMS IN PRIMARY CARE SETTINGS

There are several barriers to the collection of standardized mental health assessment data in the primary care setting. These fall into two major categories: physician resistance and client resistance.

The PCP has historically had inadequate experience and knowledge to adequately identify and treat psychiatric conditions that are common to primary care patients. In addition, practitioners are often uncomfortable talking to patients about mental health problems and believe that patients are uncomfortable talking about psychiatric issues.

Although the collection of laboratory data is clearly familiar to the PCP and intrinsic to the practice of primary care medicine, the collection of mental heath data is not routinely seen as part of business as usual in the primary care setting, and therefore is not viewed as further collection of laboratory data. Part of this problem is related to the nature of brief mental health assessment tools. Mental health assessments are often perceived as subjective: the mental health profession does not yet have a proverbial "blood test" to measure diagnoses but relies on patient and clinician perceptions to assess mental health functioning. Mental health assessments are often not perceived as "hard data." This is complicated by the fact that the assessment of mental health patients is difficult at best, and even more challenging in nonmental health settings, such as the physician's office. In fact, mental health assessment tools are *not* just like a blood test or an x-ray; results are complicated by patients' attitudes (for example, exaggeration of symptoms or minimization of symptoms), risk factors, socioeconomic factors, and functional levels. It is our hope that the training of PCPs in the use of assessment tools and in the understanding of psychiatric disorders will increase physician acceptance of psychiatric assessment.

In addition, there has been concern that patients will also resist mental health assessment: a general perception has been that patients are uncomfortable addressing mental health issues in the primary care setting (Docherty, 1997). Certainly, at times, this is true. Some patients do react negatively to questions about mental health functioning in the general medical setting and would rather focus on somatic symptoms. However, a growing body of literature is emerging that indicates that patients are comfortable completing mental health screening tools if the tools are relatively easy to complete (Chen, Broadhead, Doe, & Broyles, 1993).

Patient resistance to mental health screening appears to be more myth than reality, however. In a recent study on the reaction of patients to psychological assessment in the primary care setting, it was found that fewer than 2% of the sample objected to completing a psychological assessment tool in a medical setting, and only about 3% were embarrassed by the content of the questions (Zimmerman et al., 1996). Indeed, data are emerging that patients are comfortable talking about emotional problems in the primary care setting: in one study, 84% of patients with an assumed diagnosis of major depression and 79% of patients with an assumed diagnosis of minor depression felt that it was somewhat important to receive help from their physician (Brody, Khaliq, & Thompson, 1997).

RECOMMENDATIONS

It is clear that currently in managed care and primary care settings, the presence of mental health problems is often not routinely assessed. This is problematic for several reasons. First, people with psychopathology often present in primary care settings. In addition, psychopathology is often misinterpreted in this setting as reflective of a physical condition, and even when physical problems are the primary concern, existing psychopathology, especially when undocumented, can complicate treatment and recovery. Therefore, instituting routine assessment for mental health problems is an appropriate and necessary step. The assessment approach must be brief, flexible, and informative, and this can be accomplished in a variety of ways.

In some settings, it might be most appropriate to screen for overall level of psychological distress. Once those persons who meet some predetermined, clinically significant level of distress are identified, they can then undergo a more thorough assessment in another setting. The goal of simply identifying high levels of psychological distress might prove easier and more efficient for clinicians who do not specialize in mental health, such as general physicians and nurses. Patients with high levels of psychological distress will likely be the most difficult to treat in the immediate setting and might therefore require a team of providers, rather than only the primary care medical staff. Identifying and properly treating these patients will prove helpful to both patient and PCP. Finally, noting high distress in some individuals might prove a more straightforward task than requiring staff to identify particular symptom patterns and render a diagnosis, particularly when they are not well trained in the area.

A second approach might be to identify particular disorders or symptom patterns. While establishing a psychiatric diagnosis is a learned skill, identifying provisional or tentative clinical diagnoses using a screening assessment should be possible. Also, because more specialized assessments are often more costly, it might be preferable to identify patients with likely disorders at the screening level in order to streamline the use of assessment resources. This would then enable the next level of assessment to be more focused. An added benefit of more precise screening is that, often, only treatment for diagnosable mental disorders is covered under insurance plans. Although many people could benefit from mental or behavioral health interventions, such as stress management or smoking cessation, in times of limited resources, only those with diagnosable problems might be eligible for such treatments and more focused screening would identify these individuals sooner and direct them to the appropriate resources.

A third approach might be to screen for specific symptoms. Routine screening for psychotic symptoms, depression, and suicidality might serve to identify those who are most at risk to themselves and most costly to the system, especially if they are left untreated. The screening approach could be relatively straightforward and could potentially identify some very serious problems. Additional specific areas for which to screen include the presence of violence or abuse in the home, personal or familial substance abuse or dependence, and the quality of interpersonal relationships and general psychosocial adjustment. Functional problems at home or work might suggest that a more detailed mental health assessment is appropriate.

Each of these areas, if problematic, could have substantial impact on a patient's functioning and could cause an individual to not follow through with appropriate medical care. In those cases, additional treatment (e.g., by a team of physicians, psychologists, or other therapists) might better help and enable a person to comply with medical treatment. Current screening practices for these areas are cursory and unlikely to yield satisfactory or adequate information. If a formal assessment protocol is not implemented, standard, detailed questions regarding all these domains should be a part of all assessments. For instance, simply asking whether a person uses substances is not going to provide the quality of information necessary to recommend additional assessment or to discuss treatment options. Therefore, the implementation of a standardized screen would eliminate guessing a patient's status and would ensure that relevant domains that could impact treatment and overall health are assessed for all individuals.

CONCLUSIONS

At this point, it is clear that screening patients for psychiatric problems in the primary care setting is both cost-effective and important from a public health and an individual patient viewpoint.

Screening Is Only the First Step

Primary care staff must remember that screening is just the beginning and that often screening does not result in a firm diagnosis: in fact, it may lead to more questions than answers. For instance, a brief multidomain screening tool, such as the TOP or PRIME-MD, may not derive the final diagnosis—either because the tool is not designed for that purpose or because the tool is incapable of providing accurate diagnoses for every DSM-IV category; but such a tool can identify many complex and interrelated problems. Once the presence of mental health symptoms has been noted, a more thorough assessment is almost always necessary. Improved screening methods should not lead to the belief that identification of problems equals the ability to make final complex diagnoses or the ability to adequately treat complex mental health problems.

Prescription of Medication Alone May Not Be Sufficient or Desirable

After a mental health assessment (or even without a formal mental health assessment), the PCP often chooses to treat provisionally identified mental health disorders in the primary care setting. This may imply that physicians with inadequate training in mental health treatments are the first or only source of care. Much of this treatment, therefore, is psychopharmacological, and there is a great deal of literature indicating that primary care physicians often undermedicate psychiatric patients. In addition, research indicates that pharmacological therapy alone is not the primary treatment of choice for many psychological disorders. Finally, behavioral treatments may be preferred by some patients and may be more cost effective than pharmacotherapy. In many instances, behavioral treatments are certainly as effective as medications (Lambert & Bergin, 1994), do not have unwanted physical side effects, and may therefore be safer for some patients with complicating somatic concerns.

Further Assessment Is Almost Always Needed

In general, the staff in a primary care practice may be able to do preliminary screens for mental health problems, although they often lack the necessary expertise to provide in-depth assessment and treatment. Therefore, although there is a small but growing movement toward multidisciplinary primary care settings, for the most part, patients must be referred outside of the primary care setting to a clinic or individual practitioner for appropriate diagnostic assessment and then treatment.

Unfortunately, in today's managed care environment, there are often incentives for treating patients within the primary care setting, as opposed to referring patients for specialized care. In addition, many patients in today's environment do not have mental health coverage and must be treated in the primary care setting. Finally, even when the physician is willing to make a referral and insurance coverage is available, specialized mental health care is often unavailable, especially in rural settings. Many clinicians and patients are demanding enhanced access to mental health care for all patients. Hopefully, improved screening in primary care settings and the documentation of the need for accessible and integrated mental health services will lead to increases in availability of and access to services. The present limitations of managed care should not be a deterrent to instituting appropriate procedures.

Many clients with a broad range of mental health issues, both children and adults, are being seen only in primary care settings. Additionally, there is a preponderance of data that mental health issues are being underdiagnosed in primary care settings, and there are both financial and human costs associated with this underdiagnosis. Given these facts, it becomes imperative for medical staff in primary care settings to become more vigilant to individuals with mental health needs and to improve current practices to identify mental health problems. Instituting brief self-report screening assessments or standardized brief interviews that are psychometrically sound and patient-friendly may be the most direct and efficient route to the identification of these problems.

REFERENCES

Abdallah, T. (1998). The Satisfaction with Life Scale (SWLS): Psychometric properties in an Arabic-speaking sample. *International Journal of Adolescence and Youth, 7,* 113–119.

American Psychiatric Association. (1994). *Diagnostic and statistical manual of mental disorders* (4th ed.). Washington, DC: Author.

Anderson, E. A. (1987). Preoperative preparation for cardiac surgery facilitates recovery, reduces psychological distress and reduces the incidence of acute postoperative hypertension. *Journal of Consulting and Clinical Psychology, 55,* 513–520.

Andrykowski, M. A., Cordova, M. J., Studts, J. L., & Miller, T. W. (1998). Posttraumatic stress disorder after treatment for breast cancer: Prevalence of diagnosis and use of the PTSD Checklist—Civilian Version (PCL-C) as a screening instrument. *Journal of Consulting and Clinical Psychology, 66,* 586–590.

Baldessarini, R. J., Finkelstein, S., & Arana, G. W. (1983). The predictive power of diagnostic tests and the effect of prevalence of illness. *Archives of General Psychiatry, 40,* 569–573.

Beck, A. T., Ward, C., Mendelson, M., Mock, J. E., & Erbaugh, J. K. (1961). An inventory for measuring depression. *Archives of General Psychiatry, 4,* 53–63.

Berwick, D. M., Murphy, J. M., Goldman, P. A., Ware, J. E., Barsky, A. J., & Weinstein, M. C. (1991). Performance of a five-item mental health screening test. *Medical Care, 29,* 169–175.

Bonicatto, S., Dew, M. A., Soria, J. J., & Seghezzo, M. E. (1997). Validity and reliability of Symptom Checklist 90 (SCL-90) in an Argentine population sample. *Social Psychiatry and Psychiatric Epidemiology, 32,* 332–338.

Boulet, J., & Boss, M. W. (1991). Reliability and validity of the Brief Symptom Inventory. *Psychological Assessment, 3,* 433–437.

Broadhead, W. E., Blazer, D. G., George, L. K., & Tse, C. K. (1990). Depression, disability days and days lost from work in a prospective epidemiological survey. *Journal of the American Medical Association, 264,* 2524–2528.

Broadhead, W. E., Leon, A. C., Weissman, M. M., Barrett, J. E., Blacklow, R. S., Gilbert, T. T., Keller, M. B., & Higgins, E. S. (1995). Development and validation of the SDDS-PC screen for multiple mental disorders in primary care. *Archives of Family Medicine, 4,* 211–219.

Brody, D. S., Khaliq, A. A., & Thompson, T. L. (1997). Patients' perceptions on the management of emotional distress in primary care settings. *Journal of General Internal Medicine, 12,* 403–406.

Butcher, J. N., Dahlstrom, W. G., Graham, J. R., Tellegen, A. M., & Kaemmer, B. (1989). *MMPI-2: Manual for administration and scoring.* Minneapolis: University of Minnesota Press.

Carmin, C. N., & Klocek, J. W. (1998). To screen or not to screen: Symptoms identifying primary care medical patients in need of screening for depression. *International Journal of Medicine, 28,* 293–302.

Cassidy, L. J., & Jellinek, M. S. (1998). Approaches to recognition and management of childhood psychiatric disorders in pediatric primary care. *Pediatric Clinica North America, 45,* 1037–1052.

Chartrand, E., & Julien, D. (1994). Validation of a French-Canadian version of the Interactional Dimensions Coding System (IDCS). *Canadian Journal of Behavioural Science, 26,* 319–337.

Chen, A. L., Broadhead, W. E., Doe, E. A., & Broyles, W. K. (1993). Patient acceptance of two health status measures: The Medical Outcomes Study Short-Form General Health Survey and the Duke Health Profile. *Family Medicine, 25,* 536–539.

Cherpitel, C. J. (1997). Brief screening instruments for alcoholism. *Alcohol Health and Research World, 21,* 348–351.

Costello, E. J., Edelbrock, C., Costello, A. J., Dulcan, M. K., Burns, B. J., & Brent, D. (1988). Psychopathology in pediatric primary care: The new hidden morbidity. *Pediatrics, 8,* 415–424.

D'Avanzo, C. E., & Barab, S. A. (1998). Depression and anxiety among Cambodian refugee women in France and the United States. *Issues in Mental Health Nursing, 19,* 541–556.

Derogatis, L. R. (1977). *SCL-90-R: Administration, scoring, and procedures manual for the revised version.* Baltimore: John Hopkins University School of Medicine, Clinical Psychometrics Research Unit.

Derogatis, L. R. (1994). *SCL-90-R: Administration, scoring and procedures manual* (3rd ed.). Minneapolis, MN: National Computer Systems.

Derogatis, L. R., & Melisaratos, N. (1983). The Brief Symptom Inventory: An introductory report. *Psychological Medicine, 13,* 596–605.

Derogatis, L. R., Rickels, K., & Rock, A. F. (1976). The SCL-90 and the MMPI: A step in the validation of a new self-report scale. *British Journal of Psychiatry, 128,* 280–289.

Docherty, J. P. (1997). Barriers to the diagnosis of depression in primary care. *Journal of Clinical Psychiatry, 58*(Suppl. 1), 5–10.

Eisen, S. V., & Culhane, M. A. (1999). Behavior and Symptom Identification Scale (BASIS-32). In M. Maruish (Ed.), *The use of psychological testing for treatment planning and outcomes assessment* (pp. 759–790). Mahwah, NJ: Erlbaum.

Eisen, S. V., Dill, D. L., & Grob, M. C. (1994). Reliability and validity of a brief patient-report instrument for psychiatric outcome evaluation. *Hospital and Community Psychiatry, 33,* 242–247.

First, M. B., Spitzer, R. L., Gibbon, M., & Williams, J. B. W. (1997). *Structured Clinical Interview for DSM-IV Axis I Disorders (SCID-I), Clinician Version.* Washington, DC: American Psychiatric Press.

Fleming, M. F., Mundt, M. P., French, M. T., Manwell, L. B., Stauffacher, E. A., & Barry, K. L. (2000). Benefit–cost analysis of brief physician advice with problem drinkers in primary care settings. *Medical Care, 38,* 7–18.

Garland, M. E., Bowman, F. M., & Mandalia, S. (1999). Children with psychiatric disorders that are frequent attendees to primary care. *European Journal of Child and Adolescent Psychiatry, 8,* 34–44.

Geisinger, K. F. (1998). Psychometric issues in test administration. In J. Sandoval, C. L. Frisby, K. F. Geisinger, J. D. Scheuneman, & J. Grenier (Eds.), *Test interpretation and diversity* (pp. 17–30). Washington, DC: American Psychological Association.

Goldberg, D. P. (1972). *The detection of psychiatric illness by questionnaire.* London: Oxford University Press.

Goldberg, D. P. (1989). Screening for psychiatric disorder. In P. Williams, G. Wilkinson, & K. Rawnsley (Eds.), *The scope of epidemiological psychiatry* (pp. 108–127). London: Routledge.

Groth-Marnat, G., & Edkins, G. (1996). Professional psychologists in general health care settings: A review of the financial efficacy of direct treatment interventions. *Professional Psychology: Research and Practice, 27,* 161–174.

Hankin, J. R., Kessler, L. G., & Goldberg, I. D. (1983). A longitudinal study of offset in the use of nonpsychiatric services following specialized mental health care. *Medical Care, 21,* 1099–1110.

Hawkins, J. D., Catalano, R. F., & Miller, J. Y. (1992). Risk and protective factors for alcohol and other drug problems in adolescence and early adulthood: Implications for substance abuse prevention. *Psychological Bulletin, 112,* 64–105.

Hoffmann, F. L., Capelli, K., & Mastrianni, X. (1997). Measuring treatment outcome for adults and adolescents: Reliability and validity of BASIS-32. *Journal of Mental Health Administration, 24,* 316–331.

Holden, R. R. (1991, June). *Psychometric properties of the Holden Psychological Screening Inventory (HPSI).* Paper presented at the meeting of the Canadian Psychological Association, Ottawa, Canada.

Holden, R. R., Mendonca, J. D., Mazmanian, D., & Reddon, J. R. (1992). Clinical construct validity of the Holden Psychological Screening Inventory (HPSI). *Journal of Clinical Psychology, 48,* 627–633.

Jenkinson, C., Layte, R., & Lawrence, K. (1997). Development and testing of the Medical Outcomes Study 36-Item Short Form Health Survey Summary Scale: Scores in the United Kingdom. Results from a large-scale survey and a clinical trial. *Medical Care, 35,* 410–416.

Johnson, J., Spitzer, R., Williams, J., Kroenke, K., Linzer, M., Brody, D., deGruy, F., & Hahn, S. (1995). Psychiatric comorbidity, health status and functional impairment associated with alcohol abuse and dependence in primary care patients: Findings of the Prime-MD-1000 Study. *Journal of Consulting and Clinical Psychology, 63,* 133–140.

Joseph, R. C., & Hermann, R. C. (1998). Screening for psychiatric disorders in primary care settings. *Harvard Review of Psychiatry, 6,* 165–170.

Katz, I. (1998). What should we do about undertreatment of late life psychiatric disorders in primary care? *Journal of the American Geriatric Society, 46,* 1573–1575.

Kessler, R. C., Barber, C., Birnbaum, H. G., Frank, R. G., Greenberg, P. E., Rose, R. M., Simon, G. E., & Wang, P. (1999). Depression in the workplace. *Health Affairs, 18,* 163–171.

Klinkenberg, W. D., Cho, D. W., & Vieweg, B. (1998). Reliability and validity of the interview and self-report versions of the BASIS-32. *Psychiatric Services, 49,* 1229–1231.

Kobak, K. A., Taylor, L. H., Dottl, S. L., Greist, J. H., Jefferson, J. W., Burroughs, D., Katzelnick, D. J., & Mandell, M. (1997). Computerized screening for psychiatric disorders in an outpatient community mental health clinic. *Psychiatric Services, 48,* 1048–1057.

Kramer, T., & Garrada, M. E. (1998). Psychiatric disorders in adolescents in primary care. *British Journal of Psychiatry, 173,* 508–513.

Kraus, D. R., Jordan, J., Horan, F. P., & Crawford, J. (in press.) Validation of a treatment outcome and assessment tool: The Treatment Outcome Package. *Psychological Assessment.*

Lambert, M. J., & Bergin, A. E. (1994). The effectiveness of psychotherapy. In A. E. Bergin & S. L. Garfield (Eds.), *Handbook of psychotherapy and behavior change* (pp. 143–189). New York: Wiley.

Lechnyr, R. (1992). Cost savings and effectiveness of mental health services. *Journal of Oregon Psychological Association, 38,* 8–12.

Leon, A. C., Kelsey, J. E., Pleil, A., Burgos, T. L., Portera, L., & Lowell, K. N. (1999). An evaluation of a computer assisted telephone interview for screening for mental disorders among primary care patients. *Journal of Nervous and Mental Disease, 187,* 308–311.

Leon, A. C., Olfson, M., Weissman, M. M., Portera, L., & Sheehan, D. V. (1996). Evaluation of screens for mental disorders in primary care: Methodological issues. *Psychopharmacology Bulletin, 32,* 353–361.

Leon, A. C., Portera, L., Olfson, M., Weissman, M. M., Kathol, R. G., Farber, L., Sheehan, D. V., & Pleil, A. M. (1997). False positive results: A challenge for psychiatric screening in primary care. *American Journal of Psychiatry, 154,* 1462–1464.

Lichtenstein, E., & Glasgow, R. E. (1997). A pragmatic framework for smoking cessation implications for clinical and public health programs. *Psychology of Addictive Behavior, 11,* 142–151.

Lish, J. D., Zimmerman, M., Farber, N. J., Lush, D., Kuzma, M. A., & Plescia, G. (1995). Psychiatric screening in geriatric primary care: Should it be for depression alone? *Journal of Geriatric Psychiatry and Neurology, 8,* 141–153.

Literacy Volunteers of America. (2000, May 30). Puzzling...isn't it? [On-line]. Available: www.geocities.com/Athens/Parthenon/2594/puzzling.htm.

Maercker, A., & Schuetzwohl, M. (1998). Assessment of post-traumatic stress reactions: The Impact of Event Scale—Revised (IES-R). *Diagnostica, 44,* 130–141.

Magruder-Habib, K., Zung, W. W., & Feussner J. R. (1990). Improving physicians' recognition and treatment of depression in general medical care: Results from a randomized clinical trial. *Medical Care, 28,* 239–250.

McHorney, C. A.,Ware, J. E., & Raczek, A. E. (1993). The MOS 36-Item Short Form Health Survey (SF-36): Psychometric and clinical tests of validity in measuring physical and mental health constructs. *Medical Care, 31,* 247–263.

Miller, B., & Farber, L. (1996). Delivery of mental health services in the changing health care system. *Professional Psychology: Research and Practice, 27,* 527–529.

Mumford, E., Schlesinger, H. L., Glass, G. V., & Cuerdon, T. (1984). A new look at evidence about reduced cost of medical utilization following mental health treatment. *American Journal of Psychiatry, 141,* 1145–1158.

Narrow, W. E., Regier, D. A., Rae, D. S., Manderscheid, R. W., & Locke, B. Z. (1993). Use of services by persons with mental and addictive disorders. *Archives of General Psychiatry, 50,* 95–107.

Noh, S., & Avison, W. R. (1992). Assessing psychopathology in Korean immigrants: Some preliminary results on the SCL-90. *Canadian Journal of Psychiatry, 37,* 640–645.

Noltorp, S., Gottfries, C. G., & Norgaard, N. (1998). Simple steps to diagnosis at primary care centres. *International Clinical Psychopharmacology, 13*(Suppl. 5), S31–S34.

Olbrisch, M. (1981). Evaluation of a stress management program *Medical Care, 19,* 153–159.

Parker, T., May, P. A., Maviglia, M. A., Petrakis, S., Sunde, S., & Gloyd, S. V. (1997). PRIME-MD: Its utility in detecting mental disorders in American Indians. *International Journal of Psychiatry in Medicine, 27,* 107–128.

Peragallo, N. (1996). Latino women and AIDS risk. *Public Health Nursing, 13,* 217–222.

Perez-Stable, E. J., Miranda, J., Munoz, R. F., & Ying, Y. W. (1990). Depression in medical outpatients: Underrecognition and misdiagnosis. *Archives of Internal Medicine, 150,* 946–948.

Pinto, R. P., & Hollandsworth, J. G. (1989). Using videotape modeling to prepare children psychologically for surgery: Influence of parents and costs versus benefits of providing preparation services. *Health Psychology, 8,* 79–95.

Rinaldi, R. C. (1992). Screening for mood disorders. *Journal of Family Practice, 34,* 103–104.

Ruehlman, L. S., Lanyon, R. I., & Karoly, P. (1999). Development and validation of the Multidimensional Health Profile, Part I: Psychosocial Functioning. *Psychological Assessment, 11,* 166–176.

Russo, J., Roy-Byrne, P., Jaffe, C., Ries, R., Dagadakis, C., Dwyer-O'Connor, E., & Reeder, D. (1997). The relationship of patient-administered outcome assessments to quality of life and physician ratings: Validity of the BASIS-32. *Journal of Mental Health Administration, 24,* 200–214.

Saitz, R., Mulvey, K. P., Plough, A., & Samet, J. H. (1997). Physician unawareness of serious substance abuse. *American Journal of Drug and Alcohol Abuse, 23,* 343–354.

Schurman, R. A., Kramer P. D., & Mitchell, J. B. (1985). The hidden mental health network: Treatment of mental illness by non-psychiatrist physicians. *Archives of General Psychiatry, 42,* 89–94.

Sheehan, D.V., Lecrubier, Y., Harnett Sheehan, K., Amorim, P., Janavs, J., Weiller, E., Hergueta, T., Baker, R., & Dunbar, G. C. (1998). The Mini-International Neuropsychiatric Interview (M.I.N.I.): The development and validation of a structured diagnostic psychiatric interview for DSM-IV and ICD-10. *Journal of Clinical Psychiatry, 59*(Suppl. 20), 22–33.

Shepherd, M., Cooper, B., Brown, A. C., & Kalton, G. (1981). *Psychiatric illness in general practice.* New York: Oxford University Press.

Simon, G., & Von Korff, M. (1996). Recognition, management and outcomes of depression in primary care. In S. Vibbert & M. T. Youngs (Eds.), *Behavioral outcomes and guidelines sourcebook* (pp. F23–F29). New York: Faulkner & Gray.

Spitzer, R. L., Williams, J. B.W., Kroenke, K., Linzer, M., deGruy, F. V., Hahn, S. R., Brody, D., & Johnson, J. G. (1994). Utility of a new procedure for diagnosing mental disorders in primary care: The PRIME-MD 1000 study. *Journal of the American Medical Association, 272,* 1749–1756.

Valenstein, M., Kales, H., Mellow, A., Dalack, G., Figueroa, S., Barry, K. L., & Blow, F. C. (1998). Psychiatric diagnosis and intervention in older and younger patients in a primary care clinic: Effect of a screening and diagnostic instrument. *Journal of the American Geriatrics Society, 46,* 1499–1505.

Ware, J. E. (1999). SF-36 Health Survey. In M. Maruish (Ed.), *The use of psychological testing for treatment planning and outcomes assessment* (pp. 1227–1246). Mahwah, NJ: Erlbaum.

Ware, J. E., & Sherbourne, C. D. (1992). The MOS 36-Item Short Form Health Survey (SF-36): Conceptual framework and item selection. *Medical Care, 30,* 473–481.

Wetherell, J. L., & Arean, P. A. (1997). Psychometric evaluation of the Beck Anxiety Inventory with older medical patients. *Psychological Assessment, 9,* 136–144.

World Health Organization. (1990). *International classification of diseases, injuries and causes of death* (10th ed.). Geneva: Author.

Zimmerman, M., Lish, J. D., Farber, N. J., Hartung, J., Lush, D., Kuzma, M. A., & Plescia, G. (1994). Screening for depression in medical patients: Is the focus too narrow? *General Hospital Psychiatry, 16,* 388–396.

Zimmerman, M., Lush, D. T., Farber, N. J., Hartnung, J., Plescia, G., Kuzma, M. A., & Lish, J. (1996). Primary care patients reactions to mental health screening. *International Journal of Psychiatry and Medicine, 26,* 431–441.

Zimmerman, M., & Mattia, J. I. (1999). The reliability and validity of a screening questionnaire for 13 DSM-IV Axis I disorders (the Psychiatric Diagnostic Screening Questionnaire) in psychiatric outpatients. *Journal of Clinical Psychiatry, 60,* 677–683.

Zimmerman, M., & Mattia, J. I. (2001a). The Psychiatric Diagnostic Screening Questionnaire: Development, reliability, and validity. *Comprehensive Psychiatry, 42,* 175–189.

Zimmerman, M., & Mattia, J. I. (2001b). A self-report scale to help make psychiatric diagnoses: The Psychiatric Diagnostic Screening Questionnaire (PDSQ). *Archives of General Psychiatry, 58,* 787–794.

PART II

APPROACHES FOR SPECIFIC PSYCHOLOGICAL PROBLEMS

3

Panic Disorder and Agoraphobia

Sandra L. Baker
Marcus D. Patterson
David H. Barlow

Panic disorder (PD) with and without agoraphobia is a debilitating and costly condition that frequently leads to high utilization of health care services, as well as other costs (Ballenger, 1998; Davidson, 1996). Because effective treatments have been developed for the treatment of PD and panic disorder with agoraphobia (PDA), it is paramount that clinicians identify these patients to provide symptomatic relief and to minimize the health-related, occupational, and personal costs associated with the disorder. In this chapter we provide a review of the assessment of PD and agoraphobia, including differential diagnosis, diagnostic and psychometric measures, and practical recommendations for assessment. We then discuss strategies for linking assessment to treatment, as well as issues related to assessment of PD in primary care settings.

OVERVIEW OF PANIC DISORDER AND AGORAPHOBIA

Diagnostic Criteria for Panic Disorder

As specified in the fourth edition of the *Diagnostic and Statistical Manual of Mental Disorders* (DSM-IV; American Psychiatric Association, 1994), panic attacks are characterized by a sudden rush of fear or anxiety that includes four or more of the following physical and cognitive symptoms: (1) palpitations, pounding heart, or accelerated heart rate; (2) sweating; (3) trembling or shaking; (4) shortness of breath or smothering sensations; (5) feelings of choking; (6) chest pain or discomfort; (7) nausea or abdominal distress; (8) dizziness, unsteadiness, lightheadedness, or faintness; (9) feelings of unreality (derealization) or being detached from oneself (depersonalization); (10) numbing or tingling sensations (paresthesias); (11) chills or hot flushes; (12) fear of going crazy or losing control; and (13) fear of dying.

Panic attacks occur across all of the anxiety disorders, as well as in other psychological disorders, and in the general population. In many cases, panic attacks are triggered by spe-

cific situations, stresses, or worries. However, the hallmark symptom of PD is the experience of uncued or unexpected panic attacks that seemingly occur out of the blue, without
any obvious trigger or cue. The particular symptoms of panic vary from person to person,
and certain sensations may distress some people more than others. Further, individuals with
PD often avoid situations due to anxiety over experiencing physical sensations, which may
lead to varying degrees of agoraphobia.

To meet criteria for a diagnosis of PD, a person must have experienced recurrent unexpected or uncued panic attacks. Although the word "recurrent" is often operationally defined as meaning "two or more," individuals with PD typically have a longstanding pattern
of experiencing frequent panic attacks. In addition, panic attacks must occur abruptly and
peak within 10 minutes. The panic attacks also must be followed by a period of 1 month or
more in which the individual has persistent concern about having additional panic attacks,
worry about the consequences of the panic attacks (e.g., worries about dying, having a
heart attack, and going crazy), or a change in behavior as a result of having the panic attacks. Finally, the panic attacks may not be due to the direct physiological effects of a medical condition (e.g., hyperthyroidism) or a substance (e.g., medications and drugs of abuse),
and may not be better accounted for by another mental disorder (see later section on differential diagnosis).

Although the presence of unexpected panic attacks is necessary to make a diagnosis of
PD, patients with PD frequently report having expected or "predictable" panic attacks.
Usually, these predictable panic attacks occur in situations where the patient anticipates
having another panic attack or has previously had a panic attack. Some patients may be
quite adept at predicting their panic attacks and upon initial screening may deny having
spontaneous or unexpected panic attacks. Here, the clinician may ask the patient to think
back to his or her initial panic attacks to establish whether there is a history of unexpected
panic attacks.

Diagnostic Features of Agoraphobia

Agoraphobia is characterized by anxiety about going into certain places or situations due to
apprehension about experiencing a panic attack or panic-like symptoms, especially in contexts where escape may be difficult or help may not be accessible. Typical agoraphobic situations include driving locally or long distances; being in crowds, grocery stores, malls, movie
theaters, restaurants, churches or temples, public transportation, elevators; traveling over
bridges; and being in enclosed or open spaces. In severe cases, individuals with agoraphobia
may not leave their homes, may avoid work situations, and (very rarely) may even confine
themselves to a single room in their home due to an intense fear of experiencing panic attacks.

PD can occur with or without agoraphobia, although typically these features co-occur.
Additionally, although agoraphobia is not always accompanied by panic attacks, approximately 95% of individuals with agoraphobia who present for treatment in clinical settings
also have PD (American Psychiatric Association, 2000). When agoraphobia occurs in the
absence of a history of PD, individuals typically fear experiencing panic-like sensations or
other potentially embarrassing symptoms (e.g., vomiting, diarrhea, loss of bladder control),
but may never have experienced a full-blown panic attack. However, such individuals may
experience "limited symptom" attacks (i.e., with fewer than four symptoms).

Prevalence

Generally, the lifetime prevalence of PDA is estimated to be between 1.0% and 3.5%, with
a 1-year prevalence between 0.5% and 1.5% (American Psychiatric Association, 2000).

Higher rates of PDA have been found in women than in men. In fact, the lifetime prevalence of PDA has been found to be more than two times greater in women than in men (Katerndahl & Realini, 1993). Although PDA has been documented to occur in young children and in older adults, the median age of onset is 24 years (Burke, Burke, Regier, & Rae, 1990). The Epidemiologic Catchment Area (ECA) study found a bimodal distribution in age of onset with a peak occurring between the ages of 15 and 24 years, and another between the ages of 45 and 54 years (Eaton, Kessler, Wittchen, & Magee, 1994).

ASSESSMENT OF PANIC DISORDER AND AGORAPHOBIA

Before developing a treatment plan, it is critical that a reliable diagnosis of PD with or without agoraphobia, or of agoraphobia without a history of PD (AWOHPD), is established. Differential diagnosis is sometimes challenging because panic attacks can occur across a range of different anxiety disorders, making it difficult to distinguish PDA from other conditions. Empirically supported treatments vary somewhat across the anxiety disorders. Therefore, accurate diagnosis is important for selecting interventions that have been shown to be particularly effective for treating PD and PDA (Barlow, 2001; Craske & Barlow, 2001).

Assessment of PDA should include a number of methods, including structured and semistructured interviews, behavioral tests, self-report questionnaires, self-monitoring, and, more recently, computerized assessment. Each strategy is designed to capture particular aspects of PDA, and all of these methods may be helpful for treatment planning and ongoing evaluation. In the following section, instruments for assessing PDA are reviewed, followed by practical recommendations for selecting instruments for assessment. Because panic attacks and agoraphobia are typically linked, it is important to assess both of these features when screening for PD. This section is intended to demonstrate the range of instruments available to assess panic-related symptoms, as well as to provide an overview of their utility across a range of contexts. Many of the available instruments were developed for research on the epidemiology, descriptive psychopathology, and treatment of PD and PDA. In addition, they vary considerably with respect to their purpose, format, psychometric properties, and features measured. This review is intended to help the clinician choose the most reliable and valid instruments, as well as those that capture the aspects of the disorder that are relevant to the specific treatment being provided.

CLINICIAN-ADMINISTERED DIAGNOSTIC INTERVIEWS

The following clinician-administered diagnostic interviews include sections for diagnosing PDA, along with other anxiety, mood, and psychological disorders.

Anxiety Disorders Interview Schedule–IV (ADIS-IV)

The ADIS-IV (Brown, Di Nardo, & Barlow, 1994) is a clinician-administered, semistructured diagnostic interview that provides current DSM-IV diagnoses. In addition, a lifetime version of the interview (ADIS-IV-L; Di Nardo, Brown, & Barlow, 1994) is available. Both the ADIS-IV and ADIS-IV-L assess the full range of anxiety disorders, as well as mood disorders and other commonly comorbid conditions (e.g., somatization disorder, hypochondriasis). They also screen for the presence of substance use disorders and psychotic disorders, and they provide a full medical history. In addition to providing diagnostic information, these interviews provide data regarding the onset, course, and other features associated with anxiety disorders. All information is based on continuous ratings of severity.

The ADIS-IV is grouped into sections based on anxiety diagnosis in DSM-IV, with PDA coming first in the interview. Within these sections, questions are based on criteria from DSM-IV, and the symptoms that are most central to the disorder are queried first. There are also hierarchical decision rules in the interview, based on DSM-IV criteria. If a key diagnostic criterion for a particular disorder is not met, the clinician is instructed to skip to the next section rather than continuing to assess the remaining criteria for the disorder. In addition to providing diagnostic information, the ADIS-IV-L provides useful information about a patient's history of anxiety and mood disorders, which is often helpful for understanding the nature, course, and manifestations of the disorders and which may influence treatment outcome. However, the ADIS-IV-L is used mostly in research settings due to its length.

The ADIS-IV has been shown to have good interrater reliability for the diagnosis of PDA. Using the ADIS-IV-L, interrater agreement on the diagnosis of 362 individuals with PD with or without agoraphobia was found to be .79 (Brown, Di Nardo, Lehman, & Campbell, 2001). Interrater reliability of the ADIS-IV-L dimensional ratings was .58, .53, .86, and .83 for number of panic attacks, fear of having panic attacks, agoraphobic avoidance, and clinical severity rating (CSR), respectively. The structured format of the ADIS-IV also allows for differential diagnosis, particularly within the anxiety categories, to be made accurately.

Structured Clinical Interview for DSM-IV (SCID-IV)

The SCID-IV (First, Spitzer, Gibbon, & Williams, 1996) is another commonly used diagnostic instrument. Like the ADIS-IV, the SCID-IV is based on DSM-IV criteria and contains decision rules for making an appropriate diagnosis. Although the SCID-IV covers a broader range of diagnostic categories, it lacks detailed questions about the additional features of individual anxiety disorders, including PDA. In addition, criteria are rated as present, absent, or subthreshold; continuous ratings of symptom severity are not provided. Psychometric data are only available for a previous version of the SCID (for DSM-III-R). Williams et al. (1992) examined test–retest reliability of the SCID-III-R using both patients and nonpatients. Kappa coefficients were .58 for a current diagnosis of PD, .54 for a lifetime diagnosis of PD, .43 for a current diagnosis AWOHPD, and .48 for a lifetime diagnosis of AWOHPD. These reliability figures were lower than the reliability of many other Axis I disorders. Kappa coefficients for other Axis I disorders averaged .61 for a current and .68 for a lifetime diagnosis. Other studies have found high levels of reliability for PD diagnoses. For example, First et al. (1996) obtained a kappa of .87 for the diagnosis of panic.

Schedule for Affective Disorders and Schizophrenia—Lifetime Version, Modified for Anxiety Disorders, Updated for DSM-IV (SADS-LA-IV)

The SADS-LA-IV (Fyer, 1995) is a semistructured clinical interview that assesses a variety of psychiatric conditions, including PDA. Unlike the ADIS-IV and the SCID-IV, the SADS-LA-IV provides information in a variety of spheres that are not typically assessed in structured interviews. In particular, the organizational structure of the SADS-LA-IV does not follow that of DSM-IV but, rather, combines the criteria for anxiety disorders in the Research Diagnostic Criteria (RDC; Spitzer, Endicott, & Robins, 1978), in DSM-III and DSM-III-R (Mannuzza et al., 1989), and in DSM-IV (Fyer, 1995).

The SADS-LA was initially designed to capture relationships among diagnostic conditions and to assess for past episodes (Mannuzza et al., 1989). The SADS-LA-IV provides information on anxiety, mood, and substance use disorders, and it assesses for separation anxiety disorders in childhood, hypochondriasis, somatization disorder, antisocial personality disorder, tic disorders, and major psychotic disorders. The SADS-LA-IV was designed specifically for use in the study of anxiety disorders (Fyer, Mannuzza, Chapman, Martin, & Klein, 1995). Mannuzza et al. (1989) found that the SADS-LA was able to reliably diagnose uncomplicated PD and PD with agoraphobia, with kappa statistics of .76 and .81, respectively. Panic with limited avoidance was less reliable (kappa = .62). In general, the SADS-LA-IV has the virtue of allowing for additional information not typically queried in a structured interview, but it may be more cumbersome than other clinician-administered instruments.

SELF-RATED AND CLINICIAN-RATED MEASURES FOR PANIC DISORDER AND AGORAPHOBIA

A number of brief instruments, both self-report and clinician-administered, have proven useful in the assessment of PDA. Whereas the more comprehensive interviews reviewed earlier are designed to arrive at a diagnosis, other measures are helpful in confirming the initial diagnosis, illuminating specific aspects of the diagnosis, and assessing the severity of the condition. Table 3.1 presents a summary of self-report and clinician-rated measures for PD, including a brief description of each instrument, the number of items, and the approximate time to administer each scale.

Measures of Panic Frequency and Severity

The instruments described in this section are designed to measure the severity of panic-related symptoms. Generally, these scales are useful both for research and clinical purposes.

Panic Attack Questionnaire–Revised (PAQ-R)

The PAQ-R (Cox, Norton, & Swinson, 1992) is a detailed clinical interview that provides information on the phenomenology of panic attacks, including panic symptoms, situational triggers, and coping styles. The instrument provides both clinical and qualitative data. It provides demographic data, as well as family history of panic, course of panic attacks over time, severity of panic symptoms, expectancies about panic, perceived control, functional impairment, suicidal ideation, and coping strategies. This measure does not provide a specific score, but relevant sections are easily reviewed. Neither the PAQ-R nor its predecessor (the PAQ) has been subjected to comprehensive validation studies; however, the various sections of this measure have been derived from well-validated measures.

Panic Disorder Severity Scale (PDSS)

The PDSS (Shear et al., 1997) is a brief, clinician-rated, 7-item scale that assesses seven specific dimensions that comprise the key features of PDA, which are rated on a 5-point scale (0, none; 4, extreme). The seven items include frequency of panic, anxiety focused on future panic, distress during panic, interoceptive avoidance, situational avoidance, interference in social functioning, and interference in work functioning. The PDSS was found to have excellent interrater reliability (kappa = .87). It has fair internal consistency, with a Cronbach's

TABLE 3.1. Assessment Instruments for Panic Disorder and Agoraphobia

Instrument name	What it measures	No. of items	Administered by (self or clinician)	Time to administer (minutes)
Measures of panic frequency and severity				
Panic Attack Questionnaire—Revised (PAQ-R; Cox et al., 1992)	Phenomenology of panic attacks, including symptoms, triggers, and coping styles	*	Clinician	20–30
Panic Disorder Severity Scale (PDSS; Shear et al., 1997)	Severity of diagnosis	7	Either	5–10
Panic and Agoraphobia Scale (PAS; Bandelow, 1995, 1999)	Severity of diagnosis	13	Either	5–10
Panic-Associated Symptoms Scale (PASS; Argyle et al., 1991)	Severity of symptoms	9	Clinician	10
Panic Attack Symptoms Questionnaire (PASQ; Clum et al., 1990)	Duration of symptoms during a panic attack	36	Self	10–20
Panic–Agoraphobic Spectrum Questionnaire (P-ASQ; Cassano et al., 1997)	Behaviors associated with agoraphobia	144	Clinician	20
Cognitive measures				
Agoraphobic Cognitions Questionnaire (ACQ; Chambless et al., 1984)	Frequency of catastrophic cognitions	15	Self	5
Agoraphobic Cognitions Scale (ACS; Hoffart et al., 1992)	Degree of fear of situations	10	Self	5
Agoraphobic Self-Statement Questionnaire (ASQ; van Hout et al., 2001)	Frequency of positive and negative thoughts	25	Self	5
Cognition Checklist—Anxiety Scale (CCL-A; Taylor et al., 1997)	Anxious and depressed thoughts	26	Self	5–10
Catastrophic Cognitions Questionnaire—Modified (CCQ-M; Khawaja et al., 1994)	Catastrophic thoughts about bodily sensations and personal reactions	21	Self	10–20
Panic Appraisal Inventory (PAI; Telch, 1987)	Anticipation of panic in a variety of situations, anticipated consequences of panic, and perceived ability to cope with panic	45	Self	20–30
Panic Attack Cognitions Questionnaire (PACQ; Clum et al., 1990)	Catastrophic cognitions before, during, and after a panic attack	25	Self	10–20
Panic Belief Questionnaire (PBQ; Greenberg, 1988)	Beliefs about panic disorder	42	Self	10–20
Measure of perceived control				
Anxiety Control Questionnaire (ACQ^2; Rapee et al., 1996)	Perceived control over anxiety-related events	30	Self	10–15

TABLE 3.1. *(continued)*

Instrument name	What it measures	No. of items	Administered by (self or clinician)	Time to administer (minutes)
Measures of sensation-focused fear and vigilance				
Anxiety Sensitivity Index (ASI; Reiss et al., 1986; Peterson & Reiss, 1993)	Anxiety aroused by symptoms of fear	16	Self	5–10
Body Sensations Questionnaire (BSQ; Chambless et al., 1984)	Anxiety aroused by bodily sensations	18	Self	5–10
Body Sensations Interpretation Questionnaire (BSIQ; Clark et al., 1997)	Misinterpretations of panic	27	Self	10–15
Body Vigilance Scale (BVS; Schmidt, Lerew, & Trakowski, 1997)	Vigilance for panic-related sensations	4	Self	5–10
Measures of panic-related avoidance				
Albany Panic and Phobia Questionnaire (APPQ; Rapee et al., 1995)	Interoceptive, social, and situational avoidance	27	Self	5–10
Mobility Inventory for Agoraphobia (MI; Chambless et al., 1985)	Avoidance of agoraphobic situations	27	Self	10
Fear Questionnaire (FQ; Marks & Mathews, 1979)	Avoidance of situations related to agoraphobia, social phobia, and blood phobia	15	Self	5–10
Phobic Avoidance Rating Scale (PARS; Hoffart et al., 1989)	Agoraphobic avoidance	13	Clinician	10–15
Texas Safety Maneuver Scale (TSMS; Kamphuis & Telch, 1998)	Safety behaviors	50	Self	5–10

*The PAQ-R is a clinical interview and does not have a finite number of questions.

alpha of .65, in view of the fact that the key features of PDA vary considerably from patient to patient. The total score on the PDSS was significantly correlated with the clinical severity ratings for PD on the ADIS-IV ($r = .55$; Shear et al., 1997), although the PDSS provides more information than the ADIS-IV clinical severity rating and profiles the essential targets for treatment. Although this is not a diagnostic tool, it is a simple method for clinicians to rate the severity of panic-related symptoms in those diagnosed with PD and can, therefore, be used to track the course of the disorder. A self-report version of the PDSS is now available.

Panic and Agoraphobia Scale (PAS)

The PAS (Bandelow, 1995, 1999) has two versions: a self-report scale and a clinician-rated scale. The PAS is a 13-item measure that, much like the PDSS, was designed to assess the clinical severity of PDA. The PAS, however, is less reliable as a clinician-rated measure than the PDSS. Like several other measures, it was specifically designed for use in drug trials. It assesses a variety of aspects of PDA, including the duration, severity, and frequency of panic attacks, as well as panic-related avoidance, functional impairment, and anticipatory anxiety. Good internal consistency has been found with the self-report version of this measure (Cronbach's alpha = .88). The observer-rated measure was found to have satisfactory inter-rater reliability ($r = .78$). The PAS is highly correlated with the Panic-Associated Symptom Scale (Argyle et al., 1991) ($r = .82$).

Panic-Associated Symptoms Scale (PASS)

The PASS (Argyle et al., 1991) is a 9-item, clinician-administered instrument that was designed to measure the severity of certain key symptoms of PDA. Unlike other measures, the PASS requires that the patient first receive psychoeducation about PDA and then complete a diary of panic-related symptoms for a 1-week period. On the basis of the patient's report, the clinician completes the PASS, which includes five rating scales. The first three scales, which include situational, unexpected, and limited-symptom attacks, are rated on a 4-point scale, with regard to the frequency and intensity of panic attacks. The other two scales—anticipatory anxiety related to panic and level of distress related to panic—are rated on a 4-point scale, measuring the intensity and duration of these feelings. Based on DSM-III-R criteria, the PASS was found to have poor internal consistency, with a Cronbach alpha of .69. The PASS was also moderately correlated with the Hamilton Anxiety Rating Scale (Hamilton, 1959) ($r = .47$). The advantage of this measure is that it does not rely on retrospective reports; a disadvantage is that it has to be administered by a clinician.

Panic Attack Symptoms Questionnaire (PASQ)

The PASQ (Clum, Broyles, Borden, & Watkins, 1990) is a 36-item measure designed to assess the severity of panic attack symptoms. The measure lists 36 common panic symptoms, and patients are asked to rate the duration with which they experience these symptoms during a typical panic attack. Each item is rated on a 6-point, Likert-type scale, ranging from "did not experience this" to "protracted period" of time. Cronbach's alpha for this measure was .88, suggesting good internal consistency. With six other scales, the PASQ is now part of a larger, self-report measure known as the Comprehensive Panic Profile (CPP; Clum, 1997).

Panic–Agoraphobic Spectrum Questionnaire (P-ASQ)

The P-ASQ (Cassano et al., 1997) is a 144-item measure that focuses on behaviors associated with panic and agoraphobia. The items are grouped on the basis of seven subdomains: panic attack symptoms, anxious expectation, phobic and/or avoidant features, reassurance sensitivity, substance sensitivity, general stress sensitivity, and separation sensitivity. Interviewers indicate whether the symptoms are either present or absent. If they are present, then they are rated on a 6-point scale. In one study comparing diagnostic groups, Cassano et al. (1997) found that patients with PDA scored the highest on this measure, compared to patients diagnosed with depression or with an eating disorder. No psychometric data are available for this measure.

Cognitive Measures

The following instruments assess specific cognitions or beliefs that are often associated with PD and PDA. These instruments are useful in both clinical and research contexts.

Agoraphobic Cognitions Questionnaire (ACQ)

The ACQ (Chambless, Caputo, Bright, & Gallagher, 1984) is a 15-item, self-report measure that assesses the frequency of frightening or maladaptive thoughts about the consequences of panic and anxiety on a 5-point Likert scale. Items 1 through 14 include cognitions that are often associated with PD and agoraphobia. The scale contains six behavioral/social items and eight physiological items, such as, "I am going to throw up," "I won't be able to get to safety," and "I will not be able to control myself." The ACQ also contains an extra item, item 15, where respondents can record an "other" response. This response is not included in the mean score. The ACQ has been found to have good test–retest reliability (r = .86). Good internal consistency was suggested by a Cronbach's alpha of .80. The ACQ was also found to be highly correlated with the Body Sensations Questionnaire (Chambless et al., 1984) (r = .67).

Agoraphobic Cognitions Scale (ACS)

The ACS (Hoffart, Friis, & Martinsen, 1992) is a 10-item self-report instrument assessing perceived negative consequences of panic that was designed to be used as an outcome measure. Ratings are made on a 4-point Likert scale. Hoffart et al. (1992) found three factors underlying the scale: fear of losing control (alpha = .63), fear of bodily incapacitation (alpha = .81), and fear of embarrassing action (alpha = .74). The two subscales relevant to panic—fear of losing control and fear of bodily incapacitation—were found to be correlated with the ACQ (r = .57 and r = .70, respectively). The third subscale, related to social anxiety, was not significantly correlated with the ACQ.

Agoraphobic Self-Statement Questionnaire (ASQ)

The ASQ (van Hout, Emmelkamp, Koopmans, Bogels, & Bouman, 2001) is a 25-item self-report questionnaire in which respondents rate the frequency of positive and negative thoughts that occur during exposure to an anxiety-provoking situation. Each item is rated on a 5-point scale (0, never, to 4, continuously). In a sample of outpatients who had been diagnosed with PD, van Hout et al. (2001) found good internal consistency for both scales (alpha = .88 for the negative subscale and alpha = .87 for the positive subscale). A confirmatory factor analysis of this measure also supported the two-factor structure (van Hout et al., 2001).

Cognition Checklist (CCL)

The CCL (Taylor, Koch, Woody, & McLean, 1997) is a 26-item, self-report measure that consists of thoughts related to anxiety and depression. The CCL contains two subscales, depression (CCL-D) and anxiety (CCL-A), which assess the cognitions associated with these emotions. Patients are asked to rate the frequency of the thoughts on a 5-point Likert scale, ranging from 0 (never) to 5 (always). Items include thoughts such as "I'm going to have an accident" and "There's something wrong with me." The CCL-A was demonstrated to have good internal consistency (alpha = .89) and adequate test–retest reliability (alpha = .68). However, the CCL-A did not have good criterion validity. Specifically, CCL-A scores were compared across three groups (PD, major depression, and major depression with PD). Although the group effect was significant, the CCL-A score for the PD plus major depression group (M = 22.9, SD = 10.2) was significantly greater than that of the PD group (M = 15.1,

$SD = 10.5$), suggesting weak criterion validity. Overall, the results generally support the reliability and validity of CCL scales as research tools.

Catastrophic Cognitions Questionnaire–Modified (CCQ-M)

The CCQ-M (Khawaja, Oei, & Baglioni, 1994) is a 21-item questionnaire designed to measure catastrophic thoughts associated with PDA. There are three subscales to this measure: emotional catastrophes, mental catastrophes, and physical catastrophes. Clients are asked to rate the dangerousness of a variety of bodily and emotional reactions on a 5-point Likert scale from 1 (not at all) to 5 (extremely dangerous). Items include responses, such as "being irritable," "having a heart attack," and "unable to control thinking." Five factors were derived from this scale with good to excellent internal consistency: emotional (alpha = .94), physical (alpha = .90), mental (alpha = .91), social (alpha = .86), and bodily reactions (alpha = .87). The CCQ was also significantly correlated with the Fear Questionnaire (Marks & Mathews, 1979) ($r = .53$), the Body Sensations Questionnaire (Chambless et al., 1984) ($r = .47$), and the ACQ ($r = .34$).

Panic Appraisal Inventory (PAI)

The PAI (Telch, 1987) is a 45-item, self-report measure that was designed to assess three domains of panic appraisal: anticipation of panic, consequences of panic, and perceived ability to cope with panic. Patients are asked to rate the likelihood that they will have a panic attack in 15 different situations. Respondents are told to assume that they do not have the benefit of safety signals (e.g., companionship, medication). Patients are also asked to rate how distressed they are by 15 panic-related thoughts using a 10-point scale. Finally, they are told to rate their ability to cope with 15 different, panic-related situations. In a recent psychometric study of the PAI, Feske and de Beurs (1997) found that the instrument had five subscales derived from the three domains listed above. The "consequences of panic" domain was further divided into physical consequences, social consequences, and loss of control. These scales were highly internally consistent, with Cronbach's alphas ranging from .86 to .90. They also found that fear of physical consequences on the PAI was significantly correlated with the ACQ physical concerns ($r = .80$) and with the Body Sensations Questionnaire (Chambless et al., 1984) ($r = .44$).

Panic Attack Cognitions Questionnaire (PACQ)

The PACQ (Clum et al., 1990) is a 25-item measure designed to capture severity of panic-related thoughts at various times (e.g., before, during, and after a panic attack). It consists of 25 commonly reported catastrophic cognitions, 14 of which are taken from the ACQ. Patients are asked to rate on a 4-point Likert scale the severity of the cognitions before, during, and after a panic attack. Cronbach's alpha was reported to be .88, suggesting good internal consistency. Both the PASQ and the PACQ are included as measures in the CCP (Clum, 1997).

Panic Belief Questionnaire (PBQ)

The PBQ (Greenberg, 1988) is a 42-item questionnaire that was developed to assess a person's convictions about panic, including beliefs about panic itself and about one's ability to cope with it (e.g., "A panic attack can give me a heart attack" and "There is only so much anxiety my heart can take"). Patients are asked to rate the strength of their beliefs on a 6-point Likert scale from "totally disagree" to "totally agree." Excellent internal consistency was reported (Cronbach's alpha = .94). No other psychometric properties are available for this measure.

Measures of Perceived Control

Anxiety Control Questionnaire (ACQ²)

The ACQ² (Rapee, Craske, Brown, & Barlow, 1996) is a self-report measure of perceived control over a number of potentially threatening internal situations (sample item: "When I am put under stress, I am likely to lose control") and external situations (sample item: "Whether I can successfully escape a frightening situation is always a matter of chance with me"). The ACQ² contains 30 items that are rated on a 6-point Likert scale ranging from 0 (strongly disagree) to 5 (strongly agree). Internal consistency was good in a nonclinical sample (alpha = .89) and in a sample of individuals with anxiety disorders (alpha = .87). Good convergent and discriminant validity were also demonstrated with this measure, as well as sensitivity to change following cognitive-behavioral treatment.

Measures of Sensation-Focused Fear and Vigilance

Anxiety Sensitivity Index (ASI)

The ASI (Reiss, Peterson, Gursky, & McNally, 1986; Peterson & Reiss, 1993) is a 16-item measure of anxiety over panic-related sensations. Anxiety sensitivity (AS) refers to the belief that beyond any immediate physical discomfort, anxiety and its accompanying symptoms may cause deleterious physical, psychological, or social consequences (McNally & Lorenz, 1987; Reiss et al., 1986; Taylor, Koch, McNally, & Crockett, 1992). ASI items are rated on a 5-point Likert scale. Telch, Shermis, and Lucas (1989) found that the ASI was able to reliably distinguish panic and agoraphobia from other anxiety disorders. Cronbach's alpha has been found to be .88, suggesting good internal consistency (Peterson & Heilbronner, 1987). In their factor analysis, Zinbarg, Mohlman, and Hong (1999) found strong support for a hierarchical model of AS, consisting of three lower-level factors (AS—physical concerns, AS—mental incapacitation concerns, and AS—social concerns) loading on a single, higher-order AS construct. The ASI has also found to be highly correlated with the Body Sensations Questionnaire (r = .66) (McNally & Lorenz, 1987). Although AS was originally thought to be primarily a feature of PDA, it appears that AS is also prominent in other clinical disorders, including depression, substance abuse, and chronic pain (Asmundson, 1999; Cox, Borger, & Enns, 1999; Stewart, Samoluk, & MacDonald, 1999). Consequently, although this measure is commonly used in the assessment of PDA, further investigation is needed to critically examine the nature of anxiety sensitivity across multiple disorders and its implications for understanding PD in particular. For example, ASI appears to be useful in predicting stable withdrawal from alprazolam. In a study of discontinuation from alprazolam with and without cognitive-behavioral treatment for PDA, Bruce, Spiegel, Gregg, and Nuzzarello (1995) found that the ASI was the only significant predictor of stable withdrawal.

The ASI has been expanded and adapted in a variety of ways. The ASI–Revised 36 (Taylor & Cox, 1998a) is an expanded version of the ASI; the revised version was developed to measure more broadly the various dimensions that underlie anxiety sensitivity. The Anxiety Sensitivity Profile (ASP; Taylor & Cox, 1998b) is another expansion of the ASI that focuses on the cognitive aspects of anxiety sensitivity. In addition, the ASI has been adapted for children and adolescents and has been translated into a variety of languages.

Body Sensations Questionnaire (BSQ)

The BSQ (Chambless et al., 1984) is an 18-item measure of anxiety focused on bodily sensations. Patients are asked to rate the degree to which they experience anxiety related to specify bodily sensations (e.g., heart palpitations, pressure in the chest, numbness in arms or legs) on a 5-point Likert scale. As in the ACQ, the final item on the BSQ allows respondents to record an "other" response, which is not included in the mean score. The scale was found to be internally consistent with a Cronbach's alpha of .87. Test–retest reliability was shown to be adequate ($r = .67$), and as noted earlier, it is highly correlated with the ACQ.

Body Sensations Interpretation Questionnaire (BSIQ)

The BSIQ (Clark et al., 1997) is a self-report measure that provides a description of 27 ambiguous situations. After reading each event, the individual is asked "Why?" and responds with an open-ended interpretation of the situation. Respondents are then provided with three possible interpretations of the event, one of which is negative. They are asked to rank the three interpretations of the events in order of the likelihood that the situation would occur if the person were in that situation (1, most likely to come true; 2, second most likely to come true; 3, least likely to come true). After rating all 27 events, the individual then re-rates each belief based on the likelihood of each being true, using a 9-point scale (0, not at all likely, to 8, extremely likely).

The BSIQ has four subscales: panic body sensations, general events, social events, and other symptoms. Information about the internal consistency of the BSIQ is unavailable. However, a brief version of the BSIQ, the Brief Body Sensations Interpretation Questionnaire (BBSIQ; Clark et al., 1997), is also available, and it has more information about the psychometrics. This 14-item scale consists of two subscales: panic body sensations and external events. Clark et al. (1997) have found satisfactory internal consistency for the BBSIQ scales (alpha = .86, .90, .74, and .80, for panic body sensations rankings, panic body sensation belief rankings, external event rankings, and external event belief rankings, respectively). The panic body sensation subscale and the external events subscale have been shown to be significantly correlated with the physical concerns and the social-behavioral factors on the ACQ, respectively. The panic body sensations subscale was not significantly associated with the social-behavioral factor; the external events subscale was not significantly correlated with the physical concerns factor.

Body Vigilance Scale (BVS)

The BVS (Schmidt, Lerew, & Trakowski, 1997) is a four-item self-report measure of body vigilance, or conscious attention to internal bodily cues. Individuals rate how closely they pay attention to bodily symptoms, how sensitive they are to those sensations, how much time they spend checking for symptoms, and how much attention they pay to a range of panic sensations (e.g., heart palpitations, chest pain, and numbing). Overall, individuals with PD indicated higher levels of bodily vigilance than did nonclinical sample populations. The BVS demonstrated good internal consistency (alpha = .83, .82, and .82 for student, community, and PD samples, respectively). Adequate test–retest reliability over a 5-week interval was demonstrated in both student and PD samples ($r = .68$ and .58, respectively). The

BVS was related to anxiety sensitivity, whereas the ASI was predictive of changes in body vigilance during cognitive-behavioral treatment.

Measures of Panic-Related Avoidance

Albany Panic and Phobia Questionnaire (APPQ)

The APPQ (Rapee, Craske, & Barlow, 1995) is a 27-item measure designed to assess anxiety focused on activities and situations that produce panic-related sensations. Patients are asked to rate their degree of fear in a variety of situations on a 9-point, Likert-type scale. Examples include "playing vigorous sports on a hot day," "blowing up an airbed quickly," and "running up stairs." There are three subscales: interceptive (alpha = .87), situational agoraphobia (alpha = .90), and social phobia subscales (alpha = .91). The APPQ was compared with the Depression, Anxiety Stress Scale (DASS; Lovibond & Lovibond, 1995) and the ASI. The DASS was selected because of its ability to discriminate between depression and anxiety, which often overlap. Scores on the ASI correlated significantly more with the agoraphobia and interoceptive subscales than with the social phobia subscale. Scores on the DASS–Anxiety subscale correlated significantly less with the social phobia subscale than with the agoraphobia subscale.

Mobility Inventory for Agoraphobia (MI)

The MI (Chambless et al., 1985) is a 27-item self-report inventory that measures agoraphobic, situational avoidance and frequency of panic attacks. It is divided into four sections. The first section measures degree of avoidance of 26 situations that are commonly reported by individuals with agoraphobia. Patients are asked to separately rate avoidance of these situations for when accompanied and when alone, using a 5-point scale ranging from 1 (never avoid) to 5 (always avoid). Two subscales are derived: avoidance alone and avoidance accompanied. Both were found to have excellent internal consistency (alpha = .96 and alpha = .90, respectively). Both of these subscales were found to be significantly correlated with the agoraphobia factor on the Fear Questionnaire (see the next section) for avoidance when alone and accompanied ($r = .68$ and $r = .44$, respectively). The first part of the MI is the most commonly used and the most frequently reported in the research literature. The second part of the MI requires individuals to circle five items from the first section that cause the greatest concern or impairment. The third section asks three questions about frequency and severity of panic (e.g., frequency of panic over past 7 days, the past 3 weeks, and severity of panic during the past week). The fourth part of the MI asks the person to indicate the size of his or her safety zone, if relevant.

Fear Questionnaire (FQ)

The FQ (Marks & Mathews, 1979) was originally developed to monitor changes in phobic avoidance among individuals with agoraphobia, social phobia, and blood-injury phobia. The FQ is a 15-item rating scale in which clients are asked to rate their avoidance of a variety of situations on a 9-point scale, ranging from 0 (no avoidance) to 8 (total avoidance). The FQ is scored on three subscales, one of which measures agoraphobia. There is empirical support for the reliability and validity of FQ as a measure of agoraphobic avoidance (Cox, Swinson, & Parker, 1993). Because it targets agoraphobic avoidance, the measure alone provides very little general information on the other symptoms of PDA. The FQ has commonly been used as an outcome measure for the treatment of agoraphobia. In particular,

Cox, Swinson, Norton, and Kuch (1991) found that the FQ reliably distinguished agoraphobia and social phobia and identified patients with PDA 82% of the time.

Phobic Avoidance Rating Scale (PARS)

The PARS (Hoffart, Friis, & Martinsen, 1989) is a 13-item interview in which clinicians rate the degree to which an individual avoids a variety of situations. Items are rated on a 5-point scale (0, no avoidance, to 4, avoids the situation regularly). The PARS contains three subscales that have been found to have good to adequate internal consistency: separation avoidance (alpha = .88), social avoidance (alpha = .58), and simple avoidance (alpha = .68). In their factor-analytic study, Hoffart et al. (1989) found support for the three subscales. They also found high correlations between other measures of agoraphobic avoidance.

Texas Safety Maneuver Scale (TSMS)

The TSMS (Kamphuis & Telch, 1998) is a 50-item, self-report questionnaire that was designed to measure avoidance behaviors (safety maneuvers) that happen in situations for individuals with PD. Four option items are also included in this measure to capture "other" safety behaviors. Items are rated on 5-point scales that measure the extent to which individual use particular avoidance strategies to control their anxiety or panic. Ratings range from 1 (never to manage anxiety or panic) to 5 (always to manage anxiety or panic). Individuals are also asked to indicate whether they engage in avoidance behavior but not as a means of managing anxiety or panic.

   The TSMS consists of six subscales, all of which were found to have good to excellent internal consistency. These include agoraphobic avoidance (alpha = .90), relaxation techniques (alpha = .88), stress avoidance (alpha = .87), somatic avoidance (alpha = .77), distraction techniques (alpha = .82), and escape (alpha = .79). The TSMS and its various subscales have also been found to be significantly correlated with measures of anxiety sensitivity, agoraphobic avoidance, general anxiety, and depression (Kamphuis & Telch, 1998).

BEHAVIORAL ASSESSMENT STRATEGIES

Behavioral Assessment Tests (BATs)

Situational avoidance is an obvious behavioral sign of agoraphobia, and one way to determine the degree of agoraphobic avoidance is to observe the patient in a variety of naturalistic situations. The BAT (also known as a behavioral approach test or behavioral avoidance test) involves asking patients to enter situations that they typically avoid or that normally trigger fear. Before entering the situation, the patient is asked to rate his or her anticipatory anxiety and the fear level that he or she expects to experience in the situation. Patients are instructed that they may discontinue the BAT at any time. During or following the BAT, the patient provides an estimate of the actual fear level that was experienced. The BAT provides the clinician with an opportunity to directly observe the idiosyncratic fear-reducing responses (e.g., safety behaviors) used by the patient. Behavioral observations also may provide a basis for planning treatment (e.g., choosing relevant exposure practices) and may more completely assess agoraphobic avoidance than retrospective self-report alone.

   In addition, BATs have the advantage of actually inducing sensations associated with panic in a naturalistic setting, which can, in turn, be measured through self-report. Behavioral tests can therefore be used to capture the level of anxiety associated with particular sensations that are experienced in feared situations. Thus, a BAT may help clinicians gauge the degree of fear and avoidance associated with both sensations and situations. Ratings can then be used to track progress and to identify situations and sensations that can be utilized during exposure therapy.

Fear and Avoidance Hierarchy (FAH)

A FAH can be a useful clinical assessment tool for treatment of PDA. A FAH is typically constructed jointly by the clinician and patient and is organized around the patient's specific situational agoraphobic fears (see Craske & Barlow, 2000, for a detailed description). A list of situations from varying levels of avoidance and fear is developed, and the clinician then collaborates with the patient to rank these situations. One way of accomplishing this is to have the patient rate each situation on a 9-point scale, separately indicating his or her levels of both fear and avoidance (ranging from 0, no fear or avoidance, to 8, maximum fear or avoidance). Although no psychometrics exist for the FAH, this measure can serve as a guide to help the clinician design appropriate exercises for systematically confronting feared situations. This measure may also be used to track the progress of treatment by having the patient periodically rate the hierarchy items again, throughout the duration of treatment.

Symptom Induction Tests

Asking patients to engage in symptom induction exercises can be a helpful way of assessing the severity of an individual's symptoms, as well as identifying the exercises that might be most useful for conducting interoceptive exposure practices during treatment. Symptom induction involves provoking panic sensations by having the patient perform a variety of tasks that have been found to naturally elicit physical sensations associated with panic. Table 3.2 includes a list of exercises and the respective symptoms that they tend to trigger. We recommend that the exercises be conducted in the order presented (starting with exercises that tend to be less fear-provoking and progressing to more difficult exercises), because carry-over effects in symptoms may occur from exercise to exercise, thereby inflating the patient's fear rating for the given exercise.

These exercises may also be altered to enhance the specific symptoms that more closely mimic a patient's natural panic sensations (e.g., tying a scarf around the neck to induce choking sensations). The tasks are performed for a fixed duration, usually between 30 seconds and 2 minutes, depending on the exercise. Before carrying out the tests, patients are told that they may discontinue at any time. Patients are instructed to rate their levels of anticipatory anxiety prior to the exercise and their actual fear levels during the task. Patients are also asked to describe the physical sensations experienced during the exercise, rate the intensity of the sensations experienced, and rate the similarity of the sensations to those experienced during naturally occurring panic attacks. Interoceptive assessment procedures are useful, not only to help identify the sensations that the patient associates with fear and panic but also to visibly verify the presence of anxiety and panic and to witness the anxiety response.

Panic induction challenges may also be conducted using sodium lactate (e.g., Murray, 1987; Pitts & McClure, 1967), carbon dioxide (e.g., Sanderson, Rapee, & Barlow, 1989; Schmidt, Trakowski, & Staab, 1997; van den Hout, 1988), yohimbine (e.g., Charney, Woods, Goodman, & Heninger, 1987), caffeine (e.g., Charney, Heninger, & Jarlow, 1985; Uhde, 1990), and cholecystokinin (e.g., Bradwejn et al., 1992). These substances, most

TABLE 3.2. Symptom Induction Exercises and Associated Symptoms

Exercise	Associated symptoms
Shake head from side to side (30 seconds)	Dizziness, disorientation
Place head between legs (30 seconds) then lift quickly	Lightheadedness, blood rushing to head
Breath holding (30 seconds or as long as possible)	Shortness of breath, heart palpitations, lightheadedness, chest tightness
Run in place (1 minute) or, using stairs, take one step up and one step down	Accelerated heart rate, sweating, shortness of breath
Full body muscle tension (tense every possible muscle in the body) or hold a push-up position (1 minute)	Heaviness in the muscles, tingling sensations, weakness, trembling
Spin in a chair or while standing (1 minute)	Dizziness, faintness, nausea
Breathe through a thin straw (1 minute) (while holding nostrils together)	Shortness of breath, smothering sensations, dizziness
Hyperventilation (1 minute) (breathe rapidly and deeply through the chest)	Accelerated heart rate, dizziness, faintness, sweating, shortness of breath, dry mouth, headache, cold and hot feelings
Stare intensely in a mirror or at a spot on the wall (2 minutes)	Depersonalization, derealization

Note. From Barlow and Craske (2000). Copyright 2000 by Graywind Publications. Adapted and reproduced by permission of the publisher, The Psychological Corporation, a Harcourt Assessment Company. All rights reserved.

commonly used in laboratory settings, have been shown to induce panic attacks more frequently in individuals with PD than in normal controls. Panic induction challenges may be used to assess responses to panic-related symptoms. They may also be used to measure and evaluate treatment outcome, for example, by repeating the challenges prior to and following treatment.

PSYCHOPHYSIOLOGICAL ASSESSMENT STRATEGIES

Psychophysiological assessment involves taking various physiological measures (e.g., heart rate, blood pressure, galvanic skin response, breathing rate) while a patient is having a panic attack, is exposed to a feared situation or panic induction challenge, or while at rest. Although they are not commonly used in clinical settings, psychophysiological assessment procedures may provide important information that might otherwise go unnoticed. For example, measuring heart rate can provide data to reassure physically healthy patients that their pulse remains in a safe range, even during a panic attack. Some difficulties with using psychophysiological measures to assess a patient's emotional response include the following: (1) multiple factors affect arousal, in addition to just fear and anxiety, (2) psychophysiological measures often do not correlate well with one another or with other aspects of anxiety (e.g., a patient's subjective report), and (3) equipment for measuring psychophysiological responses is often expensive, requires special training, and may take up space that could otherwise be used differently. Thus, these methods are seldom used outside of research settings.

A wide range of physiological symptoms may also be monitored for a given individual. For example, ambulatory monitoring of heart rate and finger temperature has been used as a physiological means of corroborating self-reports of panic attacks. Recently, we experimented with using ambulatory monitoring for clinical purposes (Hofmann & Barlow, 1999). In this report, a patient who had relapsed after successful treatment became panicky after experiencing a stressful event and became concerned (once again) that her panic may reflect problems with her heart. Ambulatory physiological monitoring demonstrated that she was, in fact, overestimating her actual heart rate. In addition, and in contrast with her belief that these attacks came from "out of the blue," the increase in heart rate and respiration actually followed anxious thoughts, suggesting to the patient that she could control these events after all. Although still expensive, ambulatory physiological monitoring holds promise for the future, and pricing is becoming more reasonable. The clinician may select such measures as needed, while balancing the costs (e.g., time, money, utility) associated with additional assessment strategies.

DIARY MEASURES

One of the limitations of both structured interviews and questionnaires is that they are often retrospective in nature, and therefore may be influenced by retrospective recall biases. In the case of PDA, patients have been found to overestimate both the frequency and intensity of their panic attacks (Margraf, Taylor, Ehlers, Roth, & Agras, 1987). Self-monitoring is one means to overcome this limitation. Self-monitoring involves recording instances of anxiety and panic attacks on a daily basis, as the symptoms occur. Self-monitoring is typically used in the weeks preceding treatment, throughout the duration of treatment, and during follow-up.

In addition to providing information regarding the presence, severity, and frequency of panic attacks, monitoring also assists the clinician in determining the times and situational triggers that are most often associated with panic. These data can assist in generating a functional analysis of the attacks and in planning appropriate interventions. Patients are often unaware of the factors that trigger their panic attacks, and monitoring can be useful for illuminating these cues. Finally, monitoring of attacks is important for assessing the course and outcome of treatment.

Patients may need to be reminded of the importance of timely and accurate record keeping. In fact, the clinician may choose to interrupt treatment in the event of noncompliance in order to underscore that treatment will not be maximally effective unless the patient is willing to invest sufficient time and energy into record keeping. Monitoring can be complemented by other approaches, such as the psychophysiological assessment methods mentioned earlier. McNally (1994) suggested that self-monitoring should be intermittently combined with ambulatory physiological monitoring to provide important information beyond that obtained from retrospective reports of panic attacks. As in all assessment strategies, recordkeeping provides the clinician with collateral information that can be judged in the context of other information obtained.

Panic Attack Record (PAR)

The PAR (Barlow & Craske, 2000) is a monitoring record on which the patient reports various aspects of a panic attack soon after it occurs (see Figure 3.1). The information recorded may include the date and time of the attack, whether it was expected or unexpected, whether the person was alone or with someone else, the intensity of the panic attack, and any symptoms that were experienced (using a checklist format). Patients are asked to carry the record with them at all times so that the panic attack features can be recorded close in

Panic Attack Record | Date _____ Time Began _____ AM/PM
☐ Expected   Triggers _____
☐ Unexpected _____
_____

Maximum Fear *(circle)*

0	1	2	3	4	5	6	7	8
None		Mild		Moderate		Strong		Extreme

Symptoms
(Check all symptoms present to at least a mild degree.)

☐ Difficulty Breathing   ☐ Nausea/Abdominal Distress   ☐ Unsteadiness/Dizziness/ Faintness

☐ Racing/Pounding Heart   ☐ Chest Pain/Discomfort   ☐ Fear of Dying

☐ Choking   ☐ Hot/Cold Flashes   ☐ Fear of Losing Control/ Going Crazy

☐ Numbness/Tingling   ☐ Sweating

☐ Trembling/Shaking   ☐ Feelings of Unreality

FIGURE 3.1. Panic attack record. From Barlow and Craske (2000). Copyright 2000 by Graywind Publications. Adapted and reproduced by permission of the Publisher, The Psychological Corporation, a Harcourt Assessment Company. All rights reserved.

proximity to the time of the attack. In this way, memory of the attack is most accurate, and the patient may learn to more accurately observe the attacks as they occur.

PRACTICAL RECOMMENDATIONS FOR THE ASSESSMENT OF PANIC DISORDER AND AGORAPHOBIA

Screening for Panic Disorder and Related Symptoms

Early detection of PDA is important—not only to minimize the costs associated with the disorder but also because longer duration of the illness has been shown to be a predictor of poorer outcome (Scheibe & Albus, 1996). For effective screening, it is important for clinicians to note the characteristics that may put an individual at increased likelihood for developing PD (e.g., being female, early adulthood, a family history of PD or PDA, recent life stresses).

Although PD typically begins in young adulthood, this condition may also affect older adults and is often overlooked or misdiagnosed in this population. Anxiety disorders in older adults may be particularly difficult to diagnose due to the higher likelihood of encountering medical conditions that mimic symptoms of PDA. Identification is critical in this population to provide effective treatment and to minimize health care utilization. In addition, Eaton et al. (1994) found in the national comorbidity study that individuals with educational levels 12 years or below were more than 10 times more likely to be diagnosed with PDA than were their counterparts with 16 or more years of education. Consequently, screening for PDA in settings where patients have lower levels of education may be particularly important.

Brief Screening Instruments for Panic Disorder and Agoraphobia

Ballenger (1998) suggested a very simple screening approach for PDA—that health professionals ask one question with a high likelihood of identifying most patients with PDA:

"Have you experienced brief periods for seconds or minutes of an overwhelming panic or terror that was accompanied by racing heart, shortness of breath, or dizziness?" Although this question could lead to a positive response from people other than those with anxiety disorders, it may be a quick and useful way to begin the screening process for PDA.

Autonomic Nervous System Questionnaire (ANS)

The ANS (Stein et al., 1999) is another screening measure for PD. This is a brief, 5-item, self-report measure that was developed to be used in primary care settings. Stein and colleagues tested their screen as a two-question and a five-question measure. Patients were first asked whether "In the past 6 months, did you ever have a spell or an attack when all of a sudden you felt frightened, anxious, or very uneasy" and "In the past 6 months, did you ever have a spell or attack when for no reason your heart suddenly began to race, you felt faint, or couldn't catch your breath?" If a patient answered "yes" to either of these questions, he or she was asked three, more specific questions. The initial two questions of the screen were highly sensitive to the presence of panic (i.e., able to correctly identify people who have PD) with a range of .9 to 1.00 across three sites, but had low specificity (i.e., ability to screen out people who do not have PD) in the range of .25 to .59. When the three additional questions were added, the specificity of the measure increased only modestly (.50 to .75), but this came with a reduction in sensitivity (.78 to .88). Although the screen is useful because of its brevity and its ability to detect PD, it provides very little additional information on the associated features of the condition. Screening measures such as the ANS should not be used in the absence of additional self-report or interview-based assessments.

Primary Care Evaluation of Mental Disorders (PRIME-MD)

The PRIME-MD (Spitzer et al., 1994) is a broad-based diagnostic interview that is derived from DSM-IV criteria. It is administered in two stages. A 26-item, self-report measure is provided initially. Individuals answer "yes" or "no" to a range of symptoms across five domains: depression, anxiety, alcohol, somatization, and eating disorders. Individuals who endorse symptoms within a given domain are interviewed by a clinician using a module that corresponds to the domain. The advantage of the PRIME-MD is that it can be administered quickly, while covering a broad range of possible diagnoses. In one study, the average time that physicians spent administering the PRIME-MD was 8.4 minutes (Spitzer et al., 1994). A computer version of the PRIME-MD is now available.

Differential Diagnosis

In a clinical setting, assessment may need to be completed quickly, while still maintaining a broad scope. However, despite these pressures, a thorough assessment is important for making a differential diagnosis, in part because panic attacks occur frequently in the context of other anxiety and mood disorders, often leading to misdiagnosis and perhaps inappropriate treatment recommendations. Although a hallmark feature of PD is a tendency for patients to report worry and apprehension over the possibility of experiencing panic symptoms, this feature is sometimes present in other disorders as well, making differential diagnosis particularly difficult. Below are guidelines for distinguishing PD from other anxiety disorders. In general, it is important to consider the focus of the anxiety, whether a person's panic attacks are unexpected, and the range of situations avoided.

Social Phobia

Differentiating PDA from social phobia can often be difficult and sometimes may be appropriate to assign both diagnoses. For example, studies have suggested that as many as 46% of individuals with PDA carry an additional diagnosis of social phobia (Stein, Shea, & Uhde, 1989). Data from our Center for Anxiety and Related Disorders indicate that approximately 15% of individuals with a principal diagnosis of PDA ($N = 360$) have an additional diagnosis of social phobia (T. A. Brown, personal communication, April 28, 2000).

In other cases, however, only one of these diagnoses may be appropriate. There is often considerable overlap in the features of PDA and social phobia. Both groups may report fear of situations that are typically considered either agoraphobic (e.g., crowds, public places) or social (e.g., parties, meetings). In addition, people in either group may report concerns about embarrassing themselves when experiencing a panic attack in a public place. PDA is also characterized by the presence of unexpected panic attacks, whereas individuals with social phobia tend to experience panic attacks that are exclusively cued by social situations. In addition, whereas individuals with PDA may be concerned about the social consequences of having panic attacks, individuals with social phobia are typically also concerned about a broader range of embarrassing or humiliating consequences (e.g., saying something inappropriate, making mistakes, looking incompetent, seeming uninteresting). Furthermore, their concern over experiencing panic symptoms may be limited to those that may be noticeable to others (e.g., blushing, sweating, shaky hands, unsteady voice).

If a person has a history of unexpected panic attacks and his or her social concerns revolve exclusively around the possibility of experiencing panic attacks, a diagnosis of PD may better account for the condition. It may also be helpful to inquire about which nonsocial situations (e.g., going into enclosed places alone, driving over bridges or through tunnels) the person avoids. If the avoidance exclusively occurs in social situations, and there is no clear history of unexpected panic attacks, a diagnosis of social phobia may be more appropriate.

Generalized Anxiety Disorder

Individuals with generalized anxiety disorder (GAD) often "worry themselves into having a panic attack." In fact, up to 75% of individuals with principal diagnoses of GAD may experience an occasional unexpected or worry-induced panic attack (Barlow, 2001; Barlow & Wincze, 1998). Assessing the nature and content of the worry is essential for differentiating PD from GAD. A report of excessive worry about work, finances, health, and family matters may initially look like GAD, but if the content of the worry is exclusively about the impact of the patient's unexpected panic attacks on his or her ability to work, health, finances (due to missed days at work), and relationships (e.g., not being able to date because of panic attacks), PDA may be the most appropriate diagnosis. In contrast, if the person's panic attacks are exclusively worry-driven and his or her worries are not limited to the effects of the panic attacks, then GAD may be a more appropriate diagnosis. In other words, to assign a diagnosis of GAD, the clinician should establish the presence of worries that are distinct from concerns about panic attacks and agoraphobia. In some cases, it may be appropriate to assign both diagnoses.

Specific Phobia

Individuals with specific phobia may also express anxiety about having panic attacks, but their concern is circumscribed to a specific situation or object. Individuals with PDA, by contrast, experience unexpected panic attacks outside of any specific situation. Frequently there may be overlap between agoraphobic situations and specific phobia (e.g., driving, flying, elevators, bridges). Thus, the presence of unexpected panic attacks is important to assess. In addition, the feared consequences are often different in people with PDA and people with specific phobia. For example, for most people with a specific phobia of flying, the concern is focused on crashing. In contrast, people with PDA are more likely to fear flying because of anxiety over having a panic attack and not being able to escape from the airplane.

Obsessive–Compulsive Disorder

In obsessive–compulsive disorder (OCD), individuals may have panic attacks or avoid situations in response to obsessions (e.g., avoiding "contaminated" objects, panicking while walking on a busy street after experiencing an urge to jump in front of traffic, avoiding driving due to fear of accidentally hitting a pedestrian). In OCD, panic attacks occur exclusively in response to situational or internal triggers (e.g., obsessions). In contrast, PDA is associated with unexpected or uncued panic attacks. Both disorders may be associated with anxiety over experiencing panic attacks or uncomfortable physical sensations; however, this is often a more prominent feature of PDA than OCD.

Posttraumatic Stress Disorder

Individuals with posttraumatic stress disorder (PTSD) frequently report a fear of having panic attacks, which may or may not cue traumatic memories. In fact, in contrast to people with the other anxiety disorders, individuals with PTSD showed similar levels of anxiety sensitivity (anxiety over panic-related sensations) in response to physical sensations compared to those with PD (Taylor, Koch, & McNally, 1992). Moreover, PDA frequently occurs in the context of PTSD, and both diagnoses may be given if the criteria are met for each.

Michelson, June, Vives, Testa, and Marchione (1998) found that, among PDA patients, several trauma-related variables (e.g., history of a traumatic experience, type of trauma, age of trauma occurrence, perceived responsibility for trauma, available social support, and level of violence) were predictive of response to cognitive-behavioral treatment for PDA. These trauma variables, along with the presence of dissociative symptoms, were related to greater pretreatment psychopathology, poorer response to treatment, greater risk of relapse, and poorer maintenance of gains 1 year after treatment. Consequently, assessing for comorbid PTSD may have important implications for treatment response and maintenance of gains.

Hypochondriasis

Although people with PDA may express strong concerns about having a life-threatening disease (e.g., cardiovascular disease, brain tumor), these hypochondriacal-like beliefs may not necessarily reflect a diagnosis of primary hypochondriasis. As Otto, Pollack, Sachs, and Rosenbaum (1992) suggest, these beliefs may reflect underlying anxiety sensitivity. PDA and hypochondriasis may be distinguished on the basis of the content of these beliefs. Specifically, individuals with PDA usually misinterpret autonomic body sensations (e.g., heart rate, shortness of breath, dizziness), leading to erroneous beliefs about the danger associated with these symptoms. In contrast, individuals with hypochondriasis rarely focus on autonomic symptoms but instead misinterpret other sensations and physical manifestations on the body (e.g., lumps, skin disturbances, and headaches) as an indication of a physical illness. Furthermore, the degree of belief conviction often varies between the two disorders. Individuals with hypochondriasis tend to believe more strongly that they are ill, and are often only temporarily reassured by medical professionals. In contrast, although individuals with PDA may have strong beliefs about organic causes for their physical sensations, they are typically more likely to admit that they probably don't have a serious illness, particular when they are not in the midst of having a panic attack (Côté et al., 1996).

VARIABLES TO ASSESS DURING A CLINICAL INTERVIEW

The clinical interview should cover a range of variables, including thoughts and beliefs about the harmful nature of panic attacks, anxiety over experiencing the physical sensations of panic, and panic-related behaviors such as phobic avoidance. These factors often interact with one another and may contribute to the maintenance of the disorder. In addition, a thorough evaluation of medical conditions, cultural factors, and suicide risk is important. Each of these areas will be discussed in more detail here.

Thoughts and Beliefs Regarding Panic Attacks

When a person cannot identify an obvious external trigger to explain his or her panic-related symptoms, he or she may turn inward for an explanation, particularly when the panic attack symptoms occur suddenly and unexpectedly. The beliefs associated with panic attacks vary substantially from individual to individual. Individuals may develop fears of having a heart attack, stroke, or seizure; of suffocating, fainting, vomiting, having diarrhea, or dying; of going "crazy" or doing something uncontrolled (e.g., running, screaming, attacking someone, attempting suicide). Understanding the cognitions associated with an individual's panic attacks will help the clinician arrive at a more accurate diagnosis and will also help select specific cognitions to target during treatment with cognitive restructuring. Examples of questions that can be used to identify panic-related thoughts include "What do you think might happen if you experience a panic attack?" and "If you were to panic while in a theater and you couldn't escape, what do you imagine would happen?"

Anxiety over Experiencing Physical Sensations

Patients with PDA tend to report strong anxiety over experiencing the physical sensations associated with panic. As a result, they usually avoid situations in which they are likely to have panic attacks, as well as situations or activities that are likely to elicit physical sensations similar to their panic attacks. Table 3.3 provides a list of situations and activities that are often avoided by patients with PD because they naturally produce physical sensations. Physical sensations and associated activities that are feared or avoided by the patient should be assessed carefully. This assessment will be particularly useful for developing interoceptive and situational exposure assignments during treatment, so that patients can decrease their sensitivity to physical sensations.

Panic-Related Behaviors

Patients often engage in a variety of behaviors that they believe will protect them from having panic attacks or from suffering specific consequences during their attacks. These behaviors range from active avoidance or escape to more subtle "safety" behaviors. Examples of

TABLE 3.3. Situations and Activities That Naturally Elicit Physical Sensations

Drinking caffeinated beverages	Engaging in heated arguments
Drinking alcohol	Watching thrilling movies
Smoking	Amusement park rides
Eating spicy foods	Reading while riding in the car (to induce nausea)
Going into saunas	Aerobic exercise
Steamy showers	Doing housework rapidly
Standing in the sun	Sexual activity
Hot weather	Being in a hurry
Cold weather (enough to see breath)	Relaxation exercises

subtle avoidance and safety behaviors include efforts to distract oneself by engaging in conversation, turning up the radio, watching television, or reading a magazine. Other examples include carrying particular items such as bottled water, a paper bag (for breathing into), a mobile phone, or a talisman. Avoidance behaviors are believed to maintain fearful beliefs about panic because the individual is prevented from learning that his or her fearful beliefs would not have come true, even in the absence of these behaviors. Ultimately, these behaviors may undermine the effects of treatment if they are not identified and eliminated.

Nocturnal Panic Attacks

Nocturnal panic attacks refer to sudden, unexpected panic attacks, during which the patient awakens from sleep in a state of panic. As with daytime panic attacks, nocturnal panic attacks occur unexpectedly and without any obvious trigger. They are not cued by nightmares or by external environmental stimuli (e.g., a telephone ringing suddenly), and they do not include panic attacks that occur after the person awakens. Interestingly, they may not be exclusive to individuals with PDA but, rather, may occur across different anxiety disorders, as do daytime panic attacks.

Nocturnal panic attacks are frequently overlooked and are often misdiagnosed as primary sleep disorders (e.g., sleep apnea, parasomnias, nightmares, and sleep terrors), posttraumatic stress disorder, nocturnal epilepsy, or isolated sleep paralysis (Craske & Rowe, 1997). Consequently, inappropriate treatments may be recommended for patients who suffer from nocturnal panic attacks.

Nocturnal panic attacks usually occur as the individual enters slow-wave sleep, typically about 1 to 2 hours after falling asleep. Nocturnal panic attacks tend to occur late in stage 2 or early in stage 3 sleep (Craske & Rowe, 1997). To differentiate nocturnal panic attacks from other sleep-related disturbances, it is often useful to examine at the stage of sleep in which the symptoms occur, as well as other characteristics of the disturbance. For example, unlike nocturnal panic attacks, the symptoms of sleep apnea often occur during stages 1 and 2 of sleep and during rapid eye movement (REM) sleep (van Oot, Lane, & Borkovec, 1984). Sleep apnea (but not nocturnal panic) is associated with repeated cessations in breathing while asleep, and this occurs throughout the night and often with individuals who are not aware that they are occurring.

Night terrors (sudden awakenings in a state of confusion and physiological arousal) usually occur 30 minutes to 3 hours after falling asleep (stage 4) and are most common in children. Night terrors are also associated with sleepwalking (Hurwitz, Mahowald, Schenck, Schulter, & Bundie, 1991). People with night terrors usually return to a tranquil sleep and seldom remember the event the following day (Cameron & Thyer, 1985). In contrast, individuals with nocturnal panic attacks vividly recall the incident and usually do not return to sleep quickly. Also, nocturnal panic attacks are generally not associated with sleepwalking.

Isolated sleep paralysis is characterized by a short-lived period of paralysis that occurs when falling asleep or upon waking. Individuals may appear to be in a deep sleep, although some individuals are awake when it occurs. They also may experience frightening hallucinations, difficulty breathing, sweating, and palpitations. Nocturnal panic attacks are not associated with hallucinations or lack of voluntary movement, and individuals are generally awoken by the attack.

Finally, nocturnal seizures may be differentiated from nocturnal panic attacks by the tendency to demonstrate signs of seizure activity and EEG abnormalities, neither of which are present in nocturnal panic (Uhde, 1994).

Cultural Factors

There is evidence that cultural factors have an impact on the ways in which individuals describe their anxiety-related symptoms. Understanding anxiety within a social and cultural context may have important implications for diagnosis and treatment. In the case of PDA, clinicians should assess whether the fear reaction is truly unexpected or whether it occurs in response to situational stressors. For example, when individuals present with "agoraphobia," clinicians should identify whether the patient is avoiding situations due to a fear of hostility from others (which may trigger panic attacks or panic-like symptoms) as opposed to a fear of the panic attack itself. Once individuals are appropriately identified and diagnosed, culturally sensitive treatment programs should be developed and implemented. Ignoring issues related to a patient's culture may adversely affect the outcome of treatment or lead to premature attrition. Variables such as ethnic identity, age, education, gender roles, family background, community, traditions, language, communication styles, religion and spirituality, and acculturation should all be considered.

Cultural factors relevant to PDA will be reviewed briefly in the following sections, with a particular emphasis on the presentation of the disorder in African Americans, Cambodians, and *ataques de nervios* in Hispanic populations. Friedman (1997) provides a thorough review of the assessment and treatment of anxiety disorders across cultures.

PDA in African Americans

Despite similar rates of anxiety disorder prevalence in African American and Caucasian samples, African Americans are greatly underrepresented in treatment settings and research programs (Paradis, Hatch, & Friedman, 1994). African Americans may also have a later age of onset of PDA and may rely on different coping strategies than European Americans (Smith, Friedman, & Nevid, 1999). In an anxiety disorders clinic sample, Friedman, Paradis, and Hatch (1994) found that African American and Caucasian individuals displayed similar symptoms of PDA. However, African Americans had more needless psychiatric hospitalizations, more frequent emergency room visits, higher incidence of childhood trauma, and more life stressors. African Americans have also been shown to have a higher incidence of isolated sleep paralysis. Isolated sleep paralysis is important for health care professionals to assess in the context of PDA (Craske & Rowe, 1997), particularly in African Americans, as patients may misinterpret these symptoms as evidence of going crazy or having a stroke as a result of panic attacks. Given recent findings that fears of dying and of going crazy appear to be more common in African Americans with PDA than in European Americans with PDA (Smith et al., 1999), it is possible that incidences of isolated sleep paralysis contribute to the persistence of these beliefs.

Kyol Goeu *and "Sore Neck" in Cambodians*

Hinton, Ba, Peou, and Um (2000) found that among 89 Khmer patients surveyed in two Massachusetts psychiatric clinics, 60% were diagnosed with PD. Four main subtypes of panic attacks were suggested, including "sore neck," orthostatic dizziness, gastrointestinal upset, and effort-induced dizziness. Common triggers of panic attacks included expending effort, standing, olfactory stimuli, and feelings of hunger. The most commonly reported fear in the Khmer refugees was of death due to a rupture in a neck vessel as a result of increased blood and wind pressure, also called "sore neck syndrome." Sore neck "attacks" are characterized by headache, blurry vision, buzzing in the ear, and dizziness, as well as other common symptoms of autonomic arousal (e.g., accelerated heart rate, shortness of breath, trembling). This condition fits the classic definition for panic attacks or PD, but reflects the Khmer cultural belief of the importance of "wind overload" (*Kyol Goeu*) as a cause of symptoms (of anxiety), which could signal a blockage of important vessels (especially those in the neck) that carry blood and wind to the body.

Ataques de Nervios *in Hispanic Populations*

Ataques de nervios is a culturally specific reaction that may be diagnostically related to PD. This syndrome occurs most commonly in individuals from Puerto Rico but has also reported among Hispanic people living in the Caribbean and in other Latin American areas (Guarnaccia, Canino, Rubio-Stipec, & Bravo, 1993). Typically, *ataques de nervios* occur during severe stress (e.g., funerals, accidents, conflict in the family) (Guarnaccia, Rubio-Stipec, & Canino, 1989) and are generally culturally acceptable responses to stress. During an *ataque de nervios*, an individual may experience symptoms similar to panic, including palpitations, shaking, numbness, and heat rising to the head. Further, the person may shout, swear, or fall to the ground in convulsive movements, without recollection of the event afterward. *Ataques de nervios* may occur separately, but often coexist with PDA.

Medical and Substance-Related Factors

PDA is frequently complicated by nonpsychiatric medical problems and substance use. The clinician should assess for organic factors that (1) may directly produce somatic symptoms resembling those in panic attacks; and (2) may have caused initial panic attacks, influenced the severity of PDA, or influenced the course of treatment. Medical conditions and psychoactive substances can affect the course of PDA symptoms in complex ways. Therefore, it may be difficult to determine whether a medical condition or substance is a cause, a complicating factor, or completely independent from the PDA symptoms (Zaubler & Katon, 1996).

In order for a diagnosis of PDA to be established, medical conditions that can produce panic-like symptoms must first be ruled out. Patients with PDA may commonly present to medical settings with complaints of cardiac, neurological, or gastrointestinal problems. Ballenger (1997) maintains that PD is often misdiagnosed or unrecognized in primary care settings, and he documents several conditions that may produce panic-like symptoms, including anemia, angina, arrhythmia, chronic obstructive pulmonary disease, Cushing's disease, electrolyte disturbance, epilepsy, hyperthyroidism, hypoglycemia, parathyroid disorders, pheochromocytoma, pulmonary embolus, and transient ischemic attacks. Occasionally, these conditions are sufficient to account for the panic-like symptoms, with remediation of the medical disorder resulting in a full remission of the panic symptoms. More often, however, these conditions produce somatic symptoms that exacerbate a person's PDA symptoms. To screen for and identify these conditions, Ballenger (1997) suggests a work-up that includes (1) a complete medical, psychiatric, and social history; (2) physical and neurological examination; (3) family history; (4) medication and drug history; (5) an electrocardiogram in patients over 40 years of age; and (6) laboratory tests, including complete blood count, chemistry panel, thyroid function test, and any other tests that may be indicated from the history.

Certain medical conditions also put individuals at greater risk for the development of panic attacks and PDA. For example, asthma has been noted as a risk factor for the development of PDA, since feelings of suffocation may produce panic attacks (Carr, 1998, 1999). Consequently, asthma may contribute to the development of initial panic attacks, which, in turn, may lead to the development of PDA. The presence of PDA and anxiety may also affect the severity of asthma due to the hyperventilation that is often associated with panic. In turn, this may influence the use or overuse of asthma medications (Carr, 1998).

Controversy exists in the literature about the relationship between mitral valve prolapse (MVP) and PD. Recent studies have documented that panic attacks have no statistically significant effect on MVP (e.g., Yang, Tsai, Hou, Chen, & Sim, 1997). Further, the prevalence of PDA has been found to be no different in chest pain patients with or without MVP (Bowen, D'Arcy, & Orchard, 1991). Again, it may be more likely that symptoms of MVP increase the patient's awareness of his or her heart, which, in turn, may exacerbate panic symptoms.

The role of substance use in the development and maintenance of panic attacks and PDA should also be evaluated, because panic attacks are frequently associated with substance use disorders (Cox, Norton, Swinson, & Endler, 1990). Substances such as marijuana, cocaine, caffeine, and even general anesthetics often cause initial panic attacks, which may lead to the development of PDA (e.g., Aronson & Craig, 1986; Geracioti & Post, 1991; Louie, Lannon, & Ketter, 1989; Schnoll & Daghestani, 1986; Weller, 1985). Moreover, individuals with PD appear to be particularly sensitive to the effects of marijuana, and many will avoid smoking marijuana due to the increased anxiety that they experience (Szuster, Pontius, & Campos, 1988).

Medical Conditions and Treatment Outcome

Schmidt and Telch (1997) found that individuals with PDA who perceived their health as poor or who had comorbid medical conditions evidenced poorer rates of recovery at posttreatment and 6 months after cognitive-behavioral treatment (CBT). Medical conditions represented in the study included chronic back difficulties, hypertension, asthma, arthritis, irritable bowel syndrome, ulcer, heart conditions, cancer, migraine, diabetes, and other conditions. Interestingly, actual medical comorbidity did not predict outcome over and above beliefs about perceived health.

Special considerations may need to be made in cases of patients with particular medical conditions. For example, certain medical conditions may contraindicate the use of some interoceptive exposure exercises that might otherwise be used to induce feared physical sensations during CBT for PDA. An assessment of these medical conditions will allow for the selection of safer exercises. For instance, it is recommended that CBT be tailored for individuals with asthma. Feldman, Giardino, and Lehrer (2000) outlined a CBT program that was adapted for individuals with PDA and asthma. Treatment included cognitive restructuring techniques, modifications to interoceptive exposure, and assisting the patient to differentiate asthma from panic. Because symptom induction exercises involving breath holding could induce chest pain and risk bronchoconstriction following deep inhalation, the authors suggest "pursed lip breathing" as a safer alternative.

In addition, one aim of psychological treatment is to assist the patient to estimate the likelihood of actual medical risks versus perceived ones. Because individuals with PDA often overestimate the likelihood of medical risks (e.g., having a heart attack or stroke), they may benefit from a thorough medical assessment and education about the actual risks associated with their panic attacks.

Suicide Risk

Patients with PD frequently have concerns about dying, and it is not unusual for them to present to emergency rooms believing that they are having a heart attack. Because of their intense fear of death, it may be tempting to consider patients with PDA to be at lower risk for suicide. However, assessment of suicide risk in individuals with PDA is important, particularly because the disorder causes significant impairment in quality of life and functioning. Panic attacks, among other factors, have also been shown to be predictive of suicide risk (Clayton, 1993), and studies have found a high risk for suicidal ideation in individuals with PDA (e.g., Cox, Direnfeld, Swinson, & Norton, 1994). Weissman, Klerman, Markowitz, and Ouellette (1989) found that 20% of individuals with PD had made a suicide attempt, making this risk comparable to major depression. Further, their results indicated that individuals with PD were 18 times more likely to attempt suicide than individuals with no mental disorder.

One explanation for these findings is the high rate of comorbid Axis I disorders, including major depression, that may increase the risk for suicidal ideation among people with PDA. Likewise, comorbid personality disorders, particularly borderline personality disorder, may increase suicidal risk. In a retrospective review of patients with PDA with and without borderline personality disorder, Friedman, Jones, Chernen, and Barlow (1992) found that 25% of patients with PDA and comorbid borderline personality disorder attempted suicide, compared to 2% of individuals with PDA alone. In addition, Johnson, Weissman, and Klerman (1990) explored the risk of suicide in "uncomplicated" PDA and found that only 7% of individuals reported suicide attempts. Still, because of the high rate of comorbidity (51%; Brown, Antony, & Barlow, 1995) in patients with PDA, assessment of suicidal ideation is essential.

CHOOSING AMONG DIFFERENT ASSESSMENT STRATEGIES

Choice of assessment strategies will largely depend on the nature of the setting and the time allocated for assessment. Different settings may permit only brief periods to conduct an assessment, whereas other sites may have more flexibility. The duration of the assessment will also depend on how long the patient is able to tolerate the procedures. For example, a patient who is highly agoraphobic may be too fearful to tolerate a lengthy assessment or may require frequent breaks. Moreover, the types of assessment tools used should be influenced by the educational level and cognitive ability of the patient, which can affect the validity of the instruments. When choosing assessment instruments, cultural factors and normative data for the various measures should also be considered.

In general, one should include measures that directly assess both panic and the conditions that are commonly associated with panic that may affect treatment outcome. It is also beneficial to have self-report and behavioral measures of symptoms associated with PDA. For example, ability to tolerate symptom induction exercises may provide valuable information regarding the person's anxiety response in the face of physical sensations, over and above that of self-report. Similarly, assessing the patient's reactions in a variety of settings provides useful information about situations that influence the patient's anxiety. The clinician may choose to conduct these assessment exercises in-session, or assign them for homework. In the latter case, the patient may be asked to monitor such variables as his or her level of anxiety, the physical symptoms experienced, the intensity of the symptoms, the similarity of symptoms to those during natural panic, and his or her fearful thoughts.

In an attempt to standardize assessment procedures for research on PDA, Shear and Mazer (1994) discussed essential and recommended areas of measurement for PDA. Essential areas included (1) diagnostic assessment using a structured clinical interview to assess PDA and comorbid Axis I disorders; (2) measurement of panic attack severity, anticipatory anxiety, and phobic symptoms; (3) degree of impairment, overall severity, and improvement; (4) type and frequency of interval treatments; and (5) medical conditions. Other recommendations included the use of panic attack diaries and assessment of life events and quality of life.

RECOMMENDATIONS FOR ASSESSING ASSOCIATED FEATURES

Because PDA frequently co-occurs with other anxiety disorders, depression, and substance use disorders, it is important to assess for the presence of these comorbid conditions. Several studies have documented the relationship between PDA and major depressive disorder (MDD) (e.g., Brown et al., 1995). The prevalence of MDD in people with PD has been found to range between 50% and 65% (Baldwin, 1998; Gorman & Coplan, 1996). Keller and Hanks (1993) found that among individuals with PDA, approximately 50% to 75% had experienced at least one major depressive episode, thus highlighting the importance of assessing depression. Moreover, Basoglu et al. (1994) found that among other factors, a past history of depression was predictive of poor outcome 6 months following treatment with alprazolam and exposure.

As with depression, GAD is also commonly associated with PDA. It is important for the clinician to distinguish PD from GAD, as well as to assess for comorbid GAD. Comorbid GAD has also been found to be a strong predictor of the presence of PDA at a 2-year follow-up (Scheibe & Albus, 1997).

Substance Use Disorders

Alcohol abuse/dependence has been shown to frequently co-occur with PDA. Otto, Pollack, Sachs, O'Neil, and Rosenbaum (1992) found that 24% of individuals with PDA had comorbid alcohol dependence. One theory to account for this relationship is the self-medication hypothesis, which states that individuals self-medicate their anxiety with alcohol or other drugs to achieve symptomatic relief. Oei and Loveday (1997) have argued, based on their review, that alcohol disorders and anxiety disorders should be considered to be distinct conditions that require separate but parallel treatments when they occur together. However, research on the most effective approach to treating these comorbid conditions is clearly needed. In a series of case studies from our center, Lehman, Brown, and Barlow (1998) found that cognitive-behavioral treatment for PDA led to a subsequent decrease in alcohol abuse (early full remission) at posttreatment for all three patients. Unfortunately, one patient later relapsed.

Individuals with comorbid PDA and alcohol dependence report greater levels of avoidance behavior, depression, social anxiety, panic intensity, and interoceptive sensitivity than individuals with PDA alone (Bibb & Chambless, 1986; Chambless, Cherney, Caputo, & Rheinstein, 1987). Concurrent alcohol abuse or dependence may also undermine the effects of psychological treatment for PDA. Consequently, we recommend the standard inclusion of measures to assess alcohol use in the assessment battery.

As already mentioned, other drugs, such as marijuana and cocaine, have been associated with the onset of panic attacks and PD and should also be assessed routinely. Initial screening for drug and alcohol abuse or dependence may include brief questions about the quantity and frequency of alcohol and drug use. Clinicians may also benefit from asking patients whether they ever drink alcohol or use drugs to alleviate negative mood, such as anxiety or depression. It is important for clinicians to be aware of patients who use alcohol or other drugs to self-medicate, but who may not meet formal criteria for alcohol or substance abuse or dependence. Such behavior may still undermine the effects of treatment.

Mental health professionals should also be aware of the risks of benzodiazepine abuse in individuals with PDA and the potential influence of these drugs on treatment. Benzodiazepines may interfere with acquisition and retention of information (e.g., Barbee, Black, & Tordorov, 1992) or state dependent learning (Overton, 1991). Moreover, patients who are taking benzodiazepines may have difficulty tapering off of these medications because the symptoms of withdrawal often mimic the very symptoms of panic that the patient is trying to avoid. CBT administered concurrently with slow medication taper has been shown to be helpful for assisting these individuals to withdraw from their medications (Otto, Pollack, Meltzer-Brody, & Rosenbaum, 1992; Spiegel & Bruce, 1997). CBT also helped prevent relapse and recurrence of PD after discontinuation (Bruce, Spiegel, & Hegel, 1999).

Finally, less attention has been paid to the role of smoking in PDA. Among people who have anxiety disorders, those with PDA display the highest rates of smoking (Baker, Wiegel, Gulliver, & Barlow, 1999; Himle, Thyer, & Fischer, 1988). Considering the well-known health consequences associated with both stress and smoking, people with PDA who smoke may be at increased risk for adverse health problems. If they self-medicate their anxiety by smoking, these individuals also may have increased difficulty with smoking cessation since increased anxiety is a common withdrawal symptom when quitting smoking.

Personality Disorders

Approximately 40% to 65% of patients with PDA have a concurrent personality disorder diagnosis (Brooks, Baltazar, & Munjack, 1989). The most commonly occurring personality disorders are avoidant, dependent, and histrionic personality disorders (Chambless, Renneberg, Goldstein, & Gracely, 1992; Diaferia et al., 1993). Controversy exists with regard to the effects of PDA treatment in individuals who have comorbid personality disorders, and there is some evidence that individuals with personality disorders may improve more slowly than those without comorbid personality disorders (Marchand, Goyer, Dupuis, & Mainguy, 1998). Further, Black, Wesner, Gabel, Bowers, and Monahan (1994) found that, in response to short-term cognitive therapy, the presence of a personality disorder was a negative predictor of outcome, whereas the absence of a personality disorder was a positive predictor of recovery.

Hofmann et al. (1998) explored the effects of panic treatment (CBT or imipramine) on personality disorder characteristics in people with PD with mild or no agoraphobia. The Wisconsin Personality Disorders Inventory (Klein, Benjamin, Treece, Rosenfeld, & Greist, 1990) was used to assess personality disorder characteristics, as defined in DSM-III-R (American Psychiatric Association, 1987) personality disorders. Both treatments were effective for reducing panic symptomatology, and both had a favorable effect on most personality disorder characteristics. In contrast to previous findings, personality disorder characteristics did not predict outcome for either treatment.

SAMPLE ASSESSMENT BATTERY FOR PANIC DISORDER AND AGORAPHOBIA

Table 3.4 depicts a sample battery for assessing individuals with PDA. This battery includes strategies for thoroughly assessing various aspects of PDA, as well as associated conditions. Self-report instruments are used to supplement information obtained by the clinician. Although the length of the assessment may be a limitation for some settings, later in this chapter we discuss strategies for assessing the features of PDA in settings where the evaluation must be completed quickly (e.g., primary care settings).

To illustrate how this assessment battery can be implemented in clinical practice, we present the case of Ms. W. When she first presented at our center, Ms. W was a 34-year-old, Caucasian woman, with a 10-year history of PDA. The onset of her PDA occurred while she was in the midst of a stressful legal battle. Ms. W's primary panic-related concerns surrounded her anxiety about having a heart attack or going "crazy" during a panic attack. Consequently, the symptoms that were most distressing to Ms. W included a racing heart, dizziness, and feelings of unreality. She avoided many situations (e.g., driving, flying, public transportation, crowds, going to malls) because of her anxiety about having panic attacks. Although Ms. W could enter many of these situations when accompanied, she would not travel to any locations beyond a 5-mile radius from her home when she was alone.

Clinical Interview

The ADIS-IV was the primary instrument used for diagnostic assessment and to provide background information, much of which was outlined in the preceding section. Ms. W was assigned a principal diagnosis of PDA and additional diagnoses of GAD and a specific phobia of heights. Although Ms. W was not diagnosed with a substance use disorder based on the ADIS-IV, she reported a tendency to use alcohol to manage her anxiety during air travel.

Clinicians who do not have time to conduct a lengthy interview may instead choose to administer subsections of the ADIS-IV. These sections should be chosen carefully (e.g., using appropriate screening questions) to maximize the chances of identifying all comorbid conditions. If an abbreviated clinical interview is used, the clinician may opt to use additional self-report measures to screen for factors that may influence treatment (e.g., depressive symptoms and excessive worry). Using additional self-report measures has the benefit of assessing for potential problems without requiring additional time on the part of the clinician.

TABLE 3.4. Sample Assessment Battery for Panic Disorder with Agoraphobia

Assessment type	Measure
Diagnostic assessment interview	Anxiety Disorders Interview Schedule–IV (ADIS-IV; Brown et al., 1994)
Self-report scales for panic	Panic Disorder Severity Scale (PDSS; Shear et al., 1997)
	Anxiety Sensitivity Index (ASI; Reiss et al., 1986)
	Agoraphobic Cognitions Questionnaire (ACQ; Chambless et al., 1984)
	Anxiety Control Questionnaire (ACQ^2; Rapee et al., 1996)
	Panic Attack Record (PAR; Barlow & Craske, 2000)
Self-report scales for agoraphobia	Individualized fear and avoidance hierarchy (FAH)
	Albany Panic and Phobia Questionnaire (APPQ; Rapee et al., 1995)

Panic-Related Measures

The PDSS was selected to supplement data from the ADIS-IV and to assess PDA severity at various time points throughout treatment. The ASI was used to measure the degree of anxiety sensitivity before and after treatment, because several studies have found a positive relationship between changes in ASI scores and an individual's overall response to treatment for PDA (e.g., Baker, Vitali, Spiegel, Hofmann, & Barlow, 1998; McNally & Lorenz, 1987; Otto & Reilly-Harrington, 1999). In addition, the ACQ was chosen to assess anxious thoughts related to panic, and the ACQ[2] was selected to measure perceived control over anxiety when in a number of different situations. Finally, panic attack records were used, both to verify the presence and frequency of panic attacks and to acquire a detailed and qualitative description of the nature and context of the panic attacks.

Table 3.5 depicts pretreatment scores for Ms. W, along with a brief interpretation of the scores. Generally, Ms. W's PDA symptoms were viewed as being in the severe range, as demonstrated by her score on the PDSS, which indicated strong levels of anxious apprehension, heightened distress during panic, significant interoceptive and situational avoidance, and considerable interference with work functioning and social activities. As can be seen from the other measures, Ms. W displays strong levels of anxiety sensitivity and maladaptive thoughts and low levels of perceived control over her anxiety. These measures also served as a baseline assessment for tracking her progress over the course of treatment.

Measures of Agoraphobic Avoidance

The APPQ was selected as an objective measure of avoidance, because it is brief and because it assesses different types of avoidance (e.g., situational, interoceptive, social) that are common in PDA. In general, Ms. W reported strong levels of interoceptive and situational avoidance. An individualized FAH was also created during the first treatment session (sometimes this is provided as a homework assignment following the first session). Items on Ms. W's FAH were selected to reflect her difficulties going into situations alone versus when accompanied. A wide range of situations were selected, representing varying degrees of difficulty. Examples of specific items included driving alone for 30 minutes on a highway, driving accompanied for 30 minutes on a highway, driving alone to the supermarket across

TABLE 3.5. Assessment Results for Ms. W

Measure	Pretreatment score	Interpretation
PDSS	23	Severe range of PDA
ASI	40	Very strong levels of anxiety sensitivity
ACQ	2.86	Within range of individuals with PDA
ACQ[2]		Higher scores indicate greater perceived control;
Total score	64	Ms. W shows greater perceived control over
Reactions subscale	28	events than with her anxiety reactions
Events subscale	36	
APPQ		
Interoceptive	64	Very strong interoceptive sensitivity
Avoidance	59	Very strong avoidance levels
Social anxiety	16	Moderate levels of social anxiety

Note. PDSS, Panic Disorder Severity Scale (Shear et al., 1997); PDA, panic disorder with agoraphobia; ASI, Anxiety Sensitivity Index (Reiss et al., 1986); ACQ, Agoraphobic Cognitions Questionnaire (Chambless et al., 1984); ACQ[2], Anxiety Control Questionnaire (Rapee et al., 1996); APPQ, Albany Panic and Phobia Questionnaire (Rapee et al., 1995).

town, going to the mall with a friend during peak hours, and going to the mall alone during peak hours. The FAH items were rated again at each treatment session to assess changes in Ms. W's anxiety levels and avoidance and to help with the selection of new and challenging situations that could be used for exposure practices during subsequent treatment sessions.

Other Measures

Measures for other non-panic-related features (e.g., depression) can be included as described earlier. The ADIS-IV may be used to screen for comorbid diagnoses, and, based on this assessment, appropriate objective measures may be added to supplement the interview.

FACTORS COMPLICATING THE ASSESSMENT PROCESS

Several factors may complicate the assessment of PDA. As discussed earlier, certain medical conditions may mimic or mask a diagnosis of PDA. Thus, before assigning a final diagnosis and recommending a particular course of treatment, a proper medical evaluation should be completed. In practice, however, this is seldom necessary because most patients with PDA will have already undergone multiple medical evaluations prior to contact with a mental health professional. In fact, the National Institute of Mental Health has warned against providing excessive medical workups to patients with PDA (Wolfe & Maser, 1994, p. 52).

Due to the problems associated with retrospective self-report, it may also be useful for patients to monitor their panic attacks and associated avoidance using diaries, as discussed earlier. However, several difficulties may arise when using diaries. For example, patients may not understand fully how to use the panic diaries, may not have the cognitive ability to complete the forms, or may not be motivated to use the diaries. Discussing the rationale for using panic diaries and providing adequate instruction are essential for ensuring that patients understand the importance of the diaries and know how to complete them properly.

Accurate assessment requires that the patient record panic-related events shortly after they occur. To assist with prompt monitoring, some patients may respond favorably to the use of computerized palm-sized computers for recording episodes of panic. Finally, patients may be fearful of completing the panic diaries. That is, some patients may experience an increase in anxiety when asked to focus on their panic attacks and to record the relevant information. In this case, the patient's concerns should be appropriately addressed and normalized, and the patient should be reassured that monitoring will become easier over time.

Similar difficulties may arise when completing self-report scales, which may influence the reliability and validity of any information collected in this manner. Specifically, patients may misunderstand or misinterpret certain questions. In addition, patients' responses may be influenced by a desire to make a particular impression on the clinician or on another individual (e.g., a friend, family member, or other "safe" person) who is present while the assessment is being completed. Measures should be scanned for inconsistent responses, and these should be followed up with the patient for clarification. Clinicians may need to assist with the completion of measures for patients who have cognitive deficits or reading difficulties.

Patient motivation may also be a complicating factor during assessment. For example, patients may not fully understand the rationale for particular components of the assessment and, consequently, may be less motivated to set aside time to complete them. Anxiety related to completing assessment exercises (e.g., interoceptive induction exercises; filling out forms that require patients to focus on their anxiety) may also influence motivation and prevent the patient from completing such exercises. Finally, overall motivation for being in treatment, as well as issues related to secondary gain, may affect motivation. In general, the importance of the assessment process and compliance with the necessary exercises and forms cannot be overemphasized. The therapist may need to take a hard stance on the importance of monitoring and assessment; patients should be informed that unless they complete the assessment, the effectiveness of treatment may be compromised.

FROM ASSESSMENT TO TREATMENT

Overview of Empirically Supported Treatments

Psychological treatments for PDA have been well studied. For a thorough review of the psychological theories that underlie these treatments, see Bouton, Mineka, and Barlow (2001) and Thorn, Chosak, Baker, and Barlow (1999). For a more detailed review of psychological treatments, see Chosak, Baker, Thorn, Spiegel, and Barlow (1999) and Craske (1999). For a thorough review of medication treatments for PDA, see Nutt, Ballenger, and Lepine (1999) and Spiegel, Wiegel, Baker, and Greene (2000).

Cognitive-behavioral treatments for PDA have been demonstrated to be more effective than no treatment, nonspecific psychological interventions, and certain pharmacological treatments (Barlow, Gorman, Shear, & Woods, 2000; Clark et al., 1994; Craske, 1999; Fava, Zielezny, Savron, & Grandi, 1995). A behavioral treatment component, involving systematically confrontation of feared situations and interoceptive cues, is important for individuals with varying levels of avoidance. In general, cognitive-behavioral treatments (CBT) have received the most empirical support for the treatment of PDA, particularly the treatment developed at our center (Barlow & Craske, 1988, 2000; Craske, Barlow, & Meadows, 2000), which will be the focus of the remaining discussion.

The most comprehensive randomized clinical trial conducted on the treatment of PDA is our multisite collaborative study for the treatment of PD (Barlow et al., 2000). In this study, five treatment conditions were compared: CBT plus imipramine, CBT plus placebo, CBT alone, imipramine alone, and placebo alone. All participants were diagnosed with PD and had either mild or no agoraphobia. The results of this study indicated that both active treatments were significantly greater than placebo. CBT and imipramine had equivalent effects at posttreatment and at 6 months follow-up, although among treatment responders the quality of response was better for those who received imipramine at posttreatment. However, those who received imipramine, either alone or in combination with CBT, evidenced greater levels of deterioration 6 months following treatment than those who received CBT or CBT plus placebo. Consequently, although imipramine produced superior quality of response at acute treatment, the effects of CBT were more longlasting.

Most recently, we have been conducting an intensive CBT program across an 8-day period for patients with severe agoraphobia, called intensive sensation-focused treatment (ISFT). This treatment has been described in detail by Heinrichs, Hofmann, and Spiegel (in press). During this program, standard panic control treatment (Barlow & Craske, 1988; Craske & Barlow, 2000) is condensed into three 2- to 3-hour sessions during the first 3 days. Interoceptive exposure is a strong component of these initial days of treatment, along with cognitive restructuring. Supplemental readings are also provided. Over subsequent days, therapist-assisted situational and interoceptive exposure is conducted. Here, patients expose themselves to their most feared agoraphobic situations, and they simultaneously induce feared physical sensations. Rather than using a hierarchically based exposure format, patients begin with the most difficult situations, with the rationale that the situations that are less fear-provoking will then become easier. Exposures begin with the assistance of a therapist who ensures that the patient is conducting the exposure practices properly. However, the therapist involvement is tapered quickly so that the patient begins to do exercises on his or her own. Preliminary results from a case study of ISFT were very promising (Baker, Spiegel, & Barlow, 1999).

Linking Assessment to Treatment Planning

More than other approaches, CBT relies on assessment to inform the planning of most aspects of treatment. The following discussion will focus largely on how to use assessment to plan the course of CBT. Generally, assessment should help the clinician identify the physiological, cognitive, and behavioral features of an individual's PDA that can subsequently be targeted during treatment. Common techniques to address anxiety associated with panic attacks include cognitive restructuring, interoceptive exposure, and breathing retraining. Situational exposure is perhaps the most important component of treatment for agoraphobic avoidance. Finally, teaching a patient to use self-assessment strategies may help to facilitate the maintenance of gains following treatment. Each strategy is discussed in the following sections.

Cognitive Restructuring

It is important to know precisely which cognitions are associated with an individual's panic, and to what extent the patient believes his or her anxious thoughts. To guide the assessment of such thoughts, Cox (1996) recommends using a combination of questions from the ASI (e.g., "When I notice that my heart is beating rapidly, I worry that I might have a heart attack") and questions regarding the DSM-IV cognitive panic attack symptoms (e.g., fear of dying and fear of going crazy). Further, it is important for patients to be as specific as possible about their thoughts. For example, if a patient reports having a fear of dying, he or she should be asked questions to ascertain the expected cause of death (e.g., heart attack, suicide). Identifying the connection between fearful thoughts and panic attacks will assist the therapist in challenging a patient's panic-related misconceptions using cognitive restructuring techniques. Assessment of specific fearful predictions will assist the clinician in developing appropriate exercises to test the validity of particular anxious thoughts during treatment (e.g., using interoceptive or situational exposure). As discussed earlier, measures for panic-related cognitions include the ACQ, the CCL-A, and the PACQ.

Interoceptive Exposure

Individuals with PDA are fearful of the physical sensations associated with panic. Inducing symptoms during the assessment (using various interoceptive exercises) is useful for directly assessing the fearful cognitions that are elicited, as well as for identifying interoceptive exposure exercises that can be repeatedly practiced during treatment. During treatment, different interoceptive assessment exercises may be conducted to induce the most relevant symptoms; however, the assessment should include a wide range of exercises to detect sensitivity to physical sensations that the patient may not be aware of. During treatment, exercises that induce the most fear and that are most similar to naturally occurring panic are practiced repeatedly in a systematic manner in order to decrease the patient's sensitivity to the physical sensations of panic. For example, a patient who is most frightened of a racing heart, dizziness, and feelings of unreality could use exercises such as hyperventilation, spinning in a chair, running in place, and staring in a mirror to experience these sensations and eventually learn to respond to these feelings without fear. Interoceptive exposure exercises should also be incorporated into practices that involve exposure to feared agoraphobic situations (e.g., hyperventilating while driving, spinning in a department store).

Breathing Retraining

Patients with PDA often rely on their chest muscles for breathing (filling only the top parts of their lungs with air), rather than using their diaphragms. In addition, PDA is often associated with a tendency toward chronic hyperventilation (i.e., breathing too quickly given the aerobic demands currently placed on an individual's body), which, in turn, can lead to many of the same symptoms that are associated with panic attacks. Breathing retraining involves teaching a patient to breathe more slowly, primarily using the diaphragm. However, it is important to ensure that the patient does not rely on the breathing exercises as a safety behavior.

To assess the effect of overbreathing on a particular patient, the clinician can ask the individual to engage in voluntary hyperventilation for 90 seconds (Barlow & Craske, 2000). After the exercise, the patient describes the symptoms experienced (e.g., heart racing and dizziness). If the symptoms are qualitatively similar to those that occur during a typical panic attack, then overbreathing may be a factor in the patient's panic symptomatology. Alternatively, if the symptoms are not similar to those during panic attacks, the exercise is repeated for another 2 to 2½ minutes. If the extended exercise still does not induce panic-like feelings, then overbreathing is assumed not to be a contributing factor for the patient. In such cases, diaphragmatic breathing may be only a small component of treatment, if it is used at all.

Agoraphobic Avoidance

As discussed earlier, avoidance behavior may be either overt (e.g., leaving a situation) or subtle (e.g., distraction). Exposure-based treatments focus on helping a patient eliminate both subtle and obvious forms of avoidance. Identifying subtle avoidance strategies is often more difficult than identifying overt avoidance because patients may not be aware of their subtle avoidance behaviors. In such cases, behavioral assessment tests may provide an opportunity for the clinician to observe a patient's subtle avoidance behaviors. Identification of these safety behaviors is essential for designing situational exposure exercises that will subsequently be used during treatment. The extent to which a patient avoids particular situations and activities should influence the extent to which situational exposure is emphasized during treatment.

Using Self-Assessment to Facilitate Relapse Prevention

Teaching the patient to engage in self-assessment may be beneficial for relapse prevention. Patients can be trained to be their own therapists and to assess their progress during and following treatment. After treatment ends, if the patient experiences an increase in his or her panic symptoms, ongoing self-assessment may help identify the problem early and facilitate resuming treatment before the symptoms worsen even more.

ASSESSMENT OF OUTCOME DURING AND FOLLOWING TREATMENT

Continuing assessment throughout treatment allows the clinician to measure the effectiveness of the intervention and provides important data that can be used to make decisions about whether to continue with a particular treatment approach or to change directions. In addition to measuring the effects of treatment, continual assessment may assist the patient's attitudes toward the treatment and his or her motivation to use the treatment techniques. Motivation may shift throughout treatment, particularly when exposure practices become more difficult or when the patient has improved considerably and the problem is no longer as distressing as it was in the beginning.

At a minimum, clinicians should assess status and progress at pretreatment, midtreatment, and posttreatment. Patients may also benefit from follow-up assessments (e.g., at 3- and 6-month intervals) to track their progress and ensure that their treatment gains have been maintained. If longer-term treatments are being conducted, rather than a midtreatment assessment, clinicians may choose to assess status approximately every 4 to 6 weeks. Appropriate measures for such an assessment might include the PDSS, ASI, APPQ, or other measures. Alternatively, clinicians may opt to assess patient status on a session-by-session basis using briefer measures (e.g., the ASI and FAH). In addition, assessing residual agoraphobia may be critical for ensuring long-term maintenance of treatment gains. Residual agoraphobia has been shown to be a strong predictor of poorer outcome and greater relapse following the termination of treatment (Keller et al., 1994). Finally, in addition to using the standard measures of outcome that were reviewed previously, assessment of outcome should include measures of distress and interference (e.g., at work, in relationships, and in daily activities) related to panic attacks and avoidance.

ASSESSMENT OF PANIC DISORDER AND AGORAPHOBIA IN MANAGED CARE AND PRIMARY CARE SETTINGS

As suggested earlier, assessment is closely linked to treatment: the assessment tools that one chooses should depend in part on the goals for treatment. In primary and managed care settings, these treatment goals will have to be weighed against a variety of other factors that are often not in the clinician's control. These factors may include limits on the number of sessions and other cost-containment strategies, client heterogeneity with respect to both diagnosis and level of functioning, and heterogeneity among staff who are treating the client. Thus, the clinician will have to choose assessment tools with an eye to the treatment approaches that will be most feasible within a particular setting and for a particular client. In this section, we will outline some considerations that are relevant to the assessment of PDA in a medical setting, along with strategies for addressing these issues.

Management of PDA in primary care settings broadly includes (1) screening for PDA symptoms, (2) accurate diagnosis and differential diagnosis, (3) design and execution of a feasible treatment plan, (4) provision of ongoing support for the client, and (5) ongoing evaluation of outcome to ensure accountability for treatment delivery.

Patients with PDA are most likely to present for treatment in a medical setting and are more likely to present to physicians than psychologists. As many as 35% of patients with PDA are first seen by a general internist or family practitioner, 43% by an emergency room physician, and 35% by a mental health professional (Katerndahl & Realini, 1995). Because PDA is often not diagnosed initially in these settings, patients with PD are likely to return repeatedly for medical treatment before they are diagnosed (Ballenger, 1998) and are more likely to overuse medical services (Ballenger, 1997). In addition, misdiagnosis of panic in medical settings may be perpetuated by the comparatively low levels of reimbursement for psychological versus medical conditions and the stigma associated with psychological disorders. Given the serious consequences of PDA and the stress that it puts on the health care system, effective screening procedures are an important first step in the management of

PDA in the primary care setting. Effective screening helps set the stage for providing treatment recommendations and ultimately may reduce the need for health care.

Once a careful screening has suggested the presence of PDA, the clinician should assign a diagnosis, followed by an appropriate treatment plan. Limits to the number of sessions may constrain the clinician to choose only the most important therapeutic strategies; however, choosing appropriate interventions will be difficult without a thorough initial diagnostic assessment. A comprehensive assessment provides information about diagnosis and symptomatology. Detailed assessment is crucial for determining the best course of treatment.

Cost-containment strategies may limit the scope of one's assessment. For example, managed care companies may be reluctant to pay for lengthy diagnostic assessments because of the time that it takes to administer them. In such cases, one may need to choose briefer but less thorough and less reliable measures to verify the presence of panic that was initially suggested by the screen. As discussed previously, clinicians may need to rely more heavily on self-report instruments to minimize therapist time. Alternatively, health professionals should be proactive by attempting to influence managed care organizations by convincing them of the long-term utility and cost-effectiveness of comprehensive assessments. Rapaport and Cantor (1997) have emphasized the importance of helping to shape managed care plans by providing them with information about cost-effectiveness and outcome data in the case of PDA. Because assessment and treatment are so closely related, incomplete assessments and misdiagnosis could lead to inappropriate and perhaps ineffective treatments.

It has been suggested that standard PDA treatments are not useful in primary care settings because the clients are not "diagnostically pure." However, treatment of panic has been found to be effective even in the context of other comorbid conditions, such as GAD (Brown et al., 1995) and alcohol abuse (Lehman et al., 1998), and treatment seems to reduce the severity of these other conditions as well. Still, it is important to be aware of the specific comorbid conditions when making decisions about treatment, again pointing to the importance of careful diagnosis.

Although much of this chapter has focused on the assessment of symptom severity, primary care settings often view psychological conditions in the context of overall quality of life. Impairment levels and quality of life are often the central outcome measures in primary care environments, and thus clinicians should consider overall impairment as they judge the severity of panic. Whereas many of the measures previously reviewed provide some information on impairment, they do not provide thorough information on overall life functioning. Several scales are available to provide detailed information on functional impairment. In the case of PDA, it may be important to use scales that measure functional impairment independent of symptom severity, since one study found that measures that assess both were not predictive of disability at follow-up (Katschnig, Amering, Stolk, & Ballenger, 1996). Useful impairment measures include the Work Productivity and Activity Impairment Questionnaire (WPAI; Reily, Zbrozek, & Dukes, 1993), which evaluates the effects of symptoms on work, and the Sheehan Disability Scale (SDS; Leon, Olfson, Portera, Farber, & Sheehan, 1997), which measures levels of disability. As discussed here, assessment must always be done with an eye to how the information will be used.

A number of other measures have been used to capture impairment in medical and primary care settings. The Illness Intrusiveness Rating Scale (IIRS; Devins et al., 1983) has been used to measure the ways in which illness disrupts life functioning, particularly in areas of individual interest and involvement. The domains of functioning that are examined include health, diet, work, active recreation, passive recreation, financial situation, relationship with partner, sex life, family relations, other social relations, self-expression/improvement, religious expression, and community and civic involvement. Each item is rated for interference on a scale from 1 to 7 (1, a little, to 7, a lot). While the IIRS has been used most often to examine illness interference in the context of medical illnesses, one study examined this in the context of anxiety and PD (Antony, Roth, Swinson, Huta, & Devins, 1998). They found that individuals with anxiety disorders (social phobia, OCD, and PD) scored higher on the IIRS than did groups with other chronic illnesses. The life domains that were most affected were the areas that included social relationships, self-expression/improvement, and health. This study suggests that it may be important to examine areas and level of impairment for individuals with PD.

Another measure that has been widely used to assess health-related quality of life issues is the Short-Form Health Survey (SF-36; Ware & Sherbourne, 1992). This interview can be self-administered or it can be administered by an interviewer, whether in person or by telephone. The SF-36 includes one scale that assesses impairment on eight health dimensions related to health problems: limitations in physical activities, limitations in social activities due to emotional problems, limitations in usual role activities because of physical problems, bodily pain, general mental problems, limitations in usual role because of mental problems, vitality, and general health perceptions. One advantage of the SF-36 over other measures is that it inquires directly about impairment related to both physical and psychological conditions.

The health care provider may also need to consider who will be involved in the delivery of care to the patient. In a primary care setting, clinicians are likely to collaborate with professionals from a variety of backgrounds, including primary care physicians, psychologists, psychiatrists, nurses, psychiatric nurses, and social workers. Clinicians treating PDA will have to consider whether the health care workers involved are properly trained to deliver the treatment in the appropriate way and to track outcome. Coordination of staff from diverse backgrounds may involve providing education regarding the importance of thorough assessment and ongoing tracking to maximize success during treatment.

Because cost containment is managed care's raison d'être (Rapaport & Cantor, 1997), the feasibility of multiple patient visits and extensive assessment are central issues in the managed care system. Given the high medical costs associated with PDA, greater initial investments in assessment may be justified from a financial perspective. Appropriate treatment of PDA is likely to be cost effective by minimizing overall medical utilization and reducing impairment. Comprehensive assessment is instrumental for documenting the outcome of treatment, with respect to both improved symptom severity and improved quality of life.

CONCLUSION

In summary, thorough assessment of PD and its accompanying physical and psychological conditions is instrumental in the development of effective treatment programs. Moreover, assessment throughout the course of the treatment guides the clinician to tailor treatment appropriately and maximize the time spent in the sessions. In this chapter, we have reviewed the most commonly used and well-established measures of PD and agoraphobia. Our aim has been to facilitate the selection of measurement instruments and to provide practical recommendations for linking assessment to treatment.

REFERENCES

American Psychiatric Association. (1987). *Diagnostic and statistical manual of mental disorders* (3rd ed., rev.). Washington, DC: Author.

American Psychiatric Association. (1994). *Diagnostic and statistical manual of mental disorders* (4th ed.). Washington, DC: Author.

American Psychiatric Association. (2000). *Diagnostic and statistical manual of mental disorders* (4th ed., text rev.). Washington, DC: Author.

Antony, M. M., Roth, D. A., Swinson, R. P., Huta, V., & Devins, G. M. (1998). Illness intrusiveness in individuals with panic disorder, obsessive–compulsive disorder, or social phobia. *Journal of Nervous and Mental Disease, 186,* 311–315.

Argyle, N., Deltito, J., Allerup, P., Maier, W., Albus, M., Nutzinger, D., Rasmussen, S., Ayuso, J. L., & Bech, P. (1991). The Panic-Associated Symptom Scale: Measuring the severity of panic disorder. *Acta Psychiatrica Scandinavica, 83,* 20–26.

Aronson, T. A., & Craig, T. J. (1986). Cocaine precipitation of panic disorder. *American Journal of Psychiatry, 143,* 643–645.

Asmundson, G. J. G. (1999). Anxiety sensitivity and chronic pain: Empirical findings, clinical implications, and future directions. In S. Taylor (Ed.), *Anxiety sensitivity: Theory, research and the treatment of the fear of anxiety* (pp. 269–286). Mahwah, NJ: Erlbaum.

Baker, S. L., Spiegel, D. A., & Barlow, D. H. (1999, August). *Two-week cognitive-behavioral treatment for severe agoraphobia: A case study.* Poster presented at the annual meeting of the American Psychological Association, Boston.

Baker, S. L., Vitali, A. E., Spiegel, D. A., Hofmann, S. G., & Barlow, D. H. (1998, March). *Anxiety sensitivity and responder status across treatment for panic disorder with agoraphobia.* Poster presented at the annual meeting of the Anxiety Disorders Association of America, Boston.

Baker, S. L., Wiegel, M., Gulliver, S. G., & Barlow, D. H. (1999, August). *Smoking prevalence in anxiety disorders and major depression: Preliminary findings.* Poster presented at the annual meeting of the American Psychological Association, Boston.

Baldwin, D. S. (1998). Depression and panic: Comorbidity. *European Psychiatry, 13*(Suppl.), 65S–75S.

Ballenger, J. C. (1997). Panic disorder in the medical setting. *Journal of Clinical Psychiatry, 58*(Suppl. 2), 13–17.

Ballenger, J. C. (1998). Treatment of panic disorder in the general medical setting. *Journal of Psychosomatic Research, 44,* 5–15.

Bandelow, B. (1995). Assessing the efficacy of treatments for panic disorder and agoraphobia: I. The Panic and Agoraphobia Scale. *International Clinical Psychopharmacology, 10,* 73–81.

Bandelow, B. (1999). *Panic and Agoraphobia Scale (PAS) manual.* Seattle, WA: Hogrefe & Huber.

Barbee, J. G., Black, F. W., & Todorov, A. A. (1992). Differential effects of alprazolam and buspirone upon acquisition, retention, and retrieval processes in memory. *Journal of Neuropsychiatry, 4,* 308–314.

Barlow, D. H. (2001). *Anxiety and its disorders: The nature and treatment of anxiety and panic* (2nd ed.). New York: Guilford Press.

Barlow, D. H., & Craske, M. G. (1988). *Mastery of your anxiety and panic.* San Antonio, TX: Psychological Corporation.

Barlow, D. H., & Craske, M. G. (2000). *Mastery of your anxiety and panic (MAP-3).* San Antonio, TX: Psychological Corporation.

Barlow, D. H., Gorman, J. M., Shear, M. K., & Woods, S. W. (2000). Cognitive-behavioral therapy, imipramine, or their combination for panic disorder: A randomized controlled study. *Journal of the American Medical Association, 283,* 2529–2536.

Barlow, D. H., & Wincze, J. (1998). DSM-IV and beyond: What is generalized anxiety disorder? *Acta Psychiatrica Scandinavica, 98,* 23–29.

Basoglu, M., Marks, I. M., Swinson, R. P., Noshirvani, H., O'Sullivan, G., & Kuch, K. (1994). Pretreatment predictors of treatment outcome in panic disorder and agoraphobia treated with alprazolam and exposure. *Journal of Affective Disorders, 30,* 123–132.

Bibb, J., & Chambless, D. L. (1986). Alcohol use and abuse among diagnosed agoraphobics. *Behaviour Research and Therapy, 24,* 49–58.

Black, D. W., Wesner, R. B., Gabel, J., Bowers, W., & Monahan, P. (1994). Predictors of short-term treatment response in 66 patients with panic disorder. *Journal of Affective Disorders, 30,* 233–241.

Bouton, M. E., Mineka, S., & Barlow, D. H. (2001). A modern learning-theory perspective on the etiology of panic disorder. *Psychological Review, 108,* 4–32.

Bowen, R. C., D'Arcy, C., & Orchard, R. C. (1991). The prevalence of anxiety disorders among patients with mitral valve prolapse syndrome and chest pain. *Psychosomatics, 32,* 400–406.

Bradwejn, J., Koszycki, D., Couetoux du Tertre, A., Bourin, M., Palmour, R., & Ervin, F. (1992). The cholecystokinin hypothesis in panic and anxiety disorders: A review. *Journal of Psychopharmacology, 6,* 345–351.

Brooks, R. B., Baltazar, P. L., & Munjack, D. J. (1989). Co-occurrence of personality disorders with panic disorder, social phobia, and generalized anxiety disorder: A review of the literature. *Journal of Anxiety Disorders, 3,* 259–285.

Brown, T. A., Antony, M. M., & Barlow, D. H. (1995). Diagnostic comorbidity in panic disorder: Effect on treatment outcome and course of comorbid diagnoses following treatment. *Journal of Consulting and Clinical Psychology, 63,* 408–418.

Brown, T. A., Di Nardo, P., & Barlow, D. H. (1994). *Anxiety Disorders Interview Schedule for DSM-IV.* San Antonio, TX: Psychological Corporation.

Brown, T. A., Di Nardo, P. A., Lehman, C. L. , & Campbell, L. A. (2001). Reliability of DSM-IV anxiety and mood disorders: Implications for classification of emotional disorders. *Journal of Abnormal Psychology, 110,* 49–58.

Bruce, T. J., Spiegel, D. A., Gregg, S. F., & Nuzzarello, A. (1995). Predictors of alprazolam discontinuation with and without cognitive behavioral therapy for panic disorder. *American Journal of Psychiatry, 152,* 1156–1160.

Bruce, T. J., Spiegel, D. A., & Hegel, M. T. (1999). Cognitive-behavioral therapy helps prevent relapse and recurrence of panic disorder following alprazolam discontinuation: A long-term follow-up of the Peoria and Dartmouth studies. *Journal of Consulting and Clinical Psychology, 67,* 151–156.

Burke, K. C., Burke, J. D., Jr., Regier, D. A., & Rae, D. S. (1990). Age at onset of selected mental disorders in five community populations. *Archives of General Psychiatry, 47,* 511–518.

Cameron, O. G., & Thyer, B. A. (1985). Treatment of pavor nocturnus with alprazolam. *Journal of Clinical Psychology, 46,* 405.

Carr, R. E. (1998). Panic disorder and asthma: Causes, effects and research implications. *Journal of Psychosomatic Research, 44,* 43–52.

Carr, R. E. (1999). Panic disorder and asthma. *Journal of Asthma, 36,* 143–152.

Cassano, G. B., Michelini, S., Shear, M. K., Coli, E., Maser, J. D., & Frank, E. (1997). The Panic-Agoraphobic Spectrum: A descriptive approach to the assessment and treatment of subtle symptoms. *American Journal of Psychiatry, 154*(6 Suppl.), 27–38.

Chambless, D. L., Caputo, G., Bright, P., & Gallagher, R. (1984). Assessment of "fear of fear" in agoraphobics: The Body Sensations Questionnaire and the Agoraphobic Cognitions Questionnaire. *Journal of Consulting and Clinical Psychology, 52,* 1090–1097.

Chambless, D. L., Caputo, G., Gracely, S., Jasin, E., & Williams, C. (1985). The Mobility Inventory for Agoraphobia. *Behaviour Research and Therapy, 23,* 35–44.

Chambless, D. L., Cherney, J., Caputo, G. C., & Rheinstein, D. J. (1987). Anxiety disorders and alcoholism: A study with inpatient alcoholics. *Journal of Anxiety Disorders, 1,* 29–40.

Chambless, D. L., Renneberg, B., Goldstein, A., & Gracely, E. J. (1992). MCMI-diagnosed personality disorders among agoraphobic outpatients: Prevalence and relationship to severity and treatment outcome. *Journal of Anxiety Disorders, 6,* 193–211.

Charney, D. S., Heninger, G. R., & Jarlow, P. I. (1985). Increased anxiogenic effects of caffeine in panic disorders. *Archives of General Psychiatry, 42,* 233–243.

Charney, D. S., Woods, S. W., Goodman, W. K., & Heninger, G. R. (1987). Neurobiological mechanisms of panic anxiety: Biochemical and behavioral correlates of yohimbine-induced panic attacks. *American Journal of Psychiatry, 144,* 1030–1036.

Chosak, A., Baker, S. L., Thorn, G. R., Spiegel, D. A., & Barlow, D. H. (1999). Psychological treatment of panic disorder. In D. J. Nutt, J. C. Ballenger, & J. Lepine (Eds.), *Panic disorder: Clinical diagnosis, management and mechanisms* (pp. 203–219). London: Martin Dunitz.

Clark, D. M., Salkovskis, P. M., Hackman, A., Middleton, H., Anastasiades, P., & Gelder, M. (1994).

A comparison of cognitive therapy, applied relaxation, and imipramine in the treatment of panic disorder. *British Journal of Psychiatry, 164,* 759–769.

Clark, D. M., Salkovskis, P. M., Öst, L.G., Breitholtz, E., Koehler, K. A., Westling, B. E., Jeavons, A., & Gelder, M. (1997). Misinterpretation of body sensations in panic disorder. *Journal of Consulting and Clinical Psychology, 65,* 203–213.

Clayton, P. I. (1993). Suicide in panic disorder and depression. *Current Therapeutic Research, 54,* 825–831.

Clum, G. A. (1997). *Manual for the Comprehensive Panic Profile.* Blacksburg, VA: Self-Change Systems.

Clum, G. A., Broyles, S., Borden, J., & Watkins, P. L. (1990). Validity and reliability of the panic attack symptoms and cognitions questionnaires. *Journal of Psychopathology and Behavioral Assessment, 12,* 233–245.

Côté, G., O'Leary, T., Barlow, D. H., Strain, J. J., Salkovskis, P. M., Warwick, H. M. C., Clark, D. M., Rapee, R., & Rasmussen, S. A. (1996). Hypochondriasis. In T. A. Widiger, A. J. Frances, H. A. Pincus, R. Ross, M. B. First, & W. W. Davis (Eds.), *DSM-IV sourcebook* (Vol. 2, pp. 933–947). Washington, DC: American Psychiatric Association.

Cox, B. J. (1996). The nature and assessment of catastrophic thoughts in panic disorder. *Behaviour Research and Therapy, 34,* 363–374.

Cox, B. J., Borger, S. C., & Enns, M. W. (1999). Anxiety sensitivity and emotional disorders: Psychometric studies and their theoretical implications. In S. Taylor (Ed.), *Anxiety sensitivity: Theory, research and the treatment of the fear of anxiety* (pp. 115–148). Mahwah, NJ: Erlbaum.

Cox, B. J., Direnfeld, D. M., Swinson, R. P., & Norton, R. G. (1994). Suicidal ideation and suicide attempts in panic disorder and social phobia. *American Journal of Psychiatry, 151,* 882–887.

Cox, B. J., Norton, G. R., & Swinson, R. P. (1992). *Panic attack questionnaire—revised.* Toronto: Clarke Institute of Psychiatry.

Cox, B. J., Norton, G. R., Swinson, R. P., & Endler, N. S. (1990). Substance abuse and panic-related anxiety: A critical review. *Behaviour Research and Therapy, 28,* 385–393.

Cox, B. J., Swinson, R. P., Norton, G. R., & Kuch, K. (1991). Anticipatory anxiety and avoidance in panic disorder with agoraphobia. *Behaviour Research and Therapy, 29,* 363–365.

Cox, B. J., Swinson, R. P., & Parker, J. D. A. (1993). Confirmatory factor analysis of the Fear Questionnaire in panic disorder with agoraphobia patients. *Psychological Assessment, 5,* 325–327.

Craske, M. G. (1999). *Anxiety disorders: Psychological approaches to theory and treatment.* Boulder, CO: Westview Press.

Craske, M. G., & Barlow, D. H. (1989). Nocturnal panic. *Journal of Nervous and Mental Disease, 177,* 160–168.

Craske, M. G., & Barlow, D. H. (2000). *Mastery of your anxiety and panic (MAP-3): Agoraphobia supplement.* San Antonio, TX: Psychological Corporation.

Craske, M. G., & Barlow, D. H. (2001). Panic disorder and agoraphobia. In D. H. Barlow (Ed.), *Clinical handbook of psychological disorders: A step-by-step treatment manual* (3rd ed., pp. 1–59). New York: Guilford Press.

Craske, M. G., Barlow, D. H., & Meadows, E. (2000). *Mastery of your anxiety and panic: Therapist guide for anxiety, panic, and agoraphobia (MAP-3).* San Antonio, TX: Psychological Corporation.

Craske, M. G., & Rowe, M. K. (1997). Nocturnal panic. *Clinical Psychology: Science and Practice, 4,* 153–174.

Davidson, J. R. T. (1996). Quality of life and cost factors in panic disorder. *Bulletin of the Menninger Clinic, 60*(Suppl. A), A5–A11.

Devins, G. M., Binik, Y. M., Hutchinson, T. A., Hollomby, D. J., Barre, P. E., & Guttman, R. D. (1983). The emotional impact of end-stage renal disease: Importance of patients' perceptions of intrusiveness and control. *International Journal of Psychiatry and Medicine, 13,* 327–343.

Diaferia, G., Sciuto, G., Perna, G., Barnardeschi, L., Battaglia, M., Rusmini, S., & Bellodi, L. (1993). DSM-III-R personality disorders in panic disorder. *Journal of Anxiety Disorders, 7,* 153–161.

Di Nardo, P., Brown, T. A., & Barlow, D. H. (1994). *Anxiety Disorders Interview Schedule for DSM-IV (Lifetime Version).* San Antonio, TX: Psychological Corporation.

Eaton, W. W., Kessler, R. C., Wittchen, H. U., & Magee, W. J. (1994). Panic and panic disorder in the United States. *American Journal of Psychiatry, 151,* 413–420.

Fava, G. A., Zielezny, M., Savron, G., & Grandi, S. (1995). Long-term effects of behavioural treatment for panic disorder and agoraphobia. *British Journal of Psychiatry, 166,* 87–92.

Feldman, J. M., Giardino, N. D., & Lehrer, P. M. (2000). Asthma and panic disorder. In D. I. Mostofsky & D. H. Barlow (Eds.), *The management of stress and anxiety in medical disorders.* Boston: Allyn & Bacon.

Feske, U., & de Beurs, E. (1997). The Panic Appraisal Inventory: Psychometric properties. *Behaviour Research and Therapy, 35,* 875–882.

First, M. B., Spitzer, R. L., Gibbon, M., & Williams, J. B. W. (1996). *Structured Clinical Interview for DSM-IV Axis I Disorders—Patient Edition (SCID-I/P, Version 2.0).* New York: Biometrics Research Department, New York State Psychiatric Institute.

Friedman, S. (Ed.). (1997). *Cultural issues in the treatment of anxiety.* New York: Guilford Press.

Friedman, S., Jones, J. C., Chernen, L., & Barlow, D. H. (1992). Suicidal ideation and suicide attempts among patients with panic disorder: A survey of two outpatient clinics. *American Journal of Psychiatry, 149,* 680–685.

Friedman, S., Paradis, C. M., & Hatch, M. (1994). Characteristics of African-American and White patients with panic disorder and agoraphobia. *Hospital and Community Psychiatry, 45,* 798–803.

Fyer, A. J. (1995). *Schedule for Affective Disorders and Schizophrenia—Lifetime Anxiety Version, Updated for DSM-IV (SADS-LA-IV).* New York: Anxiety Disorders Clinic, New York State Psychiatric Institute.

Fyer, A. J., Mannuzza, S., Chapman, T. F., Martin, L. Y., & Klein, D. F. (1995). Specificity in familial aggregation of phobic disorders. *Archives of General Psychiatry, 52,* 286–293.

Geracioti, T. D., & Post, R. M. (1991). Onset of panic disorder associated with rare use of cocaine. *Biological Psychiatry, 29,* 403–406.

Gorman, J. M., & Coplan, J. M. (1996). Comorbidity of depression and panic disorder. *Journal of Clinical Psychiatry, 57*(Suppl.), 34–41.

Greenberg, R. L. (1988). Panic disorder and agoraphobia. In J. G. Williams & A. T. Beck (Eds.), *Cognitive therapy in clinical practice: An illustrative casebook* (pp. 25–49). London: Routledge.

Guarnaccia, P. J., Canino, G., Rubio-Stipec, M., & Bravo, M. (1993). The prevalence of ataques de nervios in the Puerto Rico Disaster Study. *Journal of Nervous and Mental Disease, 181,* 157–165.

Guarnaccia, P. J., Rubio-Stipec, M., & Canino, G. J. (1989). Ataques de nervios in the Puerto Rican Diagnostic Interview Schedule: The impact of cultural categories on psychiatric epidemiology. *Culture, Medicine, and Psychiatry, 13,* 275–295.

Hamilton, M. (1959). The assessment of anxiety states by rating. *British Journal of Medical Psychology, 32,* 50–55.

Heinrichs, N., Hofmann, S. G., & Spiegel, D. A. (in press). Panic disorder with agoraphobia. In F. Bond & W. Dryden (Eds.), *Handbook of brief cognitive-behavioral therapy.* Chichester, UK: Wiley.

Himle, J., Thyer, B. A., & Fischer, D. J. (1988). Prevalence of smoking among anxious outpatients. *Phobia Practice and Research Journal, 1,* 25–31.

Hinton, D., Ba, P., Peou, S., & Um, K. (2000). Panic disorder among Cambodian refugees attending a psychiatric clinic: Prevalence and subtypes. *General Hospital Psychiatry, 22,* 437–444.

Hoffart, A., Friis, S., & Martinsen, E. W. (1989). The phobic avoidance rating scale: A psychometric evaluation of an interview-based scale. *Psychiatric Developments, 1,* 71–81.

Hoffart, A., Friis, S., & Martinsen, E. W. (1992). Assessment of fear of fear among agoraphobic patients: The Agoraphobia Cognitions Scales. *Journal of Psychopathology and Behavioral Assessment, 14,* 175–187.

Hofmann, S. G., & Barlow, D. H. (1999). The costs of anxiety disorders: Implications for psychosocial interventions. In N. E. Miller & K. M. Magruder (Eds.), *Cost-effectiveness of psychotherapy: A guide for practitioners, researchers, and policy makers* (pp. 224–234). New York: Oxford University Press.

Hofmann, S. G., Shear, M. K., Barlow, D. H., Gorman, J. M., Hershberger, D., Patterson, M., &

Woods, S. W. (1998). Effects of panic disorder treatments on personality disorder characteristics. *Depression and Anxiety, 8,* 14–20.

Hurwitz, T., Mahowald, M., Schenck, C., Schulter, J., & Bundie, S. (1991). A retrospective outcome study and review of hypnosis and treatment of adults with sleep waking and sleep terror. *Journal of Nervous and Mental Disease, 179,* 228–233.

Johnson, J., Weissman, M. M., & Klerman, G. L. (1990). Panic disorder, comorbidity, and suicide attempts. *Archives of General Psychiatry, 47,* 805–808.

Kamphuis, J. H., & Telch, M. J. (1998). Assessment of strategies to manage or avoid perceived threats among panic disorder patients: The Texas Safety Maneuver Scale (TSMS). *Clinical Psychology and Psychotherapy, 5,* 177–186.

Katerndahl, D. A., & Realini, J. P. (1993). Lifetime prevalence of panic states. *American Journal of Psychiatry, 150,* 246–249.

Katerndahl, D. A., & Realini, J. P. (1995). Where do panic sufferers seek care? *Journal of Family Practice, 40,* 237–243.

Katschnig, H., Amering, M., Stolk, J. M., & Ballenger, J. C. (1996). Predictors of quality of life in a long-term followup study in panic disorder patients after a clinical drug trial. *Psychopharmacology Bulletin, 32,* 149–155.

Keller, M. B., & Hanks, D. L. (1993). Course and outcome in panic disorder. *Progress in Neuro-Psychopharmacology and Biological Psychiatry, 17,* 551–570.

Keller, M. B., Yonkers, K. A., Warshaw, M. G., Pratt, L. A., Golan, J., Mathews, A. O., White, K., Swots, A., Reich, J., & Lavori, P. (1994). Remission and relapse in subjects with panic disorder and agoraphobia: A prospective short interval naturalistic follow-up. *Journal of Nervous and Mental Disease, 182,* 290–296.

Khawaja, N. G., Oei, T. P. S., & Baglioni, A. J. (1994). Modification of the catastrophic cognitions questionnaire (CCQ-M) for normals and patients: Exploratory and LISREL analyses. *Journal of Psychopathology and Behavioral Assessment, 16,* 325–342.

Klein, M. H., Benjamin, L. S., Treece, C., Rosenfeld, R., & Greist, J. (1990). *The Wisconsin Personality Disorder Inventory.* (Available from Marjorie H. Klein, Department of Psychiatry, University of Wisconsin, School of Medicine, Madison, WI 53706)

Lehman, C. L., Brown, T. A., & Barlow, D. H. (1998). Effects of cognitive behavioral treatment for panic disorder with agoraphobia on concurrent alcohol abuse. *Behavior Therapy, 29,* 423–433.

Leon, A. C., Olfson, M., Portera, L., Farber, L., & Sheehan, D. V. (1997). Assessing psychiatric impairment in primary care with the Sheehan Disability Scale. *International Journal of Psychiatry in Medicine, 27,* 93–105.

Louie, A. K., Lannon, R. A., & Ketter, T. A. (1989). Treatment of cocaine-induced panic disorder. *American Journal of Psychiatry, 146,* 40–44.

Lovibond, S. H., & Lovibond, P. F. (1995). *Manual for the Depression Anxiety Stress Scales* (2nd ed.). Sydney: Psychology Foundation of Australia.

Mannuzza, S., Fyer, A. J., Martin, L. Y., Gallops, M. S., Endicott, J., Gorman, J., Liebowitz, M. R., & Klein, D. F. (1989). Reliability of anxiety assessment: 1. Diagnostic agreement. *Archives of General Psychiatry, 46,* 1093–1101.

Marchand, A., Goyer, L. R., Dupuis, G., & Mainguy, N. (1998). Personality disorders and the outcome of cognitive-behavioral treatment of panic disorder with agoraphobia. *Canadian Journal of Behavioural Science, 30,* 14–23.

Margraf, J., Taylor, B., Ehlers, A., Roth, W. T., & Agras, W. S. (1987). Panic attacks in the natural environment. *Journal of Nervous and Mental Disease, 175,* 558–565.

Marks, I. M., & Mathews, A. M. (1979). Brief standard self-rating for phobic patients. *Behaviour Research and Therapy, 17,* 263–267.

McNally, R. J. (1994). *Panic disorder: A critical analysis.* New York: Guilford Press.

McNally, R. J., & Lorenz, M. (1987). Anxiety sensitivity in agoraphobics. *Journal of Behavior Therapy and Experimental Psychiatry, 18,* 3–11.

Michelson, L., June, K., Vives, A., Testa, S., & Marchione, N. (1998). The role of trauma and dissociation in cognitive-behavioral psychotherapy outcome and maintenance of panic disorder with agoraphobia. *Behaviour Research and Therapy, 36,* 1011–1050.

Murray, J. B. (1987). Psychopharmacological investigation of panic disorder by means of lactate infusion. *Journal of General Psychology, 114,* 297–311.

Nutt, D. J., Ballenger, J. C., & Lepine, J. (Eds.). (1999). *Panic disorder: Clinical diagnosis, management and mechanisms.* London: Martin Dunitz.

Oei, T. P. S., & Loveday, W. A. L. (1997). Management of co-morbid anxiety and alcohol disorders: Parallel treatment of disorders. *Drug and Alcohol Review, 16,* 261–274.

Otto, M. W., Pollack, M. H., Meltzer-Brody, S., & Rosenbaum, J. F. (1992). Cognitive behavioral therapy for benzodiazepine discontinuation in panic disorder patients. *Psychopharmacology Bulletin, 28,* 123–130.

Otto, M. W., Pollack, M. H., Sachs, G. S., O'Neil, C. A., & Rosenbaum, J. F. (1992). Alcohol dependence in panic disorder patients. *Journal of Psychiatric Research, 26,* 29–38.

Otto, M. W., Pollack, M. H., Sachs, G. S., & Rosenbaum, J. F. (1992). Hypochondriacal concerns, anxiety sensitivity, and panic disorder. *Journal of Anxiety Disorders, 6,* 93–104.

Otto, M. W., & Reilly-Harrington, N. A. (1999). The impact of treatment on anxiety sensitivity. In S. Taylor (Ed.), *Anxiety sensitivity: Theory, research and the treatment of the fear of anxiety* (pp. 321–336). Mahwah, NJ: Erlbaum.

Overton, D. A. (1991). Historical context of state dependent learning and discriminative drug effects. *Behavioral Pharmacology, 2,* 253–264.

Paradis, C. M., Hatch, M., & Friedman, S. (1994). Anxiety disorders in African Americans: An update. *Journal of the National Medical Association, 86,* 609–612.

Peterson, R. A., & Heilbronner, R. L. (1987). The Anxiety Sensitivity Index: Construct validity and factor analytic structure. *Journal of Anxiety Disorders, 3,* 25–32.

Peterson, R. A., & Reiss, S. (1993). *Anxiety Sensitivity Index Revised test manual.* Worthington, OH: IDS Publishing.

Pitts, F. N., & McClure, J. N. (1967). Lactate metabolism in anxiety neurosis. *New England Journal of Medicine, 277,* 1329–1336.

Rapaport, M. H., & Cantor, J. J. (1997). Panic disorder in a managed care environment. *Journal of Clinical Psychiatry, 58*(Suppl.), 51–55.

Rapee, R. M., Craske, M., & Barlow, D. H. (1995). Assessment instrument for panic disorder that includes fear of sensation-producing activities: The Albany panic and phobia questionnaire. *Anxiety, 1,* 114–122.

Rapee, R. M., Craske, M., Brown, T. A., & Barlow, D. H. (1996). Measurement of perceived control over anxiety-related events. *Behavior Therapy, 27,* 279–293.

Reily, M. C., Zbrozek, A. S., & Dukes, E. M. (1993). The validity and reproducibility of a work productivity and activity impairment instrument. *Pharmacological Economics, 4,* 353–365.

Reiss, S., Peterson, R. A., Gursky, D. M., & McNally, R. J. (1986). Anxiety sensitivity, anxiety frequency and the prediction of fearfulness. *Behaviour Research and Therapy, 24,* 1–8.

Sanderson, W. C., Rapee, R. M., & Barlow, D. H. (1989). The influence of an illusion of control on panic attacks induced via inhalation of 5.5% carbon dioxide enriched air. *Archives of General Psychiatry, 46,* 157–162.

Scheibe, G., & Albus, M. (1996). Predictors of outcome in panic disorder: A 5-year prospective follow-up study. *Journal of Affective Disorders, 41,* 111–116.

Scheibe, G., & Albus, M. (1997). Predictors and outcome of panic disorder: A 2-year prospective follow-up study. *Psychopathology, 30,* 177–184.

Schmidt, N. B., Lerew, D. R., & Trakowski, J. H. (1997). Body vigilance in panic disorder: Evaluating attention to bodily perturbations. *Journal of Consulting and Clinical Psychology, 65,* 214–220.

Schmidt, N. B., & Telch, M. J. (1997). Nonpsychiatric medical comorbidity, health perceptions, and treatment outcome in patients with panic disorder. *Health Psychology, 16,* 114–122.

Schmidt, N. B., Trakowski, J. H., & Staab J. P. (1997). Extinction of panicogenic effects of a 35% CO_2 challenge in patients with panic disorder. *Journal of Abnormal Psychology, 106,* 630–638.

Schnoll, S. H., & Daghestani, A. N. (1986). Treatment of marijuana abuse. *Psychiatric Annals, 16,* 249–254.

Shear, M. K., Brown, T. A., Barlow, D. H., Money, R., Sholomskas, D. E., Woods, S. W., Gorman, J.

M., & Papp, L. A. (1997). Multicenter Collaborative Panic Disorder Severity Scale. *American Journal of Psychiatry, 154,* 1571–1575.

Shear, M. K., & Maser, J. D. (1994). Standardized assessment for panic disorder research: A conference report. *Archives of General Psychiatry, 51,* 346–354.

Smith, L. C., Friedman, S., & Nevid, J. (1999). Clinical and sociocultural differences in African American and European American patients with panic disorder and agoraphobia. *Journal of Nervous and Mental Disease, 187,* 549–561.

Spiegel, D. A., & Bruce, T. J. (1997). Benzodiazepines and exposure-based cognitive-behavioral therapies for panic disorder: Conclusions from combined treatment trials. *American Journal of Psychiatry, 154,* 773–781.

Spiegel, D. A., Wiegel, M., Baker, S. L., & Greene, K. A. I. (2000). Pharmacotherapy of anxiety disorders. In D. I. Mostofsky & D. H. Barlow (Eds.), *The management of stress and anxiety in medical disorders.* Boston: Allyn & Bacon.

Spitzer, R. L., Endicott, J., & Robins, E. (1978). Research diagnostic criteria. *Archives of General Psychiatry, 35,* 773–782.

Spitzer, R. L., Williams, J. B. W., Kroenke, K., Linzer, M., deGruy, F. V., Hahn, S. R., Brody, D., & Johnson, J. G. (1994). Utility of a new procedure for diagnosing mental disorders in primary care: The PRIME-MD 1000 study. *Journal of the American Medical Association, 272,* 1749–1756.

Stein, M. B., Roy-Byrne, P. P., McQuaid, J. R., Laffaye, C., Russo, J., McCahill, M. E., Katon, W., Craske, M., Bystritsky, A., & Sherbourne, C. D. (1999). Development of a brief diagnostic screen for panic disorder in primary care. *Psychosomatic Medicine, 61,* 359–364.

Stein, M. B., Shea, C. A., & Uhde, T. W. (1989). Social phobic symptoms in patients with panic disorder: Practical and theoretical implications. *American Journal of Psychiatry, 146,* 235–238.

Stewart, S. H., Samoluk, S. B., & MacDonald, A. B. (1999). Anxiety sensitivity and substance use and abuse. In S. Taylor (Ed.), *Anxiety sensitivity: Theory, research and the treatment of the fear of anxiety* (pp. 287–320). Mahwah, NJ: Erlbaum.

Szuster, R. R., Pontius, E. B., & Campos, P. E. (1988). Marijuana sensitivity and panic anxiety. *Journal of Clinical Psychiatry, 49,* 427–429.

Taylor, S., & Cox, B. J. (1998a). An expanded Anxiety Sensitivity Index: Evidence for a hierarchic structure in a clinical sample. *Journal of Anxiety Disorders, 12,* 463–483.

Taylor, S., & Cox, B. J. (1998b). Anxiety sensitivity: Multiple dimensions and hierarchic structure. *Behaviour Research and Therapy, 36,* 37–51.

Taylor, S., Koch, W. J., & McNally, R. J. (1992). How does anxiety sensitivity vary across the anxiety disorders? *Journal of Anxiety Disorders, 6,* 249–259.

Taylor, S., Koch, W. J., McNally, R. J., & Crockett, D. J. (1992). Conceptualizations of anxiety sensitivity. *Psychological Assessment, 4,* 245–250.

Taylor, S., Koch, W. J., Woody, S., & McLean, P. (1997). Reliability and validity of the Cognition Checklist with psychiatric outpatients. *Assessment, 4,* 9–16.

Telch, M. J. (1987). *The Panic Appraisal Inventory.* Unpublished manuscript, University of Texas, Austin.

Telch, M. J., Shermis, M. D., & Lucas, J. A. (1989). Anxiety sensitivity: Unitary personality trait or domain-specific appraisals. *Journal of Anxiety Disorders, 3,* 25–32.

Thorn, G. R., Chosak, A., Baker, S. L., & Barlow, D. H. (1999). Psychological theories of panic disorder. In D. J. Nutt, J. C. Ballenger, & J. Lepine (Eds.), *Panic disorder: Clinical diagnosis, management and mechanisms* (pp. 93–108). London: Martin Dunitz.

Uhde, T. W. (1990). Caffeine provocation of panic: A focus on biological mechinisms. In J. C. Ballenger (Ed.), *Neurobiology of panic disorder* (pp. 219–242). New York: Wiley-Liss.

Uhde, T. W. (1994). The anxiety disorders: Phenomenology and treatment of core symptoms and associated sleep disturbance. In M. Kryger, T. Roth, & W. Dement (Eds.), *Principles and practice of sleep medicine* (pp. 871–898). Philadelphia: Saunders.

van den Hout, M. A. (1988). The explanation of experimental panic. In S. Rachman & J. D. Maser (Eds.), *Panic: Psychological perspectives* (pp. 237–257). Hillsdale, NJ: Erlbaum.

van Hout, W. J. P. J., Emmelkamp, P. M. G., Koopmans, P. C., Bogels, S. M., & Bouman, T. K. (2001). Assessment of self-statements in agoraphobic situations: Construction and psychometric evaluations of the Agoraphobic Self-Statements Questionnaire (ASQ). *Journal of Anxiety Disorders, 15,* 183–201.

van Oot, P., Lane, T., & Borkovec, T. (1984). Sleep disturbance. In H. Adams & P. Sutker (Eds.), *Comprehensive handbook of psychopathology* (pp. 683–723). New York: Plenum Press.

Ware, J. E., & Sherbourne, C. D. (1992). The MOS 36-item short-form health survey (SF-36): I. Conceptual framework and items selection. *Medical Care, 30,* 473–483.

Weissman, M. M., Klerman, G. L., Markowitz, J. S., & Ouellette, R. (1989). Suicidal ideation and suicide attempts in panic disorder and attacks. *New England Journal of Medicine, 321,* 1209–1214.

Weller, R. A. (1985). Marijuana: Effects and motivation. *Medical Aspects of Human Sexuality, 19,* 92–104.

Williams, J. B. W., Gibbon, M., First, M. B., Spitzer, R. L., Davies, M., Borus, J., Howes, M. J., Kane, J., Pope, H. G., Rounsaville, B., & Wittchen, H. (1992). The Structured Clinical Interview for DSM-II-R (SCID): II. Multisite test–retest reliability. *Archives of General Psychiatry, 49,* 630–636.

Wolfe, B. E., & Maser, J. D., (Eds.). (1994). *Treatment of panic disorder: A consensus development conference.* Washington, DC: American Psychiatric Press.

Yang, S., Tsai, T. H., Hou, Z. Y., Chen, C. Y., & Sim, C. B. (1997). The effect of panic attack on mitral valve prolapse. *Acta Psychiatrica Scandinavica, 96,* 408–411.

Zaubler, T. S., & Katon, W. (1996). Panic disorder and medical comorbidity: A review of the medical and psychiatric literature. *Bulletin of the Menninger Clinic, 60*(Suppl. A), A12-A38.

Zinbarg, R. E., Mohlman, J., & Hong, N. N. (1999). Dimensions of anxiety sensitivity. In S. Taylor (Ed.), *Anxiety sensitivity: Theory, research and the treatment of the fear of anxiety* (pp. 83–114). Mahwah, NJ: Erlbaum.

4

Specific and Social Phobia

Randi E. McCabe
Martin M. Antony

Specific phobia is characterized by clinically significant anxiety that is associated with exposure to a specific object or situation (e.g., certain animals or insects, heights, enclosed
places), often leading to avoidance behavior. *Social phobia* (social anxiety disorder) is characterized by clinically significant anxiety associated with exposure to social or performance
situations (e.g., public speaking, writing or eating in public, meeting strangers) in which embarrassment may occur, often leading to avoidance of the feared situations. The purpose of
this chapter is to provide comprehensive coverage of the issues involved in assessment,
treatment planning, and outcome evaluation for specific and social phobias. Following a
brief overview of the disorders, an empirical review of assessment instruments for specific
and social phobia is presented, including information on clinical interviews, self-report
measures, and behavioral tests. Next, practical recommendations for the assessment of specific and social phobias are covered. This is followed by a discussion of the role of assessment in treatment planning and outcome measurement. Finally, practical issues in the assessment of specific and social phobia in managed care and primary care settings are
discussed.

OVERVIEW OF SPECIFIC AND SOCIAL PHOBIA

Diagnostic Features

This section outlines the diagnostic features of specific and social phobia as described in the
revised fourth edition of *Diagnostic and Statistical Manual of Mental Disorders* (DSM-IV;
American Psychiatric Association, 2000). In both specific and social phobias, exposure to,
or anticipation of, the feared stimulus is almost invariably associated with an immediate
fear response that may take the form of a panic attack—for example, a person with a specific phobia of dogs may have a panic attack upon seeing a dog in the neighborhood; a person with social phobia may experience a panic attack when anticipating an upcoming presentation at work).

113

Adults and adolescents with specific or social phobia recognize that their fear is excessive or unreasonable. Although childhood fears are often transient and do not cause clinically significant distress or impairment, children may exhibit clinically significant, maladaptive, and persistent fear reactions consistent with specific and social phobia. If an individual is under 18 years of age, the duration of the fear must be at least 6 months to warrant a diagnosis of specific or social phobia. In addition, children may not recognize that their fear is excessive or unreasonable. For a diagnosis of social phobia in children, the anxiety must not be limited to interactions with adults but must also occur in peer settings. In addition, there must be evidence that the child can maintain age-appropriate social relationships with familiar people. For a more extensive discussion of the assessment of childhood phobias, see King, Ollendick, and Murphy (1997).

In both specific and social phobias, the feared stimulus or situation is usually avoided or may be endured with intense dread. A diagnosis of specific or social phobia is only warranted if the fear and avoidance significantly interfere with everyday functioning (e.g., social, occupational, leisure) or if the fear and avoidance cause marked distress. For example, a person with an excessive fear of elevators who lives in a rural area where he or she never encounters elevators and who is not distressed by having this fear would not receive a diagnosis of specific phobia. Similarly, an individual who is shy and quiet upon meeting new people but who does not avoid these situations or report distress resulting from his or her shyness would not receive a diagnosis of social phobia.

For social phobia, the fear and avoidance are not limited to concern about the social impact of another mental disorder (e.g., abnormal eating behavior or low weight in anorexia nervosa) or medical condition (e.g., stuttering or tremor in Parkinson's disease) with potentially embarrassing symptoms. Finally, a diagnosis of either specific or social phobia is not assigned if the symptoms are better accounted for by the presence of another mental disorder.

DSM-IV describes five subtypes of specific phobia that are based on the types of situations feared and avoided: *animal type*—includes fears of animals and insects (e.g., cats, dogs, snakes, spiders, mice, birds); *natural environment type*—includes objects or situations in the natural environment such as storms, heights, and water; *blood–injection–injury type* (BII)—includes seeing blood or an injury, receiving an injection or an invasive medical procedure, watching or undergoing surgery, and other related medical situations; *situational type*—includes specific situations such as public transportation, tunnels, elevators, bridges, flying, driving, or enclosed places; and *other type*—includes other stimuli that do not fit into the first four types, such as fear of choking or vomiting, fears of contracting an illness, and children's fears of loud sounds or costumed characters (e.g., clowns). Specific phobia types differ in a number of important ways. For a discussion of the heterogeneity among specific phobia types, see Antony, Brown, and Barlow (1997).

For social phobia, the generalized specifier is used (e.g., social phobia, generalized) when social fears are triggered by most social situations (including both public performance and social interactional situations). Individuals with generalized social phobia tend to have increased social skills deficits and a greater severity of impairment in functioning than do individuals with nongeneralized social phobia (American Psychiatric Association, 2000).

Descriptive Characteristics

Prevalence estimates for specific phobia vary, depending on the threshold used for defining impairment or distress. According to DSM-IV, point prevalence rates range from 4% to 8.8%, and lifetime prevalence rates range from 7.2% to 11.3% and also vary across the different subtypes of specific phobia (American Psychiatric Association, 2000). Often, the fear of the specific object or situation is present for some time before it becomes significantly impairing or distressing (Antony et al., 1997). Although specific phobias may be the most prevalent anxiety disorder diagnosis, they are also the most treatable of all disorders, with as little as one session of systematic exposure to the feared situation required (for a review, see Antony & Swinson, 2000a).

For social phobia, prevalence rates also vary widely, depending on the threshold used to determine distress or impairment, as well as the range of social situations assessed (Stein, Walker, & Forde, 1994). Lifetime prevalence rates for social phobia from epidemiological and community-based studies range from 3% to 13%, whereas rates for outpatient clinics range from 10% to 20% (American Psychiatric Association, 2000).

The age of onset for specific phobia tends to vary, depending on the phobic subtype. Numerous studies have shown that animal and BII phobias have a childhood onset, whereas situational phobias such as driving phobia and claustrophobia typically begin in late adolescence or early adulthood (e.g., Antony et al., 1997; Curtis, Hill, & Lewis, 1990). Evidence regarding the age of onset for situational phobias has varied. For example, some research suggests height phobia typically begins in the midteens (e.g., Curtis et al., 1990), and other research suggests it typically begins in the mid-20s (e.g., Antony et al., 1997).

Social phobia tends to begin in adolescence, often developing from a childhood history of social inhibition or shyness. However, some individuals report an onset in early childhood. For example, approximately one-half of the participants surveyed in a large epidemiological study reported having suffered from social phobia for their entire lives or since before the age of 10 (Schneier, Johnson, Hornig, Liebowitz, & Weissman, 1992). When social phobia is untreated, its course is typically chronic and lifelong; however, there may be fluctuations in severity during adulthood (American Psychiatric Association, 2000).

Although twice as many women as men meet the criteria for specific phobia, sex differences vary across the five subtypes of specific phobia. One review indicates that sex differences are strongest for animal type phobias and smaller for BII and height phobias (Antony & Barlow, 1998). For social phobia, sex differences are less evident, with only slightly more women meeting criteria for social phobia than men (for a review, see Antony & Barlow, 1997).

Specific phobias often occur comorbidly with other anxiety disorders, mood disorders, and substance-related disorders. In addition, the presence of one subtype of specific phobia increases the likelihood that another phobia within the same subtype is also present. However, when present comorbidly, specific phobia is generally associated with less distress and impairment in functioning than is the comorbid primary disorder. It is estimated that only 12% to 30% of individuals seek professional help for their specific phobia (American Psychiatric Association, 2000).

Social phobia often co-occurs and typically precedes a number of disorders, including other anxiety disorders, mood disorders, substance-related disorders, bulimia nervosa, and avoidant personality disorder. In addition, social phobia is commonly associated with increased sensitivity to negative evaluation, difficulties with assertiveness, low self-esteem, social skills deficits, poorer social supports, and underachievement in work or school due to avoidance of speaking in groups, public speaking, speaking to authority figures, participating in class, and test anxiety (American Psychiatric Association, 2000). Social phobia has also been linked to perfectionism (e.g., Antony, Purdon, Huta, & Swinson, 1998). Avoidant personality disorder overlaps to a great degree with generalized social phobia and may be considered a more severe manifestation of generalized social phobia (Widiger, 1992). For example, the presence of both social phobia and avoidant personality disorder is associated with greater interpersonal sensitivity and poorer social skills than is social phobia alone (Turner, Beidel, Dancu, & Keys, 1986).

REVIEW OF THE EMPIRICAL LITERATURE ON ASSESSMENT MEASURES

In this section, the features and psychometric properties of some of the key measures for assessing specific and social phobia, including interview measures, self-report questionnaires, and behavioral assessment strategies, are reviewed. A more comprehensive list of measures is presented later in the chapter in Table 4.1 for specific phobia and Table 4.2 for social phobia. For a more detailed discussion of these measures and others, the reader is referred to Antony, Orsillo, and Roemer (2001).

Structured and Semistructured Interviews

Diagnostic Interviews

This section will be covered briefly given that Chapter 1 reviews these measures in detail. Within the field of anxiety disorders, the two most commonly used and extensively studied semistructured interview measures for diagnosing anxiety-related problems are the Anxiety Disorders Interview Schedule for DSM-IV (ADIS-IV; Brown, Di Nardo, & Barlow, 1994; Di Nardo, Brown, & Barlow, 1994) and the Structured Clinical Interview for DSM-IV/Axis I Disorders (SCID-IV; First, Spitzer, Gibbon, & Williams, 1996). Two versions of the ADIS-IV are available. The *standard version* assesses only current Axis I diagnoses, whereas the *lifetime version* assesses both current and lifetime Axis I diagnoses. The SCID-IV is available in an Axis I *research version* (patient and nonpatient versions) that includes current diagnoses for most disorders and lifetime diagnoses for a few disorders, as well as an Axis I *clinician version* that is shortened for clinical practice. There is also an Axis II version of the SCID-IV to assess personality disorders. The ADIS-IV lifetime version typically requires 2 to 4 hours of administration time, whereas the SCID-IV research version typically requires 1 to 3 hours of administration time.

The specific phobia and social phobia sections of the ADIS-IV include dimensional ratings of fear and avoidance for 17 objects or situations from the five types of DSM-IV specific phobias, as well as dimensional ratings of fear and avoidance for 13 social situations associated with social phobia. Current and lifetime diagnoses of specific phobia and social phobia based on the ADIS-IV have been shown to have good to excellent reliability for the specific phobia types and the generalized type of social phobia (Brown, Di Nardo, Lehman, & Campbell, 2001). Currently, there are no published studies on the psychometric properties of the SCID-IV, but previous versions for DSM-III-R have been shown to be reliable, especially for phobic disorders (for review, see Segal, Hersen, & van Hasselt, 1994).

Briefer semistructured interviews are also available for diagnostic assessment of specific and social phobia such as the Primary Care Evaluation of Mental Disorders (PRIME-MD; Spitzer et al., 1994) and the Mini-International Neuropsychiatric Interview (MINI; Sheehan et al., 1998). However, these measures do not provide as detailed an assessment of the DSM criteria for specific and social phobia as do the SCID-IV and ADIS-IV. To assess the relevant criteria for specific and social phobia, there are also structured interviews available, such as the Diagnostic Interview Schedule, Version IV (DIS-IV; Robins, Cottler, Bucholz, & Compton, 1995). However, there is evidence that fully structured interviews tend to overdiagnose a number of disorders when compared with semistructured interviews conducted by expert clinicians (e.g., Antony, Downie, & Swinson, 1998).

The ADIS-IV and the SCID-IV each have advantages and disadvantages. The SCID-IV provides a detailed assessment of a broader range of disorders than does the ADIS-IV, including eating disorders and psychotic disorders. However, the ADIS-IV provides more detailed information on each of the anxiety disorders, as well as DSM-IV diagnoses for those disorders that typically co-occur with the anxiety disorders (e.g., substance use disorders and somatoform disorders). In addition, the ADIS-IV provides more detailed information to differentiate specific and social phobias from those disorders for which there is characteristic overlap (Antony & Swinson, 2000a).

Liebowitz Social Anxiety Scale (LSAS)

The LSAS (Liebowitz, 1987) is a brief clinician-rated measure (taking approximately 10 minutes to administer) that assesses the severity of anxiety in social and performance situations. The clinician provides separate fear and avoidance ratings based on a 4-point scale for 11 social interaction situations (e.g., going to a party) and for 13 performance situations (e.g., speaking up at a meeting). The LSAS, formerly called the Liebowitz Social Phobia Scale (LSPS), has been shown to have good internal consistency, convergent validity, and discriminant validity (Heimberg et al., 1999). One limitation of the LSAS is that it does not assess the cognitive or physiological aspects of social phobia and, thus, is not a comprehensive measure of symptomatic improvement during treatment; however, it may be useful for building a treatment hierarchy (Shear et al., 2000). The LSAS has been adapted and used in self-report format (e.g., Cox, Ross, Swinson, & Direnfeld, 1998) and for computer administration (Heimberg, Mennin, & Jack, 1999).

Brief Social Phobia Scale (BSPS)

The BSPS (Davidson et al., 1991) is another clinician-rated scale that was designed to assess social phobia symptoms. The clinician provides separate fear and avoidance ratings using a 5-point Likert type scale for seven different social and performance situations: public speaking, talking to people in authority, talking to strangers, being embarrassed or humiliated, being criticized, social gatherings, and doing something while being watched. In a separate section, the clinician uses a 5-point scale to rate the severity of four different physical symptoms—blushing, palpitations, trembling/shaking, and sweating—that are experienced by the patient when exposed to or imagining being in a feared social situation. The BSPS has good reliability (e.g., test–retest, interrater, internal consistency) and validity (concurrent), as well as demonstrated sensitivity to change after treatment (Davidson et al., 1991, 1997). However, the reliability and validity data for the physiological arousal scale are not as strong (Davidson et al., 1997). The BSPS has also been adapted for computer administration (Kobak et al., 1998).

General Self-Report Measures for Specific and Social Phobia

There are many self-report measures designed to assess specific and social phobia. When possible, it is recommended that self-report measures be completed before the initial clinical interview. This will help the clinician determine, in advance, areas that may require further follow-up during the interview. The clinician should keep in mind that responses on self-report measures do not always correlate highly with actual behavioral performance (e.g., Klieger, 1987). In addition, men are more likely than women to underreport their fear on measures of specific phobia (Pierce & Kirkpatrick, 1992).

A common screening measure for phobic disorders is the Fear Survey Schedule (FSS; Geer, 1965; Wolpe & Lang, 1964, 1969, 1977), a self-report measure that was designed to assess fears of a range of specific objects and situations, including items related to specific phobia (e.g., injections, airplanes), social phobia (public speaking), and agoraphobia (e.g., crowds). Several versions of the FSS have been developed. The 51-item FSS-II (developed by

Geer, 1965) and the 72-item FSS-III and 108-item FSS-III (revised by Wolpe & Lang, 1969, 1977) have been the most popular versions and are often used to screen phobic individuals, measure fear severity, and assess treatment outcome. In addition to including items typically related to phobic disorders (e.g., animals, heights, storms, vomiting, enclosed places), both the FSS-II and the FSS-III include items unrelated to typical phobic disorders (e.g., noise of vacuum cleaners, ugly people, parting from friends, nude men and women), and for this reason, it is not an ideal diagnostic measure for specific or social phobia (Antony & Swinson, 2000a). In addition, there is conflicting evidence regarding the ability of the FSS to discriminate between different anxiety disorders (e.g., Beck, Carmin, & Henninger, 1998; Stravynski, Basoglu, Marks, Sengun, & Marks, 1995). There is still a need for further revision of the FSS to more closely assess the fears of situations and objects reported by individuals with specific phobias (Antony, 2001a). At this point, evidence suggests that the FSS-II and the FSS-III are best used only as a screening instrument for determining feared objections and situations. The clinician should bear in mind that there is a high likelihood of false positives and that scores on the FSS are not a basis for establishing a clinical diagnosis (Klieger & Franklin, 1993).

Another general fear survey measure is the Fear Questionnaire (FQ; Marks & Mathews, 1979), a self-report questionnaire that assesses the severity of common phobias, including agoraphobia, BII phobia, and social phobia, as well as related symptoms of anxiety and depression. The psychometric properties of the agoraphobia and social phobia subscales of the FQ are good (for review, see Shear et al., 2000); however, the reliability and validity of the BII subscale are less documented.

Self-Report Measures for Specific Phobia

This section provides an overview of some of the most commonly used self-report instruments for the assessment of specific phobia (for descriptions of additional measures refer to Table 4.1). A survey of measures for the assessment of specific phobia reveals a number of self-report questionnaires for targeting specific fears. This section presents some of these measures, organized by subtype of specific phobia.

Animal Type

Within the animal subtype of specific phobia, there are a variety of measures for assessing spider phobia including the Fear of Spiders Questionnaire (FSQ; Szymanski & O'Donohue, 1995), the Spider Questionnaire (SPQ; Klorman, Hastings, Weerts, Melamed, & Lang, 1974); the Watts and Sharrock Spider Phobia Questionnaire (WS-SPQ; Watts & Sharrock, 1984), and the Spider Phobia Beliefs Questionnaire (SBQ; Arntz, Lavy, van den Berg, & van Rijsoort, 1993). The SPQ is a 30-item self-report scale that assesses the verbal–cognitive component of spider fear and takes approximately 5 minutes to complete. Fearful and nonfearful spider-related statements are rated as true or false. The SPQ has excellent test–retest reliability over 3 weeks (Muris & Merckelbach, 1996) and over 1 year (Fredrikson, 1983). Data indicate that the SPQ has adequate to good internal consistency (e.g., Fredrikson, 1983; Muris & Merckelbach, 1996). There is also support for both discriminant (e.g., Fredrikson, 1983) and convergent validity (e.g., Muris & Merckelbach, 1996) of the SPQ. In addition, the SPQ has been proven to be sensitive to the effects of treatment in a number of studies (e.g., Muris & Merckelbach, 1996; Öst, 1996).

Snake phobia is commonly assessed using the Snake Questionnaire (SNAQ; Klorman et al., 1974), a 30-item self-report scale measuring the verbal–cognitive component of snake fear that takes approximately 5 minutes to complete. As in the SPQ, fearful or non-

TABLE 4.1. Self-Report Assessment Instruments for Specific Phobia

Measure	Purpose	Length (No. items)	Time[a] (minutes)	Psychometric properties[b]
Animal type				
Fear of Spiders Questionnaire (FSQ; Szymanski & O'Donohue, 1995)	Measures severity of spider phobia	18	5	Good reliability and validity; may be more sensitive measure for assessing fear in the nonphobic range (Muris & Merckelbach, 1996); treatment sensitivity documented
Spider Questionnaire (SPQ; Klorman et al., 1974)	Measures the verbal–cognitive component of spider fear	30	5	Reliability moderate to good; established validity; demonstrated treatment sensitivity
Watts and Sharrock Spider Phobia Questionnaire (WS-SPQ; Watts & Sharrock, 1984)	Assesses vigilance, preoccupation, and avoidance of spiders	43	5	Preliminary reliability and validity data promising; treatment sensitivity reported
Spider Phobia Beliefs Questionnaire (SBQ; Arntz et al., 1993)	Assesses fearful beliefs about spiders and reactions to seeing spiders	78	10–15	Good reliability and validity; established treatment sensitivity
Snake Questionnaire (SNAQ; Klorman et al., 1974)	Assesses the verbal–cognitive component of snake fear	30	5	Good reliability and support for validity; however, may yield false positives (Klieger, 1987); demonstrated treatment sensitivity
Natural environment type				
Acrophobia Questionnaire (AQ; Cohen, 1977)	Assesses the severity of anxiety and avoidance related to situations involving common heights	40	5	Adequate reliability and validity; sensitivity to treatment effects established
Blood–injection–injury type				
Blood–Injection Symptom Scale (BISS; Page et al., 1997)	Assesses anxiety, tension, and faintness associated with blood and injections	17	1–2	Internal consistency variable; limited data available for validity
Mutilation Questionnaire (MQ; Klorman et al., 1974)	Measures the verbal–cognitive features of mutilation and blood/injury fear	30	5	Reliability fair to good; established validity; demonstrated treatment sensitivity
Medical Fear Survey (MFS; Kleinknecht, Thorndike, & Walls, 1996)	Assesses five dimensions of medically related fear: injections, blood draws, sharp objects, examinations, and mutilation	50	5	Preliminary data are promising; lack of norms for clinically diagnosed individuals with BII phobias

(continued)

TABLE 4.1. (continued)

Measure	Purpose	Length (No. items)	Time[a] (minutes)	Psychometric properties[b]
Blood–injection–injury type (cont.)				
Dental Anxiety Inventory (DAI; Stouthard et al., 1993)	Measures the severity of dental anxiety	36	5–10	Good reliability and validity
Dental Cognitions Questionnaire (DCQ; de Jongh et al., 1995)	Assesses negative cognitions associated with dental treatment	38	5–7	Good reliability and validity; treatment sensitivity established
Dental Fear Survey (DFS; Kleinknecht et al., 1973)	Measures fear of dental stimuli, dental avoidance, and physiological symptoms during dental treatment	20	2–5	Established reliability and validity; treatment sensitivity documented
Dental Anxiety Scale—Revised (DAS-R; Ronis, 1994)	Measures the severity of trait dental anxiety	4	1–2	Good reliability and validity
Situational type				
Claustrophobia General Cognitions Questionnaire (CGCQ; Febbraro & Clum, 1995)	Assesses thoughts associated with claustrophobic situations	26	5	Preliminary data promising; no data available on convergent or discriminant validity
Claustrophobia Situations Questionnaire (CSQ; Febbraro & Clum, 1995)	Assesses anxiety and avoidance associated with specific claustrophobic situations	42	5–10	Preliminary data promising; no data available on convergent or discriminant validity
Claustrophobia Questionnaire (CLQ; Radomsky et al., 2001)	Measures claustrophobia, including fear of suffocation and fear of restriction	26	5–10	Good data supporting reliability and validity
Fear of Flying Scale (FFS; Haug et al., 1987)	Assesses fear associated with different aspects of flying	21	5–10	No psychometric data available; treatment sensitivity documented

[a]Approximate time for completion.
[b]For more detailed review of the psychometric properties for these measures, see Antony (2001b).

fearful snake-related statements are rated as true or false. The SNAQ has good to excellent internal consistency (Fredrikson, 1983; Klorman et al., 1974) and high test–retest reliability (Fredrikson, 1983). The SNAQ has been shown to discriminate individuals with snake phobias from both individuals with spider phobias and nonphobic students (Fredrikson, 1983), and this provides evidence for discriminant validity. In addition, SNAQ scores have been shown to significantly correlate with aversiveness ratings of slides depicting snakes (Fredrikson, 1983), which provides evidence for convergent validity. The SNAQ is also sensitive to treatment effects (Öst, 1978). However, there is evidence that the SNAQ tends to yield false positives as Klieger (1987) reported that the relationship between SNAQ scores and the tendency to avoid a caged snake during a behavioral test was not strong.

The Dog Phobia Questionnaire (DPQ; Hong & Zinbarg, 1999) is currently in development and is designed to assess the severity of dog phobia. However, there are no published measures to comprehensively assess other animal fears such as fears of insects, rodents, cats, or birds.

Natural Environment Type

There are very few published measures to assess the natural environment subtype of specific phobias. Although the Acrophobia Questionnaire (AQ; Cohen, 1977) is a popular measure designed to assess fear of heights, there are no published measures to assess fears of water and storms in adults. The AQ is a 40-item self-report scale that measures the severity of anxiety and avoidance associated with common height-related situations and takes approximately 5 minutes to complete. The AQ consists of an anxiety scale and an avoidance scale. Split-half reliability for the anxiety scale is adequate ($r = .82$), whereas split-half reliability for the avoidance scale is weaker ($r = .70$) (Baker, Cohen, & Saunders, 1973). Test–retest reliability for both the anxiety and avoidance scales is good over a 3-month period (Baker et al., 1973). There is also support for the validity of the AQ: AQ scores correlate moderately with scores on a behavioral test, and both the anxiety and avoidance scores have been shown to be sensitive to treatment effects (Cohen, 1977).

Blood–Injection–Injury Type

In contrast to the lack of measures for natural environment phobias, there are a number of measures that target specific medically related fears within the BII subtype of specific phobia. The Mutilation Questionnaire (MQ; Klorman et al., 1974) is a 30-item self-report scale that measures the verbal–cognitive component of mutilation and blood/injury fear that takes approximately 5 minutes to complete. Fearful or nonfearful statements related to blood, injury, or mutilation are rated as "true" or "false." Internal consistency findings range from fair to good across a number of nonclinical samples (Kleinknecht & Thorndike, 1990). Data from a number of studies support the validity of the MQ. For example, MQ scores are correlated with blood and injury-related items from the Fear Survey Schedule and are predictive of a history of fainting in blood/injury-related situations (Kleinknecht & Thorndike, 1990). In addition, MQ scores are related to a tendency to avoid blood/injury-related situations (Kleinknecht & Lenz, 1989) and are sensitive to treatment effects (e.g., Öst, Lindahl, Sterner, & Jerremalm, 1984).

The Medical Fear Survey (MFS; Kleinknecht, Thorndike, & Walls, 1996) is a 50-item self-report measure designed to assess the severity of medically-related fears and takes approximately 5 minutes to complete. Five subscales derived by factor analysis (Kleinknecht, Thorndike, & Walls, 1996) measure fears of injections, blood draws, sharp objects, examinations, and symptoms as intimation of illness, blood, and mutilation. Internal consistency of the scale is good to excellent, and convergent validity is also good (Kleinknecht, Kleinknecht, Sawchuk, Lee, & Lohr, 1999). Sensitivity to treatment effects has not yet been reported.

There are also numerous measures of dental fear and anxiety, including the Dental Anxiety Inventory (DAI; Stouthard, Mellenbergh, & Hoogstraten, 1993), the Dental Cognitions Questionnaire (DCQ; de Jongh, Muris, Schoenmakers, & Horst, 1995), the Dental Fear Survey (DFS; Kleinknecht, Klepac, & Alexander, 1973), and the Dental Anxiety Scale—Revised (Ronis, 1994), an updated version of the Corah Dental Anxiety Scale (CDAS; Corah, 1969).

Situational Type

For assessing fears within the situational subtype, there are a several measures to assess claustrophobia, including the Claustrophobia General Cognitions Questionnaire (CGCQ; Febbraro & Clum, 1995), the Claustrophobia Situations Questionnaire (CSQ; Febbraro & Clum, 1995), and the Claustrophobia Questionnaire (CLQ; Radomsky, Rachman, Thordarson, McIsaac, & Teachman, 2001). The CGCQ is a 26-item self-report scale that measures cognitions associated with claustrophobic situations and consists of three subscales: fear of loss of control, fear of suffocation, and fear of inability to escape. The CGCQ takes approximately 5 minutes to complete. The CSQ is a 42-item self-report scale that measures anxiety and avoidance related to specific claustrophobic situations and consists of two anxiety subscales (fear of entrapment and fear of physical confinement) and two avoidance subscales (avoidance of crowds and avoidance of physical confinement). All psychometric data for both the CGCQ and CSQ are based on a sample of 94 individuals who reported fear of enclosed places (Febbraro & Clum, 1995). Internal consistency for all subscales of both the CGCQ and CSQ is excellent. The subscales for both measures were derived by factor analysis. Data on test–retest reliability, validity, and treatment sensitivity have not yet been reported.

With the exception of the Fear of Flying Scale (FFS; Haug et al., 1987), there are no measures to assess other specific fears within this subtype, such as fears of driving, tunnels, or public transportation.

Other Type

Finally, with respect to the *other* subtype of specific phobias, there are currently no specific measures to assess fears of vomiting or choking. Fear of contracting an illness may be assessed using the Worry About Illness subscale of the Illness Attitudes Scale (IAS; Kellner, 1986, 1987). The IAS is a self-report measure that assesses fears, attitudes, and beliefs associated with hypochondriacal concerns and abnormal illness behavior.

Measures of Specific Phobia Onset

There are a number of measures to assess precipitating factors for an individual's specific phobia, including the 16-page self-report Origins Questionnaire (OQ; Menzies & Clarke, 1993) designed for determining the etiology of a phobia, and the short 9-item self-report Phobia Origins Questionnaire (POQ; Öst & Hugdahl, 1981) that measures an individual's history of experiencing a range of etiologically relevant events related to a feared object or situation.

Summary

Given the preceding review of the self-report measures for assessing specific phobia, it is evident that there is a need for more comprehensive measures to assess fears of the situations and objects that more closely relate to specific phobias as defined by DSM-IV. Such measures should assess for fears of animals other than only snakes, spiders, and dogs—for example, rodents, birds, cats, and fish. There is also a need to develop measures for fears of driving, storms, water, and other common fears.

Self-Report Measures for Social Phobia

This section provides an overview of some of the most commonly used self-report measures for the assessment of social phobia (for description of additional measures refer to Table 4.2). The majority of these measures assess the severity or intensity of social anxiety.

Two scales designed to measure social–evaluative anxiety are the Fear of Negative Evaluation (FNE) scale and the Social Avoidance and Distress Scale (SADS) (Watson & Friend, 1969). The FNE scale is designed to measure concern with social-evaluative threat and the SADS assesses distress and avoidance in social situations. Data suggest that both the FNE scale and SADS are better measures of social anxiety than of social phobia specifically, because they do not always discriminate well between social phobia and other anxiety disorders (for review, see Orsillo, 2001). However, the FNE scale, in particular, has been shown to be a highly sensitive outcome measure following cognitive behavioral group therapy for social phobia (Cox et al., 1998; Heimberg, Dodge, Hope, Kennedy, & Zollo, 1990).

Two well-validated companion scales (designed to be administered together) that are useful for the assessment of social phobia are the Social Interaction Anxiety Scale (SIAS) and the Social Phobia Scale (SPS) developed by Mattick and Clarke (1998). The SPS assesses fears of performance or of being observed by others during routine activities (e.g., eating, writing), whereas the SIAS assesses fears of more general social interaction (e.g., meeting an acquaintance). A number of studies support the reliability and validity of the SIAS and SPS (Brown et al., 1997; Mattick & Clarke, 1998; Osman, Gutierrez, Barrios, Kopper, & Chiros, 1998).

The Social Phobia and Anxiety Inventory (SPAI; Turner, Beidel, Dancu, & Stanley, 1989) is another widely used and validated measure of the somatic, cognitive, and behavioral symptoms of social phobia across a range of situations and settings (see Orsillo, 2001, for review of the psychometric properties of the SPAI). There is also a children's version of the SPAI (SPAI-C; Beidel, Turner, & Fink, 1996) that was designed to assess childhood social fears.

A more recent measure of social phobia symptoms is the Social Phobia Inventory (SPIN; Connor et al., 2000). The SPIN is a self-report scale designed to assess fear, avoidance, and physiological arousal associated with social phobia. Psychometric studies carried out in both clinical and nonclinical samples reveal the SPIN to have strong reliability (test–retest reliability and internal consistency) and validity (convergent, divergent, and construct), as well as sensitivity to change in response to pharmacological treatment (Connor et al., 2000).

A number of measures have been designed to assess public speaking anxiety more specifically. The Self-Statements during Public Speaking Scale (SSPS) (Hofmann & DiBartolo, 2000) is a 10-item questionnaire that assesses fearful thoughts associated with public speaking. The Personal Report of Confidence as a Speaker (PRCS) scale was originally developed by Gilkinson (1942) as a 104-item self-report measure of fear of public speaking. Paul (1966) shortened the PRCS to a 30-item measure that may be useful for screening or

TABLE 4.2. Self-Report (SR) and Semistructured Interview (SSI) Assessment Instruments for Social Phobia

Measure	Purpose	Format	Time[a] (minutes)	Psychometric Properties[b]
Fear of Negative Evaluation (FNE; Watson & Friend, 1969)	Assesses concerns with social-evaluative threat	30-item SR	5–10	Reliability and validity are good; demonstrated treatment sensitivity
Social Avoidance and Distress (SADS; Watson & Friend, 1969)	Assesses distress and avoidance in social situations	28-item SR	5–10	Reliability and validity are good; sensitivity to treatment effects documented
Social Interaction Anxiety Scale (SIAS; Mattick & Clarke, 1998, 1999)	Measures fears of general social interaction	19-item[c] SR	5	Good reliability and validity across a variety of samples (clinical, community, student); documented treatment sensitivity
Social Phobia Scale (SPS; Mattick & Clarke, 1998)	Measures fears of being evaluated during routine activities	20-item SR	5	Good reliability and validity across a variety of samples (clinical, community, student); treatment sensitivity established
Social Phobia and Anxiety Inventory (SPAI; Turner et al., 1989)	Empirically derived measure designed to assess the somatic, cognitive, and behavioral symptoms of social phobia	45-item SR	20–30	Reliability and validity well-documented; established treatment sensitivity
Social Phobia Inventory (SPIN; Connor et al., 2000)	Assesses symptoms of fear, avoidance, and physiological arousal associated with social phobia	17-item SR	10	Preliminary data suggest good reliability and validity (Connor et al., 2000), although reliability of physiological arousal scale weaker; sensitivity to treatment effects established

Measure	Description	Type	Time[a]	Psychometric properties[b]
Self-Statements during Public Speaking Scale (SSPS; Hofmann & DiBartolo, 2000)	Assesses positive and negative thoughts associated with public speaking	10-item SR	5–10	Psychometric properties promising (Hofmann & DiBartolo, 2000)
Brief Social Phobia Scale (BSPS; Davidson et al., 1991)	Measures symptoms of fear, avoidance, and physiological arousal associated with social phobia	18-item SSI	10–15	Preliminary data suggest good reliability and validity (Davidson et al., 1997); however, reliability and validity for the physiological arousal subscale is weak; treatment sensitivity documented
Fear of Intimacy Scale (FIS; Descutner & Thelen, 1991)	Assesses fear of intimacy with significant others	35-item SR		Good reliability and validity demonstrated in adolescents (Sherman & Thelen, 1996), college students (Descutner & Thelen, 1991), and middle-aged adult (Doi & Thelen, 1993) samples
Liebowitz Social Anxiety Scale (LSAS; Liebowitz, 1987)	Measures a wide range of performance and social difficulties related to social phobia	24-item SSI	5–10	Reliability and validity are established; documented treatment sensitivity
Social Interaction Self-Statement Test (SISST; Glass et al., 1982)	Assesses positive and negative cognitions associated with social phobia	30-item SR	5–10	Good psychometric properties; treatment sensitivity established

SR, self-report; SSI, semistructured interview (includes clinician- or observer-rated scales).

[a]Approximate time for completion.

[b]For more detailed review of the psychometric properties for these measures, see Orsillo (2001).

[c]The SIAS has 19 items, but there is also a 20-item version that has frequently been used in research.

measuring treatment outcome. The 20-item Speaking Extent and Comfort Scale (SPEACS; Lyons & Spicer, 1999) was developed to measure frequency and comfort in making conversation in general and in making conversation about the self.

How do the general social phobia measures compare to each other in terms of treatment sensitivity? One study that sought to answer this question examined a number of commonly used social phobia measures (including the FQ, FNE, SPS/SIAS, LSAS, and SPAI) to determine each measure's sensitivity to treatment change by comparing scores before and after cognitive-behavioral group therapy for social phobia (Cox et al., 1998). Findings revealed that all of the measures had satisfactory internal consistency. With respect to treatment sensitivity, strongest support was found for the SPAI and the SPS/SIAS. All measures demonstrated sensitivity to detecting treatment gains, with the exception of mixed findings for the LSAS. Whereas the Avoidance/Performance subscale of the LSAS demonstrated good treatment sensitivity, the Fear/Social subscale demonstrated poor treatment sensitivity. It is recommended that outcome studies include more than one measure of social phobia, as well as at least one older measure of social phobia, such as the FQ, to facilitate comparison with previous research (Cox et al., 1998).

Behavioral Assessment

Behavioral assessment is used to identify specific fear cues and to determine the intensity of a person's fear when exposed to the actual phobic situation. This is important because people often have difficulty identifying or remembering subtle cues that affect their fear and avoidance. In addition, individuals often overreport the amount of fear that they typically experience in a phobic situation (e.g., Klieger, 1987). Thus, behavioral assessment is an important component in a comprehensive cognitive-behavioral assessment of phobic disorders.

The most common form of behavioral assessment is the behavioral approach test— sometimes referred to as a behavioral avoidance test—or BAT. Antony and Swinson (2000a) have described two types of BAT: selective and progressive. During a *selective* BAT, the clinician selects phobic situations from a list or exposure hierarchy and instructs the patient to enter the situation for several minutes or more, provoking a moderate to high fear response. For an individual with a specific phobia of spiders, this may involve standing as close as possible to a live spider in a jar. For an individual with social phobia, this may involve sitting in the crowded waiting room or a role-played social interaction (e.g., a job interview, meeting a stranger, or a presentation). During or immediately after the BAT, the following variables may be assessed by the clinician:

1. *Cues that affect the intensity of fear experienced.* For spider phobia, these cues may include such variables as the movement, color, or size of the spider. For social phobia, these may include such variables as the number of people in the waiting room and what the people in the situation are doing (activity, eye contact, conversation). To assess these types of cues, the clinician should provide some examples for patients, illustrating how different variables can increase or decrease a person's level of fear. Then, the clinician should ask patients what types of variables seemed to increase or decrease their own fear.

2. *The intensity of the fear experienced.* This intensity can be rated on a scale of 0–100. The clinician should describe the end points of the scale (e.g., "a score of 0 would mean absolutely no fear, whereas a score of 100 would mean the most extreme fear you have ever felt"), and ask patients to remember some experiences that they would rate as a 0, 50, or 100. Then, based on the situation they just experienced, patients should be asked to rate their level of fear using the scale.

3. *The physical sensations experienced.* These sensations may include palpitations, dizziness, sweating, blushing, and shakiness. The clinician should ask patients to describe the physical sensations they experienced while in the situation. It can also be helpful to go through a list of panic symptoms to determine, in a systematic manner, the physical sensations experienced.

4. *Anxious cognitions experienced.* These cognitions may include expectations, thoughts, predictions, and beliefs—for example, "The spider will bite me" or "People will think I am incompetent." Anxious cognitions can be assessed by asking patients about their thoughts while in the situation. Some questions that may be helpful to ask include "What were you afraid would happen when _____?" and "What was going through your mind when _____?"

5. *Any anxious behaviors,* such as escape, avoidance, and distraction. These behaviors may be assessed by asking patients, "What did you do when you started to feel quite fearful in the situation?" and "Did you engage in any behaviors that helped decrease your fear level, such as looking away or distracting yourself?"

The information collected during the BAT is used not only to identify the parameters of an individual's fear but also to develop a specific cognitive-behavioral treatment plan.

A *progressive* BAT involves having the patient engage in progressively more difficult steps that involve exposure to the feared object or situation. The steps can be taken from an exposure hierarchy developed for that particular patient, or a standard hierarchy can be used. In addition to the variables outlined here, the clinician can also record how close the patient gets to the feared object or situation, how many steps were completed, and the fear rating for each step completed. See Table 4.3 for an example of a progressive BAT used in the assessment of an individual with a specific phobia of snakes.

Development of an individualized fear and avoidance hierarchy is a helpful part of the assessment process. The fear and avoidance hierarchy is useful for conducting a BAT, measuring baseline levels of fear and avoidance, measuring progress across treatment sessions, and measuring treatment outcome. During treatment, the hierarchy provides a basis for assigning exposure practices. The hierarchy should consist of 10 to 15 specific situations that the patient could realistically enter, ranging from mildly fear provoking (30 to 40 on a 100-point scale) to extremely fear provoking (100 or maximum fear and avoidance). Situations should be quite detailed, including relevant variables such as time of day, duration of exposure, and presence of other people.

TABLE 4.3. Specific Phobia of Snakes: Steps in a Behavioral Approach Test

Step[a]	Task (minimum 10 seconds)	Fear rating (0–100)
1.	Walk toward a snake in a cage (placed on a desk); closest distance from snake _____ feet	_____
2.	Touch the top of the cage	_____
3.	Touch the side of the cage	_____
4.	Lift the cage up by the handle	_____
5.	Open the top door of the cage	_____
6.	Touch the snake with a pencil	_____
7.	Touch the snake with your finger	_____
8.	Hold the snake in your hands	_____

[a]In ascending order of difficulty.

TABLE 4.4. Example of a Fear and Avoidance Hierarchy for Generalized Social Phobia

Task[a]	Fear rating (0–100)	Avoidance rating (0–100)
1. Make conversation at a family gathering	30	30
2. Go out for dinner with my spouse and eat facing the wall	40	30
3. Walk down a busy street alone wearing dark clothing and sunglasses	50	60
4. Answer the telephone	60	70
5. Ask for directions from a stranger	70	80
6. Ask a question in a meeting	70	75
7. Attend an office party without drinking alcohol	80	100
8. Go out for dinner with my spouse and eat facing other people	95	100
9. Walk alone on a busy street wearing a bright sweater and no sunglasses	95	100
10. Invite coworkers to a party in my home	100	100

[a]In ascending order of difficulty.

Variables that may affect fear can be incorporated directly into the hierarchy. For example, an early step on a social phobia hierarchy for an adult may be "asking a child for the time," and a higher step may be "asking someone my own age for the time." In addition to age, other variables that may affect fear in individuals with social phobia include (1) aspects of the target person such as sex, relationship status, perceived social status, and perceived intelligence; (2) the relationship between the target person and the patient, such as familiarity, level of intimacy, and history of conflict; (3) aspects of the patient, such as fatigue and stressors; and (4) aspects of the situation such as lighting, formality, the number of people involved, the activity involved, and the ability to use alcohol or drugs (Antony & Swinson, 2000a). See Table 4.4 for a sample hierarchy for social phobia.

PRACTICAL RECOMMENDATIONS FOR THE ASSESSMENT OF SPECIFIC AND SOCIAL PHOBIA

This section includes practical suggestions for the assessment of specific and social phobias and covers a number of issues that the clinician should be aware of during the assessment process, including initial evaluation, identifying the primary problem, defining the parameters of the fear, clinical interview, differential diagnosis, cultural differences in the expression of fear, and associated features (e.g., fainting history in BII phobia, fear of anxiety-related sensations, disgust sensitivity).

Initial Evaluation

It is important for the clinician to be aware that the assessment process itself can be quite anxiety-provoking for individuals with either specific or social phobia. For many people with specific phobia, just saying the phobic word aloud or reading it on paper can trigger an anxiety reaction or a panic attack. Thus, it is a good idea to ask the patient if discussing the phobic object or situation will lead to anxiety. If so, the clinician should explain the importance of gathering information about the individual's fears, as well as the therapeutic value of discussing the fears. Keeping in mind the importance of developing rapport to maximize therapeutic effectiveness, the clinician should carefully consider just how far the patient should be pushed in the first session.

For most people with social phobia, the assessment session itself is a phobic encounter:

sitting in the waiting room before an appointment, filling in an initial intake form in public, and meeting a clinician for the first time are situations that provoke high levels of fear. Thus, it is important for the clinician to be aware of these potential difficulties and to provide support and reassurance as needed.

Determining the Primary Problem

Often individuals with specific and social phobias present with more than one psychological disorder. Together, the clinician and the individual must make a decision regarding which problem will be treated first. Generally, the problems that should be targeted first are those that are most impairing or distressing, those for which the individual has presented for treatment and is most motivated to work on, those that are most likely to respond to treatment, and those for which treatment is most likely to lead to improvement of associated problems such as other anxiety disorders or depression (Antony & Swinson, 2000a).

Defining the Cognitive and Behavioral Features of the Individual's Fear

To plan a comprehensive treatment, it is important for the clinician to fully assess the features of a patient's fear, including fear-related cognitions, reliance on safety cues, the types of overt and subtle avoidance strategies used, and the range of situations avoided. Cognitions may include anxious thoughts, predictions, or expectations that help maintain the fear (e.g., fear of being bitten by a dog in specific phobia or fear of looking stupid in social phobia). These cognitions can be related to the situation itself or to concerns about the experience of fear or of having anxiety symptoms. Safety cues are objects or stimuli that provide a sense of security in the feared situation (Antony & Barlow, 1998) and may include such objects as carrying pepper spray (dog phobia) and carrying extra makeup to hide blushing (social phobia).

Avoidance can be overt, such as escaping a situation or not entering a situation in the first place, but it can also be subtle, such as the use of distraction or engaging in overprotective behaviors. For example, a person with a specific phobia of heights who avoids looking out of windows when in his or her apartment is engaging in subtle avoidance. A person with social phobia who avoids making eye contact, wears sunglasses or baggy, dark clothing to appear less noticeable in public is also engaging in subtle avoidance. Other subtle avoidance strategies used by individuals with social phobia may include wearing a turtleneck or scarf to hide blushing, making excuses to leave events early, overcompensating by memorizing a presentation, avoiding certain topics of conversation, and arriving at the bank with a transaction slip already filled out to avoid writing in public (Antony & Swinson, 2000a). Alcohol is another commonly reported subtle avoidance strategy used by some people who have social phobia to cope with social interaction situations, in particular. Common subtle avoidance strategies associated with specific phobia include wearing protective clothing so that spiders cannot crawl on the skin (spider phobia), staying in the basement or away from windows during a thunderstorm (storm phobia), driving only at certain times of the day and on certain roads (driving phobia), crossing the street to the opposite side to avoid a dog (dog phobia), and closing one's eyes during films with blood scenes (BII phobia; Antony & Swinson, 2000a).

Diagnosis

A number of assessment issues may arise when classifying a specific phobia according to DSM-IV criteria. Some phobias do not clearly fall into one of the DSM-IV types. For example, does a fear of the dark correspond to the natural environment type or the situational type? It has also been argued that some of the examples of each type listed in DSM-IV may be misplaced (Antony & Swinson, 2000a). For example, given the features shared by height phobias and other situational phobias, it may make more sense to have height phobias classified in the situational phobias rather than among the natural environment phobias, where they are currently listed (Antony et al., 1997). In addition, some people who have social phobia may not spontaneously report the full extent of their social fears, so it is important for the clinician to ask about a range of social and performance situations (see Table 4.5).

The criterion for specific or social phobia that requires that an individual have insight into the excessiveness of his or her fear was introduced to differentiate between phobias and delusional fears, which, by definition, are associated with a lack of such insight. However, there is evidence that some individuals with specific phobia may not recognize that their fears are excessive or unreasonable, although their beliefs are not of a delusional intensity (e.g., Jones, Whitmont, & Menzies, 1996). For example, an individual with spider phobia may consider it perfectly reasonable to sleep with a heavy comforter in summer as protection against potentially dangerous spiders.

To make an accurate diagnosis, a thorough knowledge of the DSM-IV criteria is required, in addition to careful evaluation of the following features of the problem: the focus of apprehension or anxiety and reasons for avoidance, the contexts in which the fear occurs, and the range of situations feared. For specific phobia, the focus of the fear may be anticipated harm from some aspect of the object or situation (e.g., an individual who fears driving is concerned about crashing) or concerns about the physiological (increased heart rate, shortness of breath, fainting) and emotional (e.g., fears of losing control, panicking) manifestations of fear that occur upon exposure to the phobic stimulus (e.g., an individual with a fear of heights may fear getting dizzy as well as falling). For social phobia, the focus of the anxiety is generally related to being embarrassed, humiliated, or negatively evaluated in a social or performance context (e.g., an individual with social phobia may avoid social gatherings for fear that he or she will be unable to carry on a conversation and that others will judge him or her to be anxious or stupid).

TABLE 4.5. Social Performance and Social Interaction Situations Associated with Social Phobia

Social performance situations	Social interaction situations
• Formal public speaking	• Initiating and maintaining conversations
• Participating in meetings/classes	• Meeting new people
• Eating or drinking in front of others	• Making "small talk"
• Speaking in front of others	• Talking to strangers (e.g., asking for directions or the time)
• Writing in front of others	
• Being in public situations (e.g., shopping mall, crowded bus, walking on a busy street)	• Disclosing personal information to others
• Arriving late for a meeting/class	• Being assertive (e.g., refusing an unreasonable request)
• Participating in sports or athletics (e.g., aerobics, team sport, exercising in public)	• Dating situations, intimate or sexual relations
• Performing music	• Expressing disagreement or disapproval and conflict situations
• Using public washrooms with other people nearby	• Talking on the telephone
	• Talking to people in authority (e.g., boss, teacher)
• Making mistakes in front of other people	• Going to a party or social gathering

Note. Adapted from Antony and Swinson (2000a). Copyright 2000 by the American Psychological Association. Adapted by permission.

The context of an individual's anxiety refers to the situations or variables that trigger the fear reaction. The range of situations avoided can be small or large. For specific phobia, the context is circumscribed to cues that are related to a specific situation or stimulus. An individual with a snake phobia has a clinically significant fear of snakes, and related fear cues may include grass, long green or black objects, hearing or reading the word "snake," and toy snakes, as well as pictures of snakes in books, movies, or television. This person may fear or avoid any situations related to these fear cues, including entering toy stores, walking on grass, entering the backyard with bare feet, going to the cottage or on a vacation where there is a possibility of encountering a snake. For social phobia, the context is specific to social performance and social interaction situations. The feared situations avoided can range from one situation (e.g., public speaking) to almost any situations where other people are present. See Table 4.5 for a list of situations that are often feared by individuals with social phobia.

Differential Diagnosis

To make an accurate diagnosis of specific or social phobia, it is important to rule out other disorders that may have overlapping features. For example, other anxiety disorders such as panic disorder and agoraphobia (fear of panic-related physical sensations and situations), posttraumatic stress disorder (fear of trauma-related cues), obsessive–compulsive disorder (obsessional fears such as contamination), and separation anxiety disorder (fear of situations related to separation), as well as other mental disorders such as hypochondriasis (fear of having a serious illness), eating disorders (fear of eating specific foods, unrelated to fear of choking), and psychotic disorders (fear related to a delusion), may be associated with fear and avoidance of specific stimuli and should be distinguished from specific phobia through careful assessment. Often individuals report subclinical fears of specific objects or situations that are misdiagnosed as specific phobias.

A specific phobia of contracting an illness may be distinguished from hypochondriasis by assessing the nature of the health anxiety. A specific phobia of contracting an illness is characterized by fear of stimuli that may lead to developing an illness. In contrast, hypochondriasis is characterized by worries that one has a serious disease based on the misinterpretation of bodily symptoms. For differentiating anxiety disorders from eating disorders it is helpful to assess the focus of the anxiety and the reasons for phobic avoidance. For example, an individual with a choking phobia avoids foods for fear of choking, whereas an individual with an eating disorder avoids foods because of an intense fear of gaining weight.

Social anxiety may be associated with a number of DSM-IV disorders, including eating disorders (fear of eating in public), body dysmorphic disorder (preoccupation with the erroneous belief that one has a flaw in his or her physical appearance), panic disorder (fears of embarrassment from panic symptoms), and obsessive–compulsive disorder (fear that others will notice rituals). Again, careful assessment is required to distinguish social phobia from other disorders associated with social anxiety. Patients who present with subclinical fears of public speaking or other social situations may also be misdiagnosed with social phobia.

For a number of reasons, panic disorder with agoraphobia may often be difficult to distinguish from multiple specific phobias or from social phobia. Situational phobias include situations often associated with agoraphobia (e.g., enclosed places, driving, elevators) (Antony & Barlow, 1998), and some studies suggest that situational phobias are more likely to be associated with delayed and unpredictable panic attacks (Antony et al., 1997). In addition, people who have panic disorder often report significant social anxiety (e.g., fears of embarrassment and humiliation in social situations because of anxiety symptoms), as well as avoidance of social situations. In addition to an assessment of the anxiety features described earlier, assessment of the type (e.g., cued vs. uncued) and location (e.g., the range of situations that trigger panic attacks) of panic attacks, as well as the focus of apprehension (e.g., a fear of having a panic attack on an airplane [panic disorder] vs. a fear of crashing [specific phobia of flying]), is critical for distinguishing panic disorder and agoraphobia from situational specific phobias or social phobia.

The presence of uncued, recurrent panic attacks and significant anxiety between attacks (outside of avoided situations) suggests panic disorder. For both specific and social phobias, panic attacks are typically cued, and anxiety outside of phobic situations is not typically heightened. In addition, panic disorder is often characterized by avoidance of a broader range of situations that are generally associated with agoraphobia (e.g., crowds, standing in line, public transportation, and being alone) than are either specific or social phobia. Finally, the focus of apprehension in panic disorder is specific to concerns about the possibility of panicking in the phobic situation or about the consequences of panicking (e.g., embarrassment and humiliation), whereas in specific and social phobia, other aspects of the phobic situation are a focus of apprehension as well (e.g., the dangerousness of the situation in specific phobia and the possibility of negative evaluation in social phobia). However, panic disorder may exist comorbidly with either specific or social phobia. In such a case, the criteria for both disorders should be met, such that the symptoms of one disorder are not accounted for by the other (e.g., an individual who presents with recurrent, unexpected panic attacks and concern about future attacks and who also reports a long history of anxiety in social situations for fear of negative evaluation would likely receive diagnoses of panic disorder and social phobia).

With respect to social phobia, it is important to remember that a social phobia diagnosis is not given if the social anxiety is exclusively related to the symptoms of a medical condition that may be noticed by other people. A person who has a stuttering condition and reports clinically significant anxiety and avoidance of social situations solely because of concerns related to the stuttering (e.g., being embarrassed or looking stupid) would not be given a diagnosis of social phobia but instead would be assigned a diagnosis of anxiety disorder not otherwise specified. In this case, it is important to ask if the individual would still experience anxiety in social situations if he or she did not have the symptoms of the medical condition. If the answer is "yes," then further probing of the individual's social fears is warranted and a diagnosis of social phobia may be appropriate.

The clinician must always keep in mind whether an individual's fear meets a clinical threshold for diagnosis. Anxiety disorder symptoms occur on a continuum with normal functioning. To meet full diagnostic criteria for either social phobia or specific phobia, the person must be distressed about having the problem or must experience clinically significant functional impairment (e.g., at work, in relationships, or other important areas of functioning).

Quite often, people who have depression also report avoidance of social situations. Depressed persons generally avoid social situations because of a lack of interest in socializing rather than a fear of humiliation or embarrassment. When their depression remits, their interest in socializing usually returns. However, individuals with social phobia avoid social situations because of *fear* rather than *anhedonia*. It can be useful to ask whether the individual enjoys socializing when he or she is not depressed.

Clinical Interview

A clinical interview is often the most common method of collecting information in clinical practice. Although use of a full semistructured interview is recommended, it may not always be practical. When an unstructured clinical interview is used, we recommend that it be conducted in a systematic way, assessing each of the variables outlined in Table 4.6.

TABLE 4.6. Specific and Social Phobias: Variables to Assess during a Clinical Interview

1. Presenting problem

2. DSM-IV diagnostic criteria for relevant disorders (establish principal diagnosis, differential diagnoses)

3. Onset, development, and course of problem

4. Impact on functioning (social, work/school, relational)

5. Pattern of physical symptoms (typical symptoms, frequency, intensity, physical sensations, history of fainting, panic attacks)

6. Anxiety-related cognitions (thoughts, beliefs, predictions, cognitive biases related to the phobic situation)

7. Focus of apprehension (anxiety symptoms, characteristics of phobic situation)

8. Patterns of overt avoidance (review list of common phobic situations for specific phobia or social phobia and have individual rate fear and avoidance of problematic situations)

9. Subtle avoidance strategies (overprotective behaviors, distraction, and reliance on safety cues)

10. Parameters of the fear (variables that affect the individual's fear such as the proximity of the stimulus, presence of others, etc.)

11. Family factors and social supports (family history of anxiety-related problems, symptom accommodation by family member, availability of family or close friends to assist in treatment)

12. Treatment history (treatment strategies tried and treatment responses)

13. Skills deficits (e.g., lack of assertiveness, poor eye contact, poor conversation skills, poor driving skills)

14. Relevant medical history and physical limitations

Note. Adapted from Antony and Swinson (2000a). Copyright 2000 by the American Psychological Association. Adapted by permission.

Cultural Differences

Research on cultural differences in the expression of specific and social phobias has been increasing. There is some evidence of cultural differences in the prevalence of specific phobias (e.g., Brown, Eaton, & Sussman, 1990), and a number of studies have examined the nature of social phobia in a variety of countries. Cultural differences have been found with respect to the features of social anxiety, types of situations provoking anxiety, scores on standard measures of social anxiety, and the role of early parenting (Heimberg, Makris, Juster, Öst, & Rapee, 1997; Kleinknecht, Dinnel, Kleinknecht, Hiruma, & Harada, 1997; Leung, Heimberg, Holt, & Bruch, 1994). Culturally specific diagnostic biases of clinicians in the assessment of social anxiety have also been identified (Tseng, Asai, Kitanishi, McLaughlin, & Kyomen, 1992).

To ensure accurate diagnoses, clinicians should be aware of cultural differences in presentation (verbal and nonverbal communication, use of interpersonal space, and other verbal cues such as tone and loudness) when conducting assessments with individuals from different cultures. For a review of cultural-specific issues in the assessment of anxiety, see Friedman (2001).

Assessing Associated Features

History of Fainting

The BII type of specific phobia is often associated with a vasovagal fainting response. A history of fainting in BII type situations is reported by up to 75% of people who have this fear (American Psychiatric Association, 2000). It is important to assess for a history of fainting, as this information will help determine the appropriate treatment strategies used. For example, applied muscle tension has been demonstrated to be helpful for individuals with BII phobias who report a history of fainting in the phobic situation but not for those individuals who do not report a history of fainting (e.g., Hellström, Fellenius, & Öst, 1996).

Apprehension in Response to Physical Sensations

Apprehension in response to physical sensations may play a critical role in the maintenance of anxiety and avoidance in both specific phobias (e.g., fears of choking, vomiting, dizziness, and fainting) and social phobia (e.g., fears of shaking, sweating, blushing). Research has shown that individuals with specific phobias report apprehension about experiencing uncomfortable physical sensations (e.g., Hugdahl & Öst, 1985), as well as anxiety over their physical reactions to the phobic situation (e.g., having a panic attack) (McNally & Steketee, 1985). Two psychometrically sound measures of anxiety in response to physical sensations are the 16-item self-report Anxiety Sensitivity Index (ASI; Peterson & Reiss, 1993) and the 18-item self-report Body Sensations Questionnaire (BSQ; Chambless, Caputo, Bright, & Gallagher, 1984).

Anxiety in response to physical symptoms is greater in individuals who have situational specific phobias, such as claustrophobia, than other types such as animal type phobias (Craske & Sipsas, 1992). The level of anxiety in response to physical sensations should be a factor when choosing treatment strategies. If a person reports significant apprehension in response to physical sensations, it may be helpful to incorporate an interoceptive exposure component into the treatment plan (see Antony & Swinson, 2000a).

Disgust Sensitivity

In addition to fear, people who have BII phobias and those with specific phobias of certain animals such as spiders and snakes often report feelings of disgust when confronted with phobic stimuli (Woody & Teachman, 2000). Thus, it can be helpful to measure disgust as part of a comprehensive assessment. Two psychometrically sound measures developed to assess disgust sensitivity in individuals with BII and animal fears are the Disgust Scale (DS; Haidt, McCauley, & Rozin, 1994) and the Disgust Emotion Scale (DES; Kleinknecht, Tolin, Lohr, & Kleinknecht, 1996). The 32-item DS (Haidt et al., 1994) is a measure of disgust sensitivity that assesses seven disgust-eliciting domains: food, animals, body products, sex, body envelope violations, death, and hygiene. Two additional disgust-eliciting domains (moral and interpersonal) have been added to the scale (Haidt, Rozin, McCauley, & Imada, 1997). The 30-item DES (Kleinknecht, Tolin, et al., 1996) is a factor-analytically derived scale that assesses five disgust domains: blood, injury, and injections; mutilated bodies; animals; odors; and rotting foods.

Other Relevant Dimensions

A thorough assessment of specific and social phobias should also include measures of related dimensions, such as generalized anxiety, depression, perfectionism, and functional impairment. The Depression Anxiety Stress Scales (DASS; Lovibond & Lovibond, 1995) is a 42-item measure with three subscales: depressed mood, generalized anxiety, and stress. The DASS has been proven to have excellent psychometric properties in patients with anxiety disorders (e.g., Antony, Bieling, Cox, Enns, & Swinson, 1998). Two psychometrically sound measures of perfectionism are the Frost Multidimensional Perfectionism Scale (Frost, Marten, Lahart, & Rosenblate, 1990) and the Hewitt and Flett (1991) Multidimensional Perfectionism Scale. Finally, the Illness Intrusiveness Rating Scale (IIRS; Devins et al., 1983) measures the effect of an illness and/or its treatment on 13 domains of functioning. IIRS

TABLE 4.7. Specific and Social Phobias: Sample Assessment Packages

Phobia	Measure	Purpose
Spider phobia	Spider Questionnaire (SPQ; Klorman et al., 1974)	Assess the verbal–cognitive component of spider fear
	Depression Anxiety Stress Scales (DASS; Lovibond & Lovibond, 1995)	Assess for depression, general anxiety, and stress
	Anxiety Sensitivity Index (ASI; Peterson & Reiss, 1993)	Fear of anxiety sensations
Generalized social phobia	Social Interaction Anxiety Scale (SIAS; Mattick & Clarke, 1988)	Assess fears of general social interaction (e.g., meeting an acquaintance)
	Social Phobia Scale (SPS; Mattick & Clarke, 1988)	Assess fears of performance or being observed by others during routine activities (e.g., eating, writing)
	Multidimensional Perfectionism Scale (MPS; Hewitt & Flett, 1991)	Assess dimensions of perfectionism (self-oriented, other-oriented, and socially prescribed)
	Depression Anxiety Stress Scales (DASS; Lovibond & Lovibond, 1995)	Assess for depression, general anxiety, and stress
	Anxiety Sensitivity Index (ASI; Peterson & Reiss, 1993)	Fear of anxiety sensations
	Illness Intrusiveness Rating Scale (IIRS; Devins et al., 1983)	Interference in functioning as a result of symptoms

means for anxiety disorder patients are reported by Antony, Roth, Swinson, Huta, and Devins (1998).

Other variables related to social anxiety that are relevant in the assessment of social phobia include self-consciousness (e.g., Self-Consciousness Scale, or SCS; Fenigstein, Scheier, & Buss, 1975) and shyness and sociability (e.g., Shyness Scale and Sociability Scale; Cheek & Buss, 1981; Social Reticence Scale, or SRS; Jones & Russell, 1982; and the Stanford Shyness Survey; Maroldo, Eisenreich, & Hall, 1979; Pilkonis, 1977; Zimbardo, 1977). See Table 4.7 for examples of assessment batteries for an individual with a specific phobia of spiders and for an individual with generalized social phobia.

THE ROLE OF ASSESSMENT IN TREATMENT PLANNING AND OUTCOME EVALUATION

A comprehensive assessment achieves a number of goals including (1) establishing a diagnosis and ruling out alternative diagnoses, (2) gathering baseline data on the severity and frequency of symptoms and associated problems, (3) evaluating progress in treatment, (4) evaluating treatment outcome, and (5) detecting relapse in individuals who have received treatment (Shear et al., 2000). A thorough assessment is necessary for the selection of appropriate treatment strategies. For the assessment of specific and social phobias, a multimodal approach should be taken, which may include structured, semistructured, or unstructured interviews; self-report measures; and behavioral assessment. Each of these methods provides unique information for making diagnostic and treatment decisions. This section provides an overview of empirically supported treatments for specific and social phobia, followed by a consideration of the role of assessment in choosing appropriate treatment strategies, monitoring progress, and evaluating outcome.

Overview of Empirically Supported Treatments

Specific Phobia

In contrast to treatment for other anxiety disorders, it is generally accepted that pharmacotherapy is not an appropriate treatment for specific phobias. Rather, psychological treatments, specifically those incorporating exposure to feared objects and situations, are the empirically supported treatments of choice (Antony & Barlow, 1998; Antony & Swinson, 2000a).

Exposure-based treatments have been effectively used to treat most types of specific phobia (e.g., Bourque & Ladouceur, 1980; Craske, Mohlman, Yi, Glover, & Valeri, 1995; Öst, 1996). In fact, studies indicate that for a number of phobias (e.g., animals, injections, dental treatment) a single, prolonged session (2 to 3 hours) of *in vivo* exposure may lead to clinically significant improvement in up to 90% of patients (e.g., Öst, Brandberg, & Alm, 1997; Öst, Salkovskis, & Hellström, 1991). Clinician manuals (e.g., Antony & Swinson, 2000a; Craske, Antony, & Barlow, 1997) and patient manuals (e.g., Antony, Craske, & Barlow, 1995) are available to provide detailed descriptions of the step-by-step procedures for treating specific phobias.

For individuals with BII phobia and a history of fainting, applied muscle tension has been demonstrated to be a clinically effective treatment (e.g., Kozak & Montgomery, 1981; Öst & Sterner, 1987). Applied tension involves teaching the phobic individual to tense all body muscles, which serves to increase blood pressure and prevent fainting. This strategy is combined with cognitive strategies and *in vivo* exposure. In addition, limited evidence suggests that cognitive restructuring may be useful in certain types of specific phobia (e.g., Booth & Rachman, 1992).

Social Phobia

Empirically supported treatments for social phobia include exposure-based strategies, cognitive strategies, applied relaxation, and social skills training (for review of the empirical literature, see Antony & Swinson, 2000a; Turk, Fresco, & Heimberg, 1999; Turner, Cooley-Quill, & Beidel, 1996). Exposure-based strategies include gradual *in vivo* exposure to feared situations (e.g., public speaking) and social interactions (e.g., talking to a stranger), as well as behavioral role play practices (e.g., practicing a job interview). Cognitive strategies include examining evidence regarding anxious beliefs, attributions, interpretations, and predictions. Applied relaxation involves the combination of progressive muscle relaxation with gradual situational exposure. Finally, social skills training involves improving conversational and social skills such as maintaining eye contact, using an appropriate tone of voice, awareness of nonverbal communication, ability to initiate and maintain conversation, ability to make small talk, and assertiveness skills. Treatment manuals for patients are available that provide step-by-step application of cognitive-behavioral strategies for social anxiety (e.g., Antony & Swinson, 2000b; Hope, Heimberg, Juster, & Turk, 2000).

Treatment may be delivered either individually or in groups. Cognitive-behavioral group therapy has been shown to be particularly effective for treating social phobia because the group provides opportunities for feedback and role play practices that are not as easily available in individual treatment. Research has found cognitive-behavioral group therapy involving cognitive and exposure-based strategies to be significantly more effective than supportive group therapy for the treatment of social phobia, both in the short term (immediately following treatment) and in the long term (at 3- and 6-month follow-up and at 5-year follow-up) (Heimberg et al., 1990). There is evidence that group treatment for social phobia is most effective when cognitive therapy precedes exposure treatment (Scholing & Emmelkamp, 1993).

Social skills training has been found to lead to significant improvements in both social skills and social anxiety and may be as effective as *in vivo* exposure alone (Wlazlo, Schroeder-Hartwig, Hand, Kaiser, & Münchau, 1990). However, the addition of social skills training does not yield added benefit over and above the improvements from exposure alone (Mersch, 1995).

A number of controlled clinical trials have shown that pharmacological treatment for social phobia can be quite effective (for a review, see Antony & Swinson, 2000a). Effective medications include traditional monoamine oxidase inhibitors (e.g., phenelzine), reversible inhibitors of monoamine oxidase A (e.g., moclobemide), selective serotonin reuptake inhibitors (e.g., sertraline and paroxetine), and benzodiazepines (e.g., clonazepam and alprazolam). A recent placebo-controlled trial indicates that gabapentin may also be effective for treating social phobia (Pande et al., 1999).

A meta-analysis of 24 studies examining cognitive-behavioral and pharmacological treatments for social phobia confirms that both treatments are more effective than control conditions, with SSRIs and benzodiazepines yielding the largest effect sizes among medications, and treatments involving exposure either alone or combined with cognitive strategies yielding the largest effect sizes among cognitive-behavioral interventions (Gould, Buckminster, Pollack, Otto, & Yap, 1997). However, other meta-analytic investigations comparing cognitive therapy, exposure, and the combination of cognitive therapy and exposure have led to slightly different conclusions. For example, Taylor (1996) found that, in comparison to cognitive therapy alone, exposure alone, and social skills training, only combined treatments involving cognitive therapy and exposure had significantly larger effect sizes than placebo.

Using Assessment to Choose among Treatment Strategies

The information gathered during the assessment phase is essential for both treatment planning and the selection of appropriate treatment strategies. Information obtained from the assessment provides a basis for assigning treatment priority in situations where there is more than one problem identified. For example, consider a pregnant patient who presents with symptoms consistent with a blood phobia and social phobia. Her blood phobia is preventing her from obtaining the blood work necessary for her doctor to properly monitor her pregnancy. In this case, the blood phobia would likely receive treatment priority over the social phobia because of the immediate risk to her health.

Based on information obtained during the assessment, treatment strategies are individually tailored to meet the patient's treatment needs. If the patient described previously also reported a history of fainting in the context of her blood phobia, then applied muscle tension would be the treatment of choice. Exposure exercises should be developed based on the subtle and overt avoidance behaviors reported during the assessment. Similarly, cognitive strategies are often chosen based on fear-related beliefs, predictions, interpretations, and attributions reported during the assessment process.

Using Assessment to Monitor Progress and Measure Outcome

Symptom measures are useful not only during the assessment phase, but also for objectively assessing progress during treatment. Pretreatment measures can be administered periodically during treatment to measure change from baseline. Given that exposure based strategies are the treatment of choice for both specific and social phobia (either alone or in combination with cognitive strategies), we also recommend that patients complete fear and avoidance ratings for their exposure hierarchy at the beginning of each therapy session. This only takes a few minutes and provides important information regarding progress from session-to-session. These session-by-session hierarchy ratings can also be used within therapy to choose homework assignments and to provide a clear measure of progress that the patient can observe.

Symptom measures are also useful for measuring treatment outcome. Given the dimensional nature of the fear and avoidance characterizing specific and social phobias, a comprehensive assessment should be conducted posttreatment to provide an accurate measure of outcome. It is recommended that the self-report measures given during the pretreatment assessment be repeated posttreatment to provide a multidimensional indicator of treatment efficacy. The posttreatment package should also include a measure assessing the patient's satisfaction with treatment and perceptions regarding the quality of care provided. This measure can be constructed by the clinician to ask questions about satisfaction with particular interventions or the specific treatment setting, or a more general measure can be used such as the Client Satisfaction Questionnaire–8 (CSQ-8; Nguyen, Attkisson, & Stegner, 1983).

ASSESSMENT IN MANAGED CARE AND PRIMARY CARE SETTINGS

This section considers some issues regarding the assessment of specific and social phobias that are particularly relevant in managed care and primary care settings. For managed care settings, costs are a major issue. Thus, choosing brief screening measures to assess for specific and social phobia is recommended. For example the brief 17-item self-report SPIN measures social anxiety and avoidance of social situations with a cutoff score of 19 or greater distinguishing between individuals with social phobia and psychiatric and nonpsychiatric controls (Conner et al., 2000). The SPIN appears to have good psychometric properties and sensitivity to the effects of treatment (Conner et al., 2000). Brief screening questions are also effective and efficient. To screen for specific phobias, a useful question is, "Are there any situations or objects that you are especially afraid of, like seeing blood, heights, animals or insects, or enclosed places?" To screen for social phobia, a useful question is, "Are you excessively anxious in social situations such as public speaking, meeting new people, and eating or drinking in public?"

Research has shown that brief cognitive-behavioral treatments for specific and social phobia are highly effective, with significant clinical improvements being observed in as little as one prolonged exposure session for specific phobia and typically 12 to 15 sessions of cognitive-behavioral treatment for social phobia. Thus, the short-term nature of behavioral and cognitive-behavioral treatments is conducive to minimizing costs in managed care settings. The use of progress and outcome measures in managed care settings is also crucial when a patient's need for services extend beyond that stipulated by a third-party payer. These data can be used as grounds to negotiate further services.

There are also aspects of both specific and social phobias that are particularly relevant in the primary care settings, including medical complications related to anxiety and a tendency for phobic disorders to be underrecognized in primary care settings.

Medical Complications

The avoidance that usually accompanies specific phobia may have detrimental effects on health. For example, individuals with BII type may avoid important medical and dental procedures. Or, individuals with fear of choking may avoid eating solid foods and taking oral medications (American Psychiatric Association, 2000). Socially phobic individuals may avoid scheduled medical appointments due to anxiety associated with sitting in the waiting room or speaking to authority figures.

Lack of Disorder Recognition

Despite the significant impairment and substance use associated with social phobia, research conducted by the World Health Organization Study on Psychological Problems in General Health Care (Bisserbe, Weiller, Boyer, Lépine, & Lecrubier, 1996) has shown that the level of recognition of social phobia by general practitioners in primary care settings is quite low. Bisserbe et al. (1996) found that only 53% of a sample of patients with social phobia were correctly identified by general practitioners as having a psychological disorder. When social phobia was comorbid with depression, 66% of the patients were correctly recognized as having a psychological problem. Thus, when depression is not present comorbidly, social phobia is less likely to be identified as a psychological problem.

Research has also shown that identifying social phobia in primary care settings can help primary care clinicians target those patients who need more aggressive treatment for depression, given that patients with social phobia have an increased risk of persistent depression and patients with depression and a coexisting anxiety disorder tend to have a greater severity of depression (Gaynes et al., 1999). These findings highlight the need for primary care practitioners to be trained to recognize the clinical features of social phobia and other anxiety disorders.

It has been suggested that the name "social phobia" may also play a role in its poor recognition in primary care. Liebowitz, Heimberg, Fresco, Travers, and Stein (2000) have suggested that a switch to the alternative name of social anxiety disorder, as proposed by the DSM-IV Taskforce on Anxiety Disorders, may help in the education of psychiatric and primary care physicians by conveying a more accurate picture of the pervasive and impairing nature of the disorder.

Another obstacle in the assessment and treatment of both social and specific phobias is that individuals often do not mention these concerns to their family doctor. For example, in one study, only 5% of patients with social phobia had mentioned their concerns to their family practitioners (Weiller, Bisserbe, Boyer, Lépine, & Lecrubier, 1996). Early detection and treatment of social phobia is critical for improving the clinical course and decreasing disability. Providing information to patients in the practitioner's office in the form of pamphlets or handouts may help educate patients on the nature of anxiety problems and where to get help.

Recent research has focused on the development of a training program for primary care practitioners in conducting exposure therapy for social phobia (Haug et al., 2000). The physicians expressed satisfaction with the training program and also found it useful for treating other conditions. Exposure therapy delivered by the primary care practitioner in conjunction with medication (sertraline) was found to be more effective than exposure therapy alone (Haug et al., 2000). For a more detailed review on the management issues and strategies involved in treating social phobia in the primary care setting, see Ballenger et al. (1998).

SUMMARY

This chapter examines a range of issues relevant to assessment, treatment planning, and outcome evaluation for specific and social phobias. Empirical evidence was reviewed for some of the key measures used in the assessment of these two anxiety disorders, including semistructured interviews, self-report measures, and behavioral assessment techniques. Practical recommendations for the assessment of specific and social phobia were covered, highlighting a range of issues related to the initial evaluation situation, identification of the primary problem, defining fear parameters, developing a diagnosis, and variables to assess in an unstructured clinical interview. Issues related to differential diagnosis, cultural differences, and associated features were also discussed. The range of these assessment issues underscores the necessity of conducting a carefully planned assessment based on a thorough background knowledge of the disorders.

The role of assessment in treatment planning, monitoring progress in treatment, and measuring treatment outcome was also covered. Finally, issues relevant to the assessment of specific and social phobia in managed care and primary care settings were discussed, highlighting such issues as minimizing costs by choosing brief screening measures and utilizing cognitive-behavioral interventions that have proven efficiency; medical complications related to certain specific phobias; and the problem of a lack of disorder recognition in primary care. Early detection and treatment of both specific and social phobia is crucial for improving clinical outcome and decreasing disability.

REFERENCES

American Psychiatric Association. (2000). *Diagnostic and statistical manual of mental disorders* (4th ed., text rev.). Washington, DC: Author.

Antony, M. M. (2001a). Specific phobia: A brief overview and guide to assessment. In M. M. Antony, S. M. Orsillo, & L. Roemer (Eds.), *Practitioner's guide to empirically based measures of anxiety*. New York: Kluwer Academic/Plenum.

Antony, M. M. (2001b). Measures for specific phobia. In M. M. Antony, S. M. Orsillo, & L. Roemer (Eds.), *Practitioner's guide to empirically based measures of anxiety*. New York: Kluwer Academic/Plenum.

Antony, M. M., & Barlow, D. H. (1997). Social and specific phobias. In A. Tasman, J. Kay, & J. A. Lieberman (Eds.), *Psychiatry* (pp. 1037–1059). Philadelphia: Saunders.

Antony, M. M., & Barlow, D. H. (1998). Specific phobia. In V. E. Caballo (Ed.), *Handbook of cognitive and behavioural treatments for psychological disorders* (pp. 1–22). Oxford: Pergamon.

Antony, M. M., Bieling, P. J., Cox, B. J., Enns, M. W., & Swinson, R. P. (1998). Psychometric properties of the 42-item and 21-item versions of the Depression Anxiety Stress Scales (DASS) in clinical groups and a community sample. *Psychological Assessment, 10,* 176–181.

Antony, M. M., Brown, T. A., & Barlow, D. H. (1997). Heterogeneity among specific phobia types in DSM-IV. *Behaviour Research and Therapy, 35,* 1089–1100.

Antony, M. M., Craske, M. G., & Barlow, D. H. (1995). *Mastery of your specific phobia, client manual*. San Antonio, TX: Psychological Corporation.

Antony, M. M., Downie, F., & Swinson, R. P. (1998). Diagnostic issues and epidemiology in obsessive–compulsive disorder. In R. P. Swinson, M. M. Antony, S. Rachman, & M. A. Richter (Eds.), *Obsessive–compulsive disorder: Theory, research, and treatment* (pp. 3–32). New York: Guilford Press.

Antony, M. M., Orsillo, S. M., & Roemer, L. (Eds.). (2001). *Practitioner's guide to empirically based measures of anxiety*. New York: Kluwer Academic/Plenum.

Antony, M. M., Purdon, C. L., Huta, V., & Swinson, R. P. (1998). Dimensions of perfectionism across the anxiety disorders. *Behaviour Research and Therapy, 36,* 1143–1154.

Antony, M. M., Roth, D., Swinson, R. P., Huta, V., & Devins, G. M. (1998). Illness intrusiveness in individuals with panic disorder, obsessive compulsive disorder, or social phobia. *Journal of Nervous and Mental Disease, 186,* 311–315.

Antony, M. M., & Swinson, R. P. (2000a). *Phobic disorders and panic in adults: A guide to assessment and treatment*. Washington, DC: American Psychological Association.

Antony, M. M., & Swinson, R. P. (2000b). *The shyness and social anxiety workbook: Proven techniques for overcoming your fears.* Oakland, CA: New Harbinger.

Arntz, A., Lavy, E., van den Berg, G., & van Rijsoort, S. (1993). Negative beliefs of spider phobics: A psychometric evaluation of the Spider Phobia Beliefs Questionnaire. *Advances in Behaviour Research and Therapy, 15,* 257–277.

Baker, B. L., Cohen, D. C., & Saunders, J. T. (1973). Self-directed desensitization for acrophobia. *Behaviour Research and Therapy, 11,* 79–89.

Ballenger, J. C., Davidson, J. R. T., Lecrubier, Y., Nutt, D. J., Bobes, J., Beidel, D. C., Ono, Y., & Westenberg, H. G. M. (1998). Consensus statement on social anxiety disorder from the international consensus group on depression and anxiety. *Journal of Clinical Psychiatry, 59,* 54–60.

Beck, J. G., Carmin, C. N., & Henninger, N. J. (1998). The utility of the Fear Survey Schedule-III: An extended replication. *Journal of Anxiety Disorders, 12,* 177–182.

Beidel, D. C., Turner, S. M., & Fink, C. M. (1996). Assessment of childhood social phobia: Construct, convergent, and discriminative validity of the Social Phobia and Anxiety Inventory for Children (SPAI-C). *Psychological Assessment, 8,* 235–240.

Bisserbe, J.-C., Weiller, E., Boyer, P., Lépine, J.-P., & Lecrubier, Y. (1996). Social phobia in primary care: Level of recognition and drug use. *International Clinical Psychopharmacology, 11,* 25–28.

Booth, R., & Rachman, S. (1992). The reduction of claustrophobia: I. *Behaviour Research and Therapy, 30,* 207–221.

Bourque, P., & Ladouceur, R. (1980). An investigation of various performance-based treatments with acrophobics. *Behaviour Research and Therapy, 18,* 161–170.

Brown, D. R., Eaton, W. W., & Sussman, L. (1990). Racial differences in prevalence of phobic disorders. *Journal of Nervous and Mental Disease, 178,* 434–441.

Brown, E. J., Turovsky, J., Heimberg, R. G., Juster, H. R., Brown, T. A., & Barlow, D. H. (1997). Validation of the Social Interaction Anxiety Scale and the Social Phobia Scale across the anxiety disorders. *Psychological Assessment, 9,* 21–27.

Brown, T. A., Di Nardo, P. A., & Barlow, D. H. (1994). *Anxiety Disorders Interview Schedule for DSM-IV (ADIS-IV).* Albany, NY: Graywind.

Brown, T. A., Di Nardo, P. A., Lehman, C. L., & Campbell, L. A. (2001). Reliability of DSM-IV anxiety and mood disorders: Implications for the classification of emotional disorders. *Journal of Abnormal Psychology, 110,* 49–58.

Chambless, D. L., Caputo, G. C., Bright, P., & Gallagher, R. (1984). Assessment of "fear of fear" in agoraphobics: The Body Sensations Questionnaire and the Agoraphobic Cognitions Questionnaire. *Journal of Consulting and Clinical Psychology, 52,* 1090–1097.

Cheek, J. M., & Buss, A. H. (1981). Shyness and sociability. *Journal of Personality and Social Psychology, 41,* 330–339.

Cohen, D. C. (1977). Comparison of self-report and overt-behavioral procedures for assessing acrophobia. *Behavior Therapy, 8,* 17–23.

Connor, K. M., Davidson, J. R. T., Churchill, L. E., Sherwood, A., Foa, E., & Wesler, R. H. (2000). Psychometric properties of the Social Phobia Inventory (SPIN). *British Journal of Psychiatry, 176,* 379–386.

Corah, N. L. (1969). Development of a dental anxiety scale. *Journal of Dental Research, 48,* 596.

Cox, B. J., Ross, L., Swinson, R. P., & Direnfeld, D. M. (1998). A comparison of social phobia outcome measures in cognitive-behavioral group therapy. *Behavior Modification, 22,* 285–297.

Craske, M. G., Antony, M. M., & Barlow, D. H. (1997). *Mastery of your specific phobia (therapist guide).* San Antonio, TX: Psychological Corporation.

Craske, M. G., Mohlman, J., Yi, J., Glover, D., & Valeri, S. (1995). Treatment of claustrophobias and snake/spider phobias: Fear of arousal and fear of context. *Behaviour Research and Therapy, 33,* 197–203.

Craske, M. G., & Sipsas, A. (1992). Animal phobias versus claustrophobias: Exteroceptive versus interoceptive cues. *Behaviour Research and Therapy, 30,* 569–581.

Curtis, G. C., Hill, E. M., & Lewis, J. A. (1990). *Heterogeneity of DSM-III-R simple phobia and the simple phobia/agoraphobia boundary: Evidence from the ECA study* (Report to the DSM-IV Anxiety Disorders Work-Group). Ann Arbor: University of Michigan Press.

Davidson, J. R. T., Miner, C. M., De Veaugh-Geiss, J., Tupler, L. A., Colket, J. T., & Potts, N. L. S. (1997). The Brief Social Phobia Scale: A psychometric evaluation. *Psychological Medicine, 27,* 161–166.

Davidson, J. R. T., Potts, N. L. S., Richichi, E. A., Ford, S. M., Krishnan, K. R. R., Smith, R. D., & Wilson, W. (1991). The brief social phobia scale. *Journal of Clinical Psychiatry, 52,* 48–51.

de Jongh, A., Muris, P., Schoenmakers, N., & Horst, G. T. (1995). Negative cognitions of dental phobics: Reliability and validity of the Dental Cognitions Questionnaire. *Behaviour Research and Therapy, 33,* 507–515.

Descutner, C. J., & Thelen, M. H. (1991). Development and validation of Fear-of-Intimacy Scale. *Psychological Assessment, 3,* 218–225.

Devins, G. M., Binik, Y. M., Hutchinson, T. A., Hollomby, D. J., Barré, P. E., & Guttman, R. D. (1983). The emotional impact of end-stage renal disease: Importance of patients' perceptions of intrusiveness and control. *International Journal of Psychiatry in Medicine, 13,* 327–343.

Di Nardo, P., Brown, T. A., & Barlow, D. H. (1994). *Anxiety Disorders Interview Schedule for DSM-IV.* San Antonio, TX: Psychological Corporation.

Doi, S. C., & Thelen, M. H. (1993). The Fear-of-Intimacy Scale: Replication and extension. *Psychological Assessment, 5,* 377–383.

Febbraro, G. A. R., & Clum, G. A. (1995). A dimensional analysis of claustrophobia. *Journal of Psychopathology and Behavioral Assessment, 17,* 335–351.

Fenigstein, A., Scheier, M. F., & Buss, A. H. (1975). Public and private self-consciousness: Assessment and theory. *Journal of Consulting and Clinical Psychology, 43,* 522–527.

First, M. B., Spitzer, R. L., Gibbon, M., & Williams, J. B. W. (1996). *Structured Clinical Interview for Axis I DSM-IV Disorders—Patient Edition (SCID-I/P Version 2. 0).* New York: Biometrics Research Department, New York State Psychiatric Institute.

Fredrikson, M. (1983). Reliability and validity of some specific fear questionnaires. *Scandinavian Journal of Psychology, 24,* 331–334.

Friedman, S. (2001). Cultural issues in the assessment of anxiety disorders. In M. M. Antony, S. M. Orsillo, & L. Roemer (Eds.) *Practitioner's guide to empirically based measures of anxiety.* New York: Kluwer Academic/Plenum.

Frost, R. O., Marten, P., Lahart, C., & Rosenblate, R. (1990). The dimensions of perfectionism. *Cognitive Therapy and Research, 14,* 449–468.

Gaynes, B. N., Magruder, K. M., Burns, B. J., Wagner, H. R., Yarnall, K. S. H., & Broadhead, W. E. (1999). Does a coexisting anxiety disorder predict persistence of depressive illness in primary care patients with major depression? *General Hospital Psychiatry, 21,* 158–167.

Geer, J. H. (1965). The development of a scale to measure fear. *Behaviour Research and Therapy, 3,* 45–53.

Gilkinson, H. (1942). Social fears as reported by students in college speech classes. *Speech Monographs, 9,* 131–160.

Glass, C. R., Merluzzi, T. V., Biever, J. L., & Larsen, K. H. (1982). Cognitive assessment of social anxiety: Development and validation of a self-statement questionnaire. *Cognitive Therapy and Research, 6,* 37–55.

Gould, R. A., Buckminster, S., Pollack, M. H., Otto, M. W., & Yap, L. (1997). Cognitive-behavioral and pharmacological treatment for social phobia: A meta-analysis. *Clinical Psychology: Science and Practice, 4,* 291–306.

Haidt, J., McCauley, C., & Rozin, P. (1994). Individual differences in sensitivity to disgust: Scale sampling seven domains of disgust elicitors. *Personality and Individual Differences, 16,* 701–713.

Haidt, J., Rozin, P., McCauley, C., & Imada, S. (1997). Body, psyche, and culture: The relationship between disgust and morality. *Psychology and Developing Societies, 9,* 107–131.

Haug, T., Brenne, L., Johnsen, B. H., Berntzen, D., Götestam, K. G., & Hugdahl, K. (1987). The three-systems analysis of fear of flying: A comparison of a consonant vs. a non-consonant treatment method. *Behaviour Research and Therapy, 25,* 187–194.

Haug, T. T., Hellstrom, K., Blomhoff, S., Humble, M., Madsbu, H. P., & Wold, J. E. (2000). The treatment of social phobia in general practice. Is exposure therapy feasible? *Family Practice, 17,* 114–118.

Heimberg, R. G., Dodge, C. S., Hope, D. A., Kennedy, C. R., & Zollo, L. J. (1990). Cognitive behavioral group treatment for social phobia: Comparison with a credible placebo control. *Cognitive Therapy and Research, 14,* 1–23.

Heimberg, R. G., Horner, K. J., Safren, S. A., Brown, E. G., Schneier, F. R., & Liebowitz, M. R. (1999). Psychometric properties of the Liebowitz Social Anxiety Scale. *Psychological Medicine, 29,* 199–212.

Heimberg, R. G., Makris, G. S., Juster, H. R., Öst, L.-G., & Rapee, R. M. (1997). Social phobia: A preliminary cross-national comparison. *Depression and Anxiety, 5,* 130–133.

Heimberg, R. G., Mennin, D. S., & Jack, M. S. (1999). Computer-assisted rating scales for social phobia: Reliability and validity may not be what they appear. *Depression and Anxiety, 9,* 44–45.

Hellström, R. G., Fellenius, J., & Öst, L.-G. (1996). One versus five sessions of applied tension in the treatment of blood phobia. *Behaviour Research and Therapy, 34,* 101–112.

Hewitt, P. L., & Flett, G. L. (1991). Perfectionism in the self and social contexts: Conceptualization, assessment, and association with psychopathology. *Journal of Personality and Social Psychology, 60,* 456–470.

Hofmann, S. G., & DiBartolo, P. M. (2000). An instrument to assess self-statements during public speaking: Scale development and preliminary psychometric properties. *Behavior Therapy, 31,* 499–515.

Hong, N. N., & Zinbarg, R. E. (1999, November). *Assessing the fear of dogs: The Dog Phobia Questionnaire.* Paper presented at the meeting of the Association for Advancement of Behavior Therapy, Toronto, ON.

Hope, D. A., Heimberg, R. G., Juster, H. R., & Turk, C. L. (2000). *Managing social anxiety.* San Antonio, TX: Psychological Corporation.

Hugdahl, K., & Öst, L-G. (1985). Subjectively rated physiological and cognitive symptoms in six different clinical phobias. *Personality and Individual Differences, 6,* 175–188.

Jones, M. K., Whitmont, S., & Menzies, R. G. (1996). Danger expectancies and insight in spider phobia. *Anxiety, 2,* 179–185.

Jones, W. H., & Russell, D. (1982). The Social Reticence Scale: An objective instrument to measure shyness. *Journal of Personality Assessment, 46,* 629–631.

Kellner, R. (1986). *Somatization and hypochondriasis.* New York: Praeger.

Kellner, R. (1987). *Abridged manual of the Illness Attitudes Scale.* Albuquerque: Department of Psychiatry, School of Medicine, University of New Mexico.

King, N. J., Ollendick, T. H., & Murphy, G. C. (1997). Assessment of childhood phobias. *Clinical Psychology Review, 17,* 667–687.

Kleinknecht, R. A., Dinnel, D. L., Kleinknecht, E. E., Hiruma, N., & Harada, N. (1997). Cultural factors in social anxiety: A comparison of social phobia symptoms and Taijin Kyofusho. *Journal of Anxiety Disorders, 11,* 157–177.

Kleinknecht, R. A., Kleinknecht, E. E., Sawchuk, C., Lee, T., & Lohr, J. (1999). The Medical Fear Survey: Psychometric properties. *Behavior Therapist, 22,* 109–119.

Kleinknecht, R. A., Klepac, R. K., & Alexander, L. D. (1973). Origins and characteristics of fear of dentistry. *Journal of the American Dental Association, 86,* 842–848.

Kleinknecht, R. A., & Lenz, J. (1989). Blood/injury fear, fainting, and avoidance of medically related situations: A family correspondence study. *Behaviour Research and Therapy, 27,* 537–547.

Kleinknecht, R. A., & Thorndike, R. M. (1990). The Mutilation Questionnaire as a predictor of blood/injury fear and fainting. *Behaviour Research and Therapy, 28,* 429–437.

Kleinknecht, R. A., Thorndike, R. M., & Walls, M. M. (1996). Factorial dimensions and correlates of blood, injury, injection and related medical fears: Cross validation of the Medical Fear Survey. *Behaviour Research and Therapy, 34,* 323–331.

Kleinknecht, R. A., Tolin, D. F., Lohr, J. M., & Kleinknecht, E. E. (1996, November). *Relationships between blood injury fears, disgust sensitivity, and vasovagal fainting in two independent samples.* Paper presented at the meeting of the Association for Advancement of Behavior Therapy, New York, NY.

Klieger, D. M. (1987). The Snake Anxiety Questionnaire as a measure of ophidophobia. *Educational and Psychological Measurement, 47,* 449–459.

Klieger, D. M., & Franklin, M. E. (1993). Validity of the Fear Survey Schedule in phobia research: A laboratory test. *Journal of Psychopathology and Behavioral Assessment, 15,* 207–217.

Klorman, R., Hastings, J. E., Weerts, T. C., Melamed, B. G., & Lang, P. J. (1974). Psychometric description of some specific-fear questionnaires. *Behavior Therapy, 5,* 401–409.

Kobak, K. A., Schaettle, S. C., Greist, J. H., Jefferson, J. W., Katzelnick, D. J., & Dottl, S. L. (1998). Computer-administered rating scales for social anxiety in a clinical drug trial. *Depression and Anxiety, 7,* 97–104.

Kozak, M. J., & Montgomery, G. K. (1981). Multimodal behavioral treatment of recurrent injury-scene elicited fainting (vasodepressor syncope). *Behavioural Psychotherapy, 9,* 316–321.

Leung, A. W., Heimberg, R. G., Holt, C. S., & Bruch, M. A. (1994). Social anxiety and perception of early parenting among American, Chinese American, and social phobic samples. *Anxiety, 1,* 80–89.

Liebowitz, M. R. (1987). Social phobia. *Modern Problems in Pharmacopsychiatry, 22,* 141–173.

Liebowitz, M. R., Heimberg, R. G., Fresco, D. M., Travers, J., & Stein, M. B. (2000). Social Phobia or Social Anxiety Disorder: What's in a name? *Archives of General Psychiatry, 57,* 191–192.

Lovibond, S. H., & Lovibond, P. F. (1995). *Manual for the Depression Anxiety Stress Scales* (2nd ed.). Sydney: Psychology Foundation of Australia.

Lyons, A. L., & Spicer, J. (1999). A new measure of conversational experience: The Speaking and Comfort Scale (SPEACS). *Assessment, 6,* 189–202.

Marks, I. M., & Mathews, A. M. (1979). Brief standard self-rating scale for phobic patients. *Behaviour Research and Therapy, 17,* 263–267.

Maroldo, G. K., Eisenreich, B. J., & Hall, P. (1979). Reliability of a modified Stanford shyness survey. *Psychological Reports, 44,* 706.

Mattick, R. P., & Clarke, J. C. (1998). Development and validation of measures of social phobia scrutiny fear and social interaction anxiety. *Behaviour Research and Therapy, 36,* 455–470.

McNally, R. J., & Steketee, G. S. (1985). The etiology and maintenance of severe animal phobias. *Behaviour Research and Therapy, 23,* 431–435.

Menzies, R. G., & Clarke, J. C. (1993). The etiology of fear of heights and its relationship to severity and individual response patterns. *Behaviour Research and Therapy, 31,* 355–365.

Mersch, P. P. (1995). The treatment of social phobia: The differential effectiveness of exposure in vivo and an integration of exposure in vivo, rational emotive therapy and social skills training. *Behaviour Research and Therapy, 33,* 259–269.

Muris, P., & Merckelbach, H. (1996). A comparison of two spider phobia questionnaires. *Journal of Behavior Therapy and Experimental Psychiatry, 27,* 241–244.

Nguyen, T. D., Attkisson, C. C., & Stegner, B. L. (1983). Assessment of patient satisfaction: Development and refinement of a Service Evaluation Questionnaire. *Evaluation and Program Planning, 6,* 299–313.

Orsillo, S. M. (2001). Measures for social phobia. In M. M. Antony, S. M. Orsillo, & L. Roemer (Eds.), *Practitioner's guide to empirically based measures of anxiety.* New York: Kluwer Academic/Plenum.

Osman, A., Gutierrez, P. M., Barrios, F. X., Kopper, B. A., & Chiros, C. E. (1998). The Social Phobia and Social Interaction Scales: Evaluation of psychometric properties. *Journal of Psychopathology and Behavioral Assessment, 20,* 249–264.

Öst, L.-G. (1978). Fading vs. systematic desensitization in the treatment of snake and spider phobia. *Behaviour Research and Therapy, 16,* 379–389.

Öst, L.-G. (1996). One-session group treatment for spider phobia. *Behaviour Research and Therapy, 34,* 707–715.

Öst, L.-G., Brandberg, M., & Alm, T. (1997). One versus five sessions of exposure in the treatment of flying phobia. *Behaviour Research and Therapy, 35,* 987–996.

Öst, L.-G., & Hugdahl, K. (1981). Acquisition of phobias and anxiety response patterns in clinical patients. *Behaviour Research and Therapy, 19,* 439–447.

Öst, L.-G., Lindahl, I.-L., Sterner, U., & Jerremalm, A. (1984). Exposure in vivo vs. applied relaxation in the treatment of blood phobia. *Behaviour Research and Therapy, 22,* 205–216.

Öst, L.-G., Salkovskis, P. M., & Hellström, K. (1991). One-session therapist directed exposure vs. self-exposure in the treatment of spider phobia. *Behavior Therapy, 22,* 407–422.

Öst, L.-G., & Sterner, U. (1987). Applied tension: A specific behavioral method for treatment of blood phobia. *Behaviour Research and Therapy, 25,* 25–29.

Page, A. C., Bennett, K. S., Carter, O., Smith, J., & Woodmore, K. (1997). The Blood-Injury Symptom Scale (BISS): Assessing a structure of phobic symptoms elicited by blood and injections. *Behaviour Research and Therapy, 35,* 457–464.

Pande, A. C., Davidson, J. R., Jefferson, J. W., Janney, C. A., Katzelnick, D. J., Weisler, R. H., Greist, J. H., & Sutherland, S. M. (1999). Treatment of social phobia with gabapentin: A placebo-controlled study. *Journal of Clinical Psychopharmacology, 19,* 341–348.

Paul, G. (1966). *Insight versus desensitization in psychotherapy: An experiment in anxiety reduction.* Palo Alto, CA: Stanford University Press.

Peterson, R. A., & Reiss, S. (1993). *Anxiety Sensitivity Index Revised test manual.* Worthington, OH: IDS.

Pierce, K. A., & Kirkpatrick, D. R. (1992). Do men lie on fear surveys? *Behaviour Research and Therapy, 30,* 415–418.

Pilkonis, P. A. (1977). Shyness, public and private, and its relationship to other measures of social behavior. *Journal of Personality, 45,* 585–595.

Radomsky, A. S., Rachman, S., Thordarson, D. S., McIsaac, H. K., & Teachman, B. A. (2001). The Claustrophobia Questionnaire (CLQ). *Journal of Anxiety Disorders, 15,* 287–297.

Robins, L. N., Cottler, L., Bucholz, K., & Compton, W. (1995). *The Diagnostic Interview Schedule, Version IV.* St. Louis, MO: Washington University School of Medicine.

Ronis, D. L. (1994). Updating a measure of dental anxiety: Reliability, validity, and norms. *Journal of Dental Hygiene, 68,* 228–233.

Schneier, F. R., Johnson, J., Hornig, C. D., Liebowitz, M. R., & Weissman, M. M. (1992). Social phobia: Comorbidity and morbidity in an epidemiologic sample. *Archives of General Psychiatry, 49,* 282–288.

Scholing, A., & Emmelkamp, P. M. (1993). Exposure with and without cognitive therapy for generalized social phobia: Effects of individual and group treatment. *Behaviour Research and Therapy, 31,* 667–681.

Segal, D. L., Hersen, M., & van Hasselt, V. B. (1994). Reliability of the Structured Clinical Interview for DSM-III-R: An evaluative review. *Comprehensive Psychiatry, 35,* 316–327.

Shear, M. K., Feske, U., Brown, C., Clark, D. B., Mammen, O., & Scotti, J. (2000). Anxiety disorders measures. In Task Force for the Handbook of Psychiatric Measures (Eds.), *Handbook of psychiatric measures* (pp. 549–589). Washington, DC: American Psychiatric Association.

Sheehan, D. V., Lecrubier, Y., Sheehan, K. H., Amorim, P., Janavs, J., Weiller, E., Hergueta, T., Baker, R., & Dunbar, G. C. (1998). The Mini-International Neuropsychiatric Interview (MINI): The development and validation of a structured diagnostic psychiatric interview for DSM-IV and ICD-10. *Journal of Clinical Psychiatry, 59*(Suppl. 20), 22–33.

Sherman, M. D., & Thelen, M. H. (1996). Fear of Intimacy Scale: Validation and extension with adolescents. *Journal of Social and Personal Relationships, 13,* 507–521.

Spitzer, R. L., Williams, J. B., Kroenke, K., Linzer, M., deGruy, F. V., Hahn, S. R., Brody, D., & Johnson, J. G. (1994). Utility of a new procedure for diagnosing mental disorders in primary care. The PRIME-MD 1000 study. *Journal of the American Medical Association, 272,* 1749–1756.

Stein, M. B., Walker, J. R., & Forde, D. R. (1994). Setting diagnostic thresholds for social phobia: Considerations from a community survey of social anxiety. *American Journal of Psychiatry, 151,* 408–412.

Stouthard, M. E. A., Mellenbergh, G. J., & Hoogstraten, J. (1993). Assessment of dental anxiety: A facet approach. *Anxiety, Stress, and Coping, 6,* 89–105.

Stravynski, A., Basoglu, M., Marks, M., Sengun, S., & Marks, I. M. (1995). The distinctiveness of phobias: A discriminant analysis of fears. *Journal of Anxiety Disorders, 9,* 89–101.

Szymanski, J., & O'Donohue, W. (1995). Fear of Spiders Questionnaire. *Journal of Behavior Therapy and Experimental Psychiatry, 26,* 31–34.

Taylor, S. (1996). Meta-analysis of cognitive behavioral treatment for social phobia. *Journal of Behavior Therapy and Experimental Psychiatry, 27,* 1–9.

Tseng, W.-S., Asai, M., Kitanishi, K., McLaughlin, D. G., & Kyomen, H. (1992). Diagnostic patterns of social phobia: Comparison in Tokyo and Hawaii. *Journal of Nervous and Mental Disease, 180*, 380–385.

Turk, C. L., Fresco, D. M., & Heimberg, R. G. (1999). Cognitive behavior therapy. In M. Hersen & A. S. Bellack (Eds.), *Handbook of comparative treatments of adult disorders* (2nd ed., pp. 287–316). New York: Wiley.

Turner, S. M., Beidel, D. C., Dancu, C. V., & Keys, D. J. (1986). Psychopathology of social phobia and comparison with avoidant personality disorder. *Journal of Abnormal Psychology, 95*, 389–394.

Turner, S. M., Beidel, D. C., Dancu, C. V., & Stanley, M. A. (1989). An empirically derived inventory to measure social fears and anxiety: The Social Phobia and Anxiety Inventory. *Psychological Assessment, 1*, 35–40.

Turner, S. M., Cooley-Quill, M. R., & Beidel, D. C. (1996). Behavioral and pharmacological treatment for social phobia. In M. R. Mavissakalian & R. F. Prien (Eds.), *Long-term treatments of anxiety disorders* (pp. 343–372). Washington DC: American Psychiatric Press.

Watson, D., & Friend, R. (1969). Measurement of social-evaluative anxiety. *Journal of Consulting and Clinical Psychology, 33*, 448–457.

Watts, F. N., & Sharrock, R. (1984). Questionnaire dimensions of spider phobia. *Behaviour Research and Therapy, 22*, 575–580.

Weiller, E., Bisserbe, J. C., Boyer, P., Lépine, J. P., & Lecrubier, Y. (1996). Social phobia in general health care: An unrecognized undertreated disabling disorder. *British Journal of Psychiatry, 168*, 169–174.

Widiger, T. A. (1992). Generalized social phobia versus avoidant personality disorder: A commentary on three studies. *Journal of Abnormal Psychology, 101*, 340–343.

Wlazlo, Z., Schroeder-Hartwig, K., Hand, I., Kaiser, G., & Münchau, N. (1990). Exposure in vivo vs. social skills training for social phobia: Long-term outcome and differential effects. *Behaviour Research and Therapy, 28*, 181–193.

Wolpe, J., & Lang, P. J. (1964). A Fear Survey Schedule for use in behaviour therapy. *Behaviour Research and Therapy, 2*, 27–30.

Wolpe, J., & Lang, P. J. (1969). *Manual for the Fear Survey Schedule.* San Diego, CA: Educational and Industrial Testing Service.

Wolpe, J., & Lang, P. J. (1977). *Manual for the Fear Survey Schedule* (revised). San Diego, CA: Educational and Industrial Testing Service.

Woody, S. R., & Teachman, B. A. (2000). Intersection of disgust and fear: Normative and pathological views. *Clinical Psychology: Science and Practice, 7*, 291–311.

Zimbardo, P. G. (1977). *Shyness: What it is, what to do about it.* Reading, MA: Addison-Wesley.

5

Generalized Anxiety Disorder

Laura A. Campbell
Timothy A. Brown

The assessment of generalized anxiety disorder (GAD) presents numerous challenges to the clinician. The phenomena that comprise the essential features of GAD are present to some degree both in normal human functioning and in the symptoms associated with other psychological disorders. Determining whether the patient's symptoms meet the threshold for clinical diagnosis, and successfully differentiating GAD from other disorders, requires a thorough assessment that is based on a sophisticated understanding of psychopathology. A comprehensive assessment of GAD combines information gathered from several sources, including clinical interviews, questionnaires, and self-monitoring records. This chapter aims to provide clinicians with practical information for assessing GAD in this manner and discusses the theoretical advances that have influenced current conceptualizations and methods of assessment of GAD. Guidelines for assessment of GAD within primary and managed care settings are also provided, as patients with psychological disorders are increasingly evaluated in these settings.

OVERVIEW OF GENERALIZED ANXIETY DISORDER

The Evolution of Generalized Anxiety Disorder as a Diagnostic Category

The central feature of GAD is chronic worry about a number of life matters that is judged to be excessive and uncontrollable. To assign a diagnosis of GAD, the clinician must determine that the worry has been present more days than not for at least 6 months, and that the worry is accompanied by at least three of six associated symptoms: restlessness, fatigability, concentration difficulties, irritability, muscle tension, and sleep disturbance. The diagnosis of GAD should not be assigned if the worry and associated symptoms occur exclusively during the course of a mood disorder, psychotic disorder, pervasive developmental disorder, or posttraumatic stress disorder. In addition, anxiety or worry that is attributable to another Axis I disorder (e.g., panic disorder) does not count toward a diagnosis of GAD. Finally, the symptoms cannot be due to the physiological effects of a substance (drugs of abuse or medications) or a general medical condition (e.g., hyperthyroidism).

The criteria just outlined represent the current conceptualization of GAD as described in the fourth edition of the *Diagnostic and Statistical Manual of Mental Disorders* (DSM-IV; American Psychiatric Association, 1994). Within this apparently straightforward definition exist a number of potentially difficult diagnostic issues for the clinician. For instance, worry is a nearly universal human experience; thus, the clinician must ascertain whether the patient's worry is excessive, difficult to control, and wide-ranging enough to merit a diagnosis of GAD. In addition, anxious apprehension constitutes a feature of all of the anxiety disorders in DSM-IV (Barlow, 2002), so the diagnostician must consider whether the focus of the patient's worry suggests that another, more specific anxiety disorder is present. For example, if most of the patient's concerns are related to being evaluated negatively by others, the diagnosis of social phobia may be more suitable. Yet another complication of making a diagnosis of GAD involves adhering to the hierarchical rules specified by DSM-IV. Most commonly, the diagnostician must establish that the symptoms of GAD have existed independently from depressive psychopathology for at least 6 months.

The diagnostic category of GAD has undergone substantial revision since it first appeared in the third edition of the DSM (DSM-III; American Psychiatric Association, 1980). In its first iteration, GAD was a residual category that was assigned when patients displayed anxious symptoms but did not meet criteria for any other specific anxiety or mood disorder described in DSM-III. A diagnosis of GAD was assigned if the patient presented with symptoms from at least three of four symptom clusters: motor tension, autonomic hyperactivity, apprehensive expectation, and vigilance/scanning. These symptoms must have been present for at least 1 month for the diagnosis to be given. The DSM-III criteria for GAD proved to be problematic in that diagnostic reliability was lower than that of other anxiety disorders (Di Nardo, O'Brien, Barlow, Waddell, & Blanchard, 1983).

In an effort to improve reliability and better capture the unique features of GAD, the criteria were revised in DSM-III-R (American Psychiatric Association, 1987). It was in this edition of DSM that excessive worry became the key feature of GAD. Moreover, the hierarchical rule that disallowed diagnosis of GAD in the presence of another anxiety disorder was omitted. With regard to its relationship to the mood disorders, it was specified that GAD could not be assigned if the relevant symptoms occurred exclusively within the course of a mood disorder. In order to capture the typically diffuse nature of worry in individuals with GAD, the DSM-III-R criteria required that at least two distinct spheres of worry be apparent and that the worry be "excessive and/or unrealistic" in nature. Furthermore, a more stringent 6-month duration criterion was implemented to foster a clearer boundary between GAD and other conditions such as adjustment disorders and nonpathological worry. The associated symptoms of GAD remained largely the same—that is, symptoms of motor tension, autonomic hyperactivity, and vigilance/scanning were represented. For the diagnosis to be assigned, at least 6 of 18 associated symptoms needed to be present.

Despite the redefinition of GAD in DSM-III-R, research indicated that problems remained with this diagnosis. GAD continued to have poor interrater reliability, even when structured interviews were employed (e.g., kappa = .53; Di Nardo, Moras, Barlow, Rapee, & Brown, 1993). Interviewers tended to disagree as to whether two or more distinct worry areas were present, whether the worry was excessive or unrealistic, and whether the nature of the worry was better captured by a more specific Axis I diagnosis (Di Nardo et al., 1993). In addition to reliability problems, high comorbidity rates with other Axis I disorders raised the question of whether GAD should be conceptualized as a prodromal or residual form of other disorders rather than as an independent diagnosis (Brown & Barlow, 1992; Brown, Barlow, & Liebowitz, 1994). Furthermore, the anxious apprehension that comprised the major criterion for diagnosis of GAD was present in varying forms in other anxiety and mood disorders (Barlow, 2002), which further questioned the discriminant validity of GAD.

These difficulties provoked considerable debate during the development of DSM-IV over whether GAD should be retained as a formal diagnostic category. Brown (1997) reviewed some of the principal justifications for the decision to revise but not discard the GAD category. Numerous studies had shown that patients with GAD could be distinguished from patients with other anxiety disorders and normal controls on measures of worry. Specifically, individuals with GAD appeared to have unique difficulty with controlling the worry process when compared to individuals without a GAD diagnosis (Borkovec, 1994; Sanderson & Barlow, 1990). Patients with GAD were also distinguishable from normal and patient controls on self-report scales of worry, like the Penn State Worry Questionnaire (Brown, Antony, & Barlow, 1992; Meyer, Miller, Metzger, & Borkovec, 1990).

In DSM-IV, the diagnostic criteria for GAD were refined in a further effort to improve reliability and discriminant validity. Evidence that GAD patients found it particularly difficult to control their worry led to an emphasis on the uncontrollability of the worry rather than on the number of worry areas. The DSM-IV criteria also omitted the descriptor "unrealistic" from the definition of GAD, in recognition of the fact that pathological worry may include excessive, uncontrollable worry about realistic concerns (e.g., financial trouble).

The associated symptoms criterion for GAD also underwent substantial revision in response to research that demonstrated that motor tension and hypervigilance symptoms were endorsed most frequently by individuals with GAD (Brawman-Mintzer et al., 1994; Marten et al., 1993; Noyes et al., 1992). In contrast, the DSM-III-R autonomic hyperactivity symptoms were endorsed with less relative frequency. This was consistent with laboratory data that indicated that GAD was not associated with autonomic hyperactivity but, rather, with autonomic inflexibility and low parasympathetic tone (Hoehn-Saric, McLeod, & Zimmerli, 1989; Thayer, Friedman, & Borkovec, 1996). The autonomic hyperactivity symptoms were omitted from the DSM-IV criteria for GAD, and they are now conceptualized as more indicative of panic states than of chronic worry. The DSM-IV associated symptom criterion includes only symptoms of motor tension and vigilance/scanning that were relatively common among people who received a diagnosis of GAD. A subsequent study found that these associated symptoms have high endorsement rates among individuals with GAD and higher correlations with worry than autonomic hyperactivity symptoms do (Brown, Marten, & Barlow, 1995).

Preliminary results from our center indicate that the DSM-IV revisions to the GAD diagnostic category have indeed improved its reliability (Brown, Di Nardo, Lehman, & Campbell, 2001). In our study, 362 patients presenting for assessment underwent two independent assessments with the Anxiety Disorders Interview Schedule for DSM-IV: Lifetime Version (ADIS-IV-L; Di Nardo, Brown, & Barlow, 1994). The kappa coefficient for the principal diagnosis of GAD was .67, which places it in the range of good reliability. There was also good agreement when GAD was assigned as a lifetime diagnosis (kappa = .65). When interviewers disagreed on the presence of GAD, a large portion of the time (74%) this was due to the assignment by one clinician of a mood disorder instead of GAD. Consistent with other evidence, this suggests that the mood disorders may pose a greater boundary problem for GAD than do other anxiety disorders.

Although the preceding discussion focused on the conceptualization of GAD throughout the latest editions of DSM, it should be noted that GAD is described in another widely used classification system, the 10th edition of the *International Classification of Diseases* (ICD-10; World Health Organization, 1992). In ICD-10, GAD is defined as prominent tension, worry, and apprehension about everyday events and problems that occur persistently for at least a 6-month period. The patient must also report at least 4 of 22 associated symptoms, which represent autonomic arousal, motor tension, changes in mental state, and other nonspecific physical symptoms (e.g., chest and abdomen symptoms).

Epidemiology

The most recent prevalence data for GAD come from the National Comorbidity Survey (NCS), a community-based study in which more than 8,000 individuals were evaluated with structured diagnostic interviews (Kessler et al., 1994; Wittchen, Zhao, Kessler, & Eaton, 1994). Prevalence estimates for DSM-III-R GAD were 1.6% and 5.1% for current and lifetime GAD, respectively. These estimates were made without consideration of the DSM-III-R hierarchy rules (hence, GAD was assigned even if it occurred during the course of a mood disorder). Although the hierarchy rule was ignored, the investigators reported that prevalence estimates did not change substantially when these rules were imposed. Specifically, only 8% of individuals with GAD indicated that their excessive worry occurred exclusively during episodes of other disorders. Prevalence estimates of lifetime GAD in the NCS were considerably higher when ICD-10 diagnostic rules were employed (8.9%).

The NCS reported a 2:1 female-to-male preponderance of GAD, which confirmed the gender ratios found in other community studies (Wittchen et al., 1994). GAD was also particularly common in women aged 45 and older (current 3.5%, lifetime 10.3%). Finally, being previously married, being unemployed, being a homemaker, and living in the northeastern United States were all associated with significantly higher risk of GAD.

Comorbidity

In the NCS, fully 90.4% of individuals with a lifetime history of GAD met criteria for at least one other lifetime disorder. Two-thirds of individuals with current GAD also reported symptoms that merited another current diagnosis. The disorders most likely to be comorbid with GAD were depressive disorders, panic disorder, and agoraphobia. Comorbidity was associated with a significantly greater probability of seeking professional help, which suggests that individuals who present for GAD treatment will be very likely to have multiple diagnoses. Of all the individuals who met criteria for GAD in the NCS, 21.8% were judged to have "primary" GAD (i.e., GAD was their only disorder or the disorder with the earliest age of onset).

In a study that involved a sample of patients presenting to an anxiety disorders clinic, DSM-III-R GAD was associated with one of the highest levels of comorbidity (Brown & Barlow, 1992). GAD was also the most frequently assigned additional diagnosis when another disorder was primary. Studies of patient samples have found that more than 75% of individuals with primary GAD meet criteria for another anxiety or mood disorder (Brawman-Mintzer et al., 1993; Brown & Barlow, 1992). Common additional diagnoses include panic disorder, mood disorders, social phobia, and specific phobia. Also, one study has examined the prevalence of personality disorders in individuals with anxiety disorders (Sanderson, Wetzler, Beck, & Betz, 1994). It was found that 49% of individuals with GAD also met criteria for an Axis II diagnosis.

Onset and Course

The individual with GAD often remarks that he or she has "always been a worrier." In contrast to individuals with other anxiety or mood disorders, many persons with GAD have difficulty identifying a distinct age or date of onset, or they report symptoms dating back to childhood (e.g., Noyes et al., 1992; Sanderson & Barlow, 1990). The fact that individuals often have a lifelong history of pathological worry has prompted some researchers and clinicians to describe GAD as a "characterological" disorder. Indeed, some patients report that being a worrier is a fundamental aspect of their personality. Other patients, however, are able to link the onset of their tendency to worry to specific events in their adulthood (Brown, 1997). In these cases, the onset of GAD is usually associated with a stressful life circumstance. Shores et al. (1992) found that individuals who reported an earlier age of onset for GAD (less than 25 years old) had trends for more severe anxiety and depressive symptoms.

With regard to course, GAD tends to be a chronic, sometimes lifelong, condition. Data from the Harvard/Brown Anxiety Research Program study indicated that the mean duration of GAD at the time of patients' enrollment in the study was 20 years (Yonkers, Warshaw, Massion, & Keller, 1996). In this study, remission from GAD was uncommon even in patients who received treatment during the 3-year study period. Although the course of GAD tends to be chronic rather than episodic, it has been noted that fluctuations in GAD symptoms may occur in response to the presence or absence of life stressors (Blazer, Hughes, & George, 1987).

Etiology

Early studies of the contribution of genetic factors to GAD failed to find much evidence for a specific genetic predisposition. However, many of these studies employed selection criteria for patients with GAD that have since undergone substantial revision. Two twin studies using DSM-III criteria for GAD found similar concordance rates for the presence of GAD in monozygotic and dizygotic twins, suggesting a minimal role for genetic factors in the manifestation of GAD (Andrews, Stewart, Allen, & Henderson, 1990; Torgersen, 1983). In contrast, more recent genetic studies that employed DSM-III-R criteria found stronger evidence for a genetic component to GAD. Kendler, Neale, Kessler, Heath, and Eaves (1992a) studied a large sample of female twins ($N = 1,033$) and concluded that GAD was a moderately familial disorder, with approximately 30% heritability. Interestingly, there is also compelling evidence that GAD and major depression may be phenotypic expressions of the same genetic vulnerability. In another study, Kendler et al. (1992b) examined lifetime diagnoses of GAD and MDD in their sample of female twins. They concluded that "genetic factors were important for both major depression and generalized anxiety disorder and were completely shared between the two disorders . . . so that whether a vulnerable woman develops major depression or generalized anxiety disorder is a result of her environmental experiences" (p. 716).

While the nature of these differential environmental experiences is not yet clear, evidence does suggest that stressful life events play a significant role in the onset and persistence of GAD. Blazer et al. (1987) noted that the occurrence of one or more negative life events increased the risk of developing GAD in the following year by threefold. Other theorists have posited that early experiences are significant contributors to the development of GAD, although their theories have remained largely untested. Among the theories put forth, early experiences of uncontrollability over the environment (Barlow, 2002), psychosocial trauma (Borkovec, 1994), and insecure attachment to caregivers (Borkovec, 1994) have been conceptualized as risk factors for GAD.

The genetic evidence for a shared neurobiological diathesis for both GAD and depression converges with evidence from studies of personality dimensions and their relationship to these disorders. Many studies have supported predictions of the tripartite model of anxiety and depression (Brown, Chorpita, & Barlow, 1998; Clark & Watson, 1991). The tripartite model posits that anxiety and depression share the higher-order trait of negative affect but can be distinguished by the unique traits of low positive affect (depression) and autonomic arousal (anxiety). More recently, models based on the original tripartite theory have acknowledged that autonomic arousal may have primary relevance to panic disorder and be less definitive of other anxiety disorders (Brown et al., 1998; Mineka, Watson, & Clark, 1998). Nonetheless, the overall evidence for the tripartite model suggests that negative affect may be considered a vulnerability factor for anxiety and mood disorders, including GAD.

Treatment

Although treatment is not a major focus of this chapter, certainly a number of treatments are associated with significant reduction of GAD symptoms. GAD remains a difficult disorder to treat effectively, and there is certainly room for improvement in GAD treatment outcome. The most efficacious psychosocial treatments have relied primarily on cognitive and behavioral techniques. A number of pharmacological treatments have also been tested, with moderate results.

Spiegel, Wiegel, Baker, and Greene (2000) have recently reviewed findings in the area of pharmacotherapy for GAD. They reported that benzodiazepines, azapirones (e.g., buspirone), and antidepressants have demonstrated their superiority to placebo treatment. However, there are several limitations to these drugs, including the presence of unpleasant side effects, withdrawal problems, and the fact that many patients with GAD do not experience significant alleviation of their symptoms. Moreover, certain medications (e.g., benzodiazepines) alleviate the somatic symptoms of anxiety but not necessarily excessive worry (Spiegel & Barlow, 2000). In addition, most pharmacotherapy studies have not evaluated the long-term outcome of patients treated with these interventions.

Psychosocial treatment consists of strategies that target excessive, uncontrollable worry and persistent overarousal. For the most part, cognitive interventions have been used to address excessive worry, whereas relaxation exercises have been used for reduction of overarousal and tension. These treatments have usually been administered in 12 to 15 sessions, and they include exercises for the patient to complete outside of the treatment sessions. Early studies found cognitive-behavioral treatments (CBT) to be more efficacious than no treatment but did not establish the superiority of CBT over nondirective treatments (e.g., Barlow, Rapee, & Brown, 1992; Borkovec & Mathews, 1988). In a more recent study, Borkovec and Costello (1993) found that CBT and applied relaxation (AR) were indeed superior to nondirective therapy in treating GAD. In this study, individuals who received CBT achieved the highest end-state functioning, and gains were maintained for both CBT and AR over a 6-month follow-up period. Barlow et al. (1992) also found that the moderate treatment gains in their sample were maintained over a 2-year follow-up period and that patients decreased their use of anxiolytic medications considerably as a result of treatment.

In a recent meta-analysis, Gould, Otto, Pollack, and Yap (1997) found that CBT for GAD produced moderate to large effect sizes on measures of anxiety severity. Overall effect sizes for CBT and pharmacological interventions did not differ significantly. Among the studies of CBT, treatment packages that combined cognitive and behavioral strategies produced larger effect sizes than did treatments that used only one of these approaches. As well, one advantage of CBT over medication treatment appeared to be a greater reduction in associated depressive symptoms.

PRACTICAL ISSUES IN THE ASSESSMENT OF GENERALIZED ANXIETY DISORDER

Establishing the Presence of DSM-IV Generalized Anxiety Disorder

People who ultimately receive a diagnosis of GAD experience persistent worry and tension. They may initially complain of feeling consumed by worry or about consistently worrying about unimportant matters. Individuals with GAD may recognize before treatment that they have a tendency to anticipate the worst and that their concerns are excessive or uncontrollable. Some people with GAD focus their complaint around the physical manifestations of their anxiety, stating that they always feel keyed up or experience physical discomfort in the form of muscle tension or headaches. Others may emphasize that they have difficulty falling asleep due to an inability to turn off the worry process at the end of the day. The excessive worry and tension often lead to problems in work, school, and interpersonal functioning. This life interference may finally prompt individuals with GAD to seek treatment.

Like the other anxiety disorders, GAD is characterized by a process of what Barlow (2002) has called "anxious apprehension." This involves a future-focused state in which the person anticipates and prepares for upcoming negative events. This mood state is accompanied by an attentional focus on threat-related stimuli, high negative affect, and chronic tension and overarousal. Whereas the content of the anxious apprehension is quite specific for many of the anxiety disorders (e.g., anticipation of physical catastrophe in panickers), the focus of concern is usually diffuse for patients with GAD. Borkovec (1994) has stated that GAD is associated with a diffuse perception that the world is threatening and that it will be difficult to control or cope with future negative events.

Once the clinician has established that a patient experiences significant worry and tension, he or she must decide whether the nature and level of the worry merits a clinical diagnosis of GAD. In the following paragraphs, suggestions for the clinician's inquiry are based largely on the line of questioning included in the Anxiety Disorders Interview Schedule for DSM-IV: Lifetime Version (ADIS-IV-L; Di Nardo et al., 1994). The ADIS-IV-L is a semi-structured clinical interview that is discussed in detail in a later section of this chapter. Refer to Appendix 5.1 for the initial screening and current episode inquiry included in the GAD section of the ADIS-IV-L.

The first question posed in the GAD section of the ADIS-IV-L is the screening item, "Over the last several months, have you been continually worried or anxious about a number of events or activities in your daily life?" This enables the clinician to start gathering information about the frequency, duration, and diffuseness of the worry. If the patient answers in the affirmative, the clinician should then inquire about the content of the patient's worry. An open-ended question such as, "What kinds of things do you worry about?" can provide a rough idea about the range or pervasiveness of the worry. Individuals with GAD may worry about a multitude of topics, although most of their worries can be categorized within several broad domains. At our center, we find that most GAD worries consist of the following types: minor matters, work or school, finances, family and other relationships, health (of self and others), and community and world affairs. Most patients have several areas of concern, and, in fact, the diagnosis of GAD cannot be assigned if only one area of worry is present.

Worry is a universal human experience, and many people worry about the same life matters as patients with GAD. The clinician must therefore make a judgment regarding the excessiveness of the worry. Assessing the frequency, duration, and intensity of the worry is important in this regard. In the ADIS-IV-L, several questions are used to help the clinician make a determination of excessiveness. First, the clinician inquires about how *often* the person worries about a given domain. Is the worry about family members present every day for a significant portion of the day, or is it a fleeting concern once a week before the patient telephones his or her parents? Does the person worry about being reprimanded at work most days, or only on the day he or she receives the results of a yearly evaluation? The answers to such questions help the interviewer judge both the frequency and excessiveness of the worry.

In addition, the clinician may ask whether the person would worry about a given domain even if there were no current problems associated with it. For instance, the clinician might ask, "If things are going well at work, do you still worry about it?" This aids in determining whether the worry is out of proportion to the actual likelihood of negative events. In addition, the assessor should ask about the degree of anxiety and tension that is created by the worry. Individuals with GAD often respond emphatically to this question, describing high levels of tension in relation to their major worries. A final question the clinician may ask in order to evaluate the excessiveness of the worry is: "What percentage of an average day do you feel worried?" Most individuals who receive a diagnosis of GAD report being worried more than half of the day, and some perceive the worry to be nearly incessant.

The inquiry regarding the percentage of day worried can also inform the clinician's judgment of whether or not the worry is difficult for the patient to control. If the person is worried for the majority of the day, it is likely that he or she is unable to control the worry process effectively. To further assess controllability, the clinician may ask the patient if it is difficult to stop worrying about something once he or she starts. The clinician should also inquire about the patient's ability to "put the worry aside" when the patient needs or wants to focus on something else. The question "Do these worries ever intrude when you are trying to focus on other things (e.g., leisure activities)?" is helpful at this stage of inquiry. Difficulty stopping the worry process and worries that disrupt concentration on other tasks are strong indications that the person has trouble controlling his or her worry. If the patient endorses these characteristics, the uncontrollability criterion for diagnosis of GAD would be met.

If it has been established that the patient worries about a number of life matters in a way that is excessive and difficult to control, the clinician should proceed to inquire about time course and associated symptoms. After the clinician and patient have discussed the worry in detail, the clinician may ask when the worrying started to become a problem. If the patient reports a duration of fewer than 6 months, the formal DSM-IV diagnostic criteria for GAD would not be met. The diagnostician might consider a diagnosis of anxiety disorder not otherwise specified as an alternative. Or, if the worry and tension are in direct response to a stressor (e.g., starting a new job), the diagnosis of adjustment disorder may be appropriate. Typically, by the time the individual has sought treatment, the worry and tension have been present for well over 6 months. If this is the case, the clinician must inquire, "During the last 6 months, have you been bothered by the worries you described more days than not?" Although an affirmative answer is consistent with a diagnosis of GAD, it is still necessary for the clinician to ascertain whether the course of the symptoms overlaps with the presence of a mood disorder before judging that the diagnosis of GAD is appropriate (see "Relationship of Generalized Anxiety Disorder to Depression" below).

The associated symptoms of restlessness, fatigability, difficulty concentrating or mind going blank, irritability, muscle tension, and difficulty falling or staying asleep should also be targets of inquiry. The clinician should ask how often the patient experiences each of these symptoms. Specifically, he or she will want to ascertain that at least three of these symptoms are associated with the worry and that some have been experienced more days than not for at least 6 months. The clinician will also want to get an idea of the degree to which these symptoms are experienced, as some of them may be significant enough to constitute major focuses of treatment. For instance, if the patient reports extreme muscle tension, the treatment plan might involve a muscle relaxation exercise that is introduced early in treatment.

For most psychological diagnoses to be assigned, there must be clear evidence of interference and/or distress associated with the symptoms reported. It is extremely likely that individuals with excessive, uncontrollable worry and persistent tension will be significantly distressed, especially if they are presenting for assessment and treatment. It is also quite likely that the symptoms of GAD will affect several areas of their life in a detrimental manner. During the clinical assessment of GAD, it is helpful for the clinician to determine how the patient's worry and tension affect different aspects of his or her daily life. Direct questioning about how the symptoms affect work, relationships, daily routine, and leisure activities will help the patient describe the level of interference caused by the worry and tension.

The other element of a comprehensive assessment of GAD involves establishing that the excessive worry and tension are not attributable to another Axis I disorder, the use of a substance, or a medical condition. The issue of differentiating GAD from anxiety due to other Axis I disorders is addressed in the following section. Some medical conditions that may produce symptoms resembling anxiety are cardiac conditions (e.g., mitral valve prolapse), endocrine conditions (e.g., hyperthyroidism, hypoglycemia), neurological conditions, respiratory conditions, and pregnancy (Spiegel & Barlow, 2000). Individuals who have not had a recent physical examination should be referred for one if there is a risk for any of these conditions. It should also be noted that many types of medications have side effects that may resemble symptoms of anxiety disorders. These medications include psychotropics (e.g., antidepressants), respiratory drugs, cardiovascular drugs, medications for neurological disorders, and anesthetics (Spiegel & Barlow, 2000). If the onset of the patient's generalized anxiety and worry coincided with initiation of a medication regimen, the clinician should further investigate the possibility that the problematic anxiety is due to an adverse reaction to medication.

Differential Diagnosis

One aspect of GAD assessment that can be especially challenging is distinguishing pathological worry from the normal worry that nearly all humans experience. This task is less difficult if the clinician asks sufficient questions to determine whether or not the person's symptoms meet the criteria stated in the definition in DSM-IV. As just discussed, the worry associated with GAD is excessive in its frequency, intensity, and duration and is difficult for the patient to control. Moreover, pathological worry is distinguished from normal worry in that it causes significant interference and distress. For instance, if the person reports that they cannot enjoy leisure activities or sustain relationships due to their excessive worry and tension, then a clinical diagnosis is probably warranted.

Another difficulty with diagnosis of GAD is that many of its symptoms overlap with symptoms of other anxiety and mood disorders. It has already been mentioned that the anxious apprehension that constitutes the central feature of GAD is present to some extent in most of the other anxiety disorders. Individuals with social phobia worry about embarrassing themselves in social interactions, whereas patients with panic disorder may worry about having a panic attack and losing control of the car while driving. Such patients should not receive a diagnosis of GAD because the focus of their worry is better accounted for by another anxiety disorder.

As described, individuals with GAD often worry about everyday concerns such as work, minor matters, family, relationships, and health. People with other anxiety disorders may experience anxiety in relation to these same areas. For example, an individual with social phobia may worry about work ("Will my voice shake when I comment at the meeting?"), minor matters like being on time ("If I'm late, everyone in the room will turn around and stare!"), and relationships ("She'll think I'm stupid if I call her and can't keep up the conversation."). People whose concerns always seem to trace back to a fear of negative social evaluation should not be assigned a diagnosis of GAD, even though their worries may appear similar to those in GAD. Rather, their apprehension is better captured by the more specific diagnosis of social phobia.

Similar rules apply when a patient's worries emanate from fears of the occurrence or consequences of having panic attacks. Individuals with panic disorder may worry about running errands (which would be considered a minor matter) due to the fear of panicking while far from a safe place. They may also worry about losing employment or important relationships because of the impairment associated with their recurrent panic attacks and avoidance. People with panic disorder also frequently worry about their health, because they experience physical symptoms that they misinterpret in a catastrophic fashion. They may worry that heart palpitations signal an imminent heart attack or that dizziness is a sign of an impending stroke. They may also worry about more long-term implications of having recurrent panic attacks (e.g., that they will develop heart disease). Although these individuals may worry about work, minor matters, relationships, and health, their worry is driven by the possibility of having a panic attack or by fear of the implications of their symptoms. In these cases, the diagnosis of panic disorder accounts for their apprehension, so an additional diagnosis of GAD would not be warranted. GAD should not be assigned if the focus of the excessive anxiety or worry is confined to the occurrence or implications of having a panic attack.

Discrimination between GAD and panic disorder is sometimes complicated by the presence of occasional panic attacks in individuals with GAD. Barlow (2002) reported that 73% of individuals diagnosed with DSM-III-R GAD reported experiencing at least one panic attack in their lifetime. In some cases, the clinician may judge that comorbid diagnoses of GAD and panic disorder are warranted. These would be cases in which there is persistent concern about the occurrence or consequences of panic attacks, as well as chronic worry and tension that is unrelated to panic concerns. In many cases, individuals with GAD have occasional panic attacks that do not rise to the level of clinical panic disorder. For these people, panic attacks may be the culmination of strong bouts of worry. However, patients with GAD do not demonstrate the fear of panic symptoms or apprehension about future attacks that is present in individuals with a clinical diagnosis of panic disorder. Due to this, the panic attacks do not come to constitute a separate clinical syndrome.

As mentioned, individuals with GAD often worry about their health. This occasionally introduces some ambiguity between GAD and the somatoform disorders, particularly hypochondriasis. Individuals with GAD may apply their characteristically catastrophic interpretive style to the physical symptoms they experience. For example, they may experience chest tightness and worry about the remote possibility of having emphysema. Or they may read an article about a life-threatening disease and begin to ruminate about whether they have experienced any of the symptoms of the disease, or about what would happen to them if they developed it. These ruminations about the possibility of having or developing serious illness usually differ from hypochondriacal concerns in several important ways. The first difference is with regard to belief conviction. Individuals who receive a diagnosis of hypochondriasis report a very strong belief (perhaps even absolute certainty) that they have a specific physical disease or illness. This belief is strong enough to persist for a substantial period of time (i.e., at least 6 months). In the structured interviews conducted at our center, individuals who ultimately receive a diagnosis of hypochondriasis may estimate that there is an 80% to 90% likelihood that they have a specific disease (e.g., AIDS). When confronted directly about the likelihood of having a specific disease, people with GAD rarely endorse such high levels of belief conviction. On the contrary, they are more likely to admit that having a serious illness is a remote possibility, but that they cannot help "anticipating the worst." A second element of the hypochondriasis diagnosis that is generally not shared by individuals with GAD is the experience of persistent physical symptoms that form the basis of their belief that they have a particular illness. Hypochondriacal symptoms and concerns also lead to an overutilization of medical services (i.e., frequent visits to specialists, "doctor shopping") that is not as prominent in persons with GAD. However, this distinction is somewhat complicated by findings that individuals with symptoms of GAD frequently use primary care services (Brawman-Mintzer & Lydiard, 1996).

Another anxiety disorder that is considered to have an unclear boundary with GAD is obsessive–compulsive disorder (OCD). This is mainly due to the conceptual similarity between excessive worries and obsessions. Both excessive worry and obsessions involve repetitive thoughts that are distressing to the patient and difficult to control. The definitions of worry and obsessions, however, are differentiable on a number of dimensions. Some of these distinctions were summarized by Turner, Beidel, and Stanley (1992). Obsessions are generally experienced as more intrusive than worries, and often their content seems senseless or inappropriate to the individual. Worries, on the other hand, are usually exaggerated concerns about typical life matters (e.g., work, family, minor matters). In addition, obsessions are more likely than excessive worry to provoke a distinctive behavioral reaction. These repetitive behaviors or compulsions are usually aimed at neutralizing the patient's disturbing thoughts and may fall into well-known categories, such as checking, washing, or counting. Individuals with GAD do not typically manifest these types of compulsive behaviors. Persons with GAD may exhibit "safety checking" behaviors in response to their worries (e.g., reassurance seeking, calling loved ones excessively), but this behavioral component is less prominent and usually of less concern to the patient.

Contrary to expectation, Brown, Moras, Zinbarg, and Barlow (1993) found that GAD and OCD were not difficult for clinicians to distinguish when a structured clinical interview was used. In this study, no diagnostic disagreements were the result of one interviewer assigning GAD and the other assigning OCD. Moreover, the co-occurrence of these two disorders was quite low. People who had GAD and people who had OCD were also distinguishable, for the most part, on self-report indices designed to assess the major symptoms of each disorder. Furthermore, patients with the two disorders evidenced distinct response patterns to screening questions meant to detect the presence or absence of GAD and OCD (Brown et al., 1993).

In addition to anxious apprehension being a fundamental characteristic of other disorders, many of the associated symptoms of GAD are reported by individuals with other mental disorders (i.e., they have low *specificity*). For an associated symptom to count toward a diagnosis of GAD, the clinician must determine that the symptom is not strictly the result of another Axis I condition (e.g., difficulty concentrating in social situations due to social phobia). Brown et al. (1995) determined that over 90% of patients with depression also met the associated symptom criterion for GAD. Indeed, DSM-IV GAD and major depressive disorder (MDD) share the associated symptoms of excessive fatigue, difficulty concentrating, sleep disturbance, and restlessness/agitation. The similarities between the features of GAD and the depressive disorders have been the topic of extensive scholarly discussion, and thus a separate section of this chapter is devoted to this issue.

As with many other Axis I disorders, DSM-IV requires that the clinician establish that GAD symptoms are not due to the direct physiological effects of a substance. Excessive use of alcohol or caffeine, or the use of illegal substances such as marijuana, cocaine, and amphetamines, can provoke reactions that are similar to the symptoms of anxiety disorders. The differential diagnosis between substance disorders and anxiety disorders is somewhat complicated by the fact that individuals may use substances like alcohol or marijuana to ease their anxiety and tension. In this case, the clinician must decide which problem is principal (although it is certainly possible to assign both GAD and a substance disorder). If the person's use of a substance is mainly in reaction to high levels of anxiety and tension, and the use itself does not interfere with overall functioning, it is likely that GAD would be the principal diagnosis. In other cases, the substance use is a problem in itself and, in fact, may be the most pressing problem (e.g., if the individual uses large amounts of the substance on a frequent basis). When this occurs, a substance disorder will usually be given as the principal diagnosis and will likely be the first problem to be addressed in treatment. If the onset of GAD symptoms coincides with the start of a patient's substance use, the diagnosis of substance-induced anxiety disorder should be considered.

Finally, with regard to differential diagnosis, it is important to remember to screen for medical conditions and medication reactions that may cause symptoms of GAD. A brief medical history is usually sufficient to determine whether the GAD symptoms are explained by an underlying medical condition. If the onset of generalized anxiety appears to have coincided with a new medication regimen or a medical problem, the appropriateness of a diagnosis of GAD should be questioned and a referral for medical evaluation may be necessary.

Relationship of Generalized Anxiety Disorder to Depression

The NCS found that 62.4% of people diagnosed with lifetime GAD had lifetime major depression, and 39.5% had lifetime dysthymia (Wittchen et al., 1994). Brown and Barlow (1992) reported similar estimates in a clinical sample. Due to the symptoms shared between GAD and depression, Brown (1997) has asserted that depression may pose a greater boundary problem for GAD than other anxiety disorders do. The central feature of GAD (i.e., worry or anxious apprehension) is often manifested in the rumination that is characteristic of depressive psychopathology. Furthermore, the cognitive appraisals of people who have GAD and those who have depression are similar in that negative outcomes are anticipated and self-efficacy is compromised. Finally, as noted, there is a high degree of overlap between the somatic symptoms associated with GAD and depression.

The close relationship between GAD and depression is accounted for by the aforementioned tripartite model of anxiety and depression (Clark & Watson, 1991). Excessive worry and the associated symptoms of GAD are considered manifestations of the broader trait of negative affect, which also predisposes an individual to manifest depressive symptoms. Moreover, recent research has shown that levels of negative affect are highest for persons who have GAD or depression when all anxiety and mood disorders are considered (Brown et al., 1998). The similarity of the features of GAD and depression and their frequent co-occurrence have led some theorists to argue that GAD should be considered a prodrome or associated feature of depression, rather than an independent psychopathological entity. There is some evidence that argues against this, such as confirmatory factor analysis that showed GAD and depression to be better conceptualized as separate factors than as a single "negative affect" syndrome (Brown et al., 1998). However, the fact remains that most of the time the clinician will be assessing GAD in the context of a history of depression.

Due to the evidence that excessive worry and tension may be associated features of depression, DSM-IV prohibits diagnosis of GAD when the worry and associated symptoms occur exclusively during the course of a mood disorder. Hence, it is important during a thorough assessment of GAD to establish whether the individual has experienced any periods of clinical depression. If so, careful examination of the time course of GAD and depressive symptoms should be undertaken. Unless GAD symptoms have been present at some point for 6 months without a co-occurring mood disorder, an independent diagnosis of GAD should not be assigned. In many cases, the symptoms of GAD are subsumed under the mood disorder diagnosis because they have not existed for 6 months in the absence of depression. This does not preclude administering treatment for GAD if excessive worry is the patient's primary problem and if the depressed mood seems to be reactive to the anxiety and tension. However, the official DSM-IV diagnosis for such a patient should be a mood disorder.

The following discussion of self-report measures for GAD indicates that designing scales that are specific to anxiety or depression is not an easy task. Existing scales for the assessment of anxiety and depression are highly intercorrelated (Clark & Watson, 1991; Moras, Di Nardo, & Barlow, 1992). This is yet further evidence that anxiety and depression are closely related constructs that share many features. Many questionnaires that are meant to assess anxiety are equally sensitive to depressive symptoms. This may be due to the inclusion of items that capture manifestations of negative affect, a trait that anxiety and depression share (Brown et al., 1998; Clark & Watson, 1991).

Assessment of Associated Features

There are several clinically significant features of GAD that should be explored in a thorough assessment but which are not necessary to make a diagnosis based on criteria in DSM-IV. These symptoms are typically more relevant to treatment planning than to diagnosis. Many of these associated features have been the focus of recent research on GAD and pathological worry.

Although the behavioral component of GAD is not as prominent as the behaviors associated with other anxiety disorders (e.g., compulsions in OCD and avoidance in panic disorder with agoraphobia), individuals with GAD may engage in habitual behaviors in response to their worries. Often, these behaviors alleviate anxiety in the short term but maintain worrisome thinking in the long term. In one treatment program (Craske, Barlow, & O'Leary, 1992), these types of behaviors are denoted "worry behaviors" and are directly targeted in treatment. Examples of worry behaviors are making extensive and detailed lists, calling loved ones frequently to ascertain their safety, seeking reassurance from others, and checking tasks for accuracy. To take one example, a patient may worry excessively about forgetting to do important tasks. In response to this worry, he or she may make lists that include every minor task that needs to get done. Or the patient may leave reminder notes around his or her workspace to prevent forgetfulness. These behaviors may ease anxiety on a moment-to-moment basis, because they create a greater sense of control over the feared outcome of forgetting something. However, these behaviors also serve to maintain the anxious belief that the patient is likely to forget important things and that it would be a disaster if something was forgotten. In other words, worry behaviors prevent the patient from learning that these fears are unfounded. Because reducing safety behaviors may be an important aspect of treatment, the clinician may want to inquire about them at the assessment level. The clinician may simply ask, "Is there anything that you do to reduce your anxiety about _____? How would you feel if you could not engage in that behavior?" This line of questioning may aid the clinician in developing a comprehensive treatment plan that includes modification of safety behaviors.

Individuals with GAD may have time management and problem-solving deficits that result from and/or exacerbate their worry and tension. Often, individuals with GAD feel a need to exert control over their environment and consequently have difficulty delegating and delaying completion of tasks. They may also worry so much about certain tasks that they are unable to fulfill other obligations. Furthermore, individuals with GAD may be so overwhelmed with worry that they are less able to employ effective problem-solving techniques. The clinician can ask a few screening questions during the assessment period to establish whether time management or problem-solving are issues that require intervention. For instance, one might ask, "Does your worry about these issues ever interfere with your ability to get things done? Do you often feel that you planned or wanted to do something but it did not happen because you were overwhelmed with other things?" To address problem-solving, the clinician can inquire, "Does your worrying lead to effective solutions to your problems? Do you have any other ways of solving problems when they arise? Do you feel like many of your problems are unsolvable?"

Wells and colleagues have asserted that meta-worry is a defining characteristic of GAD (e.g., Wells & Carter, 1999). Meta-worry is a cognitive process that involves appraisals of the functions and consequences of worrying. Wells and Carter (1999) reported preliminary evidence that individuals with GAD hold both positive and negative beliefs about worrying. Frequent worrying is often conceptualized as adaptive in some ways by the patient and is viewed as part of the preparation for task execution or as a method of problem-solving. In contrast, Wells and Carter (1999) also found that patients with GAD develop negative assumptions about the worry process, such as the belief that constant worry will lead to a collapse. This meta-worry may lead to avoidance of situations that trigger strong worry, which decreases the likelihood that the person will discover that his or her apprehension about everyday situations is unfounded. Wells and Carter (1999) found that meta-worry displayed a stronger relationship to pathological worry than did concerns about everyday matters.

Assessment of both positive and negative beliefs about worry may be very helpful with treatment planning. The cognitive-behavioral perspective dictates that addressing patients' dysfunctional thoughts is a crucial part of treatment. Logically, it seems that this should extend to beliefs about the purposes and consequences of worry itself. It will be difficult for an individual to substantially decrease his or her worry if strong, positive beliefs about worry as a coping strategy are held. On the other hand, negative beliefs that worry will spiral out of control and lead to a complete breakdown may also need to be challenged in order to reduce anxiety and tension in treatment. Meta-worry appears to be an important component of the symptom picture of many individuals with GAD. Assessment of this associated feature adds to the clinician's understanding of the patient's dysfunctional assumptions and facilitates treatment planning and outcome assessment. A self-report instrument for assessing meta-worry will be discussed in the next section.

The pathological worry that characterizes GAD has been postulated to serve the function of avoidance of emotionally distressing material (Borkovec, 1994; Borkovec & Hu, 1990). The tendency of individuals with GAD to "hop" from one worry to the next may prevent cognitive and emotional processing of each individual concern. People with GAD often report that they worry about a number of different things at once, which may be indicative of this "worry as avoidance" process. Clinicians may want to assess this aspect of pathological worry by inquiring whether the patient tends to worry about many things at once or whether they worry about minor matters to avoid thinking about even more unpleasant things (Borkovec & Roemer, 1995). This variable is also relevant to treatment planning in that interventions such as worry exposure (Craske et al., 1992) seek to facilitate the emotional processing of threatening material with the eventual aim of habituation.

MODES OF ASSESSMENT OF GENERALIZED ANXIETY DISORDER

Structured and Semistructured Interviews

The various revisions of the Anxiety Disorders Interview Schedule (ADIS) have been widely used to assess anxiety and mood disorders, including GAD. The latest edition of this semistructured interview, the ADIS-IV-L (Di Nardo et al., 1994), allows for a more comprehensive assessment of GAD than did previous versions of the ADIS. In addition to assessing current DSM-IV criteria for GAD, the ADIS-IV-L allows the clinician to evaluate the presence and course of lifetime GAD. Furthermore, the ADIS-IV-L elicits dimensional clinician ratings of the essential features of GAD. Clinicians rate the excessiveness of each worry area on a scale from 0 to 8 (0, no worry/tension, to 8, constantly worried/extreme tension). This rating reflects a combination of the frequency, appropriateness, and tension associated with that worry sphere. In addition, the clinician makes a separate rating that reflects the person's ability to control the worry about that aspect of their lives (0, no difficulty, to 8, extreme difficulty). The symptoms associated with GAD are also rated dimensionally by the clinician (0, none, to 8, very severe), which permits a judgment of the degree to which an individual experiences symptoms like restlessness or irritability (as opposed to simply making a "present/absent" determination for each symptom). The ADIS-IV-L then guides the assessor through a series of questions that establish the level of interference and distress associated with the GAD symptoms, rule out medication side effects and medical conditions as causes of the symptoms, and clarify the life circumstances that were present at the onset of the excessive worry and tension. See Appendix 5.1 for the actual questions from the ADIS-IV-L.

One benefit to assessment with the ADIS-IV-L is that many of its items assist in treatment planning. If the individual's primary problem is excessive worry, the ADIS-IV-L aids the clinician in determining which areas the patient tends to worry about most. Questions are also included that probe the patient's specific concerns in relation to each major worry area. Ratings of the uncontrollability of worry and the percentage of day worried help the treating clinician determine how much control the individual is able to exert over the worry process. Finally, ratings of the associated symptoms of GAD may suggest specific interventions that target these features—for example, relaxation training for muscle tension or sleep problems.

Another benefit to employing the ADIS-IV-L for assessment of GAD is that the various dimensional ratings facilitate the assignment of an overall clinical severity rating (CSR) for the diagnosis. A scale of 0 to 8 is also used for this clinician rating (0, none, to 8, very severely disturbing/disabling). The CSR can be a useful measure of treatment outcome, in that the therapist can assign a CSR for the patient's GAD at regular intervals during treatment. In general, a CSR of 4 or higher is judged to reflect the presence of a clinical level of psychopathology, whereas a CSR of 3 or lower represents a subclinical disorder.

In addition, a structured interview such as the ADIS-IV-L is a useful tool for differential diagnosis. This interview provides in-depth assessment of other anxiety disorders, mood disorders, somatoform disorders, and substance use disorders. As already discussed, it may be a challenge to distinguish many disorders in these categories from GAD. A structured clinical interview that thoroughly assesses each of these disorders increases the likelihood of achieving a valid diagnostic profile. Moreover, most individuals who receive a diagnosis of GAD are assigned at least one comorbid Axis I disorder. Presence of comorbid conditions may influence the individual's response to treatment and should therefore be a factor considered during treatment planning (Brown & Barlow, 1992). Structured interviews such as the ADIS-IV-L provide the clinician with a comprehensive diagnostic picture, including all current and lifetime comorbid diagnoses.

The ADIS-IV-L was designed with the specific purpose of thoroughly assessing the emotional disorders. There are other structured and semistructured interviews that assess a range of psychopathology using a similar format. Some of the other widely used interviews are the Structured Clinical Interview for DSM-IV Axis I disorders (SCID-I; First, Gibbon, Spitzer, & Williams, 1996), the Schedule for Affective Disorders and Schizophrenia (SADS;

Mannuzza, 1994; Schleyer, Aaronson, Mannuzza, Martin, & Fyer, 1990), and the Composite International Diagnostic Interview (CIDI; Essau & Wittchen, 1993). A main benefit of the SCID-I, SADS, and CIDI is that they assess a wider range of psychopathology than the ADIS-IV-L—for example, they provide a thorough assessment of psychotic disorders. However, the SCID-I, SADS, and CIDI rely primarily on categorical judgments made by the clinician (i.e., the presence vs. absence of a symptom or a disorder). In contrast, the ADIS-IV-L elicits dimensional ratings from the clinician that clarify the level at which the patient experiences different symptoms. As discussed, these dimensional ratings are valuable for treatment planning and outcome assessment.

Self-Report Instruments

There are many self-report inventories designed to assess anxiety, but many of them do not help the clinician distinguish between the presence of GAD versus the other anxiety disorders. As already discussed in the context of differential diagnosis, individuals with other anxiety disorders report frequent worry and symptoms of tension. Therefore, a satisfactory clinical interview should supplement the use of self-report instruments to arrive at a valid diagnosis of GAD. Nonetheless, a number of self-report questionnaires provide reliable sources of converging evidence to support the evidence for GAD that was obtained in the clinical interview. These questionnaires also have the advantage of being brief and can easily be completed by the patient throughout treatment. Hence, they are quite useful for monitoring treatment outcome.

One quantitative measure of anxiety that deserves mention, but is not actually a self-report measure, is the Hamilton Anxiety Rating Scale (HARS; Hamilton, 1959). Along with its counterpart, the Hamilton Rating Scale for Depression (HRSD; Hamilton, 1960), the HARS has been widely used in both clinical practice and research. Both Hamilton scales are administered and rated by the clinician. The original HARS consists of 13 items that assess anxious mood, tension, fears, and a variety of somatic symptoms (e.g., muscle tension, gastrointestinal symptoms). The clinician rates the level of severity of each symptom from 0 to 3, with higher numbers indicating greater severity. The HARS contains a number of somatic symptoms that are more associated with panic states and autonomic hyperactivity than chronic worry. Hence, individuals with GAD may or may not obtain significantly elevated scores on the HARS. The HARS may capture some of the significant symptoms experienced by individuals with GAD, but it is unlikely to aid in differential diagnosis between GAD and other anxiety disorders.

Another problem with the Hamilton scales is that they have not been found to discriminate well between anxiety and depression. This is partially due to the significant overlap of items between the HARS and HRSD. This problem was addressed by Riskind, Beck, Brown, and Steer (1987), who reconstructed the scales to increase the construct and discriminant validity of the original scales. Although item overlap was reduced as a result of this reconstruction, Moras et al. (1992) found that the reconstructed scales still shared considerable variance and did not distinguish anxiety patients with comorbid mood disorders from anxiety patients without comorbid depression better than the original scales did.

The State–Trait Anxiety Inventory (STAI; Spielberger, Gorsuch, Lushene, Vagg, & Jacobs, 1983) is another commonly used measure of subjective anxiety that elicits a report of symptoms experienced both acutely and in general. The trait scale is designed to capture more enduring characteristics and patterns of symptoms. As with the HARS, the STAI predominantly measures nonspecific symptoms of anxiety and is not likely to distinguish an individual with pathological worry from persons with other anxiety disorders. Bieling,

Antony, and Swinson (1998) also found that the trait scale of the STAI was as sensitive to symptoms of depression as it was to anxiety.

The Beck Anxiety Inventory (BAI; Beck & Steer, 1990) is a 21-item self-report measure of the frequency of anxiety symptoms over the past week. Analyses of the BAI indicate that it has adequate reliability and validity (Beck, Epstein, Brown, & Steer, 1988). Some factor analyses also indicate that two distinct factors emerge from the BAI that correspond to cognitive and somatic symptoms of anxiety (Beck et al. 1988; Hewitt & Norton, 1993). The BAI overlaps with depression measures somewhat less than other measures of anxiety, due to its focus on fears and symptoms of physiological hyperarousal. As discussed, these types of symptoms are more likely to occur within panic disorder and are less frequently endorsed by patients with GAD. In fact, some have contended that the BAI is better conceptualized as a measure of panic symptoms than as a measure of general anxiety (Cox, Cohen, Direnfeld, & Swinson, 1996). Due to its emphasis on autonomic hyperactivity symptoms, the BAI is not particularly useful for assessing the essential features of GAD.

The Depression Anxiety Stress Scales (DASS; Lovibond & Lovibond, 1995) consist of 42 items that patients rate while considering how they have felt over the past week (or an alternate time frame, depending on the form used). The DASS employs a scale of 0 to 3 with clear anchors (0, did not apply to me, to 3, applied to me most of the time). Analyses indicate that the DASS is a reliable and valid measure of depression, anxiety, and stress. These studies also have confirmed the three-factor structure of the DASS and have suggested that the DASS discriminates between anxiety and depression better than other commonly used measures (Antony, Bieling, Cox, Enns, & Swinson, 1998; Brown, Chorpita, Korotitsch, & Barlow, 1997; Lovibond & Lovibond, 1995). The Depression scale includes items that measure dysphoric mood, loss of self-esteem, and hopelessness. The Anxiety scale for the most part captures physiological hyperarousal, whereas the Stress scale includes symptoms of tension and irritability. The authors of the DASS (Lovibond & Lovibond, 1995) suggest that the Stress scale measures "a state of persistent arousal and tension with a low threshold for becoming upset or frustrated" (p. 342). They also note that there is no certainty that the label of "stress" is appropriate for this set of symptoms. The items that comprise the Stress scale are similar in large part to the associated symptoms of GAD. Brown et al. (1992) found that the Stress scale of an early version of the DASS differentiated patients with GAD from all other anxiety disorder groups except for patients with OCD. Therefore, the DASS may be a particularly useful measure to use as part of an assessment of GAD.

The Penn State Worry Questionnaire (PSWQ; Meyer et al., 1990) is a well-established measure of pathological worry. The PSWQ consists of 16 statements about the patient's tendency to worry that are rated on a scale of 1 to 5 (1, not at all like me, to 5, very much like me). Studies have demonstrated the high internal consistency and temporal stability of the PSWQ, as well as its good convergent and discriminant validity (Brown et al., 1992; Meyer et al., 1990). Brown et al. (1992) reported that patients with GAD scored significantly higher on the PSWQ than did individuals who received other anxiety disorder diagnoses and normal controls. A major advantage of the PSWQ is its exclusive focus on worry, which is the defining feature of GAD. This focus, along with its good psychometric properties, makes it a valuable instrument for initial assessment of GAD, as well as for assessment of treatment outcome.

A self-report measure that elicits information pertaining to all of the DSM criteria has been created by Roemer, Borkovec, Posa, and Borkovec (1995). This measure, called the Generalized Anxiety Disorder Questionnaire (GAD-Q), asks individuals to answer short questions about the nature, frequency, and duration of their worry. The GAD-Q also lists the associated symptoms of GAD and asks individuals to check off those symptoms that bother them when they are anxious. The life interference associated with the worry is rated on a scale of 0 to 8. Based on initial reliability studies, the authors of the questionnaire concluded that the GAD-Q was fairly accurate in identifying the presence of actual GAD and very accurate in identifying its absence in their undergraduate population. The instrument is recommended for selection of potential participants in analog studies of GAD and excessive worry.

The Positive and Negative Affect Scales (PANAS; Watson, Clark, & Tellegen, 1988) is a self-report instrument that may be more relevant to research on GAD and its relationship to the traits of negative and positive affect than to clinical assessment and treatment planning. It consists of 20 items that measure the two dimensions of mood on a scale of 1 to 5 (1, very slightly or not at all, to 5, extremely). When the patient is instructed to rate the degree to which they feel the emotions on the scale *in general*, the PANAS can be used as a trait measure. It may be of interest to some clinicians to use the PANAS as a treatment outcome measure, with the potential aim of distinguishing state change from change in underlying traits.

Clark, Watson, and colleagues have also developed a measure called the Mood and Anxiety Symptoms Questionnaire (MASQ; Watson, Clark, et al., 1995; Watson, Weber, et al., 1995). This questionnaire was originally designed to test the tripartite model of anxiety and depression. Psychometric studies have demonstrated that the MASQ reliably produces a three-factor structure, with factors representing General Distress, Anxious Arousal, and Anhedonic Depression (Watson, Weber, et al., 1995). The creators of the MASQ also found that the Anxious Arousal and Anhedonic Depression scales have good convergent and discriminant validity (Watson, Clark, et al., 1995). The MASQ scales appear to discriminate between patients who are primarily anxious and patients who are primarily depressed better than do most other self-report measures.

Finally, some clinicians may be interested in measuring features of GAD that have been deemed important by current theorists, as opposed to simply measuring DSM-IV symptoms of GAD. The concept of meta-worry was discussed above as a construct that may be of interest to clinicians who assess and treat GAD. Meta-worry may be assessed by using the Anxious Thoughts Inventory (ATI; Wells, 1994). The ATI consists of 22 items that elicit level of worry about health, worry about social relationships, and meta-worry. Wells (1994) reported that the ATI has adequate reliability and validity and consistently produces a three-factor structure. Cartwright-Hatton and Wells (1997) also reported on the reliability and validity of the Meta-Cognitions Questionnaire (MCQ), which assesses beliefs about worry and intrusive thoughts. Of the five subscales of the MCQ, three predicted current level of worry. These subscales were labeled Positive Beliefs about Worry, Negative Beliefs about the Controllability of Thoughts and Corresponding Danger, and Cognitive Confidence. The first two of these scales are most relevant to clinical assessment in that they reflect beliefs about worry that may be addressed during treatment in order to decrease the frequency of worry. The ATI and MCQ have been studied primarily in nonclinical settings, and thus their clinical utility remains largely untested.

During treatment of a patient with GAD, the clinician will likely wish to monitor response to treatment. At our center, we frequently use measures such as the PSWQ and the DASS to monitor changes in worry and associated symptoms across treatment sessions. To obtain the most complete information about the patient's progress, the clinician may administer these brief questionnaires before each treatment session. The minimum that we recommend for evaluation of treatment response is to obtain these measures at the first session, at mid-treatment, and at termination. The mid-treatment evaluation can be particularly helpful in clinical decision making (e.g., if no change has occurred, perhaps the treatment strategy should be altered). Providing feedback to the patients about their scores on the questionnaires can also increase motivation and/or provide a sense of accomplishment.

Self-Monitoring

Self-monitoring is crucial to the ongoing assessment of GAD symptoms. It aids in the measurement of symptom patterns, treatment compliance, and progress/outcome. At our center, we commonly use a number of self-monitoring forms throughout the course of GAD treatment. The Weekly Record of Anxiety and Depression (WRAD; see Figure 5.1) is a useful tool for the measurement of several variables. Patients use an 8-point scale to make daily ratings of their average anxiety, maximum anxiety, average depression, maximum depression, average pleasantness, degree of control over worry, and percentage of the day they felt worried.

When CBT is employed, the clinician usually instructs the patient to monitor the

Name: _____ Week ending: _____

Each evening before you go to bed, please make the following ratings, using the scale below:

1. Your AVERAGE level of anxiety (taking all things into consideration).
2. Your MAXIMUM level of anxiety, experienced at any one point in the day.
3. Your AVERAGE level of depression (taking all things into consideration).
4. Your AVERAGE level of pleasantness (taking all things into consideration).
5. Your degree of control of worry; how difficult was it to stop worrying (e.g., could you turn off, focus upon something else?).
6. The approximate percentage of the day that you felt worried: Use a 0–100% scale where 100 means worried all of the waking day and 0 means no worry at all.

Level of Anxiety/Depression/Pleasantness/Control

0————1————2————3————4————5————6————7————8
None/   Slight/   Moderate/   A lot/   As much as I
no difficulty   slight difficulty   moderate difficulty   marked difficulty   can imagine/
                                                                              extreme difficulty

Date	Average anxiety	Maximum anxiety	Average depression	Average pleasantness	Degree of control	% of day worried (0–100)

FIGURE 5.1. Weekly Record of Anxiety and Depression. A sample self-monitoring record designed to monitor GAD and depression symptoms. From Brown, O'Leary, and Barlow (2001). Copyright 2001 by The Guilford Press. Reprinted by permission.

thoughts, feelings, and behaviors associated with the experience of anxiety. We use a simple form entitled "The Three Components of Anxiety and Depression" to assist patients' monitoring of these spheres. When this form is used early in treatment, it can help the clinician plan cognitive and behavioral interventions to address the patient's unique physiological, cognitive, and behavioral reactions. As treatment progresses, this type of monitoring helps the clinician and patient evaluate progress in modifying problematic thoughts, reducing safety behaviors, and alleviating tension.

Self-monitoring is an aspect of assessment that serves many functions. From the clinician's perspective, this mode of assessment is particularly useful for treatment planning, monitoring of progress, and outcome evaluation. This mode of assessment is also quite useful to patients: it helps them understand their anxiety and ensures continual engagement in treatment. The self-monitoring measures discussed here focus on a general assessment of GAD symptoms; however, as treatment progresses, the clinician may choose to monitor more specific targets of treatment (e.g., the frequency of a particular worry behavior).

Psychophysiological Assessment

The use of psychophysiological assessment with GAD patients has been largely confined to the laboratory and is currently not part of a routine clinical assessment. In part, this is because we are still learning about the unique psychophysiology of chronic, excessive worry. Substantial research exists on the relationship between anxiety and the activity of the autonomic nervous system (ANS). Traditionally, these investigations have focused on hyperactivity of the sympathetic branch of the ANS in persons with anxiety disorders. Individuals with panic disorder, for instance, display a wide range of physical symptoms that indicate sympathetic hyperactivity (e.g., increased heart rate, sweating, hyperventilation).

Because individuals with GAD experience chronically high levels of anxiety, we might reasonably expect them to exhibit increased sympathetic arousal on psychophysiological measures. Contrary to this expectation, worry seems to be associated with an inhibition of sympathetic systems (Borkovec & Hu, 1990; Thayer et al., 1996). Chronic worriers tend to show *diminished* autonomic response to stressors, when compared to nonanxious controls, and they are slower to habituate and return to baseline (Thayer et al., 1996). This restriction of autonomic activity is apparent on measures such as heart rate variability (Hoehn-Saric et al., 1989). There has been considerable support for the hypothesis that the autonomic inflexibility observed in patients with GAD is the result of a chronically deficient parasympathetic system (Lyonfields, Borkovec, & Thayer, 1995; Thayer et al., 1996). Investigation of the psychophysiological characteristics of GAD is proving to be an exciting area of research in that autonomic inflexibility and decreased vagal (parasympathetic) tone may be useful biological markers for establishing the presence of pathological worry.

In addition, it has been found that individuals with GAD demonstrate greater muscle tension than do normal controls at baseline and in response to psychological challenge (e.g., Hoehn-Saric et al., 1989). This finding converges with self-report findings (Brown et al., 1995; Marten et al., 1993), and the evidence that relaxation training is an effective treatment for GAD (e.g., Borkovec & Costello, 1993).

CHOOSING AN ASSESSMENT STRATEGY THAT FACILITATES TREATMENT PLANNING AND OUTCOME EVALUATION: A CASE EXAMPLE

The structured interviews, questionnaires, and diary measures reviewed above provide converging sources of information that aid in diagnosis and treatment planning. Some of these assessment tools also can be easily incorporated into a patient's treatment program in a manner that enhances both treatment efficacy and clinician accountability. To illustrate this integrated approach to assessment and treatment, the case of Mr. W will be briefly considered. Mr. W is a hypothetical patient who manifests symptoms and problems that are typical of patients with GAD in our clinical setting. Mr. W's assessment began with the administration of the ADIS-IV-L interview by a trained therapist. The majority of the interview was spent discussing Mr. W's chronic worry and tension, as this was clearly his primary problem. Mr. W did not appear to meet criteria for any other anxiety disorder, but he endorsed a history of depression. The clinician carefully evaluated the time course of Mr. W's depressive episodes and his worry. Mr. W's excessive worry was longstanding and unremitting, whereas his two past depressive episodes were in response to stressful life events and were brief in duration. His symptoms of GAD had clearly been present for more than 6 months without any clinically significant symptoms of depression. Hence, the therapist assigned a principal diagnosis of GAD and noted two past major depressive episodes. The current severity of the GAD was judged to be moderate (CSR = 5).

During the ADIS-IV-L interview, the therapist gathered a substantial amount of information that was relevant to treatment planning. She learned that Mr. W's main worry areas were work, family, and minor matters and that he felt worried 75% of the day. The therapist obtained some preliminary information about Mr. W's anxious thoughts (e.g., "If I make any errors at work, I'll never get a promotion") and problems that resulted from his anxiety (e.g., "I procrastinate on long-term projects and then I feel overwhelmed"). The ADIS-IV-L also facilitated the collection of information about his associated symptoms. Mr. W was most bothered by frequent muscle tension in his shoulders and neck, and he also complained of tension headaches. He further explained that worrying at night made it difficult for him to fall asleep, which often led to daytime fatigue. Mr. W stated that he had always been a worrier and attributed his anxious temperament to family factors. He indicated that his mother had always been anxious and had "passed along" this tendency to him.

Mr. W also completed a number of self-report questionnaires that were intended to supplement the information obtained from the ADIS-IV-L. His scores of 4, 10, and 26 on the respective Depression Anxiety Stress Scales reflected a mild level of depression, a moderate level of anxiety, and a strong level of stress. As discussed in this chapter, the Stress scale of the DASS measures many of the symptoms associated with GAD. Mr. W obtained a particularly high score of 76 on the PSWQ, which demonstrated a strong tendency to worry and difficulty controlling the worry process. Finally, Mr. W's score of 11 on the Beck Depression Inventory (BDI; Beck & Steer, 1987) confirmed that he was not experiencing clinically significant depressive symptoms at the time of the assessment, although his score was somewhat elevated due to items that reflected symptoms that are shared by GAD and mood disorders (e.g., irritability, fatigue).

Mr. W's therapist reviewed the information from the ADIS-IV-L and questionnaires prior to the first treatment session. The data from the interview suggested that a relaxation intervention would be helpful for Mr. W's associated symptoms. The therapist elected to try progressive muscle relaxation with the aim of decreasing Mr. W's muscle tension and headaches. She also predicted that relaxation exercises would help Mr. W fall asleep at night. Due to the prominence of these symptoms for Mr. W, the therapist decided that she would try this intervention early in the course of treatment.

The information obtained during the ADIS-IV-L also suggested that there was a substantial cognitive component to Mr. W's GAD. His thinking was characterized by overestimations of the likelihood of negative events, such as the probabilities that he would lose his job and that his wife would leave him. Mr. W was also a self-proclaimed "perfectionist" and tended to consider most issues in an all-or-nothing manner (e.g., one mistake meant he would be viewed unfavorably). Mr. W's therapist judged that these patterns of thinking were an important aspect of her patient's anxiety, and therefore she planned to incorporate cognitive restructuring exercises into the treatment.

Another problem area that the therapist learned of during the interview was Mr. W's tendency to procrastinate. Although this might be the result of Mr. W's maladaptive thinking, the therapist decided to further evaluate Mr. W's time management during the early treatment sessions. If time management appeared to be an independent problem, the therapist would consider implementing an intervention to specifically target this area.

At the first treatment session, the therapist presented her formulation of Mr. W's problem and outlined her tentative treatment plan. Mr. W agreed that he would benefit from working on all of the problems that the therapist had identified. Further questioning about time management revealed that Mr. W had difficulty sticking to agendas and being assertive when others infringed on his time at work. He also had a habit of occupying himself with smaller, less important tasks in order to avoid working on longer-term projects. He and the therapist agreed that developing a time management "system" would be helpful. At the end of the first treatment session, the therapist sent Mr. W home with some self-monitoring forms that would serve to continue the assessment process. These forms included the WRAD (see Figure 5.1) and the Three Components of Anxiety (TCA; Craske et al., 1992), which enables the patient to record thoughts, feelings, and behaviors associated with anxiety.

Mr. W's self-monitoring records provided valuable supplementary information to the initial assessment data. His WRAD indicated that he consistently felt the highest levels of anxiety and the lowest degrees of control on Wednesdays and Thursdays. When questioned about this, Mr. W indicated that he met with his supervisor on Thursday afternoons to review the status and progress of his projects. This event caused Mr. W a great deal of anticipatory anxiety, mainly because he feared that he would not meet his supervisor's expectations and might even be fired. The therapist gathered that it would be important to target Mr. W's thoughts about his weekly meeting during the phase of treatment focused on cognitive restructuring. Mr. W's WRAD also revealed that he had quite low pleasantness ratings on most days. The therapist decided to have Mr. W deliberately schedule more pleasant and relaxing activities in a further effort to relieve some of his tension.

The TCA form that Mr. W completed also provided information relevant to treatment planning. As expected, Mr. W's most common physical symptoms were muscle tension and headaches, and his anxious thoughts were focused on the possible occurrence of negative events. The TCA form further revealed a variety of behaviors associated with Mr. W's anxiety, including checking memos at work several times before sending them out and seeking reassurance from his wife in response to his worries. Upon reviewing the TCA forms, Mr. W and his therapist had a discussion about safety behaviors and planned to work on modifying them during a later stage of treatment.

At mid-treatment, Mr. W had been practicing progressive muscle relaxation for 4 weeks and had been using cognitive restructuring techniques for 3 weeks. His WRAD self-monitoring forms indicated that his average and maximum anxiety levels had decreased somewhat, although he still reported worrying 40% to 50% of the day. At this point, his therapist also asked him to complete the DASS and PSWQ scales again. Mr. W's score on the PSWQ had decreased to 65, but still reflected clinically significant levels of worry. His score on the DASS Stress scale had decreased considerably to a 10, possibly due to the reduction of overall tension that accompanied his mastery of the initial phases of progressive muscle relaxation. The steady decreases in Mr. W's symptoms of tension and worry (as reflected by his WRAD ratings and his DASS and PSWQ scores) suggested that he was responding positively to cognitive-behavioral strategies. Therefore, his therapist opted to continue with the interventions she had planned at the outset of treatment.

At the end of treatment, Mr. W was reevaluated by an independent therapist at the clinic to determine how he had responded to treatment. This second therapist administered a shorter version of the ADIS-IV-L that focused only on recent symptoms. He also asked Mr. W to complete the DASS and PSWQ. After a full course of treatment, Mr. W had only subclinical symptoms of GAD, and he did not meet criteria for any other mental disorder. The severity of his GAD symptoms was judged to be mild (CSR = 2). He no longer reported difficulties with muscle tension or sleep, and his headaches were much less frequent. Mr. W now estimated that he spent less than 10% of the day worrying, and he no longer felt that his worrying was interfering with his productivity. His DASS scores were in the mild range for each of the scales (0 for Depression, 2 for Anxiety, and 8 for Stress), and his PSWQ score of 50 reflected a mild to moderate tendency to worry. Although Mr. W still had residual symptoms of GAD after treatment, his worry and tension were no longer causing him substantial distress or interference in his life.

The case of Mr. W illustrates how assessment can be successfully integrated with treatment planning and outcome evaluation. It further demonstrates that the process of assessment does not cease once treatment begins. In contrast, self-monitoring forms and questionnaires continue to provide clinicians with relevant information throughout treatment. Self-monitoring forms, in particular, may lead clinicians to initiate interventions that had not been anticipated at the outset of treatment. In this manner, continual assessment contributes to the delivery of optimal treatment for a patient's individual problems.

GENERALIZED ANXIETY DISORDER IN PRIMARY AND MANAGED CARE SETTINGS

A substantial proportion of individuals with GAD seek help for their anxiety in primary care settings (Wittchen et al., 1994). There is evidence that GAD is three times more prevalent in individuals presenting to primary care clinics than in the general population (Shear & Schulberg, 1995). Individuals also frequently seek help for medical conditions that are associated with stress, such as irritable bowel syndrome and atypical chest pain (Spiegel & Barlow, 2000). The remainder of this chapter will focus on special issues to be considered when assessing GAD in primary care and managed care settings.

Streamlining Assessment of Generalized Anxiety Disorder

Assessment of GAD within a primary or managed care setting presents an additional challenge in that the assessment process needs to be streamlined substantially in these environments. Screening questions that reliably distinguish individuals with pathological worry from other groups would be very valuable to clinicians who work in these settings. Research to date on the assessment of GAD provides some hints as to which questions might be helpful in determining whether the clinician should proceed with further assessment of the patient's anxiety and worry.

Barlow (2002) reported that one question was particularly effective in distinguishing patients with GAD from individuals who received diagnoses of other anxiety disorders. This simple question was, "Do you worry excessively about minor things?" About half of the patients with other anxiety disorders answered "yes" to this question, whereas all of the patients with GAD responded affirmatively. In a later study, Sanderson and Barlow (1990) found that a larger portion of patients with GAD than patients with other anxiety disorders reported excessive worry about minor matters. It is important to note that in one study an affirmative response to "Do you worry excessively about minor matters?" could *not* confirm a diagnosis of GAD, although a negative response nearly always indicated an absence of clinically significant GAD (Di Nardo, 1991).

Another option for primary care clinicians is to draw on the introductory questions that are used in structured interviews to screen for the presence of pathological worry. For example, questions from the CIDI include the following: "Has there ever been a period in your life lasting 6 months or more when most of the time you felt worried or anxious? Did you ever have many different worries on your mind at the same time?" (Wittchen et al., 1994). The ADIS-IV-L, on the other hand, includes questions such as, "Over the past several months, have you been continually worried or anxious about a number of events or activities in your daily life?" and "On an average day, what percentage of the day do you feel worried?" (Di Nardo et al., 1994). Barlow (2002) indicated that most patients who ultimately received a diagnosis of GAD reported worrying for more than half the day, and the primary or managed care clinician may wish to investigate the patient's anxiety further if the patient endorses this level of worrying.

The time constraints associated with primary care and managed care settings make differential diagnosis difficult. However, because the features of GAD are commonly present in other psychological disorders, the clinician will need to make some preliminary differential judgments. Asking "What kinds of things do you usually worry about?" is a simple query that can begin the process of deciding whether the patient's worry is attributable to a more specific anxiety disorder. The clinician should be attuned to reports of apprehension about experiencing physical symptoms (panic disorder), worry about negative social evaluation (social phobia), worry about having a specific physical disease (hypochondriasis), worry about gaining weight (eating disorders), concerns that are accompanied by compulsive behavior (OCD), anxiety that follows a traumatic experience (PTSD), and worry that is the direct result of substance use or a medical condition. Further questioning may be necessary if any of these focuses of worry arise in the patient's description. Due to its frequent comorbidity with pathological worry, the level of depression should also be investigated. The primary care clinician may ask, "Have you been feeling down or depressed recently, or do you find yourself losing interest in your usual activities?" Affirmative answers to these types of questions are a signal that the clinician should probe further to determine whether a mood disorder diagnosis is warranted, and whether GAD symptoms have been present independently of clinical depression for at least 6 months.

Finally, performing a quick assessment of the level of interference associated with the anxiety and worry may also aid in clinical decision making. The primary care clinician may ask if the worry ever interferes with the person's ability to focus on other things or if the worry and tension seem to interfere with work or social functioning. Worry and tension that interfere significantly in these areas would most likely indicate a need for further evaluation or a referral to a mental health provider for treatment.

Two Interviews for Assessing Generalized Anxiety Disorder in Primary Care

Recently, a number of brief interviews have been developed to facilitate identification of mental health problems in primary care settings. Two of the more popular interviews are the Primary Care Evaluation of Mental Health Disorders (PRIME-MD; Spitzer et al., 1994) and the Mini-International Neuropsychiatric Interview (MINI; Sheehan et al., 1998). Each of these interviews includes a self-report symptom checklist that the patient completes before he or she meets with the primary care physician. The PRIME-MD and MINI also contain a clinician-administered interview that is used to follow up on problem areas identified by the patient. The main advantage of this type of interview is reduced time for administration: an average of 8.4 minutes for the PRIME-MD and 15 minutes for the MINI (Spitzer et al., 1994; Sheehan et al., 1998).

Both the PRIME-MD and the MINI allow the clinician to assess for GAD. The patient portion of the PRIME-MD includes such items as "During the past month, how often have you been bothered by worrying about a lot of different things?" which serve as an indication that the clinician should administer the GAD section of the interview. The MINI has a similar format. The clinician-administered portions of the PRIME-MD and MINI are comprised of closed-ended ("yes" or "no") questions that address each of the DSM-IV symptoms of GAD. Diagnosis simply requires a symptom count.

Overall, interviews such as the PRIME-MD and MINI have adequate reliability and validity (Spitzer et al., 1994; Sheehan et al., 1998). However, they present some problems with respect to the assessment of GAD. First, although both the PRIME-MD and MINI assess for depression, they do not obtain detailed information about the onset of GAD and depression symptoms. Therefore, they do not enable the clinician to adhere to the DSM-IV hierarchical rules regarding GAD and mood disorders. In addition, Spitzer et al.'s (1994) reliability and validity analyses reported relatively low reliability, sensitivity, and positive predictive value of GAD diagnoses made with the PRIME-MD. Sheehan et al. (1998) reported better reliability and validity estimates when GAD diagnoses assigned with the MINI were compared to diagnoses obtained using the SCID. However, when the MINI was compared to the CIDI, once again the reliability and positive predictive values of GAD diagnoses obtained with the MINI were found to be low (Sheehan et al., 1998). Further, the "yes–no" format of the clinician-administered portions of the PRIME-MD and MINI do not facilitate the probing that is often necessary to discriminate the worry and tension associated with GAD from similar symptoms that result from other psychological disorders.

The two primary care interviews discussed here have proven to be useful in identifying patients who may benefit from appropriate pharmacotherapy or a referral to a mental health professional (Sheehan et al., 1998; Spitzer et al., 1994). However, they have limitations in regard to obtaining a reliable and valid diagnosis of GAD. Although some patients in primary care may meet the symptom count for GAD, this diagnosis needs to be considered in the context of lifetime and current depression and other psychological disorders. If a diagnosis of GAD is made on the basis of the PRIME-MD or MINI, we recommend that the mental health professional undertake further assessment to determine if this diagnosis is indeed appropriate.

Providing Evidence of Treatment Adherence and Outcome

The need to provide documentation of treatment integrity, adherence, and outcome will be increasingly common as managed care transforms the provision of mental health care (e.g., Barlow, 1996). This chapter reviewed several modes of assessment that can be employed in evaluating symptoms of GAD over the course of treatment. In primary care and managed care settings, where lengthy clinical interviews may not be possible, self-report questionnaires and self-monitoring measures are particularly useful. For the assessment of excessive, uncontrollable worry, a measure such as the PSWQ should be used. Moreover, diary measures such as the WRAD allow the patient to record the percentage of the day spent worrying, which is another index of worry that should change with effective treatment. The WRAD also includes a rating for the degree of control the patient had over their worrisome thinking, allowing the clinician to monitor change in this essential feature of GAD.

For assessment of a broad range of symptoms that may be associated with GAD, a questionnaire measure such as the DASS would be appropriate. The somatic symptoms of GAD are captured well by scores on the Stress subscale of this measure. The DASS also provides the advantage of assessing the depressive symptoms that are so often comorbid with GAD. Other brief measures such as the BDI serve the same purpose. In the discussion of structured interviews, the notion of a clinical severity rating (CSR) was introduced. If the clinician assigns a CSR to the patient's diagnosis of GAD, he or she may also reevaluate the CSR at regular intervals throughout treatment. The clinician rating of symptom severity complements the self-report data that is obtained from questionnaires and diary measures.

Combining the use of questionnaire, self-monitoring, and clinician-rated measures provides a comprehensive picture of progress throughout treatment. The self-monitoring measures can also serve as measures of treatment compliance and integrity. For example, different monitoring forms can be used as documentation of the different skills that the patient is engaged in throughout therapy (e.g., cognitive restructuring, relaxation training). The degree to which the patient records treatment-relevant activities also demonstrates the level of compliance with therapist instruction.

Possible Pitfalls of Rapid Assessment

As emphasized at the beginning of this chapter, the assessment of GAD presents many challenges to the clinician and requires a comprehensive understanding of a wide range of psychopathology. Distinguishing symptoms of GAD from normal worry in response to stressors and from anxiety associated with other psychological disorders are two determinations that may necessitate a considerable degree of inquiry. In primary care and managed care settings where assessment must be streamlined, there is a greater risk for incomplete assessment or even misdiagnosis. Using abbreviated assessment procedures (e.g., relying heavily on questionnaires) may lead to a failure to recognize that the patient's anxiety and worry are best explained by a more specific anxiety disorder or by primary depression. Patients with many different presenting problems obtain high scores on measures such as the PSWQ, DASS, and more general measures of anxiety (e.g., BAI, STAI). Brief assessment may also fail to capture the comorbidity that more often than not is an important context to GAD. We recommend that self-report instruments not be used independently to arrive at a diagnosis; on the contrary, careful inquiry by a clinician is necessary to make a reasonable judgment that a patient suffers from GAD. This ensures that the patient will be recommended to the specific treatment that is likely to work best for him or her.

Additional Roles of Assessment in Primary and Managed Care Settings

As economic factors begin to exert more influence over mental health practice, clinicians are increasingly under pressure to provide interventions that are not just effective but efficient. A properly conducted assessment can be a valuable aspect of brief interventions for psychological problems such as GAD. Inquiry about the relationships between the patient's worrisome thinking, physical symptoms, and behavior can lay the foundation for educating patients about the likely causes of their symptoms. In this sense, assessment can be considered part of the psychoeducation that is an important component of many effective treatment strategies. Understanding the nature of anxiety and worry can help put some patients at ease about the physical symptoms they experience as a result of their chronic anxiety. Asking the right questions during the assessment may also help the patient recognize patterns that can be changed with the goal of alleviating symptoms. Finally, a thorough assessment in a primary care setting can reassure the patient that his or her symptoms are recognizable as an anxiety disorder, that anxiety disorders are common, and that effective treatments exist. Patients may be referred to self-directed treatments (e.g., Craske et al., 1992) or to a mental health care provider who specializes in the treatment of disorders like GAD.

SUMMARY

GAD is a relatively common anxiety disorder that is characterized by a chronic course and substantial impairment in important areas of functioning. Advances in our conceptualization of GAD across editions of the DSM have been accompanied by improvements in the methods of assessment and treatment of this disorder. This chapter provided guidelines for a thorough clinical interview that aids in establishing the presence of GAD and differentiating it from other psychological disorders. Establishing the precise focus of the patient's worry and investigating the possible presence of current and lifetime depression are important facets of an adequate assessment of GAD. Numerous self-report questionnaires and self-monitoring methods are available to add to information gathered at the initial assessment and to evaluate progress throughout treatment. Specific measures were identified (e.g., PSWQ and DASS) that assess important features of GAD. These brief self-report instruments may be especially useful in primary and managed care settings, where there may be considerable time constraints on the assessment process. Suggestions for streamlining assessment procedures were presented, with the caution that a less comprehensive assessment may fail to differentiate GAD from other Axis I conditions and may overlook the comorbidity that usually accompanies GAD. A thorough assessment of GAD and its associated features is integral to treatment planning and outcome evaluation in both primary care and more specialized settings.

REFERENCES

American Psychiatric Association. (1980). *Diagnostic and statistical manual of mental disorders* (3rd ed.). Washington, DC: Author.

American Psychiatric Association. (1987). *Diagnostic and statistical manual of mental disorders* (3rd ed., rev.). Washington, DC: Author.

American Psychiatric Association. (1994). *Diagnostic and statistical manual of mental disorders* (4th ed.). Washington, DC: Author.

Andrews, G., Stewart, S., Allen, R., & Henderson, A. S. (1990). The genetics of six neurotic disorders: A twin study. *Journal of Affective Disorders, 19,* 23–29.

Antony, M. M., Bieling, P. J., Cox, B. J., Enns, M. W., & Swinson, R. P. (1998). Psychometric properties of the 42-item and 21-item versions of the Depression Anxiety Stress Scales in clinical groups and a community sample. *Psychological Assessment, 10,* 176–181.

Barlow, D. H. (1996). Health care policy, psychotherapy research, and the future of psychotherapy. *American Psychologist, 51,* 1050–1058.

Barlow, D. H. (2002). *Anxiety and its disorders: The nature and treatment of anxiety and panic* (2nd ed.). New York: Guilford Press.

Barlow, D. H., Rapee, R. M., & Brown, T. A. (1992). Behavioral treatment of generalized anxiety disorder. *Behavior Therapy, 23,* 551–570.

Beck, A. T., Epstein, N., Brown, G., & Steer, R. A. (1988). An inventory for measuring clinical anxiety: Psychometric properties. *Journal of Consulting and Clinical Psychology, 56,* 893–897.

Beck, A. T., & Steer, R. A. (1987). *Manual for the revised Beck Depression Inventory.* San Antonio, TX: Psychological Corporation.

Beck, A. T., & Steer, R. A. (1990). *Manual for the Beck Anxiety Inventory.* San Antonio, TX: Psychological Corporation.

Bieling, P. J., Antony, M. M., & Swinson, R. P. (1998). The State–Trait Anxiety Inventory, Trait version: Structure and content re-examined. *Behaviour Research and Therapy, 36,* 777–788.

Blazer, D. G., Hughes, D., & George, L. K. (1987). Stressful life events and the onset of generalized anxiety disorder syndrome. *American Journal of Psychiatry, 144,* 1178–1183.

Borkovec, T. D. (1994). The nature, functions, and origins of worry. In G. Davey & F. Tallis (Eds.), *Worrying: Perspectives on theory, assessment, and treatment* (pp. 5–34). New York: Wiley.

Borkovec, T. D., & Costello, E. (1993). Efficacy of applied relaxation and cognitive-behavioral therapy in the treatment of generalized anxiety disorder. *Journal of Consulting and Clinical Psychology, 61,* 611–619.

Borkovec, T. D., & Hu, S. (1990). The effect of worry on cardiovascular response to phobic imagery. *Behaviour Research and Therapy, 28,* 69–73.

Borkovec, T. D., & Mathews, A. M. (1988). Treatment of nonphobic anxiety disorders: A comparison of nondirective, cognitive, and coping desensitization therapy. *Journal of Consulting and Clinical Psychology, 56,* 877–884.

Borkovec, T. D., & Roemer, L. (1995). Perceived functions of worry among generalized anxiety disorder subjects: Distraction from more emotional topics? *Journal of Behavior Therapy and Experimental Psychiatry, 26,* 25–30.

Brawman-Mintzer, O., & Lydiard, R. B. (1996). Generalized anxiety disorder: Issues in epidemiology. *Journal of Clinical Psychiatry, 57*(Suppl. 7), 3–8.

Brawman-Mintzer, O., Lydiard, R. B., Crawford, M. M., Emmanuel, N., Payeur, R., Johnson, M., Knapp, R. G., & Ballenger, J. C. (1994). Somatic symptoms in generalized anxiety disorder with and without comorbid psychiatric disorders. *American Journal of Psychiatry, 151,* 930–932.

Brawman-Mintzer, O., Lydiard, R. B., Emmanuel, N., Payeur, R., Johnson, M., Roberts, J., Jarrell, M. P., & Ballenger, J. C. (1993). Psychiatric comorbidity in patients with generalized anxiety disorder. *American Journal of Psychiatry, 150,* 1216–1218.

Brown, T. A. (1997). The nature of generalized anxiety disorder and pathological worry: Current evidence and conceptual models. *Canadian Journal of Psychiatry, 42,* 817–825.

Brown, T. A., Antony, M. M., & Barlow, D. H. (1992). Psychometric properties of the Penn State Worry Questionnaire in a clinical anxiety disorders sample. *Behaviour Research and Therapy, 30,* 33–37.

Brown, T. A., & Barlow, D. H. (1992). Comorbidity among anxiety disorders: Implications for treatment and DSM-IV. *Journal of Consulting and Clinical Psychology, 60,* 835–844.

Brown, T. A., Barlow, D. H., & Liebowitz, M. R. (1994). The empirical basis of generalized anxiety disorder. *American Journal of Psychiatry, 151,* 1272–1280.

Brown, T. A., Chorpita, B. F., & Barlow, D. H. (1998). Structural relationships among dimensions of the DSM-IV anxiety and mood disorders and dimensions of negative affect, positive affect, and autonomic arousal. *Journal of Abnormal Psychology, 107,* 179–192.

Brown, T. A., Chorpita, B. F., Korotitsch, W., & Barlow, D. H. (1997). Psychometric properties of the Depression Anxiety Stress Scales in clinical samples. *Behaviour Research and Therapy, 35,* 79–89.

Brown, T. A., Di Nardo, P. A., Lehman, C. L., & Campbell, L. A. (2001). Reliability of DSM-IV anxiety and mood disorders: Implications for the classification of emotional disorders. *Journal of Abnormal Psychology, 110,* 49–58.

Brown, T. A., Marten, P. A., & Barlow, D. H. (1995). Discriminant validity of the symptoms constituting the DSM-III-R and DSM-IV associated symptom criterion of generalized anxiety disorder. *Journal of Anxiety Disorders, 9,* 317–328.

Brown, T. A., Moras, K., Zinbarg, R. E., & Barlow, D. H. (1993). Diagnostic and symptom distinguishability of generalized anxiety disorder and obsessive-compulsive disorder. *Behavior Therapy, 24,* 227–240.

Brown, T. A., O'Leary, T. A., & Barlow, D. H. (2001). Generalized anxiety disorder. In D. H. Barlow (Ed.), *Clinical handbook of psychological disorders: A step-by-step treatment manual* (3rd ed., pp. 137–188). New York: Guilford Press.

Cartwright-Hatton, S., & Wells, A. (1997). Beliefs about worry and intrusions: The meta-cognitions questionnaire and its correlates. *Journal of Anxiety Disorders, 11,* 279–296.

Clark, L. A., & Watson, D. (1991). Tripartite model of anxiety and depression: Psychometric evidence and taxonomic implications. *Journal of Abnormal Psychology, 100,* 316–336.

Cox, B. J., Cohen, E., Direnfield, D. M., & Swinson, R. P. (1996). Reply to Steer and Beck: Panic disorder, generalized anxiety disorder, and quantitative versus qualitative differences in anxiety assessment. *Behaviour Research and Therapy, 34,* 959–961.

Craske, M. G., Barlow, D. H., & O'Leary, T. A. (1992). *Mastery of your anxiety and worry.* San Antonio, TX: Psychological Corporation.

Di Nardo, P. A. (1991). *MacArthur reanalysis of generalized anxiety disorder.* Unpublished manuscript.

Di Nardo, P. A., Brown, T. A., & Barlow, D. H. (1994). *Anxiety Disorders Interview Schedule for DSM-IV: Lifetime Version.* San Antonio, TX: Psychological Corporation.

Di Nardo, P. A., Moras, K., Barlow, D. H., Rapee, R. M., & Brown, T. A. (1993). Reliability of DSM-III-R anxiety disorder categories using the Anxiety Disorders Interview Schedule—Revised (ADIS-R). *Archives of General Psychiatry, 50,* 251–256.

Di Nardo, P. A., O'Brien, G. T., Barlow, D. H., Waddell, M. T., & Blanchard, E. B. (1983). Reliability of DSM-III anxiety disorder categories using a new structured interview. *Archives of General Psychiatry, 40,* 1070–1074.

Essau, C. A., & Wittchen, H.-U. (1993). An overview of the Composite International Diagnostic Interview. *International Journal of Methods in Psychiatry, 3,* 79–85.

First, M. B., Gibbon, M., Spitzer, R. L., & Williams, J. B. W. (1996). *User's guide for the Structured Clinical Interview for DSM-IV Axis I Disorders: Research version.* New York: Biometrics Research.

Gould, R. A., Otto, M. W., Pollack, M. H., & Yap, L. (1997). Cognitive-behavioral and pharmacological treatment of generalized anxiety disorder: A preliminary meta-analysis. *Behavior Therapy, 28,* 285–305.

Hamilton, M. (1959). The assessment of anxiety states by rating. *British Journal of Medical Psychology, 32,* 50–55.

Hamilton, M. (1960). A rating scale for depression. *Journal of Neurology, Neurosurgery, and Psychiatry, 23,* 56–62.

Hewitt, P. L., & Norton, R. (1993). The Beck Anxiety Inventory: A psychometric analysis. *Psychological Assessment, 5,* 408–412.

Hoehn-Saric, R., McLeod, D. R., & Zimmerli, W. D. (1989). Somatic manifestations in women with generalized anxiety disorder: Psychophysiological responses to psychological stress. *Archives of General Psychiatry, 46,* 1113–1119.

Kendler, K. S., Neale, M. C., Kessler, R. C., Heath, A. C., & Eaves, L. J. (1992a). Generalized anxiety disorder in women: A population-based twin study. *Archives of General Psychiatry, 49,* 267–272.

Kendler, K. S., Neale, M. C., Kessler, R. C., Heath, A. C., & Eaves, L. J. (1992b). Major depression and generalized anxiety disorder: Same genes, (partly) different environments? *Archives of General Psychiatry, 49,* 716–722.

Kessler, R. C., McGonagle, K. A., Zhao, S., Nelson, C. B., Hughes, M., Eshleman, S., Wittchen, H.-U., Kendler, K. S. (1994). Lifetime and 12-month prevalence of DSM-III-R psychiatric disorders in the United States. *Archives of General Psychiatry, 51,* 8–19.

Lovibond, P. F., & Lovibond, S. H. (1995). The structure of negative emotional states: Comparison of the Depression Anxiety Stress Scales (DASS) with the Beck Depression and Anxiety Inventories. *Behaviour Research and Therapy, 33,* 335–343.

Lyonfields, J. D., Borkovec, T. D., & Thayer, J. F. (1995). Vagal tone in generalized anxiety disorder and the effects of aversive imagery and worrisome thinking. *Behavior Therapy, 26,* 457–466.

Mannuzza, S. (1994). *Schedule for Affective Disorders and Schizophrenia: Lifetime Version, Modified for the Study of Anxiety Disorders (Updated for DSM-IV).* New York: Anxiety Disorders Clinic, New York State Psychiatric Institute.

Marten, P. A., Brown, T. A., Barlow, D. H., Borkovec, T. D., Shear, M. K., & Lydiard, R. B. (1993). Evaluation of the ratings comprising the associated symptom criterion of DSM-III-R generalized anxiety disorder. *Journal of Nervous and Mental Disease, 181,* 676–682.

Meyer, T. J., Miller, M. L., Metzger, R. L., & Borkovec, T. D. (1990). Development and validation of the Penn State Worry Questionnaire. *Behaviour Research and Therapy, 28,* 487–495.

Mineka, S., Watson, D., & Clark, L. A. (1998). Comorbidity of anxiety and unipolar mood disorders. *Annual Review of Psychology, 49,* 377–412.

Moras, K., Di Nardo, P. A., & Barlow, D. H. (1992). Distinguishing anxiety and depression: Reexamination of the reconstructed Hamilton scales. *Psychological Assessment, 4,* 224–227.

Noyes, R., Woodman, C., Garvey, M. J., Cook, B. L., Suelzer, M., Clancy, J., & Anderson, D. J. (1992). Generalized anxiety disorder vs. panic disorder: Distinguishing characteristics and patterns of comorbidity. *Journal of Nervous and Mental Disease, 180,* 369–379.

Riskind, J. H., Beck, A. T., Brown, G., & Steer, R. A. (1987). Taking the measure of anxiety and depression: Validity of the reconstructed Hamilton scales. *Journal of Nervous and Mental Disease, 175,* 474–479.

Roemer, L., Borkovec, M., Posa, S., & Borkovec, T. D. (1995). A self-report diagnostic measure of generalized anxiety disorder. *Journal of Behavior Therapy and Experimental Psychiatry, 4,* 345–350.

Sanderson, W. C., & Barlow, D. H. (1990). A description of patients diagnosed with DSM-III-R generalized anxiety disorder. *Journal of Nervous and Mental Disease, 178,* 588–591.

Sanderson, W. C., Wetzler, S., Beck, A. T., & Betz, F. (1994). Prevalence of personality disorders in patients with anxiety disorders. *Psychiatry Research, 51,* 167–174.

Schleyer, B., Aaronson, C., Mannuzza, S., Martin, L. Y., & Fyer, A. J. (1990). *Schedule for Affective Disorders and Schizophrenia: Lifetime Version, Modified for the Study of Anxiety Disorders (Revised).* New York: Anxiety Disorders Clinic, New York State Psychiatric Institute.

Shear, M. K., & Schulberg, H. C. (1995). Anxiety disorders in primary care. *Bulletin of the Menninger Clinic, 59,* A73–A85.

Sheehan, D. V., Lecrubier, Y., Sheehan, K. H., Amorim, P., Janavs, J., Weiller, E., Hergueta, T., Baker, R., & Dunbar, G. C. (1998). The Mini-International Neuropsychiatric Interview (M. I. N. I.): The development and validation of a structured diagnostic psychiatric interview for DSM-IV and ICD–10. *Journal of Clinical Psychiatry, 59*(Suppl. 20), 22–33.

Shores, M. M., Glubin, T., Cowley, D. S., Dager, S. R., Roy-Burne, P. P., & Dunner, D. L. (1992). The relationship between anxiety and depression: A clinical comparison of generalized anxiety disorder, dysthymic disorder, panic disorder, and major depressive disorder. *Comprehensive Psychiatry, 33,* 237–244.

Spiegel, D. A., & Barlow, D. H. (2000). Generalized anxiety disorders. In M. G. Gelder, J. J. Lopez-Ibor, & N. C. Andreasen (Eds.), *New Oxford textbook of psychiatry* (pp. 785–794). Oxford, UK: Oxford University Press.

Spiegel, D. A., Wiegel, M., Baker, S. L., & Greene, K. A. (2000). Pharmacological management of anxiety disorders. In D. I. Mostofsky & D. H. Barlow (Eds.), *The management of stress and anxiety in medical disorders* (pp. 36–65). Boston: Allyn & Bacon.

Spielberger, C. D., Gorsuch, R. L., Lushene, R., Vagg, P. R., & Jacobs, G. A. (1983). *Manual for the State–Trait Anxiety Inventory.* Palo Alto, CA: Consulting Psychologists Press.

Spitzer, R. L., Williams, J. B. W., Kroenke, K., Linzer, M., deGruy, F. V., Hahn, S. R., Brody, D., & Johnson, J. G. (1994). Utility of a new procedure for diagnosing mental disorders in primary care: The PRIME-MD 1000 study. *Journal of the American Medical Association, 272,* 1749–1756.

Thayer, J. F., Friedman, B. H., & Borkovec, T. D. (1996). Autonomic characteristics of generalized anxiety disorder and worry. *Biological Psychiatry, 39,* 255–266.

Torgersen, S. (1983). Genetic factors in anxiety disorders. *Archives of General Psychiatry, 40,* 1085–1089.

Turner, S. M., Beidel, D. C., & Stanley, M. A. (1992). Are obsessional thoughts and worry different cognitive phenomena? *Clinical Psychology Review, 12,* 257–270.

Watson, D., Clark, L. A., & Tellegen, A. (1988). Development and validation of brief measures of positive and negative affect: The PANAS scales. *Journal of Personality and Social Psychology, 54,* 1063–1070.

Watson, D., Clark, L. A., Weber, K., Assenheimer, J. S., Strauss, M. E., & McCormick, R. A. (1995).

Testing a tripartite model: II. Exploring the symptom structure of anxiety and depression in student, adult, and patient samples. *Journal of Abnormal Psychology, 104,* 15–25.

Watson, D., Weber, K., Assenheimer, J. S., Clark, L. A., Strauss, M. E., & McCormick, R. A. (1995). Testing a tripartite model: I. Evaluating the convergent and discriminant validity of anxiety and depression symptom scales. *Journal of Abnormal Psychology, 104,* 3–14.

Wells, A. (1994). A multi-dimensional measure of worry: Development and preliminary validation of the Anxious Thoughts Inventory. *Anxiety, Stress, and Coping: An International Journal, 6,* 289–299.

Wells, A., & Carter, K. (1999). Preliminary tests of a cognitive model of generalized anxiety disorder. *Behaviour Research and Therapy, 37,* 585–594.

Wittchen, H.-U., Zhao, S., Kessler, R. C., & Eaton, W. W. (1994). DSM-III-R generalized anxiety disorder in the National Comorbidity Survey. *Archives of General Psychiatry, 51,* 355–364.

World Health Organization. (1992). *International statistical classification of diseases and related health problems* (10th ed.). Geneva: Author.

Yonkers, K. A., Warshaw, M. G., Massion, A. O., & Keller, M. B. (1996). Phenomenology and course of generalised anxiety disorder. *British Journal of Psychiatry, 168,* 308–313.

APPENDIX 5.1. GAD SECTION OF ADIS-IV-L: INITIAL INQUIRY AND CURRENT EPISODE

Generalized Anxiety Disorder

I. INITIAL INQUIRY

1a. Over the last several months, have you been continually worried or anxious about a number of events or activities in your daily life?

   YES ___ NO ___

   If NO, skip to 1b.

   What kinds of things do you worry about? _____

   _____

   Skip to 2a.

b. Have you *ever* experienced an extended period when you were continually worried or anxious about a number of events or activities in your daily life?

   YES ___ NO ___

   If NO, skip to 3.

   What kinds of things did you worry about? _____

   _____

   When was the most recent time this occurred? _____

2a. Besides this current/most recent period of time when you have been persistently worried about different areas of your life, have there been other, separate periods of time when you were continually worried about a number of life matters?

   YES ___ NO ___

   If NO, skip to 3.

b. So prior to this current/most recent period of time when you were worried about different areas of your life, there was a considerable period of time when you were not having these persistent worries?

   YES ___ NO ___

c. How much time separated these periods? When did this/these separate period(s) occur?

   _____

3. Now I want to ask you a series of questions about worry over the following areas of life.

If patient does not report current or past persistent worry (i.e., NO to 1a. and 1b.), inquire about CURRENT areas of worry only. If patient reports current or past persistent worry, (i.e., YES to either 1a. or 1b.), inquire about both CURRENT and PAST areas of worry. Particularly if there is evidence of *separate* episodes, inquire for the presence of prior *discrete* episodes of disturbance (e.g., "Since these worries began, have there been periods of time when you were not bothered by them?"). Use the space below each general worry area to record the specific content of the patient's worry (including information obtained previously from items 1a. and 1b.). Further inquiry will often be necessary to determine whether areas of worry reported by patient are unrelated to a co-occurring Axis I disorder. If it is determined that an area of worry can be subsumed totally by another Axis I disorder, rate this area as "0." Use comment section to record clinically useful information (e.g., data pertaining to the discreteness of episodes, coexisting disorder with which the area of worry is related).

From Di Nardo, Brown, and Barlow (1994). Copyright 1994 by Graywind Publications. Adapted and reproduced by permission of the publisher, The Psychological Corporation, a Harcourt Assessment Company. All rights reserved.

For each area of worry, make separate ratings of excessiveness (i.e., frequency and intensity) and perceived uncontrollability using the scales and suggested queries below.

Excessiveness:

0 _____ 1 _____ 2 _____ 3 _____ 4 _____ 5 _____ 6 _____ 7 _____ 8

| No worry/ no tension | Rarely worried/ mild tension | Occasionally worried/ moderate tension | Frequently worried/ severe tension | Constantly worried/ extreme tension |

Controllability:

0 _____ 1 _____ 2 _____ 3 _____ 4 _____ 5 _____ 6 _____ 7 _____ 8

| Never/ no difficulty | Rarely/ slight difficulty | Occasionally/ moderate difficulty | Frequently/ marked difficulty | Constantly/ extreme difficulty |

Excessiveness:

How often do/did you worry about _____? If things are/were going well, do/did you still worry about _____? How much tension and anxiety does/did the worry about _____ produce?

Uncontrollability:

Do/did you find it hard to control the worry about _____ in that it is/was difficult to stop worrying about it? Is/was the worry about _____ hard to control in that it will/would come into your mind when you are/were trying to focus on something else?

	Current			Past	
	Excessiveness	Controllability	Comments	Excessiveness	Controllability
a. Minor matters (e.g., punctuality, small repairs)					
b. Work/school	___	___	___	___	___
c. Family	___	___	___	___	___
d. Finances	___	___	___	___	___
e. Social/interpersonal	___	___	___	___	___
f. Health (self)	___	___	___	___	___
g. Health (significant others)	___	___	___	___	___
h. Community/world affairs	___	___	___	___	___
i. Other	___	___	___	___	___
j. Other	___	___	___	___	___

II. CURRENT EPISODE

If evidence of a discrete past episode, preface inquiry in this section with: **Now I want to ask you a series of questions about this *current* period of worry over these areas that began roughly in** _____ (specify month/year).

List principal topics of worry: _____
_____

1. **During the past 6 months, have you been bothered by these worries more days than not?**
   YES ____ NO ____

2. **On an average day over the past month, what percentage of the day did you feel worried?**
   _____ %

3. **Specifically, what types of things do you worry might happen regarding _____** (inquire for each principal area of worry)?
   _____
   _____
   _____

4. **During the past 6 months, have you often experienced _____ when you worried? Has _____ been present more days than not over the past 6 months?** (Do not record symptoms that are associated with other conditions such as panic, social anxiety, etc.)

   0 _____ 1 _____ 2 _____ 3 _____ 4 _____ 5 _____ 6 _____ 7 _____ 8
   None   Mild   Moderate   Severe   Very severe

		Severity	More days than not	
a.	Restlessness; feeling keyed up or on edge	____	Y	N
b.	Being easily fatigued	____	Y	N
c.	Difficulty concentrating or mind going blank	____	Y	N
d.	Irritability	____	Y	N
e.	Muscle tension	____	Y	N
f.	Difficulty falling/staying asleep; restless/unsatisfying sleep	____	Y	N

5. **In what ways have these worries and the tension/anxiety associated with them interfered with your life (e.g., daily routine, job, social activities)? How much are you bothered about having these worries?**
   _____
   _____

   Rate interference: _____   distress: _____
   0 _____ 1 _____ 2 _____ 3 _____ 4 _____ 5 _____ 6 _____ 7 _____ 8
   None   Mild   Moderate   Severe   Very severe

6. **Over this entire current period of time when you've been having these worries and ongoing feelings of tension/anxiety, have you been regularly taking any types of drugs (e.g., drugs of abuse, medication)?**
   YES ____ NO ____
   Specify (type; amount; dates of use): _____
   _____

7. During this current period of time when you've been having the worries and ongoing feelings of tension/anxiety, have you had any physical condition (e.g., hyperthyroidism)?

        YES ____ NO ____

Specify (type; date of onset/remission): _____

_____

8a. For this current period of time, when did these worries and symptoms of tension/anxiety become a problem in that they occurred persistently, you were bothered by the worry or symptoms and found them hard to control, or they interfered with your life in some way? (Note: if patient is vague in date of onset, attempt to ascertain more specific information, e.g., by linking onset to objective life events.)

_____

Date of onset: _____ Month _____ Year

b. Can you recall anything that might have led to this problem?

_____

_____

_____

c. Were you under any type of stress during this time?

        YES ____ NO ____

What was happening in your life at the time?

_____

_____

Were you experiencing any difficulties or changes in:

(1) **Family/relationships?** _____

(2) **Work/school?** _____

(3) **Finances?** _____

(4) **Legal matters?** _____

(5) **Health** (self/others)? _____

9. Besides this current period of worry and tension/anxiety, have there been other, separate periods of time before this when you have had the same problems?

        YES ____ NO ____

If YES, go back and ask 2b. and 2c. from INITIAL INQUIRY.

6

Obsessive–Compulsive Disorder

Steven Taylor
Dana S. Thordarson
Ingrid Söchting

OVERVIEW OF OBSESSIVE–COMPULSIVE DISORDER

Defining Features

Obsessive–compulsive disorder (OCD) is defined by the presence of obsessions, compulsions, or both (American Psychiatric Association, 1994). Obsessions are intrusive thoughts, images, or impulses that the sufferer finds upsetting or repugnant. Common obsessions include intrusive thoughts of contamination with germs, recurrent doubts that one has turned off the stove, and abhorrent thoughts of harming loved ones. OCD sufferers often fear and try to avoid stimuli that trigger obsessions.

Compulsions are repetitive, intentional behaviors that the person feels compelled to perform, often with a desire to resist. Compulsions are typically performed to avert some feared event or to reduce distress, and behaviors may be performed in response to an obsession, such as repetitive handwashing in response to obsessions about contamination. Alternatively, compulsions may be performed in accordance with certain rules, such as checking that the door is locked four times before leaving the house. Compulsions may be overt (e.g., washing or checking) or covert (e.g., thinking a "good" thought to undo or erase a "bad" thought). Compulsions are either clearly excessive or not realistically connected to what they are designed to prevent.

Insight

"Insight" in OCD is defined as the degree to which sufferers recognize that their obsessions and compulsions are unreasonable and due to a psychiatric disorder (American Psychiatric Association, 1994). Insight varies along a continuum, ranging from good insight to overvalued ideation (poor insight) to frank delusions (extremely poor insight). In their calmer moments, OCD sufferers with good insight are able to recognize, for example, that their concerns with contamination are excessive or that repeated checking of door locks is unnecessary. OCD sufferers with poor insight are only barely able to acknowledge the possibility that their obsessions and compulsions are due to a mental disorder: they believe that their obsessional concerns and compulsive behaviors are generally reasonable and appropriate. People suffering from delusions believe that their obsessions and compulsions are entirely reasonable and appropriate. In terms of DSM-IV, the latter people would be diagnosed as having OCD comorbid with either delusional disorder or psychotic disorder not otherwise specified (American Psychiatric Association, 1994). OCD sufferers with overvalued ideation are diagnosed as having OCD with poor insight. An OCD sufferer's insight may change over time, and so diagnoses may change accordingly.

Prevalence and Course

OCD is one of the most common anxiety disorders. Its lifetime prevalence in North America has been estimated at 2.3%, with a similar prevalence in other countries (Weissman et al., 1994). OCD tends to be chronic if untreated, and symptoms wax and wane in severity, often in response to stressful life events. OCD is commonly comorbid with other disorders, including other anxiety disorders, mood disorders, eating disorders, and substance use disorders (American Psychiatric Association, 1994).

GOALS OF ASSESSMENT

Assessment is, in part, a conceptually driven venture, where theories of the causes and treatment of OCD determine what is important to assess. There are many theories of OCD, which lead to different treatments. In planning and evaluating most treatments, it is important to assess the symptoms and associated features of OCD, including an assessment of any comorbid psychopathology. Establishing the appropriate diagnoses is also important. Although diagnostic evaluations are insufficient on their own, they provide valuable information. The task of assessing DSM-IV Axes I and II encourages the clinician to look beyond the patient's most salient problems. This helps the clinician identify psychiatric problems that might otherwise be missed (Wittchen, 1996).

This chapter has three aims. First, we review assessment instruments that can be used in planning and evaluating most OCD treatments, whether they be psychological treatments or pharmacotherapies. Second, we discuss the common problems in implementing these instruments and offer some solutions. Third, to illustrate the integration of assessment and treatment planning, we describe the role of assessment in cognitive-behavioral therapy for OCD.

INSTRUMENTS FOR ASSESSING OBSESSIVE–COMPULSIVE DISORDER

The major clinical features of OCD are obsessions, compulsions, OC-related fear and avoidance, and insight into the irrationality of obsessions and compulsions. In this section we review four groups of measures that assess one or more of these features: screening instruments, structured interviews, self-report measures, and behavioral assessments. Due to space limitations, we selectively review the most well-established measures and the newer, promising ones. Psychometrically flawed instruments or lesser-used measures will not be reviewed. These have been examined elsewhere (Taylor, 1995, 1998).

Our focus is on the measures that are most useful in routine clinical practice with adult patients. This includes some but not all the scales often used in treatment outcome studies.

Although measures of global functioning and global disability are commonly used in outcome studies (e.g., Guy, 1976; Insel et al., 1983; Sheehan, 1983), they are too broad to be of much value for routine clinical practice. More specific measures are needed for the clinician to assess the precise nature of the patient's problems (Taylor, 2000a). For example, rather than assess global impairment due to OCD, it is more useful to know precisely how the patient's functioning is most impaired. Some patients can function adequately outside the house, only to be severely impaired by contamination obsessions and cleaning compulsions once they return home.

Screening Instruments

Because OCD is easily overlooked during a cursory medical or psychiatric evaluation, screening instruments are quite useful. Patients presenting with anxiety or mood symptoms as their chief problems can also receive a brief screen for OCD and other disorders. Positive responses to the screening measure are followed by a more detailed evaluation using a structured diagnostic interview. Two screening instruments have been developed for assessing OCD in primary care clinics (including managed care settings) and in psychiatric settings. The computerized Symptom Driven Diagnostic System for Primary Care (SDDS-PC; Weissman et al., 1998) screens for major depression, alcohol and drug dependence, three anxiety disorders (generalized anxiety disorder, panic disorder, OCD), and suicidal ideation and attempts. The SDDS-PC consists of a brief computerized questionnaire and a short diagnostic interview, administered by a nurse or clinical assistant. Answers to interview questions are typed into the computer by the interviewer, yielding a one-page computer-generated summary of the diagnostic information.

Weissman et al. compared SDDS-PC diagnoses to those obtained from a reliable structured clinical interview, the SCID-IV (Structured Clinical Interview for DSM-IV; see the next section). Unfortunately, for the diagnosis of OCD, the agreement between the SDDS-PC and the SCID-IV was poor (kappa = .28). Weissman et al. proposed that the lack of agreement was due to the delay between the two assessments (up to 4 days). This explanation is implausible because OCD symptoms tend to be stable over such short intervals (O'Connor, Todorov, Robillard, Borgeat, & Brault, 1999; van Balkom et al., 1998).

A more promising screening instrument is a computerized, telephone-administered version of the Primary Care Evaluation of Mental Disorders (PRIME-MD; Kobak et al., 1997). The PRIME-MD assesses mood disorders, four anxiety disorders (generalized anxiety disorder, panic disorder, social phobia, and OCD), alcohol abuse and dependence, and two eating disorders (binge eating disorder and bulimia nervosa). This instrument takes about 10 minutes to complete. The patient dials a toll-free telephone number, listens to a series of "yes"/"no" questions read by the computer over the phone, and responds by pressing a number on a Touch-Tone phone. The computer program uses branching logic in which affirmative responses to the screening questions are followed up by further questions on the disorder(s) in question. Compared to diagnoses obtained by clinicians using the SCID-IV, the PRIME-MD showed good reliability in diagnosing OCD (kappa = .64).

In summary, two screening instruments have been developed for diagnosing OCD. Preliminary results are particularly encouraging for the PRIME-MD. This instrument is quick, comprehensive, easy to use, and acceptable to most patients. A further advantage is that the PRIME-MD screens for a number of disorders, including those commonly comorbid with OCD. A disadvantage is that a specialized computer program is required.

Structured Interviews

Diagnostic Instruments

The two most widely methods for assessing OCD and other anxiety disorders are the Anxiety Disorders Interview Schedule for DSM-IV (ADIS-IV; Di Nardo, Brown, & Barlow, 1994) and the Structured Clinical Interview for DSM-IV (SCID-IV; First, Spitzer, Gibbon, & Williams, 1996). These instruments are reviewed in Chapter 1. Both can be used to establish a diagnosis of OCD, with the ADIS-IV yielding considerably more detailed information. However, as detailed information regarding OCD symptoms is better achieved using the YBOCS (see the next section), the simplicity of the SCID-IV is preferable if the YBOCS is also completed.

Yale–Brown Obsessive Compulsive Scale (YBOCS)

Structured interviews have been developed to assess the severity of various aspects of OCD, such as obsessions, compulsions, avoidance, and insight. The most widely used interview is the YBOCS (Goodman, Price, Rasmussen, Mazure, Delgado, et al., 1989; Goodman, Price, Rasmussen, Mazure, Fleischmann, et al., 1989; Goodman, Rasmussen, et al., 1989), which was designed to assess symptom severity and response to treatment for patients diagnosed with OCD. The YBOCS consists of three sections. The first contains definitions and examples of obsessions and compulsions, which the interviewer reads to the patient. The second contains a symptom checklist, consisting of more than 50 common obsessions and compulsions. The interviewer asks the patient whether each of these symptoms occur currently and whether they have occurred in the past. The interviewer and patient then collaboratively generate a short list of the most severe obsessions, compulsions, and OCD-related avoidance behaviors.

The third section of the YBOCS consists of 10 core items and 11 investigational items. The latter were included on a provisional basis and require further evaluation. The core items assess five parameters of obsessions (items 1–5) and compulsions (items 6–10). The parameters are (1) time occupied/frequency, (2) interference in social or occupational functioning, (3) associated distress, (4) degree of resistance, and (5) perceived control over obsessions or compulsions. Thus, the YBOCS assesses symptom parameters independent of symptom content.

Each core item of the YBOCS is rated by the interviewer on a 5-point scale, ranging from 0 (none) to 4 (extreme). The rater must determine whether the patient is presenting with real obsessions or compulsions, and not symptoms of another disorder such as a paraphilia. All items are accompanied by probe questions, and written definitions accompany each point on the scale of 0 to 4. Items are rated in terms of the average severity of each parameter over the past week. To illustrate, item 1 assesses the average time spent on all obsessions over the past week. The accompanying rating scale ranges from 0 (no obsessions) to 4 (extreme, greater than 8 hours/day or near constant intrusions). Scores on the 10 core items are summed to yield scores for the obsessions subscale, the compulsions subscale, and the total score on the 10-item YBOCS (i.e., the YBOCS-10).

The YBOCS investigational items assess the following: amount of time free of obsessions and compulsions (items 1b and 6b, respectively), insight into the irrationality of obsessions and compulsions (item 11), degree of OCD-related avoidance (item 12), degree of indecisiveness (item 13), overvalued sense of personal responsibility (item 14), obsessional slowness/inertia (item 15), and pathological doubting (item 16). These items are rated on a scale of 0 to 4 as are those used for the 10 core items. In addition, three global judgments are made by the interviewer at the end of the interview: global severity (item 17), global improvement since last assessment (item 18), and reliability of information obtained from the patient (item 19).

Most studies evaluating the YBOCS have focused on the YBOCS-10. This measure has excellent interrater reliability (Goodman, Price, Rasmussen, Mazure, Fleishmann, et al., 1989; Jenike et al., 1990; Price, Goodman, Charney, Rasmussen, & Heninger, 1987; Woody, Steketee, & Chambless, 1995), acceptable internal consistency (Goodman, Price, Rasmussen, Mazure, Fleishmann, et al., 1989; Richter, Cox, & Direnfeld, 1994; Woody et al., 1995), and good test–retest reliability over intervals of at least 2 weeks (Kim, Dysken, & Kuskowski, 1990, 1992; Kim, Dysken, Kuskowski, & Hoover, 1993; Woody et al., 1995). The YBOCS-10 was intended for use with patients diagnosed with OCD, and there has been only one study of its criterion-related validity. Rosenfeld, Dar, Anderson, Kobak, and Greist (1992) found that patients with OCD had higher YBOCS-10 scores than did patients with other anxiety disorders and normal controls. The YBOCS-10 has good convergent validity with other OCD measures (Black, Kelly, Myers, & Noyes, 1990; Goodman, Price, Rasmussen, Mazure, Delgado, et al., 1989; Kim et al., 1990, 1992; Richter et al., 1994; Woody et al., 1995) and is sensitive to treatment-related changes in OCD symptoms (Taylor, 1995).

A limitation of the YBOCS concerns its discriminant validity. The YBOCS-10 is highly correlated with measures of depression and with measures of general anxiety (Goodman, Price, Rasmussen, Mazure, Delgado, et al., 1989; Hewlett, Vinogradov, & Agras, 1992; Price et al., 1987; Richter et al., 1994). Research that directly compares the YBOCS to other OCD measures is needed to determine whether the discriminant validity of the YBOCS is any different from that of other OCD measures. A second limitation is that the arrangement and description of symptoms in the symptom checklist seems to miss some important symptoms (such as doubts or thoughts of terrible things happening to loved ones), which can be confusing to interviewers who are not experienced in assessing OCD. A further limitation is that the interview-administered YBOCS can be time-consuming, with interviews taking an average of 40 minutes per patient (Rosenfeld et al., 1992). However, the time taken to complete the YBOCS is justified, given the wealth of information it provides. In particular, it alerts the interviewer to obsessions and compulsions that the OCD sufferer may not have recognized or reported initially.

In summary, the YBOCS—consisting of the symptom checklist, YBOCS-10, and 11 investigational items—provides a good deal of useful information for assessment and treatment planning. With the exception of discriminant validity, the YBOCS-10 generally has good psychometric properties. The psychometric properties of the symptom checklist and investigational items remain to be investigated. Nevertheless, the checklist is useful for assessment and treatment planning because it assesses a wide range of obsessive and compulsive phenomena.

Self-Report and Computerized Versions of the YBOCS

Recent studies have shown that computerized and self-report versions of the YBOCS have good psychometric properties and yield roughly similar scores to the interviewer-administered version (Baer, Brown-Beasley, Sorce, & Henriques, 1993; Rosenfeld et al., 1992; Steketee, Frost, & Bogart, 1996; Warren, Zgourides, & Monto, 1993). However, compared to their scores on the interview versions, respondents tend to obtain higher scores on the self-report version (Steketee, Frost, & Bogart, 1996), and possibly on the computerized versions. This would occur if respondents confuse obsessions and compulsions with other phenomena, such as worries. We will return to this problem later in the chapter.

Although the self-report and computerized forms of the YBOCS are not substitutes for the interview version, they still play a useful role in assessment. Self-report and computerized versions are quick to complete, so they can be administered each week during therapy in order to monitor treatment progress (Herman & Koran, 1998; Marks et al., 1998).

Dimensional Yale–Brown Obsessive–Compulsive Scale (DYBOCS)

James F. Leckman and colleagues (Leckman, personal communication, September 23, 1998) have recently begun work on the DYBOCS, which is a variation of the YBOCS. The DYBOCS provides scores on five dimensions of OC symptoms: (1) harmful, somatic, sexual, or religious obsessions, and their related compulsions; (2) symmetry, ordering, counting, or arranging obsessions and compulsions; (3) contamination obsessions and cleaning compulsions; (4) hoarding and collecting obsessions and compulsions; and (5) "miscellaneous" obsessions and compulsions that are not included in the other dimensions (e.g., superstitious behaviors, obsessions and compulsions about lucky or unlucky numbers, obsessions consisting of intrusive nonsense sounds). The first four dimensions were based on a factor-analytic study of the YBOCS symptom checklist (Leckman et al., 1997).

The interview yields four scores for each dimension: degree of distress, time spent occupied with symptoms, degree of impairment due to symptoms, and overall severity of that dimension. Once all five dimensions are rated, the interviewer makes a global rating of OCD severity and lists the patient's three most severe OC symptoms. The interviewer also notes what the patient fears to be the consequences of not performing the compulsions and rates how strongly the patient believes that the feared consequences will occur. Compared to the original YBOCS, the DYBOCS is more labor-intensive, both for the patient and clinician. Further research is needed to evaluate the reliability and validity of the DYBOCS and to determine whether the additional information makes the DYBOCS superior to the original scale.

Interviews for Assessing Insight in OCD

The degree of insight displayed by OCD sufferers has proved to be an inconsistent predictor of treatment response. Some studies reported that poor insight predicted poor treatment outcome (Foa, 1979; Foa et al., 1983), whereas other studies found that insight was unrelated to outcome (Lelliott & Marks, 1987; Lelliott, Noshirvani, Basoglu, Marks, & Monteiro, 1988; Salkovskis & Warwick, 1985). The inconsistencies may be partly due to differences in the psychometric properties of the methods used to assess insight. It is only recently that reliable and valid methods have been developed. Accordingly, further research is needed to determine the prognostic significance of insight. In the meantime, the clinician would be wise to err on the side of caution—to be prepared to deal with problems of treatment compliance and outcome for patients with poor insight.

There are three promising interview measures of insight in OCD: the YBOCS item 11 (i.e., one of the investigational items; Goodman, Price, Rasmussen, Mazure, & Delgado, 1989; Goodman, Price, Rasmussen, Mazure, & Fleishmann, 1989; Goodman, Rasmussen, et al., 1989), the Brown Assessment of Beliefs Scale (BABS; Eisen et al., 1998), and the Overvalued Ideation Scale (OVIS; Neziroglu, McKay, Yaryura-Tobias, Stevens, & Todaro, 1999). Preliminary tests of reliability and validity are encouraging for all three scales (e.g., Eisen et al., 1998; Neziroglu et al., 1999). The main difference among these measures is the amount of time they require to complete and the amount of information they yield. Item 11 from the YBOCS takes the least amount of time and yields the least information. It is simply a rating of insight on a scale of 0 to 4, ranging from 0, "excellent insight," to 4, "no insight, delusional."

The BABS is a 7-item scale designed to assess insight in a range of psychiatric disorders, including OCD. Its items assess several aspects of insight, including the strength and persistence of beliefs, whether the patient is aware that other people do not hold the same beliefs, and whether the patient has attempted to test his or her beliefs. The OVIS contains 11 items to assess similar aspects of insight. The BABS and OVIS take 10 to 30 minutes to administer, compared to a few minutes required for the YBOCS item 11. For the busy clinician, an important question is whether the additional information from the BABS and OVIS makes a difference to treatment planning and evaluation. Researchers have yet to address this question. In the meantime, the clinician might prefer the simpler single-item YBOCS measure of insight.

Self-Report Inventories

A great many self-report inventories have been developed to assess the major symptoms of OCD. These include the self-report versions of the YBOCS and DYBOCS described earlier in this chapter. In the following sections, we review additional measures. Our focus is on the best measures identified in previous reviews (Taylor, 1995, 1998) and on the some of the most promising new developments in self-report assessment of OCD symptoms. Each of the following inventories is brief, requiring 10 to 20 minutes to complete.

Maudsley Obsessional Compulsive Inventory (MOCI)

The MOCI (Hodgson & Rachman, 1977) consists of four factorially derived subscales: (1) washing compulsions (i.e., OC-related washing compulsions and contamination fears), (2) checking compulsions, (3) obsessional slowness/repetition, and (4) excessive doubting/conscientiousness. Factor-analytic studies have generally replicated all subscales except the slowness subscale (Taylor, 1995). When used with clinical samples, all but the slowness subscales have acceptable internal consistencies (Taylor, 1995).

Test–retest reliability has been reported only for the MOCI total scale. In the absence of treatment, scores are reliable (stable) over a period of at least 6 months (Emmelkamp, Kraaijkamp, & van den Hout, 1999; Hodgson & Rachman, 1977; Sternberger & Burns, 1990). The total scale and subscales generally show good criterion-related validity, in that they discriminate patients with OCD from patients with other disorders and from normal controls (Emmelkamp et al., 1999; Hodgson, Rankin, & Stockwell, 1979, unpublished, cited in Rachman & Hodgson, 1980). The total scale and washing and checking subscales have been tested in terms of convergent and discriminant validity. The measures have performed well on these tests, and the MOCI total scale also has been shown to be sensitive to treatment effects (Taylor, 1995).

In summary, the MOCI total scale has generally acceptable psychometric properties, as do both of its washing and checking subscales. The other subscales require further investigation. The MOCI subscales were developed on the basis of factor analysis, and subsequent studies support the factorial distinction between all but the slowness subscale. The latter has poor internal consistency, which is not surprising given its heterogeneous item content. Two of its items assess ruminations, two items assess compulsive counting and the need for routine, and only three items directly assess obsessional slowness.

Although the MOCI total scale has adequate psychometric properties, it also has important limitations. The MOCI does not assess some common compulsions such as hoarding and covert rituals. It provides a limited assessment of obsessional ruminations (two items). The MOCI also does not assess important parameters of OCD, such as interference and resistance to compulsions. Interference only can be inferred by the number of symptoms endorsed by the respondent.

Padua Inventory

The Padua Inventory (Sanavio, 1988) contains four subscales that assess the severity of the following symptoms of obsession–compulsion: checking, contamination fears, mental dyscontrol (impaired control of mental activities), and fear of behavioral dyscontrol (urges and worries about losing control of one's behavior). The original Padua Inventory was strongly correlated ($rs > .55$) with distress proneness (neuroticism and trait anxiety) (Taylor, 1998). This appears to be because some items of the Padua Inventory measure worry proneness rather than obsessions (Freeston et al., 1994). Accordingly, Burns, Keortge, Formea, and Sternberger (1996) revised the Padua Inventory, primarily with the purpose of deleting items that assess worry. The result was five content-related subscales: obsessional thoughts about harm to oneself or others, obsessional impulses to harm oneself or others, contamination obsessions and washing compulsions, checking compulsions, and dressing and grooming compulsions. The subscales of the revised Padua Inventory have good internal consistency, test–retest reliability (over at least 6 months), criterion-related validity, and discriminant validity (Taylor, 1998). Convergent validity and sensitivity to treatment effects remain to be evaluated. The original Padua Inventory performed well on these indices, and so the same is likely to apply to the revised version. In summary, available data indicate that the revised Padua Inventory has good psychometric properties and is one of the most comprehensive self-report measures of OCD.

Obsessive–Compulsive Inventory (OCI)

The OCI (Foa, Kozak, Salkovskis, Coles, & Amir 1998) is a new inventory that assesses the frequency and distress associated with the following seven symptom domains: washing, checking, doubting, ordering, obsessing (i.e., having obsessional thoughts), hoarding, and mental neutralizing. Each item is rated on two scales of 0 to 4, one assessing symptom frequency and the other assessing degree of associated distress. A strength of the OCI is that this brief inventory is broad in its coverage of OC symptoms. Preliminary data (Foa et al., 1998) indicate that the total scale and its seven subscales have acceptable internal consistency and good test–retest reliability over at least 2 weeks. The total scale and subscales have generally performed well on tests of criterion-related validity; people with OCD tend to have higher scores than people with other disorders and higher than scores of normal controls. An exception is the hoarding subscale, which was weakest in terms of criterion-related validity. The OCI total scale has adequate convergent and discriminant validities (Foa et al., 1998). These validities have yet to be examined for the subscales. Sensitivity to treatment effects also remains to be examined.

Vancouver Obsessional–Compulsive Inventory (VOCI)

The VOCI (Thordarson, Radomsky, Rachman, Shafran, & Sawchuk, 1997) is another new measure of OC symptoms that is currently undergoing validation. It contains 55 items, each rated on a 5-point Likert-type scale. Originally construed as a revision of the MOCI, the

VOCI now comprises six factor-analytically derived subscales: Checking, Contamination, Indecisiveness/Perfection/Mistakes, Obsessions, Routine/Slowness/Counting, and Hoarding. Preliminary results suggest that it is a promising new measure of OCD symptoms, with factorial and criterion-related validity built in during scale development.

Behavioral Avoidance Tests (BATs)

BATs were originally developed to assess fear and avoidance in people with circumscribed fears or phobias (Lang & Lazovik, 1963). In these tasks the person is asked to approach as close as possible to a feared stimulus. The distance of closest approach is recorded as a measure of avoidance, and self-reported levels of distress at particular distances are used to assess fear. The Subjective Units of Distress Scale (SUDS) is commonly used to measure fear. Here, the person provides a rating of his or her fear or distress on a scale of 0 to 100, where 0 = no fear/distress and 100 = extreme fear/distress.

Several types of BATs have been developed to assess OC-related fear and avoidance (see Taylor, 1998, for a review). One of the most comprehensive methods is the multi-step–multitask BAT (Steketee, Chambless, Tran, Worden, & Gillis, 1996). For a given patient the assessor identifies three tasks that are difficult or impossible to perform without significant anxiety or rituals (e.g., switching off electrical appliances without checking). Each task is then broken down into three to seven steps that are intended to provoke steadily increasing levels of discomfort. For example, the patient might be asked to drive on progressively busier streets without checking. The patient is told that the BAT is not a test of courage and that he or she is free to refuse any or all of the task.

Several different measures can be incorporated into the multistep–multitask BAT. Steketee, Chambless, et al. (1996) reported using several measures, including SUDS, measures of avoidance (3-point scale, ranging from 0, no avoidance, to 2, complete avoidance of the entire task), and frequency of rituals (3-point scale, ranging from 0, no rituals, to 2, extensive rituals).

The multistep–multitask BAT has good convergent and discriminant validity and is sensitive to detecting treatment-related changes in OCD (Steketee, Chambless, et al., 1996; Woody et al., 1995). Test–retest reliability and criterion-related (known groups) validity have yet to be examined. However, it is likely that the BAT will have good criterion-related validity for many types of exposure tasks. This is because, by definition, only people with OCD will display significant fear, avoidance, and rituals in response to classic OC-related stimuli such as "contaminants," door locks, and so forth. However, it also is likely that there will be conditions in which the BAT does not discriminate between diagnostic groups. For example, a BAT consisting of driving on increasingly busier streets may evoke fear in people with OCD, as well as in people with other disorders such as agoraphobia.

BATs can be either used in the clinic or given to patients as homework assignments (where the patient records his or her levels of fear, avoidance, etc.). BATs are well suited for assessing fear and avoidance of "contaminated" stimuli associated with washing compulsions. It is more difficult to design behavioral avoidance tasks for patients with other types of compulsions, such as checking or ordering rituals. However, Steketee, Chambless et al.'s (1996) instruction guide facilitates the construction of such tasks by providing detailed guidelines and examples. A major disadvantage of BATs is that they are time-consuming to implement.

Comment

Among the most promising screening instruments for OCD is the PRIME-MD. For patients who screen positive for OCD, a DSM-IV diagnosis can be established by means of a structured clinical interview such as the SCID-IV or the ADIS-IV. For assessment of OCD symptoms, the YBOCS has the advantage of being comprehensive, with generally good psychometric properties; it can be used to assess treatment outcome before and after treatment, and to assess insight in OCD. The self-report version of the YBOCS can be used to monitor progress during treatment.

Other measures, such as other interviews for assessing insight, and the other self-report measures of OCD, also provide valuable information for treatment planning and evaluation. At the present time, however, it is not clear whether the interviews for assessing insight are more useful from the YBOCS insight item. BATs and self-report inventories, such as the revised Padua Inventory and the Obsessive–Compulsive Inventory, also provide the clinician with valuable information. Further research is needed to determine whether these measures can be used instead of the YBOCS. At present, this seems unlikely because the YBOCS is more comprehensive than other OC measures. It is also unclear whether questionnaires or BATs provide information that can usefully supplement data obtained from the YBOCS. Given that no measure has perfect psychometric properties, one clinically useful strategy is to use the YBOCS interview in addition to a questionnaire such as the Padua Inventory. Confidence in the accuracy of the assessment is suggested when the two instruments provide similar results. Additional measures are also useful to attain a comprehensive assessment of the patient's problems. These include interviews with the patient's significant others to obtain their perspective on the patient's symptoms. Such interviews can also be used to assess the way in which symptoms influence the patient's relationships, and the way that significant others might inadvertently perpetuate the patient's problems (e.g., by performing cleaning rituals for the patient).

Assessment of the patient's problems can also be supplemented by other questionnaires and interviews. To assess the patient's general level of distress, the Beck Anxiety Inventory (Beck & Steer, 1993a) can be administered, along with the Beck Depression Inventory (Beck & Steer, 1993b) or the Beck Depression Inventory–II (Beck, Steer, & Brown, 1996). Several questionnaires and interviews have been developed to assess personality disorders. Compared to structured interviews, questionnaires tend to overdiagnose personality disorders (Zimmerman, 1994), which can result in misdirected treatment plans. One of the most efficient structured interviews for DSM-IV personality disorders is the Structured Clinical Interview for DSM-IV, Axis II (First, Spitzer, Gibbon, Williams, & Lorna, 1994). It comes with a personality questionnaire in which the patient endorses the presence or absence of personality disorder traits. The clinician reviews the completed questionnaire for responses that indicate personality pathology. These responses are then probed with a structured interview. The interview typically requires fewer than 40 minutes (First et al., 1995).

Assessment can be further informed by the clinician's incidental observations during the interview. The interviewer may notice avoidance behavior (e.g., not touching doorknobs and not taking materials you give them), checking, or reassurance-seeking. Such observations provide suggestive information about the patient's symptoms and degree of impairment. Signs of impaired mental status (e.g., loose associations) or a peculiar, rather than anxious, social presentation can be important clues that OCD may not be the primary problem and that organic or psychotic disorders should be ruled out.

Comprehensive assessment takes time but usually pays off in terms of developing a good treatment plan. An assessment battery consisting of the SCID-IV (for Axis I), the SCID-II (for Axis II), and the YBOCS requires about 4 hours of interview time and may be supplemented by other measures such as the Padua Inventory and the Beck Inventories. If the clinician cannot spare this amount of time, then the SCID-II could be dropped. However, in doing this the clinician runs the risk of failing to detect personality disorders and thereby failing to plan appropriate treatment. If assessment time is limited to 60 to 90 minutes, the interviewer could complete the YBOCS and the OCD and Major Depression sections of the SCID and could give the patient questionnaires (e.g., Padua and BDI) to take home.

PRACTICAL ISSUES IN THE ASSESSMENT OF OBSESSIVE–COMPULSIVE DISORDER

Despite the usefulness of many of the measures described in this chapter, each has its limitations. The purpose of the following sections is to review some of the clinical problems that arise when using structured interviews and self-report measures to assess OCD. Two particular issues are important: (1) procedural difficulties in administering the measures, and (2) problems in distinguishing obsessions and compulsions from related phenomena—that is, problems of ensuring that a given measure is, in fact, assessing obsessions and compulsions in a given respondent.

Procedural Problems

Reluctance to Describe Symptoms

There are several reasons why people with OCD sometimes have difficulty describing their obsessions and compulsions. Some patients are embarrassed about their symptoms or are afraid that the interviewer will think they are dangerous or psychotic. The clinician needs to be sensitive to these concerns and appropriately empathic about the difficulties patients often have in describing personally repugnant or humiliating symptoms. The assessment is facilitated if the interviewer does not appear shocked or disturbed by the patient's symptoms. Structured interviews such as the YBOCS can further help put the patient at ease. As the patient is taken through the symptom checklist, he or she often comes to realize that other people have similar symptoms, and that the interviewer has encountered these symptoms before. Patients who remain reluctant to describe their symptoms can usually be persuaded to describe them in general terms (e.g., a thought of doing a terrible thing). It can be helpful for the interviewer to give case examples from the literature of horrific obsessions that were experienced by highly conscientious, moral people. Educating patients as to the nature of obsessions and how they are distinguished from, for example, sadistic fantasies can be comforting.

The belief in thought–action fusion (Shafran, Thordarson, & Rachman, 1996) can also make patients reluctant to describe their obsessions. Some patients believe that having a particular thought (e.g., an obsession that their spouse will be killed in an accident) increases the likelihood that the event will actually occur; therefore, discussing the obsession with the interviewer increases the risk that something terrible will happen. When thought–action fusion interferes with assessment, the problem usually can be overcome by gently but persistently encouraging the patient to describe his or her obsessions, at least in general terms as described above. If necessary, the patient can engage in neutralizing compulsions (e.g., replacing a harm-related obsession with a "good" thought). For the purposes of pretreatment assessment, it is acceptable for the patient to perform such compulsions. When treatment is initiated, the patient is encouraged to increasingly refrain from ritualizing.

When assessing patients who are reluctant to describe their symptoms, it is more important to complete the interview in an empathic way than to risk alienating or excessively frightening the patient with demands for precise examples of their symptoms (e.g., verbatim obsessions) at the assessment stage. Most patients will be able to more fully disclose the exact nature of their symptoms as their trust and comfort level increase in therapy.

Contamination Fears

Assessment problems may also arise when patients with contamination fears are concerned about handling questionnaires and writing materials and therefore have difficulty completing the assessment. Again, persistent, empathic encouragement is typically all that is needed. If necessary, one can remind the patient that he or she can always engage in cleaning rituals after completing the questionnaires. One of our patients, for example, would wipe down the questionnaires with disinfectant. At the pretreatment assessment, it was better to have the patient perform such a compulsion than to have him or her refuse to complete the questionnaires because of contamination fears.

Lack of Awareness or Minimization of Symptoms

A further problem concerns the person's awareness of the severity of his or her compulsions. To illustrate, a patient may not realize that he or she engages in frequent reassurance seeking. An interview with a significant other can be illuminating. Patients whose OCD is longstanding may have incorporated their symptoms so fully into their lives that they are unaware of the degree to which they are impaired. For example, some OCD sufferers with severe contamination concerns may, in fact, do very little washing because their avoidance is so extensive (e.g., they rarely leave the house) and may report that their OCD does not interfere with their lives because they spend little time doing compulsions. A useful assessment strategy is to have the person describe in as much detail as possible their day; from this description the interviewer can often find avoidance or compulsions that the sufferer finds so "normal" that he or she has ceased to notice them. This is also useful for patients who tend to give vague information as to the nature and frequency of their symptoms.

Another assessment problem is that patients sometimes attempt to minimize their symptoms. For example, people with hoarding compulsions may present for treatment at the urging of people living with them, who are no longer able to tolerate living in a house cluttered with hoarded belongings. Some hoarders do not regard their compulsions as problematic and may be reluctant to participate in assessment and treatment. When symptom minimization is suspected, it can be useful to conduct a home visit along with interviewing significant others. See Frost and Steketee (1999) for further discussion on special issues in the assessment and treatment of hoarding compulsions.

Problems Completing the Assessment in a Reasonable Time

Indecisiveness, intolerance of ambiguity, and a need for reassurance are characteristic features of OCD (Rachman & Hodgson, 1980). Occasionally, these features interfere with the assessment of OCD by greatly increasing the amount of time required to complete the assessment. For example, some patients are circumstantial in their descriptions of their symptoms, in an attempt to provide the interviewer with "all" the details, or to make sure they have expressed themselves in precisely the correct way so as not to be misinterpreted. These problems, when they arise, can often be addressed by patience and prompting. Strategies include (1) gently but persistently encouraging the patient to make short, concise responses; (2) reminding the patient of the time constraints, how many questions are left, and asking their permission for you to, in the interest of time, interrupt them and move on; and (3) asking more closed rather than open-ended questions. The YBOCS symptom checklist can be particularly challenging with some patients who seem to be reluctant to deny any symptom on the checklist outright. With these patients, it can be helpful to immediately follow up affirmative responses to checklist items with an inquiry such as "Is this a major problem for you?" In this way, symptoms that are unlikely to represent clinical obsessions or compulsions can be quickly eliminated. Patients who complete self-report measures may repeatedly ask for clarification of the meaning of questions and may repeatedly check their answers. For self-report measures, we encourage the patient to write down the first response that comes to mind, telling them it is often the most accurate response, and we discourage repeated checking of answers. These simple strategies are generally effective in completing interviews and questionnaires within a reasonable period of time.

Distinguishing Obsessions and Compulsions from Related Phenomena

The purpose of this section of the chapter is not to provide a complete list of differential diagnoses; this can be found in DSM-IV (American Psychiatric Association, 1994) and in the YBOCS interview protocol (Goodman, Rasmussen, et al., 1989). Instead, we focus on some of the more common diagnostic difficulties.

Distinguishing Obsessions from Other Recurrent Thoughts

In some cases it can be difficult to distinguish obsessions from worries. Obsessional doubts and ruminations often have a worry-like quality to them (e.g., repetitive obsessional thoughts such as "What if I didn't lock the door?" or thoughts of a loved one being killed in an accident). Obsessions and worries have some similarities—for example, both are uncontrollable and excessive. To complicate matters, people with excessive worry (i.e., those with generalized anxiety disorder) often engage in subclinical rituals, particularly checking compulsions (Brown, Moras, Zinbarg, & Barlow, 1993; Schut, Castonguay, Plummer, & Borkovec, 1995). Although obsessions can sometimes be very difficult to distinguish from worries, in most cases experienced clinicians can reliably distinguish between the two (Brown et al., 1993), and respondents can distinguish worries from obsessions once they are given definitions of these phenomena (Wells & Morrison, 1994). In a review of the literature on obsessions and worries, Turner, Beidel, and Stanley (1992) identified several ways in which worries differ from obsessions. These criteria can aid in the accurate identification of obsessions:

1. Compared to obsessions, worries are more frequently perceived (by the sufferer) as being triggered by an internal or external event.
2. The contents of worries are typically related to normal experiences of everyday living (e.g., family, finances, work), whereas the content of obsessions frequently include themes of contamination, religion, sex, and aggression (but themes of illness and harm coming to loved ones can characterize both worries and obsessions).
3. Worries typically occur as thoughts rather than images (i.e., verbal/linguistic representations), whereas obsessions can take a variety of forms (thoughts, images, impulses).
4. Although worries and obsessions are both experienced as uncontrollable, worries tend not to be resisted as strongly as obsessions, nor are worries as intrusive as obsessions.
5. The content of worries, compared to obsessions, is less likely to be regarded by the person as "unacceptable" (i.e., less likely to be ego-dystonic).

Intrusive thoughts in posttraumatic stress disorder can be distinguished from obsessions in that the former are typically memories of the traumatic event. By definition, memories are of events that have already occurred, and therefore such thoughts, no matter how recurrent or unpleasant, are not senseless or ego-dystonic and cannot be classified as obsessions. Thoughts of substance acquisition or use in substance use disorders, or sexual thoughts in paraphilias, are not ego-dystonic and therefore not obsessions; rather, they may be considered part of the craving phenomenon. The person with OCD craves nothing and gets no pleasure from their thoughts (occasional sexual arousal in response to true sexual obsessions can occur, but it is typically very distressing rather than pleasurable). The person with a paraphilia or "sexual addiction" is erotically attracted to the content of the thought, even if he wishes he were not; the person with a sexual obsession is disgusted by his thoughts and has no desire to act upon them.

Distinguishing Compulsions from Other Repetitive Behaviors

Tics and compulsions can be difficult to distinguish. They differ primarily in that compulsions are usually purposeful, meaningful behaviors, often performed in response to an obsession, and usually intended to prevent or reduce perceived threat. In contrast, tics (including tics seen in Tourette syndrome) are purposeless actions that are largely involuntary, although in some cases they can be suppressed. Unlike the majority of compulsions, tics are not performed to prevent some feared consequence. It can be difficult to distinguish compulsions that are performed to relieve discomfort at things not feeling "just right" from complex motor tics. Nevertheless, with compulsions there is usually an external circumstance which is not "just right." In addition, if they are prevented from performing the compulsion, sufferers may discover that there are underlying feared consequences of not performing compulsions.

As with tics, repetitive problematic behaviors such as hair-pulling (trichotillomania), skin-picking, and nail-biting are not used to avert a feared outcome. Occasionally, however, hair-pulling and skin-picking are done with a compulsive-like motivation, such as a strong need to have a perfectly straight hairline in a patient with other OC concerns about symmetry. In these cases, the repeated behavior can be better conceptualized as an OCD compulsion rather than as a habit or impulse control disorder.

So-called compulsive behaviors such as gambling, overeating, stealing, excessive shopping, and "sexual addiction" are positively reinforcing, even if the person wishes they did not do these behaviors to such excess. These may be distinguished from compulsions in that they are typically pleasurable activities that preoccupy the person (the problem being in their excessiveness) who feels a craving to engage in them. Compulsions, on the other hand, are not typically experienced as pleasurable and are typically performed to reduce anxiety or to avert a feared outcome.

Comment

Clinical assessment involves art and science. The science involves the construction of reliable, valid assessment instruments. The art involves drawing on one's clinical experience and other skills to help people with OCD overcome difficulties in completing the assessment measures. Anticipating these difficulties can help the clinician prepare to resolve them. Empathy, encouragement, and prompting can go a long way toward helping patients complete the assessment measures. Armed with information from these measures, the clinician is in a better position to plan treatment and to evaluate its efficacy. In addition, distinguishing obsessions and compulsions from topographically similar phenomena is essential to ensure that the patient is receiving the best possible treatment for their difficulties. While some aspects of empirically validated treatments for OCD can be helpful for problems such as worries, tics, and impulse-control disorders, it is preferable to find alternate, sharper treatments developed specifically for these problems.

INTEGRATING ASSESSMENT, TREATMENT PLANNING, AND OUTCOME EVALUATION

Particular drug treatments and psychological therapies are effective in reducing OCD (van Balkom et al., 1994). Effective pharmacotherapies include serotonin reuptake inhibitors (e.g., clomipramine, fluoxetine, fluvoxamine, sertraline, and paroxetine). Effective psychological treatments consist of behavioral or cognitive-behavioral therapies that use some form of exposure and response prevention. These psychological treatments tend to be as effective as drug treatments for OCD, and most studies suggest that efficacy is not enhanced by combining psychological and drug therapies (Hohagen et al., 1998; Kobak, Greist, Jefferson, Katzelnick, & Henk, 1998; O'Connor et al., 1999; van Balkom & van Dyck, 1998; van Balkom et al., 1994).

In the following discussion we illustrate how assessment can be integrated into one form of OCD treatment: cognitive-behavioral therapy (CBT). To place the discussion in context, we first describe the rationale and interventions used in this treatment. Then we describe how assessment methods can be used to develop a cognitive-behavioral case formulation, which contains a working hypothesis about the patient's problems, and a treatment plan. The case example described in the following sections is a composite of several patients we have treated, constructed according to Clifft's (1986) guidelines for protecting patient privacy and confidentiality.

CBT for Obsessive–Compulsive Disorder

Rationale

The major element of behavioral treatment for OCD is exposure and response prevention, which involves exposing patients to distressing but harmless stimuli (e.g., asking the patient to touch a "contaminated" object such as a trash can), and then helping the patient prevent themselves from engaging in their compulsions (e.g., refraining from hand washing). (See Steketee, 1993, for a detailed description and examples of exposure and response prevention for OCD). Although exposure and response prevention is among the most powerful OCD treatments, there is ample room for improving efficacy (Stanley & Turner, 1995). Accordingly, especially since the development of cognitive-behavioral theories of OCD (e.g., Salkovskis, 1985) cognitive interventions have been added to this treatment, resulting in CBT for OCD.

Theoretical Underpinnings

One of the most promising CBT approaches is based on Salkovskis's (1985, 1989, 1996, 1999) cognitive-behavioral model of OCD. This model begins with the observation that intrusions (i.e., intrusive thoughts, images, or impulses) are commonplace experiences; more than 80% of the general population have had intrusions at some time (Rachman & de Silva, 1978; Salkovskis & Harrison, 1984). Normal intrusions develop into clinical obsessions when the person appraises the intrusions as implicating a threat for which he or she is personally responsible. To illustrate, consider a religious person who experiences an intrusive, blasphemous thought (e.g., "The Pope is a pedophile"). The person might appraise the intrusion as odd, harmless, and personally irrelevant mental flotsam. In this case, the intrusion would be regarded as insignificant, and the person would have no reason to dwell on it further. Alternatively, the person might appraise the intrusion as threatening and blame himself or herself for its occurrence ("I'll be damned to hell for having such thoughts!"). If this occurred then the person would become distressed about the intrusion and would strive to neutralize it.

Neutralizing activities may include overt compulsions (e.g., repeatedly touching a religious object), covert compulsions (e.g., replacing the "bad" thought with "good" thoughts such as a mental prayer), or both. Neutralizing activities can also be conceptualized as including avoidance of stimuli that trigger obsessions (e.g., a person with blasphemous obsessions may avoid churches). Attempts to suppress intrusions may cause them to increase in frequency (Wegner, 1994). Neutralizing activities also become reminders of intrusions, thereby maintaining them (Salkovskis, 1996). Neutralizing activities tend to persist and tend to be excessive because (1) they temporarily remove the unwanted intrusions and so relieve distress (negative reinforcement), and (2) they prevent the person from learning that the appraisals and beliefs are unrealistic. In this way, according to Salkovskis's cognitive-behavioral theory of OCD, intrusions escalate into obsessions and OCD develops. For further details, see Salkovskis (1985, 1989, 1996, 1999).

OCD-related appraisals of intrusive thoughts, which lead to distress and neutralizing, are thought to arise from dysfunctional beliefs, such as longstanding beliefs about personal responsibility, and beliefs about the prevalence of danger. Building on the work of Salkovskis and others, the Obsessive Compulsive Cognitions Working Group (1997) recently developed a comprehensive list of OCD-related beliefs (see Table 6.1). Because of their influence in shaping appraisals, these beliefs are hypothesized to play a causal role in producing obsessions and compulsions. Therefore, the beliefs are important targets of CBT. For the CBT practitioner, these beliefs and their associated appraisals are currently best assessed via an unstructured clinical interview. Efforts at developing self-report measures of these cognitions are currently under way (Obsessive Compulsive Cognitions Working Group, 2001), and may eventually become useful clinical aids.

Treatment Procedures

As in more traditional behavior therapy for OCD, CBT usually involves exposure and response prevention exercises, although these exercises are used as behavioral experiments to test appraisals and beliefs. To illustrate, consider a patient who has recurrent images of close friends and relatives being assaulted, and a compulsion to repeatedly telephone friends and family to warn them. This patient is found to hold a belief about thought–action fusion, such as "Thinking about people who are close to me being assaulted will make such an assault actually occur." To challenge this belief, the patient and therapist can devise a test that pits this belief against a more realistic belief (e.g., "My thoughts have no influence on the occurrence of assaults"). A behavioral experiment might involve deliberately bringing on thoughts of family members and friends being assaulted and then evaluating the consequences. Methods derived from Beck's cognitive therapy (e.g., Beck & Emery, 1985) are also used to challenge OCD-related beliefs and appraisals.

Developing a Cognitive-Behavioral Case Formulation

CBT is not administered by simply following a treatment manual. The clinician first needs to develop an understanding of the patient's problems and then to use this knowledge to plan a suitable treatment. Accordingly, a case formulation is developed. This consists of a model of the causes of the patient's problems and a plan for overcoming them. The formu-

TABLE 6.1. Consensus from the Obsessive Compulsive Cognitions Working Group (1997): Important OCD-Related Beliefs

Belief domains	Definitions and examples
Overimportance of thoughts	The belief that the occurrence of a thought implies something very important. Included in this domain are beliefs that reflect thought–action fusion. That is, beliefs that the mere presence of a "bad" thought can produce a "bad" outcome. Examples: "Having a bad thought is the same as doing a bad deed." "Having violent thoughts means I will lose control and become violent."
Importance of controlling one's thoughts	Overvaluation of the importance of exerting complete control over intrusive thoughts, images, and impulses and the belief that this is both possible and desirable. Examples: "I should be able to gain complete control of my mind if I exercise enough will power." "I would be a better person if I gained control over my thoughts."
Perfectionism	The tendency to believe that (1) there is a perfect solution to every problem, (2) doing something perfectly (i.e., mistake free) is possible and necessary, and (3) even minor mistakes have serious consequences. Examples: "It is important to keep working at something until its done just right." "For me, failing partly is as bad as failing completely."
Inflated responsibility	Belief that one has the power which is pivotal to bring about or prevent subjectively crucial negative outcomes. These outcomes are perceived as essential to prevent. They may be actual, that is, having consequences in the real world, and/or at a moral level. Such beliefs may pertain to responsibility for doing something to prevent or undo harm, and responsibility for errors of omission and commission. Examples: "I often think I am responsible for things that go wrong." "If I don't act when I foresee danger, I am to blame for any bad consequences."
Overestimation of threat	Beliefs indicating an exaggerated estimation of the probability or severity of harm. Examples: "I believe the world is a dangerous place." "Small problems always seem to turn into big ones in my life."
Intolerance for uncertainty	This domain encompasses three types of beliefs: (1) beliefs about the necessity for being certain, (2) beliefs that one has a poor capacity to cope with unpredictable change, and (3) beliefs about the difficulty of adequate functioning in inherently ambiguous situations. Examples: "It is possible to be absolutely certain about the things I do if I try hard enough." "I cannot tolerate uncertainty."

lation seeks to explain the four *P*'s of clinical causation: the *predisposing, precipitating, perpetuating,* and *protective* factors in the patient's problems. Predisposing factors are diatheses or vulnerability factors, such as dysfunctional beliefs laid down early in life. Precipitating factors are those stimuli or circumstances that trigger the problems. For example, a home burglary could trigger checking compulsions in a person who has a preexisting, inflated sense of personal responsibility. Perpetuating factors are those that maintain the problems, such as compulsions and other neutralizing activities that prevent dysfunctional appraisals and beliefs from being disconfirmed. Protective factors prevent problems either from developing or from getting worse. To illustrate, a patient's fear of negative evaluation may lead him or her to voluntarily refrain from performing compulsions when other people are present. This fear causes the person to undergo, in social situations, a naturalistic form of exposure and response prevention, thereby preventing the compulsions from consuming the patient's entire waking hours. Protective factors need not be present in every case.

The case formulation is built on the information obtained from the pretreatment assessment. In the following sections, we present a case formulation approach designed specifically for understanding and treating OCD. This approach was derived from the work of Persons (1989; Persons & Tompkins, 1997) and Taylor (2000a). We also show how assessment methods can be used to develop such a formulation. The components of the formulation are summarized in Table 6.2.

Problem List

The task of constructing a case formulation begins by assembling a list of the patient's major problems. Each of the assessment instruments reviewed earlier in this chapter provides important information for assembling a problem list. The SCID-IV (for Axis I) and the YBOCS are particularly useful. To keep the list within manageable limits, only the 10 most serious problems are retained on the list, beginning with the chief problem (Persons & Tompkins, 1997). The following is the problem list of Mrs. K, a 31-year-old married mother of 3-year-old twins, who was a full-time homemaker.

1. Recurrent, intrusive thoughts of mutilating her children
2. Fear of actually harming her children
3. Repeated checking on their safety, including seeking reassurance from her husband that she had not harmed them
4. Fear and avoidance of knives and other household implements that could harm the children
5. Repeated doubts about having run over a pedestrian while driving
6. Fear and avoidance of driving
7. Compulsions to repeatedly retrace driving routes to check whether she had struck a pedestrian
8. Persistent depressed mood (without suicidal urges, plans, or intent)

TABLE 6.2. Components of the Cognitive-Behavioral Case Formulation

Component	Description
1. Problem list	A list of the patient's difficulties, beginning with the chief problem.
2. Problem context	Symptoms and disorders, current stimuli (objects, people, events, situations), and historical factors associated with the patient's problems. These provide clues about the causes of the patient's problems.
3. Dysfunctional beliefs	Dysfunctional beliefs about self, world, or future. Some of these beliefs may be causing the patient's current problems.
4. Working hypothesis	A model specifying links between components 1 to 3, including the predisposing, precipitating, and perpetuating factors for all the problems on the problem list. Protective factors (if any) are also described. The working hypothesis emphasizes cognitive and behavioral mechanisms, although other factors are also considered.
5. Treatment plan	Derived from the working hypothesis, the treatment plan contains an outline of treatment goals and a description of the methods for attaining them.
6. Treatment obstacles	A list of predicted or actual obstacles to successful treatment, along with a list of strategies for overcoming them. Strategies for overcoming the obstacles are based on either the working hypothesis or, if the obstacles arise unexpectedly, a specific formulation of the new difficulties.

Although depression was the least severe of Mrs. K's problems, it was her stated reason for seeing her primary care physician, and was also the reason for her referral for CBT. The primary care physician did not use a screening interview; instead, he relied on a brief unstructured interview. Mrs. K did not reveal her OC problems during that interview because she feared that "My doctor would think I was crazy and take away my children." It was not until Mrs. K received a SCID-IV interview from a CBT therapist that her OC symptoms were revealed as her major problems.

The therapist need not attempt to remedy all the problems on the problem list. The therapist, in consultation with the patient, might decide to address only a few of them (Persons, 1989). The decision depends on a number of factors, including the patient's goals, the number of treatment sessions available, and whether the problems are amenable to CBT. Interrelationships among problems, as specified in the case formulation, also determine which problems are most important to treat. Sometimes the successful treatment of some problems (e.g., obsessions and compulsions) can lead to reductions in others (e.g., depression).

Problem Context

A thorough assessment is conducted in order to understand the context of the patient's problems. Contextual variables are those that co-occur, or are correlated with the patient's current problems. Contextual variables include current symptoms and disorders, current stimuli (objects, people, events, situations) associated with the problems, and personal and family history. Contextual factors provide clues about the causes of the patient's current problems.

Current Symptoms and Disorders

Mrs. K met DSM-IV criteria—as assessed by the SCID-IV for Axes I and II—for OCD and dysthymic disorder. According to the SCID-II, no personality disorder was present. The YBOCS interview suggested that Mrs. K's most severe OC problems were harming obsessions and associated compulsions, fears, and avoidance (i.e., problems 1 to 4 on the problem list). These symptoms troubled her for 3 to 8 hours per day. Scores on the YBOCS (Table 6.3) also suggested that her OCD was of moderate severity. According to information elicited from the YBOCS item 11, Mrs. K appeared to have reasonably good insight into her OCD. During her calmer moments, she realized that her harming concerns were unrealistic. She had never harmed her children or anyone else, and she was deeply concerned for the well-being of others.

Table 6.3 also shows Mrs. K's scores on other assessment instruments. Scores on the Padua Inventory were used as a consistency test (for comparison with the YBOCS). Mrs. K had elevated Padua scores on scales that assess checking compulsions and obsessional thoughts of harm befalling herself or others. Scores on the other scales were in the normal range. These results are broadly consistent with the information obtained from the YBOCS. Note, however, that the YBOCS provided more detailed information. It showed that Mrs. K suffered only from specific types of harming obsessions, namely, intrusive thoughts about harming her children and about harming pedestrians while driving. She did not have obsessional thoughts about herself being harmed. Similarly, the YBOCS showed that her checking compulsions were circumscribed, limited to checking regarding her children and pedestrians.

According to her responses on the Beck Anxiety Inventory (Table 6.3), Mrs. K suffered from mild anxiety over the past week, with prominent symptoms including fear of losing control and fear of the worst happening. These fears arose whenever her obsessions oc-

TABLE 6.3. Mrs. K's Pretreatment Scores

Measure	Score	Interpretation of score	Reference for interpretation
Yale–Brown Obsessive–Compulsive Scale, interview version			Goodman, Price, Rasmussen, Mazure,
Obsessions subscale	10	OCD range	Delgado, et al. (1989);
Compulsions subscale	13	OCD range	Steketee, Chambless, et al.
Total (10-item) scale	23	OCD range	(1996)
Padua Inventory, Washington State University revision			Burns et al. (1996)
Contamination obsessions and washing compulsions	1	Normal range	
Dressing and grooming compulsions	2	Normal range	
Checking compulsions	13	OCD range	
Obsessional thoughts of harm to self or others	9	OCD range	
Obsessional impulses to harm to self or others	4	Normal range	
Beck Anxiety Inventory	11	Mild anxiety	Beck & Steer (1993a)
Beck Depression Inventory	17	Mild-to-moderate depression	Beck et al. (1996)

curred. Mrs. K's score on the Beck Depression Inventory suggested mild to moderate depression over the past week, with prominent symptoms consisting of sadness, low self-esteem, feeling that she had failed as a person, and feelings of guilt. The responses to the Beck inventories are broadly consistent with results obtained from the SCID-IV interview for Axis I, which suggested that OCD was Mrs. K's only anxiety disorder and that she suffered from a mood disorder of mild intensity (i.e., dysthymic disorder rather than major depression). Note that the SCID-IV for Axis I provides more detailed information than do the Beck inventories. The SCID-IV revealed that although Mrs. K's depression was not severe, it had been longstanding (3 years). The Beck inventories, when used in the assessment and treatment of OCD, are most valuable as quick ways of assessing the patient's level of general distress. Due to their brevity, these inventories can also be used to monitor the patient on a weekly basis. Thus, they are useful for monitoring progress during treatment.

To summarize, the results from Mrs. K's questionnaires were consistent with the results obtained from the structured interviews, although the latter provided more detail. The information was also corroborated by the patient's sister, who accompanied Mrs. K to the assessment interview. The sister was independently interviewed after Mrs. K had been assessed. The consistent pattern of information increased our confidence in the accuracy of the assessment of Mrs. K's symptoms and disorders.

Current Stimuli Associated with the Patient's Problems

Information obtained from the structured interviews—supplemented, where necessary, by additional interview questions—indicated that there were several stimuli that appeared to lead to, if not trigger, Mrs. K's intrusions and associated fears. According to her own report, horrific thoughts of harming her children were particularly likely to occur under the following circumstances: (1) when she was in close contact with her children (e.g., while feeding or bathing them); (2) while handling sharp kitchen utensils such as kitchen knives, particularly when the children were playing nearby; and (3) whenever she encountered violence-related news items (e.g., a television news segment on armed robberies).

Mrs. K attempted to avoid these stimuli, to the point that she completely avoided watching television and reading newspapers. Mrs. K had daily contact with her children, which repeatedly triggered harming intrusions. She attempted to cope with these problems by repeatedly performing checking rituals and by removing all sharp objects from the house.

With regard to her intrusive doubts and fears about running over pedestrians while driving, Mrs. K reported that these symptoms were more likely to occur (1) whenever she saw pedestrians while she was driving, (2) when driving on rough or bumpy road surfaces ("Was that a pothole or did I just run over someone?"), and (3) whenever she realized that she had been daydreaming while driving ("I might have struck a pedestrian without realizing it"). Mrs. K either attempted to avoid driving under these circumstances or retraced her driving route to check whether she had hit someone.

Particular interactions with her husband were also associated with increases in the frequency and severity of OC symptoms. Mrs. K had numerous arguments with her husband, usually about the management of their finances. At these times, Mrs. K felt particularly anxious, and her intrusive thoughts and compulsions increased in frequency. Regarding stimuli associated with her depression, Mrs. K reported that conflicts with her husband were followed by transient worsening of her mood. Her mood also tended to be especially low when she had time to herself alone, such as when her husband would take the children out for the day. At those times, Mrs. K ruminated over her problems and despaired about ever overcoming them.

Personal and Family History

Information on the patient's personal and family history was obtained from the structured interviews, supplemented by an unstructured interview after the YBOCS had been completed. Mrs. K was an only child raised in a small rural town. She described her father as an alcoholic who was physically and verbally abusive. The father deserted the family when she was 8 years old. She described her mother, a devout Catholic, as an unhappy, irritable person who often found fault with others.

Mrs. K recalled being shy as a child. Although she had always been "slow to warm up" in social situations, Mrs. K recalls that her shyness abated as she grew older, particularly during her years attending high school. At that time, she socialized more frequently, and her social circle expanded to the point that she had several close friends. Mrs. K reported that she has always been perfectionistic. Throughout her childhood and adolescence, she took great pride in keeping her room neat and tidy, and teachers frequently praised the high quality of her neatly written schoolwork and her conscientiousness in completing homework assignments.

In addition to longstanding perfectionistic tendencies, Mrs. K had appeared to have mild (subclinical) OCD symptoms during her late childhood and adolescence. She had occasional periods of intrusive thoughts of harm befalling her mother, which she attempted to remove by thinking "good" thoughts (e.g., thinking the word "gold"). During periods of stress, she also sometimes engaged in compulsive checking on the safety of her mother (e.g., creeping into her mother's bedroom at night to check that she was still breathing).

Mrs. K completed grade 11 and then obtained a clerical job in town. She married the first man she dated, when she was 27 years old, and she and her husband then moved to a nearby city, where he obtained employment as a factory worker. With the move to the city, she lost contact with most of her friends. At age 28, Mrs. K gave birth to twin girls and since then remained a full-time homemaker. Mrs. K described her marriage as "adequate," although she reported that her husband often criticized her management of the household.

Mrs. K's mood disorder and current OC problems developed soon after the birth of her children. Since then, she has felt overwhelmed with the responsibilities of motherhood, socially isolated, and dysphoric. Obsessions about harming her children steadily increased in frequency since the arrival of her children. Her concerns about running over pedestrians developed somewhat later, as she was required to increasingly use the family car for grocery shopping and other errands. At the time of assessment, Mrs. K had received no previous treatment for OCD, and she knew little about the disorder.

Dysfunctional Beliefs

The problem context provides one of the main sources of information for developing a working hypothesis. The other source comes from assessing beliefs associated with the patient's problems. Some of these beliefs may be dysfunctional or maladaptive. Such beliefs interact with precipitating factors (e.g., stressors) to contribute to the patient's problems. Cognitive-behavioral formulations of OCD (Obsessive Compulsive Cognitions Working Group, 1997; Salkovskis, 1996) provide useful guidelines as to which beliefs are likely to be associated with which particular problems. Mrs. K held the following dysfunctional beliefs about the importance of her thoughts and about the importance of controlling these cognitions:

1. "Terrible thoughts lead to terrible actions."
2. "Having horrible thoughts means that I subconsciously want to do awful things."
3. "I am a bad person for having awful thoughts."
4. "People will reject or punish me if they learn of my terrible thoughts."
5. "I must try very hard to keep bad thoughts out of my mind."
6. "If something is worth doing, it should be done perfectly."

These beliefs were identified during the course of conducting the YBOCS interview. Although the YBOCS does not assess dysfunctional beliefs in much detail, pertinent information can readily be elicited by incorporating additional questions into the YBOCS interview. Questions that are particularly useful in identifying dysfunctional OCD-related beliefs are those that ask patients to describe what bothers or worries them the most about their intrusions, what they think the intrusions might lead to, and what they think will happen if they don't perform compulsions or if they fail to avoid intrusion-triggering stimuli. The following interview fragment shows how questioning was used to elicit details of some of Mrs. K.'s beliefs:

CLINICIAN: From what you've been saying, it sounds like the thoughts of harming your children are your biggest problems.

PATIENT: Yes, that's right.

CLINICIAN: What bothers you the most about those thoughts?

PATIENT: I'm worried that, subconsciously, I might really want to hurt my children.

CLINICIAN: Is there anything else about the thoughts that worries you?

PATIENT: Yes, I worry that they mean I could lose control, just like my dad used to lose control when he was angry.

CLINICIAN: Have you ever had the thoughts at times when there was no chance that you could possibly harm your children?

PATIENT: Yes, the thoughts happen when my husband takes the kids out on weekends, to give me a break from them.

CLINICIAN: What's that like for you?

PATIENT: It's still bad. I worry that my bad thoughts might somehow cause bad things to happen to the kids. I know it sounds silly, but that's what I think sometimes.

CLINICIAN: Have you told anyone else about this problem?

PATIENT: No, I could never do that. People would think I was a basket case.

CLINICIAN: That must be difficult for you to try to deal with this problem on your own. What do you do to cope?

PATIENT: I try to distract myself by thinking positive thoughts. I also try to avoid things that bring on the thoughts, such as kitchen knives.

CLINICIAN: Is that something that you have to do?

PATIENT: I'm not sure, but I don't want to take any chances. The only solution I can see is to try harder to keep these bad thoughts out of my mind.

Observe that this brief interview elicited five of the six dysfunctional beliefs. To further assess dysfunctional beliefs, the clinician can ask the patient to make ratings of belief strength, using a scale that ranges from 0, do not believe at all, to 100, completely believe. Mrs. K's ratings for her dysfunctional beliefs were in the range of 60 to 80 (i.e., moderately strong beliefs). Ratings such as these can be obtained throughout treatment to assess whether the CBT interventions are reducing the strength of dysfunctional beliefs.

Working Hypothesis

The working hypothesis is the heart of the case formulation, where the therapist synthesizes the available information to create a model of the predisposing, precipitating, perpetuating, and protective factors in the patient's problems. It is crucial that the patient understands and agrees with the formulation and that the therapist is receptive to modifications or revisions suggested by the patient. The working hypothesis is "theory in progress," and it may change over time as information accumulates.

The working hypothesis should attempt to account for all the patient's current problems, while being as parsimonious as possible. The hypothesis is guided by the cognitive models of OCD (Salkovskis, 1996) and other disorders (e.g., Beck & Emery, 1985; Wells, 1997). Mechanisms that might account for the problems include dysfunctional beliefs, belief-maintaining behaviors (e.g., escape or avoidance), operant reinforcement contingencies, and skills deficits (Persons, 1989; Salkovskis, 1996, 1999; Wells, 1997). Cognitive and behavioral mechanisms might not account for all the problems. Biological factors also may be contributory.

The process of establishing DSM-IV diagnoses enables the clinician to begin to organize or group together the patient's problems. The problem list should be examined to identify themes among problems. This can help identify common underlying factors (Persons, 1989). One should also look for correlations among the problem contexts, beliefs, behaviors, and symptoms (Persons & Tompkins, 1997). These associations can provide clues about the factors that precipitate and perpetuate the problems.

Predisposing Factors

The working hypothesis describes the factors that predispose patients to developing their current problems. Although biological (e.g., genetic) diatheses may play a role, cognitive-behavioral formulations emphasize the role of dysfunctional beliefs (e.g., Beck & Emery, 1985; Salkovskis, 1996, 1999; Wells, 1997). To understand the predisposing factors, it is important to identify the patient's dysfunctional beliefs and to identify the factors that shaped these beliefs. These beliefs can be acquired by verbal instruction from significant others, by observational learning, and by other (e.g., traumatic) experiences.

Mrs. K's pretreatment assessment suggest that her six dysfunctional beliefs (listed above) were longstanding, having been present since at least her early adolescence. These beliefs appeared to predispose Mrs. K toward her current OC problems. As discussed earlier here, beliefs about the overimportance of thoughts, and beliefs about the need to control her thoughts, are hypothesized to be predisposing factors for the development of OCD (Obsessive Compulsive Cognitions Working Group, 1997; Salkovskis, 1996). Mrs. K's belief that she is a bad person for having bad thoughts also predisposes her to experience self-blame, guilt, and depression whenever she experienced thoughts she labeled as "bad." Her belief in the need to do things perfectly was similarly likely to lead to self-blame, guilt, and depression whenever she believed she "failed" at some personally important task, such as caring for her children. Thus, Mrs. K's dysfunctional beliefs appeared to be predisposing factors for her current problems.

How did these beliefs arise? Information obtained about her personal and family history offered several clues. Mrs. K had often observed her father "lose control" whenever he was angry and intoxicated, by becoming verbally and physically abusive. This may have contributed to Mrs. K's belief that "bad" (e.g., angry) thoughts lead to bad actions. Mrs. K's religious upbringing (due largely to the influence of her mother) also may have contributed to the development of some dysfunctional beliefs. Mrs. K vividly recalled her mother lecturing her about how "wholesome people don't have wicked thoughts" and how people with bad thoughts will be punished, "either in this life or in the next one." Mrs. K recalled that after her father deserted the family, her mother often railed about what a bad person he was and how he liked to inflict misery on others. These learning experiences may have contributed to the patient's belief that bad thoughts somehow reflect the person's true (e.g., subconscious) motivation.

Mrs. K's belief that things must be done "perfectly" may have been acquired directly from her mother, herself a perfectionistic, fault-finding person. Moreover, the patient learned early in life that she could avoid her mother's criticism by doing things "perfectly" (e.g., by keeping her room and her belongings neat and tidy). Thus, operant conditioning (negative reinforcement) seemed to have contributed to the development of Mrs. K's perfectionistic beliefs.

In summary, several learning experiences during childhood appeared to contribute to the development of Mrs. K's dysfunctional beliefs. In turn, these beliefs appeared to predispose her toward the current problems for which she sought treatment. These predisposing factors were identified largely by means of careful questioning during the structured interviews. As we have seen, the sorts of questions to ask were based on cognitive-behavioral models of OCD and other disorders.

Precipitating Factors

Precipitating factors trigger the patient's problems. These factors are assessed by inquiring about the circumstances surrounding the onset of the patient's problems. Cognitive-behavioral case formulations propose that problem onset or exacerbation arise when dysfunctional beliefs interact with stressors such as aversive or demanding life events. The birth of Mrs. K's children was such an event. Although Mrs. K had long experienced mild (subclinical) OC symptoms, her problems with OCD and dysthymia began in earnest with the arrival of her twin daughters. From the day the children were born, Mrs. K was concerned about inadvertently harming the babies (e.g., "What if I dropped one while nursing her?"). These concerns took the form of intrusive harm-related thoughts.

The children's frequent crying and tantrums also made Mrs. K irritable, and at times she wished she had never become pregnant. The crying and tantrums also led Mrs. K to have intrusive thoughts of smothering them with a pillow, so she might finally get some peace and quiet. Mrs. K's preexisting dysfunctional beliefs led her to appraise these intrusions as "horrible thoughts" and that "perhaps I subconsciously want to harm my children." The intrusions were profoundly distressing, and rapidly escalated into clinical obsessions with associated compulsions. Thus, OCD was precipitated.

Having little contact with other women with children, Mrs. K lacked clear guidelines on what was "good enough" parenting. As a result of her belief that things should be done perfectly, she worried that she was not performing adequately in her role as a mother. In fact, she regarded her harming obsessions as evidence that she was a "potentially dangerous mother." This self-view was extremely upsetting for her and appears to have played a role in precipitating her dysthymic disorder.

Soon after the birth of her children, Mrs. K was increasingly required to use the family car—for shopping errands, to take the children for medical checkups, and to drive her husband to and from work. Her self-confidence had deteriorated as a result of her perceived failure as a parent, and this loss of confidence seemed to generalize to her performance in other spheres of her life, such as driving. Mrs. K began to experience concentration difficulties, as a result of her frequent intrusions and because of sleep deprivation associated with caring for her children. These concentration difficulties further undermined her confidence as a driver, especially after she nearly struck a pedestrian on a crosswalk. This near-miss, along with her eroding confidence as a driver, precipitated doubts about whether she had accidentally struck someone. This led to checking compulsions (retracing her driving route) and, where possible, avoidance of driving.

Perpetuating Factors

According to Salkovskis (1996, 1999), obsessions are maintained by neutralizing strategies, such as compulsions and avoidance. These strategies prevent dysfunctional beliefs from being disconfirmed, thereby perpetuating OCD. Mrs. K believed that if she did not strive to suppress her harming intrusions and avoid sharp objects, then she was "bound to harm the children." Her neutralizing strategies prevented her from learning that "bad" thoughts need not translate into harmful actions.

Her checking compulsions (e.g., checking on the children's safety; seeking reassurance from her husband; retracing her driving routes) were maintained by negative reinforcement (immediate reduction in distress) and by positive reinforcement (increased confidence that a feared outcome had not occurred).

Mrs. K's depression was maintained by ongoing self-criticism about her inability to control her unwanted thoughts and about her perceived failure as a parent. Her husband's frequent criticism of the way Mrs. K. managed the household also appeared to maintain her self-criticism and associated depression.

Protective Factors

For many psychiatric disorders, social support is a protective or buffering factor; the greater the support, the lesser the severity of the problems. Social support exerts its effects in many ways. It lessens isolation and feelings of stigmatization that may arise from having a psychiatric disorder, and it may be protective because it enables the person to be exposed to corrective information (e.g., information about the prevalence of intrusive thoughts, and about the realistic expectations for good parenting). Mrs. K had low social support and therefore did not have the benefit of this protective factor.

The patient's current living circumstances required her to drive and to have close, daily contact with her children. These requirements prevented her avoidance from becoming more widespread. If, for some reason, she was unable to have access to a car, then her confidence as a driver might further erode, leading to more intrusive doubts about harming pedestrians and associated checking compulsions. Similarly, if she had a housekeeper that took care of many of the child-care responsibilities (e.g., preparing meals and bathing the children), then Mrs. K's confidence in her parenting abilities might have further eroded, leading to greater concerns about harming the children and an associated increase in intrusive harm-related thoughts and associated symptoms.

Treatment Plan

When the therapist and the patient have agreed on a working hypothesis, a treatment plan, derived from the working hypothesis, is discussed. The plan has two components: a statement of goals and a description of how to achieve these goals (Persons & Tompkins, 1997). Goals should be specific and clearly defined. For example, Mrs. K and her therapist agreed that a realistic goal would be to be able to drive without retracing her route. Clearly stated goals better tell the therapist how to intervene and make it easier to monitor treatment progress. As mentioned earlier, treatment goals might include only a few of the problems on the problem list. The relative severity of problems and the patient's reasons for seeking treatment are important considerations. If the purpose of treatment is to correct the causes of the problems, then the working hypothesis provides important information about which goals to pursue (Persons, 1989). The working hypothesis for Mrs. K suggested that important goals included reducing the strength of her dysfunctional beliefs and replacing them with more adaptive beliefs. The working hypothesis suggested that this should reduce her OCD and dysthymia.

A detailed description of the interventions used in CBT for OCD is beyond the scope of this chapter; see Salkovskis (1985, 1989, 1999) and Taylor (2000b) for details. Instead, we will summarize the interventions used in Mrs. K's therapy. Her treatment consisted of the following:

- *Psychoeducation:* Information about the nature and treatment of OCD, including information about the cognitive-behavioral model. Sharing the case formulation with the patient plays an important role in this psychoeducation.
- *Parenting education:* Information about realistic standards for childrearing. Mrs. K was encouraged to enroll her children in a parent-participation preschool. The latter required her to take an active role in organizing preschool activities and brought her in contact with other mothers. This not only increased her social support but also provided her with corrective information about what was "good enough" parenting.
- *Graduated exposure and response prevention exercises:* These were initially focused on Mrs. K's obsessions about her children and then later on her driving obsessions. Exposure and response prevention exercises included exposure to real stimuli, as well as imaginal exposure (e.g., deliberately calling to mind her harming obsessions). The exercises began with mildly anxiety-evoking tasks (e.g., using a butter knife in the presence of her children), then graduating to more frightening tasks (e.g., using a carving knife when the children were nearby). The exercises were pre-

sented as behavioral experiments, intended to test beliefs derived from her dysfunctional beliefs. For example, for the belief "bad thoughts lead to bad actions," an initial behavioral experiment was for Mrs. K to imagine her children catching the measles within the next week and then to assess whether or not this occurred. The experiment was conducted, and the results supported a benign, more realistic alternative belief, "Bad, unwanted thoughts are simply mental garbage."

- *Cognitive restructuring exercises* (e.g., Beck & Emery, 1985; Taylor, 2000b): These were used as additional means of reducing Mrs. K's dysfunctional beliefs. They included strategies specially designed to reduce her perfectionistic beliefs (e.g., Antony & Swinson, 1998).

- *Spousal support:* Mrs. K.'s husband was asked to attend a number of treatment sessions so that he could be educated about the nature and treatment Mrs. K's problems and to enlist his support. The couple were informed that Mrs. K's reassurance-seeking about the safety of the children was a form of compulsion that maintained her obsessions and associated fears. Accordingly, Mrs. K agreed that she would attempt to refrain from seeking reassurance and that her husband would attempt to refrain from reassuring her. If she asked for reassurance, Mr. K was instructed to tell her that it was "doctor's orders" that he not reassure her.

- *Maintenance:* Toward the end of treatment, a posttreatment maintenance program was devised, and Mrs. K was educated in methods of relapse prevention. (For a discussion of these strategies, see Öst [1989] and Taylor [2000a].)

Treatment Obstacles

Sometimes obstacles can be predicted from the working hypothesis and treatment plan. If obstacles arise unexpectedly, then the therapist attempts to develop a hypothesis specifically to explain the difficulties. Expectations the patient holds about therapy can be a source of treatment obstacles. When expectations are unfulfilled, the patient may become demoralized and drop out of treatment. These include expectations about one's performance (e.g., "I must be completely successful in all my homework assignments") and expectations about the effects of therapy (e.g., "It is possible to be completely free of anxiety") (Persons, 1989). Mrs. K's case formulation suggested three major obstacles: (1) arranging for child-care so that she could attend therapy sessions (Mrs. K would likely refuse treatment if she was unable to arrange suitable child-care, because she would take this as further evidence that she was a "bad" mother), (2) her perfectionistic expectations about her performance in therapy, and (3) ongoing criticism from her husband (an exacerbating factor in her problems) and his possible nonadherence to the "no reassurance" intervention. The first two obstacles were reviewed with Mrs. K during her first treatment session. Problem-solving was used to help her find a solution to the first potential obstacle, and perfectionism treatment strategies (e.g., Antony & Swinson, 1998) were used to address the second potential obstacle. Regarding the third possible obstacle, a number of conjoint sessions were arranged so that the patient and her husband could discuss these issues and plan for ways of addressing them. Mrs. K's relationship with her husband was periodically reviewed (via an unstructured interview) throughout treatment. If relationship problems continued, then it was planned to implement a course of Behavioral Couples Therapy (Baucom & Epstein, 1990).

Role of Assessment in Treatment

Testing the Formulation

Testing the accuracy of the formulation is an ongoing process, in which the therapist looks for evidence for and against the working hypothesis (Persons, 1989). One of the first steps is to share the formulation with the patient. To limit the chances that the patient will simply acquiesce with the therapist' hypotheses es, the patient should be asked to think of specific examples that either support or challenge the formulation. The therapist also can test the formulation by reviewing naturally occurring changes in the patient's problems to see if these are consistent with the formulation.

Treatment interventions, if properly administered, also provide pertinent information for testing the formulation. For Mrs. K, for example, it was predicted that attempting to suppress her harming obsessions maintained their frequency. To test this hypothesis, Mrs. K was asked to suppress the obsessions on some days (e.g., via distraction), and not suppress on other days (cf. Salkovskis, 1999). She recorded the frequency of obsessions each day, and learned that frequency was higher when she suppressed than when she did not attempt to suppress the obsessions. This not only supported the formulation but also persuaded Mrs. K that she could reduce the frequency of her obsessions by not suppressing them.

Monitoring Changes over the Course of Treatment

The self-report YBOCS is a quick and informative means of assessing the severity of the patient's OCD symptoms over the past week. It takes about 5 minutes to complete. The therapist can supplement the information obtained from this scale by asking the patient to describe his or her symptoms over the past week. Mrs. K completed the self-report YBOCS along with the BDI, at the beginning of each session. The latter was administered to assess the severity of her dysthymic disorder. As mentioned earlier, it was predicted that her depression would abate as her OCD diminished. The BDI was used to assess this prediction. In each session Mrs. K was also asked to rate the strength of her dysfunctional beliefs (on the scale of 0 to 100 described earlier) to assess whether the CBT interventions were having the intended effect of reducing these beliefs.

Specific symptoms were also monitored, depending on the nature of the homework assignment. For example, one of Mrs. K's assignments was to drive without retracing her route. Each week she was asked to record, in a notebook, the number of driving trips she had completed, along with the number of times she had retraced her route or performed any similar form of checking such as imagining herself retracing her route.

Clinical Status at the End of Treatment

To assess changes from pre- to posttreatment, it is useful to administer the interview version of the YBOCS before and after therapy, along with other measures that are used. For example, Mrs. K completed the Padua Inventory, the Beck Depression and Anxiety Inventories, and ratings of the strength of dysfunctional beliefs before and after treatment. Previously published norms (e.g., see the references cited in Table 6.3) can be used to assess whether the patient's scores have reliably changed and moved into the normal range. There are many ways of assessing these outcome variables, and there is much debate as to the best way to assess them (see the special series on assessing clinically significant change, published in *Behaviour Research and Therapy*, 1999, Vol. 37, No. 12). A useful, clinically expedient method is to regard scores as falling within the normal range if they are within 2 standard deviations of the mean score for normal controls.

For a more complete assessment, the Structured Clinical Interviews for Axes I and II (i.e., the SCID-IV and SCID-II) can be administered before and after treatment to assess treatment-related changes in comorbid disorders. Additional measures can be included as needed. Mrs. K, for example, could have completed a self-report measure of marital satisfaction. However, this extends the amount of time required for assessment. Often, variables such as marital satisfaction can be adequately assessed (at least for clinical purposes) by a brief clinical interview.

To assess long-term follow-up (e.g., 3 or 6 months after the end of therapy), patients can be invited back to the clinic or contacted by telephone and reassessed with the SCID-IV. During that assessment, the therapist can evaluate the maintenance of treatment-related gains and, if necessary, implement additional interventions.

Comment

There is no single "correct" way of developing a cognitive-behavioral case formulation. A useful method is one that provides a systematic way of developing a model of the causes and cures of the patient's problems. The method outlined in this chapter is one approach for understanding and treating OCD.

SUMMARY AND CONCLUSIONS

OCD is common, yet often overlooked, especially in cursory clinical evaluations. Screening tools can reduce this problem. One of the most useful screening instruments is the Primary Care Evaluation of Mental Disorders. Patients screening positive on this measure can be assessed in more detail with a structured diagnostic interview, such as the Structured Clinical Interview for DSM-IV.

Although the selection of additional assessment instruments depends to some extent on the clinician's theory of OCD and the nature of the treatment being offered, there are a number of assessment instruments that are generally useful. These include the Yale–Brown Obsessive Compulsive Scale and the Padua Inventory. Other assessment instruments can be added, depending on the nature of the comorbid disorders identified by the structured diagnostic interview. If a comorbid mood disorder is identified, for example, the Beck Depression Inventory could be used to monitor the patient's mood.

The assessment methods discussed in this chapter, particularly the structured interviews, are useful for developing a case formulation of the causes of the patient's problems and to develop a treatment plan. Once treatment has been initiated, assessment continues throughout the course of therapy in order to evaluate treatment-related changes in symptoms and in the putative causes of the symptoms (e.g., dysfunctional beliefs). In this way, assessment plays a vital role in the treatment of OCD.

ACKNOWLEDGMENT

Preparation of this chapter was supported in part by a grant to Steven Taylor from the British Columbia Health Research Foundation.

REFERENCES

American Psychiatric Association. (1994). *Diagnostic and statistical manual of mental disorders* (4th ed.). Washington, DC: Author.

Antony, M. M., & Swinson, R. P. (1998). *When perfect isn't good enough: Strategies for coping with perfectionism*. Oakland, CA: New Harbinger.

Baer, L., Brown-Beasley, M. W., Sorce, J., & Henriques, A. (1993). Computer-assisted telephone administration of a structured interview for obsessive–compulsive disorder. *American Journal of Psychiatry, 150,* 1737–1738.

Baucom, D. H., & Epstein, N. (1990). *Cognitive behavioral marital therapy.* New York: Brunner/Mazel.

Beck, A. T., & Emery, G. (1985). *Anxiety disorders and phobias: A cognitive perspective.* New York: Basic Books.

Beck, A. T., & Steer, R. A. (1993a). *Manual for the Beck Anxiety Inventory.* San Antonio, TX: Psychological Corporation.

Beck, A. T., & Steer, R. A. (1993b). *Manual for the Beck Depression Inventory.* San Antonio, TX: Psychological Corporation.

Beck, A. T., Steer, R. A., & Brown, G. K. (1996). *Manual for the Beck Depression Inventory–II.* San Antonio, TX: Psychological Corporation.

Black, D. W., Kelly, M., Myers, C., & Noyes, R. (1990). Tritiated imipramine binding in obsessive–compulsive volunteers and psychiatrically normal controls. *Biological Psychiatry, 27,* 319–327.

Brown, T. A., Moras, K., Zinbarg, R. E., & Barlow, D. H. (1993). Diagnostic and symptom distinguishability of generalized anxiety disorder and obsessive–compulsive disorder. *Behavior Therapy, 24,* 227–240.

Burns, G. L., Keortge, S. G., Formea, G. M., & Sternberger, L. G. (1996). Revision of the Padua Inventory for obsessive compulsive disorder symptoms: Distinctions between worry, obsessions, and compulsions. *Behaviour Research and Therapy, 34,* 163–173.

Clifft, M. A. (1986). Writing about psychiatric patients: Guidelines for disguising case material. *Bulletin of the Menninger Clinic, 50,* 511–524.

Di Nardo, P., Brown, T. A., & Barlow, D. H. (1994). *Anxiety Disorders Interview Schedule for DSM-IV.* San Antonio, TX: Psychological Corporation.

Eisen, J. L., Phillips, K. A., Baer, L., Beer, D. A., Atala, K. D., & Rasmussen, S. A. (1998). The Brown Assessment of Beliefs Scale: Reliability and validity. *American Journal of Psychiatry, 155,* 102–108.

Emmelkamp, P. M. G., Kraaijkamp, H. J. M., & van den Hout, M. A. (1999). Assessment of obsessive–compulsive disorder. *Behavior Modification, 23,* 269–279.

First, M. B., Spitzer, R. L., Gibbon, M., & Williams, J. B. W. (1996). *Structured Clinical Interview for DSM-IV Axis I—Patient edition.* New York: Biometrics Research Department, New York State Psychiatric Institute.

First, M. B., Spitzer, R. L., Gibbon, M., Williams, J. B. W., Davies, M., Borus, J., Howes, M. J., Kane, J., Pope, H. G., & Rounsaville, B. (1995). The Structured Clinical Interview for DSM-III-R personality disorders (SCID-II): Part II. Multi-site test–retest reliability study. *Journal of Personality Disorders, 9,* 92–104.

First, M. B., Spitzer, R. L., Gibbon, M., Williams, J. B. W., & Lorna, B. (1994). *Structured Clinical Interview for DSM-IV Axis II Personality Disorders (SCID-II) (Version 2.0).* New York: Biometrics Research Department, New York State Psychiatric Institute.

Foa, E. B. (1979). Failures in treating obsessive–compulsives. *Behaviour Research and Therapy, 17,* 169–176.

Foa, E. B., Grayson, J. B., Steketee, G. S., Doppelt, H. G., Turner, R. M., & Latimer, P. R. (1983). Success and failure in the behavioral treatment of obsessive–compulsives. *Journal of Consulting and Clinical Psychology, 51,* 287–297.

Foa, E. B., Kozak, M. J., Salkovskis, P. M., Coles, M. E., & Amir, N. (1998). The validation of a new obsessive–compulsive disorder scale: The Obsessive–Compulsive Inventory. *Psychological Assessment, 10,* 206–214.

Freeston, M. H., Ladouceur, R., Rhéaume, J., Letarte, H., Gagnon, F., & Thibodeau, N. (1994). Self-report of obsessions and worry. *Behaviour Research and Therapy, 32,* 29–36.

Frost, R. O., & Steketee, G. (1999). Issues in the treatment of compulsive hoarding. *Cognitive and Behavioral Practice, 6,* 397–407.

Goodman, W. K., Price, L. H., Rasmussen, S. A., Mazure, C., Delgado, P., Heninger, G. R., & Charney, D. S. (1989). The Yale–Brown Obsessive Compulsive Scale: II. Validity. *Archives of General Psychiatry, 46,* 1012–1016.

Goodman, W. K., Price, L. H., Rasmussen, S. A., Mazure, C., Fleishmann, R. L., Hill, C. L., Heninger, G. R., & Charney, D. S. (1989). The Yale–Brown Obsessive Compulsive Scale: I. Development, use, and reliability. *Archives of General Psychiatry, 46,* 1006–1011.

Goodman, W. K., Rasmussen, S. A., Price, L. H., Mazure, C., Heninger, G. R., & Charney, D. S. (1989). *Manual for the Yale–Brown Obsessive Compulsive Scale (revised).* New Haven, CT: Connecticut Mental Health Center.

Guy, W. (1976). *ECDEU assessment manual for psychopharmacology* (DHHS Publication No. ADM 76-338). Washington, DC: U.S. Government Printing Office.

Herman, S., & Koran, L. M. (1998). *In vivo* measurement of obsessive–compulsive disorder using palmtop computers. *Computers in Human Behavior, 14,* 449–462.

Hewlett, W. A., Vinogradov, S., & Agras, W. S. (1992). Clomipramine, clonazepam, and clonidine treatment of obsessive–compulsive disorder. *Journal of Clinical Psychopharmacology, 12,* 420–430.

Hodgson, R. J., & Rachman, S. (1977). Obsessional–compulsive complaints. *Behaviour Research and Therapy, 15,* 389–395.

Hohagen, F., Winkelmann, G., Raeuchle, H. R., Hand, I., Koenig, A., Muenchau, N., Hiss, H., Kabisch, C. G., Kaeppler, C., Schramm, P., Rey, E., Aldenhoff, J., & Berger, M. (1998). Combination of behaviour therapy with fluvoxamine in comparison with behaviour therapy and placebo: Results of a multicentre study. *British Journal of Psychiatry, 173*(Suppl. 35), 71–78.

Insel, T. R., Murphy, D. L., Cohen, R. M., Alterman, I., Kilton, C., & Linnoila, M. (1983). Obsessive–compulsive disorder: A double blind trial of clomipramine and clorgyline. *Archives of General Psychiatry, 40,* 605–612.

Jenike, M. A., Hyman, S., Baer, L., Holland, A., Minichiello, W. E., Buttolph, L., Summergrad, P., Seymour, R., & Ricciardi, J. (1990). A controlled trial of fluvoxamine in obsessive–compulsive disorder: Implications for a serotonergic theory. *American Journal of Psychiatry, 147,* 1209–1215.

Kim, S. W., Dysken, M. W., & Kuskowski, M. (1990). The Yale–Brown Obsessive–Compulsive Scale: A reliability and validity study. *Psychiatry Research, 34,* 99–106.

Kim, S. W., Dysken, M. W., & Kuskowski, M. (1992). The Symptom Checklist-90 Obsessive–Compulsive Subscale: A reliability and validity study. *Psychiatry Research, 41,* 37–44.

Kim, S. W., Dysken, M. W., Kuskowski, M., & Hoover, K. M. (1993). The Yale-Brown Obsessive Compulsive Scale and the NIMH Global Obsessive–Compulsive Scale (GOCS): A reliability and validity study. *International Journal of Methods in Psychiatric Research, 3,* 37–44.

Kobak, K. A., Greist, J. H., Jefferson, J. W., Katzelnick, D. J., & Henk, H. J. (1998). Behavioral versus pharmacological treatments of obsessive–compulsive disorder: A meta-analysis. *Psychopharmacology, 136,* 205–216.

Kobak, K. A., Taylor, L., Dottl, S. L., Greist, J. H., Jefferson, J. W., Burroughs, D., Mantle, J. M., Katzelnick, D. J., Norton, R., Henk, H. J., & Serlin, R. C. (1997). A computer-administered telephone interview to identify mental disorders. *Journal of the American Medical Association, 278,* 905–910.

Lang, P. J., & Lazovik, A. D. (1963). Experimental desensitization of a phobia. *Journal of Abnormal and Social Psychology, 66,* 519–525.

Leckman, J., Grice, D. E., Boardman, J., Zhang, H., Vitale, A., Bondi, C., Alsobrook, J., Peterson, B. S., Cohen, D. J., Rasmussen, S. A., Goodman, W. K., McDougle, C. J., & Pauls, D. L. (1997). Symptoms of obsessive–compulsive disorder. *American Journal of Psychiatry, 154,* 911–917.

Lelliott, P. T., & Marks, I. M. (1987). Management of obsessive–compulsive rituals associated with delusions, hallucinations and depression. *Behavioural Psychotherapy, 15,* 77–87.

Lelliott, P. T., Noshirvani, H. F., Basoglu, M., Marks, I. M., & Monteiro, W. O. (1988). Obsessive–compulsive beliefs and treatment outcome. *Psychological Medicine, 18,* 697–702.

Marks, I. M., Baer, L., Greist, J. H., Park, J. M., Bachofen, M., Nakagawa, A., Wenzel, K. W., Parkin, J. R., Manzo, P. S., Dottl, S. L., & Mantle, J. M. (1998). Home self-assessment of obsessive–compulsive disorder: Use of a manual and a computer-conducted telephone interview—Two UK–US studies. *British Journal of Psychiatry, 172,* 406–412.

Neziroglu, F., McKay, D., Yaryura-Tobias, J. A., Stevens, K. P., & Todaro, J. (1999). The Overvalued

Ideas Scale: Development, reliability and validity in obsessive–compulsive disorder. *Behaviour Research and Therapy, 37,* 881–902.

Obsessive Compulsive Cognitions Working Group. (1997). Cognitive assessment of obsessive–compulsive disorder. *Behaviour Research and Therapy, 35,* 667–681.

Obsessive Compulsive Cognitions Working Group. (2001). Development and initial validation of the Obsessive Beliefs Questionnaire and the Interpretation of Intrusions Inventory. *Behaviour Research and Therapy, 39,* 987–1006.

O'Connor, K., Todorov, C., Robillard, S., Borgeat, F., & Brault, M. (1999). Cognitive behaviour therapy and medication in the treatment of obsessive compulsive disorder: A controlled study. *Canadian Journal of Psychiatry, 44,* 64–71.

Öst, L.-G. (1989). A maintenance program for behavioral treatment of anxiety disorders. *Behaviour Research and Therapy, 27,* 123–130.

Persons, J. B. (1989). *Cognitive therapy in practice: A case formulation approach.* New York: Norton.

Persons, J. B., & Tompkins, M. A. (1997). Cognitive-behavioral case formulation. In T. D. Eells (Ed.), *Handbook of psychotherapy case formulation* (pp. 314–339). New York: Guilford Press.

Price, L. H., Goodman, W. K., Charney, D. S., Rasmussen, S. A., & Heninger, G. R. (1987). Treatment of severe obsessive–compulsive disorder with fluvoxamine. *American Journal of Psychiatry, 144,* 1059–1061.

Rachman, S., & de Silva, P. (1978). Abnormal and normal obsessions. *Behaviour Research and Therapy, 16,* 233–248.

Rachman, S., & Hodgson, R. J. (1980). *Obsessions and compulsions.* Englewood Cliffs, NJ: Prentice Hall.

Richter, M. A., Cox, B. J., & Direnfeld, D. M. (1994). A comparison of three assessment instruments for obsessive–compulsive symptoms. *Journal of Behavior Therapy and Experimental Psychiatry, 25,* 143–147.

Rosenfeld, R., Dar, R., Anderson, D., Kobak, K. A., & Greist, J. H. (1992). A computer-administered version of the Yale–Brown Obsessive–Compulsive Scale. *Psychological Assessment, 4,* 329–332.

Salkovskis, P. M. (1985). Obsessional–compulsive problems: A cognitive-behavioural analysis. *Behaviour Research and Therapy, 25,* 571–583.

Salkovskis, P. M. (1989). Cognitive-behavioural factors and the persistence of intrusive thoughts in obsessional problems. *Behaviour Research and Therapy, 27,* 677–682.

Salkovskis, P. M. (1996). Cognitive-behavioral approaches to the understanding of obsessional problems. In R. M. Rapee (Ed.), *Current controversies in the anxiety disorders* (pp. 103–133). New York: Guilford Press.

Salkovskis, P. M. (1999). Understanding and treating obsessive–compulsive disorder. *Behaviour Research and Therapy, 37,* S29–S52.

Salkovskis, P. M., & Harrison, J. (1984). Abnormal and normal obsessions: A replication. *Behaviour Research and Therapy, 22,* 549–552.

Salkovskis, P. M., & Warwick, H. M. (1985). Cognitive therapy of obsessive–compulsive disorder: Treating treatment failures. *Behavioural Psychotherapy, 13,* 243–255.

Sanavio, E. (1988). Obsessions and compulsions: The Padua Inventory. *Behaviour Research and Therapy, 26,* 169–177.

Schut, A. J., Castonguay, L. G., Plummer, K., & Borkovec, T. D. (1995, November). *Compulsive checking behaviors in generalized anxiety disorder.* Paper presented at the 29th meeting of the Association for Advancement of Behavior Therapy, Washington, DC.

Shafran, R., Thordarson, D. S., & Rachman, S. (1996). Thought–action fusion in obsessive compulsive disorder. *Journal of Anxiety Disorders, 10,* 379–391.

Sheehan, D. V. (1983). *The anxiety disease.* New York: Scribner's.

Stanley, M. A., & Turner, S. M. (1995). Current status of pharmacological and behavioral treatment of obsessive–compulsive disorder. *Behavior Therapy, 26,* 163–186.

Steketee, G. S. (1993). *Treatment of obsessive compulsive disorder.* New York: Guilford Press.

Steketee, G. S., Chambless, D. L., Tran, G. Q., Worden, H., & Gillis, M. M. (1996). Behavioral avoidance test for obsessive–compulsive disorder. *Behaviour Research and Therapy, 34,* 73–83.

Steketee, G., Frost, R., & Bogart, K. (1996). The Yale–Brown Obsessive Compulsive Scale: Interview versus self-report. *Behaviour Research and Therapy, 34,* 675–684.

Sternberger, L. G., & Burns, G. L. (1990). Compulsive Activity Checklist and the Maudsley Obsessional–Compulsive Inventory: Psychometric properties of two measures of obsessive–compulsive disorder. *Behavior Therapy, 21,* 117–127.

Taylor, S. (1995). Assessment of obsessions and compulsions: Reliability, validity, and sensitivity to treatment effects. *Clinical Psychology Review, 15,* 261–296.

Taylor, S. (1998). Assessment of obsessive–compulsive disorder. In R. P. Swinson, M. M. Antony, S. Rachman, & M. A. Richter (Eds.), *Obsessive–compulsive disorder: Theory, research, and treatment* (pp. 229–257). New York: Guilford Press.

Taylor, S. (2000a). *Understanding and treating panic disorder: Cognitive-behavioural approaches.* Chichester, UK: Wiley.

Taylor, S. (Ed.) (2000b). Special series. Treatment of obsessive–compulsive disorder: Progress, prospects, and problems. *Cognitive and Behavioral Practice, 6,* 342–426.

Thordarson, D. S., Radomsky, A. S., Rachman, S., Shafran, R., & Sawchuk, C. N. (1997, November). *The Vancouver Obsessional Compulsive Inventory (VOCI).* Paper presented at the annual convention of the Association for Advancement of Behavior Therapy, Miami Beach, FL.

Turner, S. M., Beidel, D. C., & Stanley, M. A. (1992). Are obsessional thoughts and worry different cognitive phenomena? *Clinical Psychology Review, 12,* 257–270.

van Balkom, A. J. L. M., de Hann, E., van Oppen, P., Spinhoven, P., Hoogduin, K. A. L., & van Dyck, R. (1998). Cognitive and behavioral therapies alone versus in combination with fluvoxamine in the treatment of obsessive compulsive disorder. *Journal of Nervous and Mental Disease, 186,* 492–499.

van Balkom, A. J. L. M., & van Dyck, R. (1998). Combination treatments for obsessive–compulsive disorder. In R. P. Swinson, M. M. Antony, S. Rachman, & M. A. Richter (Eds.), *Obsessive–compulsive disorder: Theory, research, and treatment* (pp. 349–366). New York: Guilford Press.

van Balkom, A. J. L. M., van Oppen, P., Vermeulen, A., van Dyck, R., Nauta, M., & Vorst, H. (1994). A meta-analysis on the treatment of obsessive compulsive disorder: A comparison of antidepressants, behavior, and cognitive therapy. *Clinical Psychology Review, 14,* 359–381.

Warren, R., Zgourides, G., & Monto, M. (1993). Self-report versions of the Yale–Brown Obsessive–Compulsive Scale: An assessment of a sample of normals. *Psychological Reports, 73,* 574.

Wegner, D. M. (1994). Ironic processes of mental control. *Psychological Review, 101,* 34–52.

Weissman, M. M., Bland, R. C., Canino, G. J., Greenwald, S., Hwu, H.-G., Lee, C. K., Newman, S. C., Oakley-Browne, M. A., Rubino-Stipec, M., Wickramaratne, P. J., Wittchen, H.-U., & Yeh, E.-K. (1994). The cross national epidemiology of obsessive compulsive disorder. *Journal of Clinical Psychiatry, 55*(Suppl. 3), 5–10.

Weissman, M. M., Broadhead, W. E., Olfson, M., Sheehan, D. V., Hoven, C., Conolly, P., Fireman, B. H., Farber, L., Blacklow, R. S., Higgins, S., & Leon, A. C. (1998). A diagnostic aid for detecting (DSM-IV) mental disorders in primary care. *General Hospital Psychiatry, 20,* 1–11.

Wells, A. (1997). *Cognitive therapy of anxiety disorders: A practice manual and conceptual guide.* Chichester, UK: Wiley.

Wells, A., & Morrison, A. P. (1994). Qualitative dimensions of normal worry and normal obsessions: A comparative study. *Behaviour Research and Therapy, 32,* 867–870.

Wittchen, H.-U. (1996). Critical issues in the evaluation of comorbidity of psychiatric disorders. *British Journal of Psychiatry, 168*(Suppl.), 9–16.

Woody, S. R., Steketee, G., & Chambless, D. L. (1995). Reliability and validity of the Yale–Brown Obsessive Compulsive Scale. *Behaviour Research and Therapy, 33,* 597–605.

Zimmerman, M. (1994). Diagnosing personality disorders: A review of issues and research methods. *Archives of General Psychiatry, 51,* 225–245.

7

Exposure to Trauma in Adults

Brett T. Litz
Mark W. Miller
Anna M. Ruef
Lisa M. McTeague

In this chapter, we review briefly the epidemiology of exposure to trauma in adults and de-scribe the complex symptoms of posttraumatic stress disorder (PTSD) from a cognitive-behavioral perspective. We also describe the associated clinical features of PTSD and the co-morbid disorders that are commonly linked to trauma exposure and PTSD. We then review clinical assessment methods and make recommendations for screening, diagnostic evalua-tion, evaluating trauma and PTSD in primary care settings, and measuring clinical outcome.

THE PHENOMENOLOGY AND EPIDEMIOLOGY OF TRAUMA

Exposure to potentially traumatizing events (PTEs) puts anyone at risk for developing post-traumatic adjustment problems. An event or context is considered potentially traumatizing if it is unpredictable, uncontrollable, and a severe or catastrophic violation of fundamental beliefs and expectations about safety, physical integrity, trust, and justice. Examples of PTEs include direct life threats, physical injury, observing violence and extreme suffering, and sexual assault. A person exposed to PTEs is likely to experience a traumatic stress reac-tion, which entails extreme activation of the physiological and psychological resources that are designed to mobilize the person to respond to threat. The traumatic stress reaction en-tails a variety of negative affects (e.g., dread, horror), intense feelings of vulnerability and loss of control, and a sense of depersonalization and derealization (e.g., Herman, 1992a; Horowitz, 1986; Rothbaum, Foa, Riggs, Murdock, & Walsh, 1992; Weiss et al., 1995).

While PTEs are extraordinary, they are not rare. Epidemiological studies reveal that risk for exposure to PTEs across the lifespan is an unfortunate part of the human condition. In one study, 68% of women reported at least one PTE over the lifespan (Resnick, Kil-patrick, Dansky, Saunders, & Best, 1993), while in another, both men and women reported a similar rate of exposure to PTEs (Norris, 1992). Kessler, Sonnega, Bromet, Hughes, & Nelson (1995) reported in the National Comorbidity Survey that 60% of men and 51% of women report exposure to at least one PTE in their lifetime. In another large study, 89% of adults in an urban area reported exposure to at least one PTE (Breslau et al., 1998). Reports of childhood sexual abuse, a particularly destructive and severe trauma, are also alarmingly high. In one study, 27% of women and 16% of men reported at least one incidence of childhood sexual abuse (Finkelhor, Hotaling, Lewis, & Smith, 1990). Childhood experiences with assaultive violence, in particular, have been shown to increase the risk for exposure to PTEs and PTSD in adulthood (e.g., Breslau, Peterson, Kessler, & Schultz, 1999). Generally, men report more frequent exposure to physical violence and witnessing violence, while women report more experience with sexual victimization (e.g., Bernat, Ronfeldt, Calhoun, & Arias, 1998). Taken as a whole, these studies underscore the ubiquity of exposure to PTEs over the lifespan.

Exposure to PTEs is not limited by culture and socioeconomic status. For example, 54% of female American college students reported some form of sexual victimization experience (Koss, Gidycz, & Wisneiwski, 1987), and a recent questionnaire study in a large American university estimated the prevalence rate of exposure to at least one PTE in young men and women to be 84% (Vrana & Lauterbach, 1994).

Most individuals exposed to PTEs experience an immediate traumatic stress reaction, which understandably disrupts normal functioning for at least a short period (e.g., Rothbaum et al., 1992). For example, it is normal for a sexual assault survivor to be stunned, fatigued, and depleted and to experience the aftereffects of sustained arousal, including impairments of memory and cognition, sleep disturbance, and emotional lability. When exposed to reminders (e.g., when discussing the crime with emergency room personnel, law enforcement, and family members), the person is likely to recall the horrifying visceral details of the experience with severe negative affect. The person who was recently traumatized is also expected to be motivated to avoid the feelings that arise when recalling the trauma and the situations that serve as reminders of their experience. He or she needs to be allowed to find a balance between stark recognition and vivid recall and finding safety and comfort (e.g., Herman, 1992a; Horowitz, 1986).

In part, the manner in which immediate posttraumatic reactions are coped with by the individual and how others respond determines risk for chronic posttraumatic maladjustment. Secondary prevention interventions, such as disaster mental health, critical incident stress debriefing, and other prevention programs are designed to reduce risk in the critical immediate posttraumatic period (e.g., Foa, Hearst-Ikeda, & Perry, 1995; Myers, 1989). If a person exposed to trauma is particularly avoidant; copes poorly with arousal symptoms (e.g., uses alcohol to self-medicate); fails to disclose his or her experience to significant others; or is exposed to a recovery environment that is particularly harsh, rejecting, or demanding of premature disclosure—in all these cases, the person is less likely to recover adaptively.

A number of psychological processes can account for the shift from normal response to PTEs and chronic disorder. For example, attempts to suppress and avoid thoughts and feelings about a trauma are draining of cognitive resources and increase arousal (e.g., Gross and Levenson, 1993, Pennebaker, Barger, & Tiebout, 1989). Selective attention to threatening information in the environment serves to confirm beliefs about danger and vulnerability (e.g., Litz and Keane, 1989; McNally, 1998), and avoidance behavior can become habitual due to negative reinforcement (e.g., Keane, Zimering, & Caddell, 1985). Significant others' negative responses can also serve to further motivate avoidance behavior and reinforce maladaptive beliefs, usually about shame (e.g., Janoff-Bulman, 1989). While the intensity, degree of life threat, and other characteristics of the trauma and the person's peritraumatic response are the best predictors of posttraumatic pathology (e.g., Kulka et al., 1988; Weiss et al., 1995), these variables account for approximately 30% of the variance in outcome in most multivariate studies. The literature has revealed a variety of demographic, individual difference characteristics, and learning history variables that also affect outcome (e.g., King, King, Foy, Keane, & Fairbank, 1999). For example, for individuals exposed to PTEs in adulthood, intelligence (e.g., Macklin et al., 1998), age, exposure to PTEs in childhood, and personality variables such as hardiness are risk factors that have been shown to affect adaptation to PTEs (e.g., Foy, Osato, Housecamp, & Neumann, 1992; Green, 1993; Kilpatrick, Veronen, & Best, 1985; King , King, Gudanowski, & Vreven, 1995). In addition, it appears that if the recovery environment is filled with financial, marital, family, and physical demands, there is greater risk for chronic PTSD (e.g., Norris & Uhl, 1993).

THE PTSD SYNDROME

Some individuals exposed to trauma fail to recover spontaneously and experience lingering symptoms that mirror their initial reaction to the event. These individuals develop an acute stress disorder or reaction that greatly interferes with their ability to return to their normal family and their social and work routines (e.g., Koopman, Classen, Cardena, & Spiegel, 1995). Within a month or so, such acute reactions usually remit, and the person returns to his or her pretrauma routine, having restored a state of homeostasis. For others, this acute reaction fails to remit and symptoms persist, becoming chronic, often debilitating PTSD (e.g., Harvey & Bryant, 1998).

An invariant pattern of positive and negative symptoms was observed in soldiers exposed to the horrors of World Wars I and II (e.g., Dollard & Miller, 1950; Freud, Fereneczi, Abraham, Simmel, & Jones, 1921), but the characteristic symptoms of PTSD were not codified in the diagnostic nosology until 1980. Although debate continues about the necessary and sufficient symptoms of PTSD and the threshold required for a diagnosis (e.g., Davidson & Foa, 1991), at present, a set of 17 symptoms or repertoires of characteristic responses have been identified as posttraumatic sequelae (DSM-IV; American Psychiatric Association, 1994). The current iteration of the PTSD syndrome classification sets forth a rough operational definition of what constitutes a traumatic event (Criterion A), requiring exposure to a PTE and a peritraumatic emotional response (fear, helplessness, or horror). The symptoms of PTSD are aggregated into three separate classes: reexperiencing phenomena (Criterion B), avoidance and emotional numbing symptoms (Criterion C), and hyperarousal disturbances (Criterion D). A diagnosis of PTSD requires that the person report a Criterion A traumatic event, at least one Criterion B, reexperiencing symptom, at least three Criterion C, avoidance and emotional numbing symptoms, and at least two Criterion D, hyperarousal symptoms. In addition, symptoms need to be present for at least a month, and they need to cause significant distress or functional impairment.

According to the cognitive-behavioral perspective, there is a primacy of conditioned emotional responses in PTSD (e.g., Keane, Zimering, & Caddell, 1985). By virtue of the intensity of the peritraumatic response, a wide variety of internal and external cues are capable of triggering trauma memory activation. This hyperaccessibility occurs because of the potency and variety of conditioned stimuli and the self-relevance and multidimensional nature of the memory (e.g., Chemtob, Roitblat, Hamada, Carlson, & Twentyman, 1988; Litz & Keane, 1989). The emotional responses that are triggered during trauma memory activation serve to mobilize defensive behavior (e.g., escape or avoidance), which, if effective, is highly negatively reinforcing. In PTSD, defensive behavior becomes routine and overlearned and thwarts the sustained emotional processing of trauma memory (Foa, Steketee, & Rothbaum, 1989). In this cognitive-behavioral framework, the reexperiencing symptoms of PTSD (e.g., intrusive thoughts and feelings about the trauma) are conceptualized as cued trauma memory reactivations. These symptoms are prototypical of the PTSD syndrome and are the modal targets in treatment, which entails a combination of sustained exposure to trauma cues and avoidance response prevention, along with applying stress management to cope adaptively with situations that trigger trauma memories (e.g., Fairbank & Nicholson, 1987; Foa and Rothbaum, 1998; Keane, 1997).

In our view, the most parsimonious explanation for the complex, seemingly distinct Criterion C and Criterion D symptoms of PTSD is that they are causally linked to cued trauma memory activation. For example, so-called emotional-numbing symptoms are considered phasic emotional-processing deficits that arise subsequent to cued trauma memory activation (Litz et al., 2000). Hyperarousal symptoms such as irritability and concentration difficulties also arise from states of cued trauma memory activation. It is difficult to remain focused on foreground activities when the background emotional state is trauma-related, and it is hard to cope with additional demands when resources are devoted to cope with trauma memory activation.

The psychological scarring associated with certain traumas is so vast that return to pre-trauma capacities is almost impossible. Examples of such events are surviving internment in a concentration camp and incest or other forms of repeated sexual abuse in childhood. The term "complex PTSD" has been used to describe a syndrome of changes in personality that stem from the effects of such horrendous trauma (Herman, 1992b; Roth, Newman, Pelcovitz, van der Kolk, & Mandel, 1997). Although the construct of complex PTSD is in need of refinement conceptually, and requires careful empirical examination, there is consensus in the literature that some individuals exposed to trauma manifest traits that are traumatogenic, yet they are not represented in the PTSD syndrome. For example, adults who were physically and sexually abused in childhood report lifelong problems with self-care, self-perception, and emotional self-regulation (e.g., Roth, Lebowitz, & DeRosa, 1997). Such problems have recently been recognized as affecting treatment outcome (e.g., Ford & Kidd, 1998) and requiring specialized treatments (e.g., Linehan, 1993).

EPIDEMIOLOGY OF PTSD

The prevalence rates of PTSD vary due to differences in samples, sampling strategies, assessment methods, and caseness definitions. However, the best estimate of the risk for PTSD in the general population comes from the National Comorbidity Survey, which yielded a lifetime prevalence rate of 8% (Kessler et al., 1995). In another national study, 17.9% of survivors of crime met criteria for a lifetime diagnosis of PTSD, and 6.7% were diagnosed with current PTSD (Resnick et al.,1993). In another large epidemiological study, 24% of women exposed to trauma reported current PTSD (Breslau, Davis, Andreski, & Peterson, 1991).

Some groups are particularly at risk for exposure to PTEs and subsequent PTSD. Examples of especially at risk groups are soldiers exposed to a war zone (e.g., Kulka et al., 1990), emergency medical technicians, police, firefighters, and members of communities or geographical regions that have been affected by natural and man-made disasters (e.g., Davidson & Baum, 1986; Green, 1991). Veterans of the Vietnam War have been extensively studied. The National Vietnam Veterans Readjustment Study (NVVRS) found prevalence rates of current PTSD to be 15.2% and 8.5% for male and female war-exposed veterans, respectively (Kulka et al., 1990). The NVVRS found lifetime prevalence rates of 30.6% for male veterans and 26.9% for female veterans. It should be emphasized that the casualties of war are not just soldiers, but large groups of civilians. A recent study in Sri Lanka, the site of civil war since 1983, estimated that 94% of the population had been exposed to at least one war-zone stressor, and 27% had current PTSD (Somasundaram & Sivayokan, 1994). In many war-torn regions of the world (e.g., Cambodia, the former Yugoslavia, and Somalia), exposure to violence affects nearly all who live in the society. For these special at-risk groups, primary prevention of PTSD is important, when feasible (e.g., special didactics and training for soldiers). After-action screening for exposure to trauma and posttraumatic difficulties in large groups is also important, and the results of these screenings should trigger a referral for secondary prevention when indicated.

COMORBIDITY AND ASSOCIATED FEATURES OF PTSD

Research has shown that individuals exposed to PTEs are at risk for the development of a variety of psychiatric disorders, in addition to PTSD (e.g., Sierles, Chen, McFarland, & Taylor, 1983; Weaver & Clum, 1993). When epidemiologists identify PTSD as the index or primary disorder, they find a very high prevalence of additional Axis I and Axis II disorders (e.g., Keane & Wolfe, 1990; Kessler et al., 1995; Kulka et al., 1990). However, it is of note that in the national comorbidity study, the rates of comorbidity in the community were no higher for PTSD than for other Axis I disorders (Kessler et al., 1995). Individuals who are in treatment or who are seeking treatment for PTSD report particularly high rates of comorbid disorders, most often substance use disorders and major depression (e.g., Kilpatrick, Best, et al., 1985; Orsillo et al., 1996).

The suffering associated with PTSD extends beyond the signs and symptoms of the disorder and formal comorbid psychiatric conditions. People with PTSD also present clinically with a variety of functional disturbances and problems that often require attention in treatment. The additional problems may reflect personal or environmental deficits that created greater vulnerability to chronic PTSD, or they may be the collateral result of having PTSD.

The associated clinical problems reported in empirical studies of patients with PTSD include: (1) problems with the availability and quality of social supports (e.g., Keane, Scott, Chavoya, Lamparski, & Fairbank, 1985); (2) suicidal and parasuicidal behaviors (e.g., Kilpatrick, Best, et al., 1985); (3) family and marital problems (e.g., Carroll, Rueger, Foy, & Donahoe, 1985; Jordan et al., 1992); (4) disturbances in sexual functioning and in the quality of emotional connection with significant others (e.g., Resick, Calhoun, Atkeson, & Ellis, 1981; Steketee & Foa, 1987); (5) coping deficits (Nezu & Carnevale, 1987; Solomon, Mikulincer, & Avitzur, 1988; Solomon, Mikulincer, & Flum, 1988); and (6) poor quality of life, somatic complaints and physical health problems (e.g., Litz, Keane, Fisher, Marx, & Monaco, 1992; Shalev, Bleich, & Ursano, 1990; Zatzick, et al., 1997). When there are multiple traumas across the lifespan or when trauma occurs early in development, researchers have observed deficits in self-care, affect regulation, and distortions in perceptions of legitimacy and agency (Herman, 1992b; McCann & Pearlman, 1990; Roth, Lebowitz, & DeRosa, 1997).

The presence of comorbid problems in patients with PTSD requires a treatment approach that is designed to target trauma-related symptoms and other adjustment problems, sometimes serially, other times in parallel (e.g., Flack, Litz, & Keane, 1998). However, several studies have shown that deficits in functional capacities and quality of life are uniquely associated with PTSD, which suggests that if PTSD symptoms are targeted successfully in treatment, many comorbid problems may well diminish (e.g., Zatzick et al., 1997).

GOALS FOR THE ASSESSMENT OF TRAUMATIZED ADULTS

Given the disruptive influence of trauma across the lifespan, the heterogeneity of symptom expression, and the complex clinical problems that result from exposure to trauma, a careful and detailed clinical assessment is critical. Fortunately, there are many resources available to assist clinicians in evaluating traumatized individuals and conceptualizing their difficulties. In the field of trauma, the last decade has seen a proliferation of empirical research in the measurement of trauma and PTSD. At present, there are at least three major edited volumes on the assessment of PTSD (Briere, 1997; Carlson, 1997; Wilson & Keane, 1997), and a number of excellent critical reviews of the assessment literature (e.g., Resnick, Kilpatrick, & Lipovsky, 1991; Sutker, Uddo-Crane, & Allain, 1991; Weathers & Keane, 1999). The field of traumatic stress has evolved to such an extent that there is now a prescriptive gold standard method for diagnosing PTSD (e.g., Keane, Weathers, and Foa, 2000).

Assigning a diagnosis of PTSD is a necessary but by no means sufficient task in the assessment of traumatized adults. There are a number of reasons why this is the case. First, given the heterogeneity of the PTSD syndrome, a diagnosis of PTSD alone does not lead to straightforward decisions about treatment. Second, as summarized here, exposure to trauma affects multiple areas of psychosocial functioning, but the information conveyed by a diagnosis of PTSD says little about the other areas of patients' lives that may be adversely affected by, or interact with, the condition (e.g., Litz, Penk, Gerardi, & Keane, 1992; Litz & Weathers, 1994).

Following, we list the major goals for the assessment of treatment-seeking traumatized adults. The necessary content areas to cover for specific clinical or research situations will vary according to the assessment context (e.g., screening large numbers of individuals exposed to a PTE, case–control research), the needs of individual patients, and clinical resources.

Establish the Presence and Extent of Trauma

To render a decision about the presence of PTSD, the clinician must first establish the presence of a Criterion A event. Although DSM-IV provides a clearer operational definition of trauma than past frameworks, it is still not perfect. The definition reads as follows: "The person experienced, witnessed, or was confronted with an event or events that involved actual or threatened death or serious injury, or a threat to the physical integrity of self or others, [and] the person's response involved intense fear, helplessness or horror" (American Psychiatric Association, 1994, pp. 427–428). The phrase "threat to the physical integrity of self or others" is particularly ambiguous and subject to interpretation. In addition, there are individuals who are exposed to an unequivocal PTE and report severe PTSD symptoms that are referenced to the specific event, but who report being numb or stunned peritraumatically. Finally, the DSM requires a categorical judgment about exposure to trauma, which fails to take into account important dimensional features of a traumatic event and the person's response at the time of the event (e.g. duration, extent of degradation, degree of life threat). Unfortunately, there is no standard, widely used trauma-exposure measure that yields the necessary categorical and dimensional information about PTEs and peritraumatic response. If a clinician decides to employ one of the available measures of PTEs, additional inquiry about the extent of trauma is necessary, as is clinical judgment about experiences that fail to readily meet the DSM-IV Criterion A.

When interviewing patients about their exposure, the clinician should ask, at a minimum: What was going on in your life at the time that this event occurred? What occurred directly prior to the event, and how were you feeling? What happened during the event; what were you seeing, hearing, sensing, feeling; and what did you try to do? What happened afterward? What were the responses of those around you? Given the high base rates for multiple traumatic events across the lifespan, the clinician should inquire about the patient's exposure to trauma during his or her entire life. If a patient reports a number of PTEs, the clinician must render a judgment about which event will be referenced when evaluating various PTSD symptoms. If a patient presents with multiple traumas across the lifespan, for diagnostic purposes, the symptoms of PTSD should be referenced specifically to the event initially reported. In some instances, the clinician may choose to refer to the worst (most severe) event, to the most recent, or to the most recent and most severe event.

Diagnostic Assessment of PTSD

Whenever possible, we recommend the use of a structured clinical interview to diagnose PTSD. This allows clinicians to make judgments about the validity of patients' appraisals of their symptoms; to assist patients in answering questions about various complex cognitive, emotional, and behavioral phenomena; and to determine whether there is a link between traumatic experiences and PTSD symptomatology. We recommend the use of diagnostic instruments (interviews or paper-and-pencil tests) that measure the severity of each symptom as described in DSM, provide a total continuous severity score, and empirically determine the cutoff for diagnosis that is derived from the total severity score. A test that provides a continuous severity score for specific PTSD symptoms, clusters of symptoms (e.g., reexperiencing symptoms), and total severity is particularly useful for monitoring treatment outcome. It also provides the clinician with information about the relative degree of distress for those patients that fail to meet the relatively arbitrary categorical case definition of PTSD stipulated in the current DSM, even though they are seeking posttraumatic treatment. Nevertheless, each instrument should also provide an empirically derived decision rule or cutoff for PTSD caseness that is based on the categorical DSM definition of PTSD. Particularly attractive instruments pay attention to linking the emotional-numbing and hyperarousal symptoms to a specific trauma and to establishing the proper temporal relationship between the trauma and the onset of these problems.

All instruments used to measure PTSD rely on self-report and are subject to biases, inaccuracies, distortions, and judgmental heuristics that are endemic to the appraisal process. Individuals with PTSD may have a particularly difficult time providing accurate frequency and intensity information about private events, many of which are not processed in a sustained, effortful way because of avoidance maneuvers. Whenever possible, a multimethod approach is recommended to increase the validity of diagnostic decisions. In the ideal case, an assessment would entail a clinical interview, the administration of at least one paper-and-pencil measure, an interview with a significant other who is familiar with the patient (e.g., Litz, Penk, et al., 1992). In most clinical contexts, a multimethod approach entails administration of an interview and at least one questionnaire. Multiple sources of data about symptoms provide information about the degree of convergence of symptom reports or the concordance between a patient's report and that of significant others.

Screen for Coexisting Psychiatric Diagnoses and Problem Areas

There are a number of ways to screen for the presence of comorbid disorders. A particularly useful method of screening for psychopathology is the initial semistructured screening and history section of the Structured Clinical Interview for DSM-IV (SCID; First, Spitzer, Gibbon, & Williams, 1996). This introductory section provides the clinician with a structure that frames the presenting complaint in the life-course context and screens for other significant problems that may need intervention (medical and psychological). Probe questions are provided to evaluate etiological and controlling factors responsible for problems (e.g., family history) and previous coping and treatment efforts (e.g., treatment history, suicidal or other self-destructive behaviors, history of treatment noncompliance). If a patient reports specific problems that warrant further inquiry, specific modules of the SCID can be used to evaluate Axis I pathology. If the interview suggests the presence of Axis II pathology, the clinician can administer the SCID-II questionnaire, which is a screening instrument for Axis-II disorders (SCID-II; First, Spitzer, Gibbon, & Williams, 1997). Another attractive feature of the initial section of the SCID is that it allows the clinician to inquire about a variety of areas of functional impairment and to establish a rough time line for their onset. This is useful for establishing a temporal link between problem areas and exposure to trauma. Finally, the open-ended format of the initial section of the SCID allows the clinician to assess resources (individual and social/familial) that could shed light on issues relevant to treatment planning and estimating prognosis (e.g., compliance).

A time-saving, but less comprehensive, alternative is to administer a broad-spectrum screening questionnaire, such as the Symptom Checklist-90—Revised (SCL-90-R; Derogatis et al., 1983), or the briefer 53-item Brief Symptom Inventory (BSI; Derogatis, 1993). Another alternative is the Minnesota Multiphasic Personality Inventory (MMPI-2; Butcher et al., 1989), which is particularly attractive because this scale has an embedded, empirically derived PTSD scale (Keane, Malloy, & Fairbank, 1984), and it has response bias and validity indicators that can contextualize a patient's approach to the assessment. The clinician should inquire about problem areas that exceed the clinical cutoffs on these tests by using appropriate modules of diagnostic instruments (e.g., the SCID, First et al., 1996; SCID-II, First et al., 1997; or the Diagnostic Interview Schedule [DIS; Robins, Cottler, Bucholz, & Compton, 1995]).

Put Traumatic Events in a Lifespan Context

There is growing evidence that pretrauma learning history and posttrauma events affect the trajectory of posttraumatic adjustment (e.g., King et al., 1999). It is important for clinicians to inquire about salient developmental events and posttrauma complications (e.g., Keane, Zimering, & Caddell, 1985). The goal here is to evaluate significant events across the lifespan that have may have colored adaptation to trauma or which contribute to the maintenance of PTSD and associated maladaptive behaviors. The clinician should also inquire about strengths that the person possesses currently or that were once part of their repertoire, which can be useful in treatment planning.

At present, there is no formal structured or semistructured instrument to examine developmental issues that are germane to adjustment to trauma. The clinician needs to facilitate a patient's narrative account of life experiences that have a thematic connection to a given trauma. Several heuristic guidelines are available for this task (see Roth, Lebowitz, & DeRosa, 1997; Lebowitz & Newman 1996). Important areas to address in an interview in reference to pre- and posttrauma experiences are the following:

1. History of extreme or overwhelming stress, especially violence and/or sexual abuse. Questions about how previous extreme stressors were appraised and managed can provide data on a person's specific coping style.
2. Family/home environment (e.g.: Was there any history of mental illness or substance abuse in the family? How did role models cope with stress? How were feelings expressed in the home?).

3. History of academic, social, and/or occupational impairment or deficits (e.g.: Were there any antisocial behaviors?).
4. History of head injury or other experiences that may have influenced cognitive functions.
5. The person's relative cognitive and behavioral strengths (e.g.: What part of a person's behavioral repertoire can be augmented or enhanced in treatment?).
6. Significant others' responses to the trauma.

Evaluate Compensation-Seeking Status and Litigation Status

There are two ways that traumatized individuals can be involved with the legal system: they may seek compensation or damages for the physical and psychological scars of trauma, or they may claim that a history of trauma and PTSD affected their psychological state, with the result that they committed a crime (Keane, 1995; Sparr & Pitman, 1998). Assessment behavior is affected by compensation seeking or litigation (e.g., Fairbank, McCaffrey, & Keane, 1985; Hyer, Fallon, Harrison, & Boudewyns, 1987). The assessor should also keep in mind that all diagnostic instruments are prone to elicit overendorsement of PTSD symptoms because they have face value. In addition, with the exception of the MMPI-2 (Butcher et al., 1989), no PTSD measure has the capacity to evaluate response bias (Litz, Penk, et al., 1992). At a minimum, at some point in the assessment of trauma survivors, clinicians need to inquire about a patient's attempts to get compensation for their trauma or victimization experiences or their legal status generally. The clinician can provide a useful service by helping the patient separate compensation and treatment issues from the clinician's role as treatment provider. A discussion of secondary gain issues in the beginning stages of the assessment can also improve the reliability of self-report data.

Evaluate Motivation and Readiness for Change of Various Aspects of the PTSD Syndrome and Other Problem Areas

One overlooked function of the assessment of traumatized adults is the determination of motivation and readiness for change and the prognosis for success or failure. The treatment of chronic PTSD is arduous, and many patients will experience a downturn in the symptoms before they get better. In addition, homework assignments are routine, and a clinician should evaluate motivational factors that may affect compliance. For many reasons, individuals who suffer from PTSD may not be motivated to adhere to a treatment program. For example, patients may have had a history of failure experiences in treatment and thus they have very low efficacy and outcome expectations, both of which have been shown to mediate behaviors that are conducive to positive treatment outcome. Some patients with chronic PTSD have learned ways of relating to others and ways of constructing ideas about themselves so that, however painful, the trauma and being a victim has become a defining characteristic, which is difficult to modify. This is typically borne from a history of not being sufficiently recognized and validated for suffering and fundamental unmet needs posttrauma.

REVIEW OF EMPIRICAL LITERATURE ON ASSESSMENT MEASURES

The 1990s will be remembered as the decade of the development and refinement of trauma and PTSD assessment instruments. Although several measures appeared earlier—for example, the Impact of Event Scale (Horowitz, Wilner, & Alvarez, 1979), which holds the distinction of being the first PTSD scale and which predates even the inclusion of the disorder in DSM-III—the vast majority of the more than two dozen PTSD instruments that exist today were published in the 1990s. One drawback from the rapid growth in the number of instruments is that the PTSD assessment literature has become glutted with generally analogous measures. As a result, clinicians and researchers face a daunting task in selecting measures for a given purpose.

Therefore, a primary objective of this section is to assist in evaluating the existing measures along several important criteria and to offer recommendations regarding the use of PTSD instruments for clinical practice. We first review three types of assessment measures designed to diagnose PTSD: (1) clinician-administered PTSD interviews, (2) self-report (paper-and-pencil) questionnaire measures of PTSD symptomatology or PTSD criteria B–D, and (3) psychophysiological techniques. This review is followed by a discussion of measures that are designed to evaluate potentially traumatizing events and trauma.

Special Psychometric Considerations in the Evaluation of PTSD Measures

Reliability

Although the majority of readers of this text are familiar with psychometric evaluation of psychological tests, we provide an overview in order to contextualize some of the unique psychometric issues in the PTSD field. Psychological instruments are traditionally evaluated largely on the basis of their reliability and validity. The reliability of an instrument is the extent to which various parts of a test measure the same construct (internal consistency), yield the same results when utilized repeatedly under similar conditions (test–retest reliability), and, in the case of interviews or rating scales, have a concordance between different raters (interrater reliability). Some types of reliability are arguably more important for the evaluation of PTSD assessment instruments than others. For the structured clinical interview, for example, demonstration of interrater reliability is of utmost importance. Typically, the degree of agreement between two raters is quantified using the kappa statistic, which provides an index of chance-corrected agreement. Test–retest reliability is also important, irrespective of whether the format is interview or self-report, but determining the most appropriate test–retest interval is a matter of some controversy because of the fluctuating nature of PTSD symptomatology. When short test–retest intervals (i.e., less than 1 week) are used, bias is introduced from the respondent's memory of prior responses. Longer test–retest intervals (i.e., 1 month or more) introduce multiple sources of variability and confound the measurement of reliability with true symptom variation.

The internal consistency of an instrument is typically quantified by calculating the average item–total correlation and/or Cronbach's alpha. In the case of PTSD instruments, however, it is not entirely clear that these measures provide the most appropriate index of internal consistency. When a unidimensional personality trait is evaluated, it is essential that all items on a scale that taps that construct are highly intercorrelated. In contrast, PTSD as defined in DSM-IV is a syndrome comprised of four clusters of symptoms (i.e., reexperiencing, strategic avoidance, emotional numbing, and hyperarousal), which conceptually and statistically are multidimensional in nature (cf. King & King, 1994). Although the exact factor structure of the PTSD syndrome remains an issue of some controversy and has been a focus of DSM-III-R and DSM-IV revisions, research supports the multidimensionality of the disorder. In light of this, demonstrating the internal consistency of a total PTSD scale may be less important than demonstrating the internal consistency of items that measure its underlying dimensions.

Validity

Assessing the validity of an instrument involves evaluating evidence that supports inferences made on the basis of test scores. Validity is a multifaceted concept. Evidence pertaining to the validity of a measure is accumulated in many ways, including evaluation of the content validity of the instrument, the quality of the method employed in the validation studies, criterion-related validity, and convergent and discriminant validity of the measure. Content validity concerns the extent to which items on a measure provide full and equal coverage of all important facets of the construct that is being measured. An important issue related to the content validity of a PTSD measure is whether it is referenced directly to the DSM definition of the disorder and assesses all 17 symptoms. A number of empirically derived PTSD scales (e.g., the MMPI–PTSD Scale; Keane et al., 1984) were not designed to assess the full range of symptoms. Other scales, such as the Mississippi Scale (Keane, Caddel, & Taylor, 1988) may emphasize the evaluation of certain features of the disorder while not specifically assessing others. Still other measures assess phenomena that are believed to be associated with the disorder but perhaps are not specifically indexed by the DSM (e.g., Trauma Symptom Inventory; Briere, Elliot, Harris, & Cotman, 1995).

Although the validity of a measure is ultimately judged by considering evidence accumulated from multiple sources, the quality of the method employed in the published validation studies represents an important factor. The quality of the validation work can be evaluated on the basis of a number of factors that influence generalizability, including the population from which the validation sample was drawn and the size of that sample. The method used for establishing the criterion-related validity of the measure is also important. Criterion-related validity is assessed by determining the relationship between scores on the test and some independent, nontest criterion. In the field of PTSD, the "gold-standard" criterion has been the clinician-determined diagnosis derived by structured clinical interview, but some validation studies have used other criteria, including scores on other previously validated self-report questionnaires—which in our opinion is not satisfactory.

The validity of a measure can also be judged by examining the extent to which scores on the test correlate highly with variables that they, in principle, should correlate highly with (convergent validity) and, conversely, correlate poorly with factors that they should not be associated with (discriminant validity). PTSD measures can be judged on the degree to which they covary with other measures of PTSD or related symptomatology (i.e., general anxiety, depression) and yet diverge from scores on measures of other symptomatology that are unrelated to the syndrome of PTSD (e.g., schizophrenia, antisocial personality disorder). Although demonstrating discriminant validity is challenging due to the heterogeneity of the PTSD syndrome and high rates of comorbidity, valid measures should reliably discriminate individuals with PTSD from psychiatric controls (i.e., samples with psychiatric conditions other than PTSD). This type of validation is rare, unfortunately.

PTSD assessment instruments can also be evaluated in terms of factors that contribute to their diagnostic utility. In this context, it is important to specify the time frame on which the assessment is based. Some questionnaires contain instructions for respondents to evaluate their symptomatology within a specific time frame (i.e., during the last week or last month); others do not designate a precise time frame, leaving it unclear whether respondents are to refer to their current or lifetime symptomatology.[1] Similarly, some measures

---

[1]It is convention to specify symptoms that have been present within the past month as *current* symptomatology and those that have not been present in the past month but were present previously as present during the *lifetime*. DSM-IV, however, does not articulate a distinction between current and lifetime symptomatology.

provide for specification of the time of symptom onset and facilitate the DSM-based classification of symptomatology as acute, chronic, or delayed onset.

PTSD instruments also vary in terms of whether they are designed to provide categorical diagnoses or dimensional measures of symptomatology, or both. Most dimensional measures assess each symptom using a Likert-type severity scale. One exception is the Penn Inventory (Hammarberg, 1992), modeled after the Beck Depression Inventory (BDI; Beck, 1988), which is comprised of items consisting of four graded statements reflecting increasing levels of psychopathology. Only the Clinician-Administered PTSD Scale (CAPS; Blake et al., 1990) assesses symptom frequency and intensity separately, although this scale introduces considerable complexity in defining decision rules for caseness.

Another issue relevant to evaluating the clinical utility of an instrument is its capacity to accurately discriminate individuals with and without the disorder (i.e., discriminative validity). Many PTSD measures solely provide a continuous measure of symptomatology and can only serve as a diagnostic tool if appropriate cutoff scores have been defined through prior validation work (for review of this process, see Weathers, Keane, King, & King, 1997). A related consideration is whether the cutoff scores derived from work with one population (e.g., male combat veterans) will generalize to other populations (e.g., female sexual assault survivors). Other measures such as the PTSD Checklist (PCL; Weathers, Litz, Herman, Huska, & Keane, 1993) permit diagnostic decisions using the DSM-IV PTSD symptom criteria.

Structured PTSD Interviews

Structured clinical interviews are formalized interview procedures designed to improve the reliability and validity of clinical diagnoses by specifying the kind of diagnostic information that is sought, the content and order of the interviewer's questions, and the rules that govern the making of diagnostic decisions. Watson and colleagues (Watson, 1990; Watson, Juba, Manifold, Kucala, & Anderson, 1991) suggested that PTSD interviews can be evaluated in terms of the extent to which they (1) correspond with current diagnostic criteria (i.e., DSM-IV; American Psychiatric Association, 1994), (2) provide both dichotomous and continuous data about each symptom and the disorder as a whole, and (3) possess adequate reliability and validity. In addition, Blake (1994) has suggested that PTSD interview measures should also be evaluated in terms of the extent to which they (4) provide explicit behavioral anchors for rating each symptom and (5) delineate the time frame for which diagnostic status is being assessed. In this section, we briefly review seven of the most widely used structured interviews for the assessment of PTSD using these criteria.

Anxiety Disorders Interview Schedule (ADIS-IV)

The ADIS-IV (Di Nardo, Brown, & Barlow, 1994) is a comprehensive interview designed to assess the full range of anxiety disorders (and affective disorders) in detail. The PTSD module of the ADIS-IV has an "initial inquiry" section that attempts to establish Criterion A. The response to the Criterion A-2 query about peritraumatic emotional response does not lead to a skip-out, which is clinically appropriate in many instances, but does not formally adhere to the decision rules in DSM. The rest of the PTSD module covers the 17 symptoms of PTSD in a straightforward manner, adhering closely to the language of DSM-IV. Unfortunately, the PTSD module of the ADIS-IV does not provide behavioral referents or anchors, so the patient is left to interpret the meaning of descriptors of symptoms. A relative strength of the ADIS-IV PTSD is that it requires the onset of emotional numbing and hyperarousal symptoms to be after the traumatic event. The ADIS-IV also provides continuous ratings of frequency and intensity of distress, which is particularly useful in treatment planning and monitoring outcome. However, the authors fail to provide recommendations for cutoff points that define a symptom's clinical significance for diagnostic purposes (e.g.: Does a symptom count toward the diagnosis if it is endorsed rarely and/or associated with mild distress?). In addition, the authors fail to provide a recommendation for a total-score cutoff that defines caseness, based on empirical research. Research on the psychometric properties of the ADIS-PTSD module is promising. Blanchard, Gerardi, Kolb, and Barlow (1986) found diagnostic agreement between the ADIS (DSM-III version) and a clinical diagnosis of PTSD in 40 of 43 cases (kappa = .86). The ADIS is the leading interview for the assessment of the full spectrum of anxiety disorders (Di Nardo, Moras, Barlow, Rapee, & Brown, 1993) and is an excellent choice for assessments when the comorbidity or differential diagnosis of PTSD with other anxiety disorders is at issue.

Clinician-Administered PTSD Scale (CAPS)

The CAPS (Blake et al., 1995) assesses the 17 DSM-IV symptoms of PTSD, as well as five associated features of the syndrome: trauma-related guilt over acts of commission or omission, survivor guilt, reductions in awareness of one's surroundings, derealization, and depersonalization. The CAPS also provides ratings of the impact of symptoms on social and occupational functioning, the status of PTSD symptoms relative to an earlier assessment, estimated validity of the overall assessment, and overall PTSD severity. The clinician assesses the severity of each symptom on the dimensions of frequency and intensity using 5-point Likert scales. For screening purposes, a scoring rule that counts symptoms as present when frequency is rated as 1 or greater (occurred at least once during the designated time frame) and intensity is rated as 2 or greater (at least moderately intense or distressing) is recommended (Weathers, Ruscio, & Keane, 1999). The presence of each symptom is determined by adding the frequency and intensity ratings. Each symptom query incorporates standard prompts, follow-up questions, and behavioral anchors.

In a major validation study, the CAPS was administered by independent clinicians to 60 service-seeking Vietnam veterans on two different occasions, 2 to 3 days apart (Weathers et al., 1992; see Weathers & Litz, 1994). Test–retest reliability for three pairs of raters ranged from .77 to .96 for the three symptom clusters and from .90 to .98 for all 17 items. Against a SCID-PTSD diagnosis, a CAPS total score of 65 was found to have good sensitivity (.84), excellent specificity (.95), and a kappa coefficient of .78. With regard to validity, the CAPS showed strong correlations with the Mississippi Scale (MS; Keane et al., 1988) (.70) and the PK Scale of the MMPI (.84) and moderate correlation with the Combat Exposure Scale (CES; Keane et al., 1989) (.42). Keane et al. (1998) found evidence that the CAPS may be more reliable than the PTSD module of the SCID.

Diagnostic Interview Schedule (DIS)

The DIS (Robins, Helzer, Croughan, & Ratcliff, 1981) was designed to be administered by trained, nonclinician interviewers. Versions of the DIS PTSD module have been employed in several epidemiological studies of PTSD, including the Epidemiologic Catchment Area survey (Helzer, Robins, & McEvoy, 1987), the Vietnam Experience Study (Centers for Disease Control, 1988), and the NVVRS (Kulka et al., 1988, 1990). The interview consists of a series of questions with dichotomous ("yes"/"no") scoring options for each DSM symptom. One standard question is provided for each PTSD symptom, and there are no follow-up questions or rating anchors. A weakness of the DIS PTSD module has to do with a skip-out that occurs very early in the administration process. In the normal interview sequence, if the respondent endorses exposure to a potentially traumatic event, then the interviewer reads a brief statement describing some of the key symptoms of PTSD and asks the respondent if he or she has experienced any of these symptoms in response to the trauma. If the respondent does not respond affirmatively to this initial query, the PTSD module is discontinued. We believe that this early summary question may reduce the sensitivity of the measure and contribute to false negatives in diagnostic decision making. Data on the psychometric performance of the DIS-PTSD module is limited, and what is available, unfortunately, is not encouraging. In the clinical examination subsample of the NVVRS, 440 participants were assessed by lay interviewers using the DIS and by clinicians using the SCID as the diagnostic criterion. In relation to the SCID, the DIS-PTSD module achieved a sensitivity of only 21.5, a specificity of 97.9, and a kappa of .26. Thus, the DIS might be appropriate to *confirm* a PTSD diagnosis, but its screening function is questionable.

PTSD Interview (PTSD-I)

The PTSD interview (Watson et al., 1991) assesses PTSD as defined by DSM-III-R. The interview begins with the interviewer making an initial determination about whether the respondent meets Criterion A. If so, for the assessment of Criteria B–E, the interviewer reads each item to the interviewee, who uses a 7-point scale to rate himself or herself on the item. In other words, in this interview it is the interviewee, not the interviewer, who rates the severity of symptomatology; the PTSD-I does not appear to include provisions for the clinician to influence the ratings. The rating scale does not distinguish between dimensions of intensity and frequency but instead includes pairs of items ranging from "no/never" to "extremely/always"; the interviewee decides whether to rate the severity or frequency of a given symptom. Watson suggests the use of a cutoff of 4, corresponding to a rating of "somewhat/commonly," to indicate the presence of a symptom. However, no empirical basis for the criterion is provided (such as the Receiver Operating Characteristic [ROC] analysis technique used to determine the optimal cutoff for a given test, as described by Weathers et al., 1997). Despite this, Watson et al. (1991) reported evidence of excellent reliability and validity for the PTSD-I. The alpha coefficient was .92. Test–retest reliability over a 1-week interval was .95, with 87% diagnostic agreement between the two administrations. Using the PTSD module of the DIS as a gold standard, the PTSD-I achieved specificity, sensitivity, and concordance coefficients of .89, .94, and .94, respectively.

PTSD Symptom Scale—Interview Version (PSS-I)

The PSS-I (Foa, Riggs, Dancu, & Rothbaum, 1993) is a 17-item interview in which each symptom is rated using a single question per symptom. Interviewers rate the severity of each symptom over the past 2 weeks on a 4-point Likert-type scale (from 0, not at all, to 3, very much). A total severity score is obtained by summing ratings over all 17 items. A PTSD diagnosis is obtained by following the DSM-IV algorithm for symptoms rated 1 or higher. The PSS-I has several noteworthy features. The instructions and formatting are simple and easy to understand, which promotes uniformity of usage (interrater reliability, greater internal consistency). The items reflect DSM-IV, but the authors chose to operationally define some symptoms in novel ways, perhaps to make them easier to interpret. On this point, it is interesting to consider the necessity of using DSM as a guide, rather than as the definitive index of the necessary and defining features of posttraumatic pathology. The PSS-I has good psychometric properties. Foa et al. (1993) reported an alpha coefficient of .85 for all 17 items and an average item-scale correlation of .45. Test–retest reliability for the total severity score was .80, and the kappa coefficient for a diagnosis of PTSD was .91. Using a

SCID-based PTSD diagnosis as the criterion, the PSS-I had a sensitivity of .88, a specificity of .96, and an efficiency of .94.

In sum, the strengths of the PSS-I are that it yields continuous and dichotomous scores, is very easy to administer, and has good reliability and validity for assessing PTSD. The disadvantages are that it includes only a single prompt for each question, its ratings anchors are not behaviorally referenced, the severity rating scale has wording that confounds frequency and intensity, and it assess symptoms over a 2-week period—an interval that may be too conservative and deviates somewhat from the 1-month convention.

Structured Clinical Interview for DSM-IV (SCID-PTSD Module)

The PTSD module of the SCID (First et al., 1996) was the original "gold standard" interview in the field of PTSD assessment. Because the SCID was designed to assess most major psychiatric disorders, it features the ability to readily assess comorbid psychopathology and includes the opportunity to assess the current presence of each of the 17 DSM diagnostic criteria. A standard prompt question is provided for each symptom, and interviewers rate the presentation of the criterion item as absent, present, subthreshold (i.e., criterion is almost met), or lacking adequate information for assessment. The scale is insensitive to severity of symptomatology and does not specifically assess frequency or intensity. For a symptom to meet criterion, it is to be "persistently experienced," but this is not well defined.

Data pertaining to the interrater reliability of the SCID-PTSD module is found in the report from the National Vietnam Veterans Readjustment Study (NVVRS; Kulka et al., 1990) which reported interrater reliability coefficients of .94 for lifetime diagnoses and .87 for current PTSD. Schnurr, Friedman, and Rosenberg (1993) obtained 100% interrater agreement in SCID-PTSD modules of six full and six subthreshold PTSD Vietnam veterans. In the NVVRS, the SCID was positively associated with other measures of PTSD, including the Mississippi Scale (kappa = .53) and the PK scale of the MMPI (kappa = .48). It had good sensitivity (.81) and excellent specificity (.98), when evaluated against a composite diagnosis of PTSD (Kulka et al., 1991; Schlenger et al., 1992). Following the SCID protocol, if criteria are not met at any stage, the interview is discontinued. The primary limitation of the SCID is that it yields essentially dichotomous data at the item level and thus is not well suited for quantifying or detecting changes in symptom severity.

Structured Interview for PTSD

The Structured Interview for PTSD (SI-PTSD) was developed by Davidson and colleagues (Davidson, Smith, & Kudler, 1989). It provides a series of initial prompt questions and follow-up questions that clarify the initial question with concrete behavioral examples. The severity of each symptom is rated on a scale of 0 to 4 and gathers information for making lifetime and current diagnostic decisions. Descriptors are provided for ratings scale anchors to clarify the meaning of a given rating. Symptoms are considered clinically significant if they are rated as 2 or higher. The psychometric properties of the instrument are strong. Using the SCID as criterion, Davidson et al. (1989) reported diagnostic agreement in 37 of 41 cases studied, yielding a kappa coefficient of .79. In terms of reliability, the SI-PTSD achieved an alpha of .94, test–retest reliability of .71, and 100% diagnostic agreement.

Summary and Recommendations for PTSD Interviews

In this section we reviewed seven structured clinical interviews for the assessment of PTSD. Four of the interviews (CAPS, PTSD-I, PSS-I, SI-PTSD) are stand-alone instruments that are designed exclusively for the assessment of PTSD. The other three (ADIS, DIS, SCID) are individual modules of more comprehensive psychiatric diagnostic systems. One important way in which the interviews differ from one another is whether individual symptoms are assessed dichotomously (present or absent) or continuously (using a multipoint Likert-type scale). Four of the seven interviews (ADIS-IV, CAPS, PSS-I, SI-PTSD) provide continuous ratings of severity for each symptom, the others rely on a dichotomous coding scheme.[2] Continuous rating scales provide a more sensitive metric for the assessment of symptomatology and possess several advantages over scales based on dichotomous items. For research purposes, a continuous measure lends itself better to correlational analysis and for the testing of hypotheses about PTSD in relation to other constructs. For clinical purposes, a continuous measure of symptom severity is more useful for detecting change in symptomatology over time and for the assessment of treatment effects. Although we recognize that a dichotomous assessment may be appropriate for screening or epidemiological sampling purposes, we focus our recommendations on those measures that provide continuous scores.

Although five of the seven measures that we reviewed were originally designed or have been revised to reflect the criteria in DSM-IV, we found no evidence that such a revision has been undertaken for Davidson et al.'s (1989) Structured Interview for PTSD. Although it may be true that diagnostic criteria in DSM-III-R and DSM-IV yield nearly identical results when using a common metric (Weathers et al., 1999), we recommend the use of scales based on DSM-IV criteria and urge investigators to make timely revisions to their measures as the DSM evolves.

The CAPS and the PSS-I are the only DSM-IV-based interviews that provide continuous measures of symptomatology based on the interviewer's ratings. Both scales possess excellent psychometric properties, and there is ample published evidence of their reliability and validity. The distinction between these measures comes down to the breadth of coverage and the depth of the assessment. The PSS-I is simple and efficient, and it can be administered in 15 minutes or less. In contrast, the CAPS assesses DSM symptoms, as well as associated features; it separates symptom severity into the dimensions of intensity and frequency; and each symptom query includes standard prompts, follow-up questions, and behavioral anchors. The CAPS is the more elaborate and sophisticated of the two instruments, but it is also substantially more time-intensive and generally takes at least 1 hour to administer. Therefore, our recommendation would be that when a detailed, comprehensive PTSD assessment is indicated, the CAPS is the instrument of choice. When administration time is a limiting factor, the PSS-I is probably the most useful.

Self-Report (Paper-and-Pencil) Measures of PTSD Symptomatology

Paper and pencil measures of PTSD are widely used to screen for PTSD and to provide dimensional data on symptom severity and extent of impairment. These tests are also used in large-scale epidemiology studies to estimate the prevalence of PTSD. In this section, we review an inclusive set of 15 peer-reviewed and published self-report measures of PTSD symptomatology. Table 7.1 provides a comparison of these instruments in terms of their design and psychometric properties.

One dimension on which the scales differ is whether the measure is referenced directly to the DSM criteria for PTSD. Of the 13 measures, 3 (PCL; PSS-SR; Purdue PTSD Scale—

---

[2]The PTSD-I also provides a continuous symptoms severity scale but differs from the CAPS, PSS-I, and SI-PTSD in that the ratings are made by the *interviewee* rather than the clinician—a feature that is likely to negatively impact on the reliability of the measure and negate the primary advantage of the clinical interview over self-report instruments (i.e., that the data are based on the observations of a trained clinician/observer).

TABLE 7.1. Psychometric Properties of PTSD Symptom Scales

| Scale | DSM referenced? | Measures associated features? | Number of items | Validation sample | Reliability | | Criterion validity (self-report or interview) | Assessment time frame | Measures symptom severity? | Measures symptom frequency? | Diagnosis using validated total score cutoff? | Diagnosis using DSM criteria? |
					Test–retest	Internal consistency						
Civilian Mississippi (Keane et al., 1988)	No	Yes	39	668 community	Unspecified	$r = .39$ $\alpha = .86–.91$	Self-report	Unspecified	Yes	No	Yes	No
Civilian Mississippi—Revised (Norris & Perilla, 1996)	No	Yes	30	404 hurricane survivors, 56 community	.84 1 week	$\alpha = .86–.88$	Unspecified	Unspecified	Yes	No	No	Yes
Crime-related SCL-90 PTSD Scale (Saunders, Arata, & Kilpatrick, 1990)	No	Yes	28	355 community females	Unspecified	$\alpha = .93$	Both	Unspecified	Yes	No	Yes	No
Impact of Event Scale (IES; Weiss & Marmar, 1997)	No	Yes	15	430 emergency personnel, 206 earthquake survivors	.57–.92 for sub-scales	$\alpha = .79–.92$ for subscales	Unspecified	1 week	Yes	No	No	No
Los Angeles Symptom Checklist (King, King, Leskin, & Foy, 1995)	No	Yes	43	600+ including veterans, child abuse survivors, psychiatric outpatients, battered women, high-risk adolescents	.90–.94 2 weeks	$\alpha = .94–.95$	Both	Unspecified	Yes	No	No	Yes
Mississippi Scale for Combat-Related PTSD (Keane et al., 1988)	No	Yes	35	326 combat veterans	.97 1 week	$r = .58$ $\alpha = .94$	Both	Unspecified	Yes	No	Yes	No
MMPI-PTSD (PK) Scale (Keane et al., 1984)	No	Yes	46	200 combat veterans	.94 2–3 days	$\alpha = .95–.96$	Both	Unspecified	No	No	Yes	No

(continued)

TABLE 7.1. (continued)

Scale	DSM referenced?	Measures associated features?	Number of items	Validation sample	Reliability Test-retest	Internal consistency	Criterion validity (self-report or interview)	Assessment time frame	Assessment Measures symptom severity?	Measures symptom frequency?	Diagnosis using validated total score cutoff?	Diagnosis using DSM criteria?
Modified PTSD Symptom Scale–Self-report (MPSS-SR; Falsetti, Resnick, & Kilpatrick, 1993)	Yes	No	17	286 community and treatment samples	Unspecified	α = .92–.93 frequency α = .94–.95 severity r = .09–.78 frequency r = .21–.84 severity	Interview	2 weeks	Yes	Yes	Yes	Yes
PTSD Checklist (PCL; Weathers et al., 1991)	Yes	No	17	123 veterans, 111 bone marrow transplants, 40 motor vehicle accident and sexual assault survivors	.96 2–3 days	r = .62–.87 α = .97	Both	1 month	Yes	No	Yes	Yes
Penn Inventory for PTSD (Hammarberg, 1992)	No	Yes	26	257 veterans	.94 2–8 days	r = .74–.75 α = .94–.96	Both	1 week	Yes	No	Yes	No
PTSD Symptom Scale (PSS-SR; Foa et al., 1993)	Yes	No	17	118 sexual and nonsexual assault survivors	.74 1 month	r = .60 α = .91	Both	1 or 2 weeks	Yes	No	No	Yes
Purdue PTSD Scale—Revised (Lauterbach & Vrana, 1996)	Yes	No	17	491 college students, 35 counseling center clients	.72 2 weeks	r = .59 α = .91	Self-report	1 month	No	Yes	No	Yes
Trauma Symptom Checklist–40 (Elliot & Briere, 1992)	No	Yes	40	2,963 professional women	Unspecified	α = .90	Self-report	2 months	No	Yes	No	No
Trauma Symptom Inventory (Briere et al., 1995)	No	Yes	100	370 psychiatric patients	Unspecified	α = .87	Self-report	6 months	No	Yes	No	No
War-Related SCL-90 PTSD Scale (Weathers, 1996)	No	Yes	25	301 combat veterans	Unspecified	r = .67–.83 α = .97	Both	Unspecified	Yes	No	Yes	No

[a]r = item–total correlations; α = Cronbach alpha coefficients.

Revised (PPTSD-R; Lauterbach & Vrana, 1996) provide a point-to-point correspondence between individual items and the DSM-IV criteria for PTSD. The advantage of these scales is that they permit diagnostic classification using the DSM algorithm, and they provide a continuous measure of syndrome severity. The non-DSM-referenced scales, in contrast, do not readily lend themselves to diagnostic classification using the DSM algorithm and typically only allow computation of a single score to reflect overall symptom severity (from which a cutoff is empirically derived to define caseness). Most of these scales assess associated features that are not included in the DSM description of PTSD and therefore assess a comparatively broader domain of content. Some scales were exclusively derived empirically from the items of broader measures of psychopathology (i.e., SCL-90, MMPI). The content tapped by the items in the embedded empirically derived PTSD measures often reflect general distress and functional impairment, rather than syndrome-specific problems, making scale scores difficult to interpret.

The 35-item MS (Keane et al., 1988) is a noteworthy example of a measure that is not directly referenced to the DSM criteria for PTSD. This scale was designed to capture combat-related PTSD and related problems experienced by Vietnam veterans. The MS has been shown to have superior psychometric characteristics in numerous assessment studies employing veterans. However, although 23 of its items correspond to symptoms defined in DSM, some symptoms are not represented (B-1, C-1, C-3, and D-6). In some instances, the MS employs multiple items to assess certain symptoms (there are four items assessing C-6 and three items assessing D-1). Twelve items on the MS assess associated features not described in DSM-IV, such as substance abuse, suicidality, and depression. Similarly, the 100-item Trauma Symptom Inventory (TSI; Briere et al., 1995), covering the largest content domain of the PTSD scales is comprised of nine subscales that assess the core symptoms of PTSD plus a variety of other associated phenomena, including dissociation, dysfunctional sexual behavior, intrusive experiences, impaired self-reference, sexual concerns, and tension-reduction behavior. These two scales are useful in treatment planning because they tap a variety of domains of functioning that are often impaired in trauma populations.

Self-report measures of PTSD also differ from one another in terms of the time-frame on which the assessment is based. As indicated in Table 7.1, six of the scales instruct respondents to evaluate the extent to which they have experienced symptomatology within a specific time frame, ranging from during the past week (Penn Inventory; Hammarberg, 1992) to within the past 6 months (TSI; Briere et al., 1995). Seven measures do not specify a time frame for the self-reported assessment. As noted, DSM-IV only specifies that symptoms must persist for more than 1 month to meet diagnostic criteria; it does not specify the time frame during which symptoms must be present to be considered current. Nonetheless, drawing on the precedent established by the SCID, it has become convention to use a monthly time frame for the assessment of current symptomatology. Although the ideal time frame for symptom assessment may vary depending on the context in which the measure is being used (i.e., in diagnostic assessments vs. as repeated measures of symptom change), we see no compelling reason for a questionnaire not to specify the time frame of the assessment in its instructions.

With the exception of the MMPI–PTSD Scale (PK; Keane et al., 1984), which is comprised of "true"/"false" statements, all of the scales assess either symptom severity or frequency on a Likert-type scale. Unfortunately, the psychometric pros and cons of assessing symptom severity versus symptom frequency are unclear. Frequency and severity are likely to be confounded, regardless of which dimension is supposed to be assessed. That is, judgments of the degree of distress evoked by a given symptom are likely to be influenced by the frequency with which the symptom occurs, and vice versa. One possible solution to this problem is to allow the respondent to make a more precise distinction between the two dimensions by assessing frequency and intensity separately. The Modified PTSD Symptom Scale—Self-Report (MPSS-SR; Falsetti, Resnick, & Kilpatrick, 1993; Falsetti, Resnick, Resick, & Kilpatrick, 1993) is the only self-report scale that does this. Considerably more research is needed, however, to evaluate whether individuals suffering from posttrauma problems can make valid distinctions between frequency and intensity in the self-reports of PTSD symptomatology.

At this point, it is difficult to distinguish self-report measures of PTSD in terms of their psychometric properties. As Table 7.1 indicates, most of the self-report measures of PTSD symptomatology have good psychometric qualities. All of the measures have demonstrated good internal consistency, and for most of the measures there is evidence of good test–retest reliability. The various instruments have been validated on a wide range of samples, and we would encourage would-be users of the scales to select measures that have been validated on a sample comparable to the one with which it is intended to be used. For screening purposes, we recommend scales that adhere to the current DSM symptomatology (e.g., the PCL). However, the embedded scales are particularly attractive when screening for a wide variety of psychopathology, particularly the PK scale, which affords the user the application of the validity scales of the full MMPI.

After reviewing this literature, it has become clear that what is needed are studies that directly compare utility of various instruments. Many of the scales developed in the last 10 years have been created in a vacuum, with no effort to compare the new scale to any of the existing ones. For a new PTSD measure to contribute substantially to the clinical and research literature, it should possess incremental clinical usefulness and validity. To demonstrate this, investigators should directly evaluate the unique features of the new instrument and compare it against existing instruments that are the closest and most psychometrically sound competitors. To our knowledge, all of the relative utility, "horse-race" type studies have been conducted on Vietnam veterans and may not be generalizeable to other populations (e.g., Kulka et al., 1988; Watson, Juba, & Anderson, 1989; Weathers et al., 1996). Nevertheless, these studies have revealed the MS to be the most reliable and valid self-report measure of war-related PTSD. Psychometric studies comparing the various instruments in other types of trauma would make an important contribution to this area.

Psychophysiological Assessment of PTSD

Research on the clinical use of psychophysiological measures in the assessment of PTSD has generated a body of literature unrivaled in magnitude by such research on the other anxiety disorders. Blanchard and Buckley (1999) identified 31 studies conducted since 1960 that have specifically addressed the question of whether people with PTSD are more physiologically reactive to trauma-related stimuli than are people without PTSD. This issue pertains to DSM-IV symptom B-5, "physiological reactivity on exposure to internal or external cues that symbolize or resemble an aspect of the traumatic event." Most of these studies have employed some form of a trauma-related challenge task that involves either presentation of audio and/or visual stimuli reminiscent of the trauma or some variant of the script-driven imagery paradigm advanced originally by Peter Lang and his colleagues (e.g., Lang, 1979). The typical assessment protocol involves recording autonomic (i.e., heart rate, blood pressure, and skin conductance) and facial electromyographic responses during exposure to neutral and trauma-related conditions. The largest and arguably most methodologically rigorous study of this type was conducted by the Department of Veterans Affairs (Keane et al., 1998). It tested the ability of psychophysiological responding to predict SCID-based PTSD diagnosis in a sample of over 1,300 male Vietnam veterans. Results revealed that an equation derived to predict PTSD status on the basis of four physiological variables that correctly classified approximately two-thirds of veterans with a current PTSD diagnosis.

Unfortunately, because the Keane et al. (1998) study failed to correctly classify one-third of the veterans with a current PTSD diagnosis, these results suggest that psychophysiological measures have limited use in confirming the diagnosis of PTSD when used as the sole index. Numerous variables may account for the imperfect association between physiological responding and PTSD in this and other studies that have reported similar results, including the following: participant compliance with protocol demands; the appropriateness of trauma cue stimuli; biological influences such as age, sex, race, and fitness level; the presence of pharmacological agents (i.e., benzodiazepines, beta-adrenergic blockers); and even personality traits that influence the emotional response to aversive stimuli (e.g., antisocial characteristics; Miller, Kaloupek & Keane, 1999). Given the array of factors that influence the psychophysiological response to trauma-related stimuli in individuals with PTSD, we are not optimistic about the prospect of improving the performance of psychophysiological tests for the clinical diagnostic assessment of PTSD much beyond the level achieved by Keane et al. (1998).

We are substantially more optimistic, however, about the use of psychophysiological methods for within-subject assessment of the treatment process and treatment outcome, and several preliminary treatment studies of this type have produced promising results. First, Shalev, Orr, and Pitman (1992) used systematic desensitization in the treatment of three individuals with PTSD and found that physiological responding to trauma-related imagery diminished from pre- to posttreatment with reductions in PTSD symptomatology. Second, in a single case study, Fairbank and Keane (1982) reported reductions in heart rate and skin conductance during trauma-related imagery, both within and between sessions. Third, Boudewyns & Hyer (1990) treated 51 cases of combat-related PTSD with either exposure-based therapy or conventional counseling. Although there were no group differences on physiological measures in terms of treatment, results did reveal that patients who showed reductions in physiological arousal posttreatment exhibited greater posttreatment improvement at a 3-month follow-up.

In sum, research on the use of psychophysiological methods for the clinical assessment of PTSD suggests that they have limited value as a diagnostic tool. In view of the findings by Keane et al. (1998) and the practical issues associated with conducting such assessments (software and hardware costs and specialized skills required), we see little rationale for encouraging the increased utilization of psychophysiological assessments for diagnostic purposes. In contrast, there is room for growth in the area of the psychophysiological assessment of treatment process and outcome. Psychophysiological methodologies also hold great promise for evaluating the cognitive, affective, and biological mechanisms that underlie posttraumatic psychopathology (e.g., Litz et al., 2000).

Measures of Potentially Traumatic Events (PTEs) and Criterion A

Compared to the amount of attention that has been devoted to the development of measures of PTSD symptomatology, the assessment of exposure to potentially traumatic events and trauma history has been a comparatively neglected area of study until recently. In this section we describe five self-report instruments and three interviews that have been developed recently and have begun to fill this void. Not included in this section are measures that detail the experiences of specific trauma populations such as refugees, survivors of natural disasters, and survivors of sexual abuse.

Establishing the psychometric soundness of self-report trauma histories presents a challenge. In terms of validity, it is difficult, if not impossible, in many circumstances to obtain external corroboration of the events that are reported. Investigators have generally focused on establishing the construct validity of PTE measures by demonstrating an association between the total number of events on a trauma inventory and symptom severity on a PTSD scale or demonstrating concurrent validity by comparing the rates of trauma endorsement between two or more measures. Evidence of reliability has typically taken the form of test–retest correlations. At a minimum, investigators need to demonstrate adequate temporal consistency. Internal consistency is not applicable to event measures because the experience of one event does not necessarily imply (covary with) the experience of another.

Potentially Traumatizing Events Checklists

Paper-and-pencil checklists of PTEs are useful clinically. They allow the clinician to screen for a variety of PTEs over the lifespan, even though the patient may be presenting with a clear focal trauma. In addition, checklists allow patients to endorse experiences that they may have difficulty initially admitting to a clinician in person.

The Traumatic Life Events Questionnaire (TLEQ; Kubany et al., 2000) is a 22-item measure that assesses exposure to a wide variety of PTEs. The scope of coverage and definition of "traumatic" is the widest of the measures reviewed here; it includes items to assess childhood sexual abuse by peers, stalking, miscarriages, abortions, childhood witnessing of family violence, and illnesses of loved ones. Using a "yes" or "no" format, respondents are asked if they experienced intense fear, helplessness, or horror at the time of the event. Kubany et al. (2000) found that test–retest stability varied, depending on the type of trauma being reported. Across several samples with test–retest intervals that varied from 1 week to 2 months, reports of accidents other than motor vehicle accidents were associated with the lowest temporal consistency (kappa < .40). The strongest stability was observed for items that assessed childhood physical abuse (kappas = .63 to .91), witnessing family violence (.60 to .79), childhood sexual abuse by someone more than 5 years older (.70 to .90), and stalking (.59 to .84). The overall average kappa across samples and TLEQ events was .60 (*N* = 204).

The Stressful Life Events Screening Questionnaire (SLESQ; Goodman, Corcoran, Turner, Yuan, & Green, 1998) is a 13-item self-report screening measure that assesses lifetime exposure to a variety of PTEs. Respondents are asked to indicate whether an event occurred, and, if so, additional information (depending on the question) is requested, including the age at which the event occurred, a brief description of the incident stating whether there were injuries or deaths, whether the participant's life was in danger, and, when appropriate, information about the perpetrator. Goodman et al. (1998) reported a median kappa of .73 for reporting on specific events across a 2-week test–retest interval (*N* = 66). Unfortunately, there is no assessment of peritraumatic emotional response, which is necessary for a formal diagnosis of PTSD (Criterion A-2).

The Traumatic Events Questionnaire (TEQ; Vrana & Lauterbach, 1994) asks respondents whether they have experienced any of 11 specific traumatic events. For each item endorsed positively, the respondent is asked to provide more detail, including the number of times that the event occurred and his or her age at the time of the event. The respondent is also asked to indicate whether he or she was injured and if life threat was involved and to rate how "traumatic" the experience was for them at the time and is for them now on a 7-point Likert-type scale. Vrana and Lauterbach reported 2-week test–retest correlations of .91 for the total number of events endorsed on the measure and a mean correlation of .80 for the specific events assessed (*N* = 51).

The Trauma History Questionnaire (Green, 1996) is a self-report scale consisting of 24 items to assess PTSD Criterion A events, as well as other stressful life events (i.e., serious illness, spanked or pushed hard enough by a family member to cause injury). Each item is followed by probes assessing the frequency of the event and the respondent's age at the time of the trauma. There is no assessment of Criterion A-2. Green reported an average test–retest correlation across items over a 2- to 3-month interval (*N* = 25) of .68.

In summary, the self-report measures of PTEs differ primarily with regard to the scope of events that are assessed and whether there is an attempt to assess both the exposure and the subjective reaction components of Criterion A. The range of experiences assessed varies from the relatively circumscribed list of 10 experiences that would clearly meet Criterion A-1 (exposure to an event that involved the threat of death or serious harm to self or others; American Psychiatric Association, 1994) assessed by the Traumatic Stress Schedule, to the much more inclusive list of experiences assessed by the TLEQ, which includes those that would not meet Criterion A-1. Three of the five measures assess Criterion A-2 (exposure to trauma evoked fear, helplessness, or horror in the individual; American Psychiatric Association, 1994).

Interviews That Evaluate Potentially Traumatizing Experiences

The Potential Stressful Events Interview (PSEI; Falsetti, Resnick, Kilpatrick, & Freedy, 1994) is a multifaceted, comprehensive interview that is designed to provide a detailed assessment of traumatic and other stressful life experiences. It is comprised of four modules assessing PTEs, low-magnitude life stressors, objective characteristics of the PTEs, and subjective peritraumatic reactions. The first module is a 35-page interview that assesses exposure to low-magnitude stressors (i.e., marital conflict, financial problems, death of family members) and high-magnitude events, including sexual assault, physical assault, homicide, combat, disaster, accidents, and chemical/radiation exposure. This is followed by nine probe questions to determine objective characteristics of the PTEs identified in the first module. Finally, the respondent uses a 15-item checklist to describe emotions that he or she experienced at the time of the event and a 10-item checklist to describe accompanying physical sensations. Administration time is 90 to 120 minutes; test–retest reliability is not reported.

The second PTE interview, the Evaluation of Lifetime Stressors (ELS; Krinsley et al., 1993), provides a comprehensive, multidimensional assessment of PTEs across the lifetime using a questionnaire and follow-up interview. This two-stage process is likely to lead to the most clinically useful and comprehensive information about lifespan traumas. The excellent screening questionnaire covers a wide variety of lifespan PTEs and potentially damaging developmental experiences and indirect signs of early trauma. The response options in the ELS are particularly appealing. Respondents are asked whether the event happened ("yes"/"no") and whether or not they are unsure if the event happened. The ELS interview is designed to follow up and confirm PTEs endorsed on the checklist (and items endorsed as "unsure"). Like the PSEI, the ELS interview features the assessment of both objective and subjective aspects of trauma experience. The ELS interview has multiple and varied opportunities for respondents to report traumatic experiences, as it uses both broad and detailed questions. For all reported events, information regarding threat, injury, emotional response, frequency, and duration is collected. Data on the test–retest reliability of the ELS indicate that reliability varies considerably, depending on the event endorsed, with kappas ranging from .45 to .91 for events that meet both criteria A-1 and A-2 of PTSD, with a median kappa of .63.

Finally, the Traumatic Stress Schedule (TSS; Norris, 1990, 1992) is a brief interview that inquires about 10 types of PTEs, ranging from criminal victimization to exposure to environmental hazards. For each PTE, there are probes designed to permit quantification of loss (the tangible loss of persons or property), scope (the extent to which persons other than the respondent were affected by the incident), threat to life and physical integrity, blame (i.e., attributions of causality), and familiarity (i.e., previous exposure to comparable experiences). Criterion A-2 is not assessed in the TSS, and reliability data are unavailable.

Both the PSEI and the ELS are superb, comprehensive, clinically useful face-valid measures of lifespan PTEs. We endorse the ELS because of its sensitive two-stage evaluation and its coverage of subtle signs of early abuse. These interviews are very time intensive, however, so for a brief screening interview the TSS provides a good alternative.

PRACTICAL RECOMMENDATIONS FOR ASSESSING TRAUMATIZED ADULTS

Interviewing Individuals about Their Exposure to Trauma

Clinicians and clinical researchers need to exercise caution and care when interviewing patients about traumatic experiences. Although it is necessary to determine that an individual has been exposed to a Criterion-A event in order to inquire about the presence of PTSD symptoms, the clinician needs to do so judiciously. It may prove necessary to probe for details of events that patients have avoided thinking about for a long time, which can unearth feelings of intense vulnerability and negative affect. It is important for clinicians to anticipate and address concerns about safety, reluctance to reveal the intricacies of traumatic events, and embarrassment and shame. It is understandably difficult for patients to discuss a trauma with a person with whom they do not have a trusting relationship (e.g., Ruch, Gartrell, Ramelli, & Coyne, 1991). In addition, it is quite common for the assessment process to reactivate painful memories and feelings, which can be particularly damaging if they are unanticipated. Therapists should also bear in mind that sometimes patients will not show negative emotional reactions but will use avoidance maneuvers. In many respects, this is to be expected in an assessment context where a working alliance is just forming.

The manner in which therapists handle discussion about traumatic events can serve to build trust, and trust is a crucial element in the treatment of PTSD. It is imperative to foster a safe and responsive interpersonal context for exploring intensely emotional material. It is important at the outset of an evaluation of trauma to provide accurate expectations about the process and to educate patients along the way. It is useful to assume that patients have not shared or focused on the details of their trauma and that the assessment will be a painful process. In an assessment, the therapist needs to be respectful of patients' need to avoid focusing on painful elements of their traumatic memories. However, to conduct a valid evaluation of trauma and PTSD, there must be a measured, empathic inquiry into past traumatic events. Therapists should watch carefully for signs of emotional reaction and go only as far as they need to. If all goes well, patients will feel understood and can learn early on that they can control the amount and depth of self-disclosure, as well as their emotional response. On some occasions, when a patient's recall of a trauma is triggered in such a stark manner, they may experience a very intense emotional reaction accompanied by a sense of loss of control. In these instances it is important for the therapist to stop the inquiry and give the patient an opportunity to recoup a sense of control.

Sensitivity to the stress that the assessment process can provoke for patients is especially important for those patients at risk for maladaptive coping (e.g., substance abuse, violence, self-destructive behavior). The clinician should monitor the emotional reactions of patients during assessment, as well as inquire how they intend to cope. There are times when the clinician will need to provide the patient with some anxiety management strategy during the assessment (e.g., slow diaphragmatic breathing). At other times, it is important to allow time at the end of a session for the patient to return to baseline before leaving the office.

These interventions during assessment are alliance building. They also educate the patient about the predictable effects of trauma memory reactivation and the need for self-care.

In general, the assessment process can be a time where the clinician can begin to educate the patient about the effects of trauma and PTSD.

Evaluating Appropriateness for Trauma-Focused Exposure Therapy

Exposure therapy for PTSD entails thorough, careful, sustained and repeated emotional processing of trauma-related memories. The goal is to reduce (or extinguish) conditioned emotional responses to trauma-related cues (e.g., Boudewyns & Shipley, 1983; Keane, Gerardi, Quinn, & Litz, 1992; Lyons & Keane, 1989). Clinicians should keep in mind several prerequisites to effective exposure therapy for PTSD as they make decisions about use of this treatment. These include a very good therapeutic relationship and working alliance; a patient's accurate expectations about the process and course of exposure therapy, in both the short term and the long run (e.g., typically there is an exacerbation of symptoms before the patient gets better); therapist training and skill level; and therapist confidence in the model. Confidence in the extinction model is particularly important because patients need reassurance and therapists need to remain empathically present but calm in the face of intense emotional responses. In addition, therapists need to be prepared to listen to stories of great human tragedy and suffering, which can be stressful.

Since exposure therapy is a very invasive and demanding intervention, clinical decision making about its appropriateness is part of a comprehensive assessment of trauma and PTSD. When polled, expert clinicians on average reported applying exposure therapy in approximately 60% of their PTSD cases (Litz, Blake, Gerardi, & Keane, 1990). Some patients with PTSD are not appropriate for exposure therapy because they have difficulty meeting the boundary conditions of exposure (e.g., they have difficulty imagining, or intense arousal is medically contraindicated). During the course of exposure therapy, patients are at risk for becoming more symptomatic, so therapists should be concerned about relapse into a comorbid condition, such as substance dependence, and about dropout potential, which can be particularly destructive (Litz et al., 1990). In these cases, exposure therapy could be considered after treatment gains are made in other problem areas.

Target Selection Issues

After collecting all the structured and semistructured interview data and the psychometric information, the clinician is faced with the most important task in the assessment process: case conceptualization and selecting and prioritizing targets for intervention. Usually, rendering a decision about a PTSD diagnosis is routine. Even if those who have been exposed to a trauma fail to meet the formal diagnostic criterion for PTSD, they may still require interventions that target their unique trauma-related adaptation. This, of course, depends on how the case is conceptualized.

An effective case conceptualization requires clinical decision making that is rooted in theory about the effects of trauma on human behavior, a detailed functional analysis of the person's unique repertoire of trauma-related problems, a clear sense of the various interventions that target specific types of posttraumatic problems and comorbid difficulties, and an evaluation of the appropriateness of the various treatment options for the patient's current circumstances. There are several heuristic guidelines that a clinician can apply. First, any problems with safety need to be the primary target for intervention (e.g., self-harm of any kind, risk for violence). Second, if comorbid problems are sufficiently severe, the clinician should consider addressing these before targeting trauma-related problems, keeping in mind that it is likely that the so-called comorbid problems are either exacerbated by or the result of a traumatic life experience. In the latter instance, the clinician should look for a functional relationship between the comorbid problem behaviors and specific PTSD symptoms and then expect collateral positive change in PTSD symptoms if the other problem is addressed successfully. For example, comorbid major depression may be a pressing problem that hinders motivation for trauma-focused therapy. Depressed behavior is often functional in that it serves to reduce the frequency of exposure to trauma-related cues and feeling states, which is highly negatively reinforcing. If cognitive therapy is used to treat the depression, usually trauma-related themes are processed, such as shame about how the trauma was coped with, repeated failure experience after the trauma, and subsequent helplessness and hopelessness.

Third, clinicians should evaluate the relative intensity and frequency of specific clusters of PTSD problems, with the goal of determining the predominant trauma-induced pathology. For example, in cases where there is a preponderance of reexperiencing symptoms—combined with intact social supports, motivation and readiness for change, and accurate expectations for change—it would be inappropriate not to consider exposure therapy. Alternatively, when the assessment results yield a symptom picture that is dominated by withdrawal, pervasive avoidance, isolation, and restrictions in a range of emotional activities, the clinician should consider focusing on cognitive and skills-based efforts to increase interpersonal risk-taking and opportunity for success experience through in vivo exercises. Increases in social contacts and the greater expression of emotion may lead a patient to recall more details of the trauma that can then be addressed through exposure therapy.

PTSD ASSESSMENT IN THE PRIMARY CARE SETTING

Assessment of Mental Health Disorders in Primary Care

For the majority of people, the main avenue to mental health services is through their primary care physician. Almost one-half of office visits that result in mental health diagnoses are to nonpsychiatric physicians (Broadhead et al., 1995). Also, research has shown that a large percentage of people who go to their primary care doctor for regular visits have a mental health diagnosis: prevalence estimates range from 9% to as high as 35% (Broadhead et al., 1995).

Unfortunately, physicians tend to underdiagnose mental health problems in their patients. General practitioners often have poorer results than checklists or psychiatric interviews in diagnosing existing disorders (e.g., Vasquez-Barquero et al., 1997). In a study in Finland, one-quarter of patients in primary care had mental disorders (as demonstrated by their scores on the SCL-25, a short form of the SCL-90; Derogatis, Lipman & Covi, 1973), but general practitioners identified only 40% of these cases (Joukamaa, Lehtinen, & Karlsson, 1995). Even when a psychological disorder is detected in the primary care setting, the general practitioner often will undertreat the problem or overtreat it with medications, without clear psychiatric indications for doing so (Broadhead et al., 1995).

A number of explanations have been proposed for the underdiagnosis of psychological problems in primary care. These include physicians' stereotypes of who is mentally ill (Marks, Goldberg, & Hillier, 1979); time restrictions (Weissman et al., 1995); insufficient physician training in mental health assessment (American Psychological Association, 1994); physicians' underappreciation of the impact of mental health problems on physical health and services utilized; deliberate miscoding of mental health problems as physical ones, for a variety of reasons (Rost, Smith, Matthews, & Guise, 1994); patient resistance to a mental health diagnosis (Olfson, 1991; Orleans, George, Houpt, & Brodie, 1985; Von Korff & Meyers, 1987) and to receiving help from their physicians with interpersonal problems

(Steinert & Rosenberg, 1987); and patients' somatic presentation of mental distress (de-Gruy, 1996). These barriers to adequate assessment of mental health problems can become even more formidable when a patient is suffering from a severe and persistent disorder like PTSD. As Mechanic (1997) points out, serious mental illnesses are more difficult to manage, more stigmatized, and potentially more disruptive to a physician's routines.

Patients who have experienced trauma often avoid seeking help because of feelings of shame and guilt, especially if they have been sexually or physically abused. Those who do seek treatment may present with complaints of anxiety or depression and do not report trauma histories unless they are specifically asked for them (Zimmerman & Mattia, 1999). In one national survey, 92% of women who were physically abused by a partner did not discuss these incidents with their physicians (Pearse, 1994). It is clear that physicians cannot rely on traumatized patients to introduce the subject of their trauma histories and resultant difficulties but, instead, must actively seek this kind of information. This active questioning becomes particularly important when a patient reports chronic pain or many symptoms, or is overusing health care services (Drossman et al., 1990). Unfortunately, doctors may feel uncomfortable asking their patients about trauma; they are anxious about delving into highly personal issues and fearful of having to manage a patient's distress if they were to do so. Even in the setting of a Veterans Administration (VA) clinic or medical center, where one would expect more familiarity with the symptoms of trauma, clinicians may not always detect noncombat PTSD. Veterans view combat trauma as more courageous and laudable, while their experiences of sexual and physical abuse lead to shame and fear (Grossman et al., 1997). The direct questioning needed to elicit abuse histories is not yet common practice in VA facilities.

Many arguments can be made for the importance of improved primary care assessment of PTSD. Patients with mental disorders have more physical health problems, are more debilitated in general, and enjoy a lower quality of life than those who do not experience such difficulties. In an examination of the association between psychiatric disorders and chronic medical conditions, only anxiety disorders (not depression or substance use disorders) were uniquely associated with chronic medical conditions (Hankin et al., 1982). In a study of anxiety disorders in primary care, PTSD was the most common anxiety disorder; 17% of the study group met criteria for PTSD (Fifer et al., 1994). Patients with untreated anxiety scored significantly lower on measures of general health perceptions and physical functioning than those without anxiety. Such a difference is equivalent to the effect of a healthy person developing a serious illness or debilitating physical problem.

Individuals with symptoms of PTSD are at elevated risk for health problems, and it has been suggested that PTSD may mediate between trauma and physical health (e.g., Friedman & Schnurr, 1995). In a sample of nontreatment-seeking firefighters with and without PTSD, the PTSD group was found to have statistically higher rates of cardiovascular, respiratory, musculoskeletal, and neurological symptoms (McFarlane, Atchison, Rafalowicz, & Papay, 1994). Veterans with PTSD also report more physical symptoms than do those without the disorder (Litz, Keane, et al., 1992). PTSD also has been associated with specific medical conditions such as chronic pain, gastrointestinal disorders, and fibromyalgia (Leskin, Ruzek, Friedman, & Gusman, 1999).

In addition to experiencing more physical health problems, patients with PTSD are known to use more services and cost the health care system more money and time than people without PTSD. In general, failure to recognize a mental disorder leads to undertreatment, greater impairment, and longer duration of illness (Weissman et al., 1995). Even without an established diagnosis of PTSD, trauma exposure itself is known to be related to increased health care utilization and substantial cost (Solomon & Davidson, 1997). Although people with PTSD tend to overuse the health care system, they underuse mental health services (Solomon & Davidson, 1997). Since the chronic health complaints of patients with PTSD lead many to seek medical care rather than mental health treatment, medical costs could be reduced by providing psychological services for somatizing patients or those who have a significant psychological component to their medical conditions (e.g., Groth-Marnat & Edkins, 1996).

For most trauma survivors, their point of entry is their general practitioner's office or the emergency room (Leskin et al., 1999); this is another strong rationale for assessing PTSD in the primary care setting. Visits to the emergency room and follow-up appointments with physicians after traumatic events such as motor vehicle accidents, rape, and episodes of physical violence offer an opportunity to intervene early and perhaps lessen the psychological impact of the trauma. The medical procedures associated with serious illnesses and injuries, such as major surgery or cancer treatment, may themselves be a source of trauma and PTSD (e.g., Jacobsen et al., 1998); the medical appointment is also the logical setting to evaluate the impact of these events.

Efforts have been made to improve the detection of mental health problems in primary care settings, so proper referrals can be made and patients can receive the treatment they need. Pallack, Cummings, Dorken, and Henke (1995) argued that physicians should not have to determine the cause of a patient's emotional problems—whether a medical condition or a side effect is causing a patient's emotional distress, or whether emotional distress may be driving the presentation of physical symptoms. They argued that it is cost-effective to increase access to mental health services because properly referred patients would be less likely to use medical resources unnecessarily.

Efforts to Improve Screening in Primary Care

Unfortunately, although screening instruments for primary care settings have been developed for many mental health disorders, PTSD has not been a component of most of these measures. In several large studies that have been carried out in medical settings, an initial sample of patients were screened with a broad measure of psychological distress; a subsample who report or show symptoms that may be indicative of one or more disorders receive a full interview (Vasquez-Barquero et al., 1997).

The PRIME-MD 1000 study (Primary Care Evaluation of Mental Disorders; Spitzer et al., 1994) used such a screening process. Some 1,000 patients filled out a screening measure with 26 "yes"/"no" questions about possible symptoms; positive responses were followed up with appropriate structured interview modules, based on criteria from DSM-III-R, that were administered by their primary care physician (physicians received a 1- to 3-hour training session on the instrument). In this manner, 18 possible mental disorders were assessed in mood, anxiety, somatoform, and alcohol-related categories. Physicians reported an average time of 8.4 minutes to complete the evaluation.

PRIME-MD mental health diagnoses agreed well with those of independent mental health professionals; for the diagnosis of any disorder, the alpha was .71 and the overall accuracy rate was 88%. Of the 287 patients given a mental health diagnosis, 48% had not been recognized to have that diagnosis by their physician before the evaluation, and 62% of the 125 patients with diagnoses who were not already being treated received a new treatment or referral.

The Symptom-Driven Diagnostic System for Primary Care (SDDS-PC) Validation Study (Broadhead et al., 1995; Weissman et al., 1995) is another large-scale (N = 937) study of mental health screening in primary care settings. Like the PRIME-MD, it uses a two-step process of a self-administered screening (16 "yes"/"no" items), followed by in-depth modules based on six diagnostic categories in DSM-IV; major depression, generalized anxiety disorder, panic disorder, obsessive–compulsive disorder, alcohol and drug abuse and dependence, and suicidal ideation or attempts. Appropriate modules, each of which took 5 minutes or less to complete, were placed in the patient's chart to be administered by their physician. Completion of the modules produced a one-page summary sheet that identified the disorders and symptoms, and this sheet was then used by the physician to confirm final diagnoses and make treatment recommendations.

Of the patients who received a positive diagnosis by the physician interview, 76.4% also tested positive on the SCID-P, administered independently by a mental health professional. Physicians found the instruments useful, but 26% thought the procedure was too time-consuming, and 80% believed that reimbursement would be necessary for routine use. The modules were originally intended to be physician-administered, but in response to the physician feedback, modules were later computerized and given by nurses (Weissman et al., 1995). Physicians in the study usually offered counseling and a return visit ("watchful waiting") to diagnosed patients. Referral to a mental health professional or the prescription of psychotropic medications was less frequent.

Other mental health screening studies include the World Health Organization Collaborative Study (Kessler, Andrews, Mroczek, Ustun, & Wittchen, 1998) and a study being carried out at Kaiser Permanente Oakland Medical Center (Miller & Farber, 1996). The World Health Organization screening uses the Composite International Diagnostic Interview Short Form (CIDI-SF; Kessler et al., 1998). The interview contains screening scales for eight DSM-III-R disorders and is based on data from the National Comorbidity Survey, but PTSD was not assessed (it is not included in the short form of the DIS). The Kaiser Permanente study began with a screening (which did not include symptoms specific to PTSD); when patients reported or showed symptoms, mental health counselors were available in the clinic to see them on a scheduled or drop-in basis per physician referral. Physicians were provided with ongoing didactic training and a case conference on recognition and treatment of psychosocial variables in primary care (Miller & Farber, 1996).

The use of a two-phase procedure in these studies overcomes the criticisms leveled at past screening methods (Broadhead et al., 1995), which often were limited to a single disorder when multiple disorders were possible and which failed to include diagnostic criteria. Both the PRIME-MD and the SDDS-PC are excellent examples of effective screening and assessment methods for mental health problems in a primary care setting, and they can serve as a model for PTSD screening, with a few additional considerations.

Screening for PTSD in Primary Care Settings

Even more than querying about symptoms of depression or substance abuse, identifying trauma exposure requires the right balance of directness and sensitivity. As Green, Epstein, Krupnick & Rowland (1997) point out, one or two quick questions to evaluate trauma exposure usually will not be effective, for several reasons. First, using words like "rape" or "incest" can lead to underreporting of trauma (Resnick, Falsetti, Kilpatrick, & Freedy, 1996). More detailed questions are needed, with descriptive language that does not rely on words that are both nonspecific and "loaded." Second, patients are unlikely to respond to open-ended questions about traumatic events, and if they are given some examples of possible events, they are unlikely to mention occurrences that are not on the list.

The best approach is to inquire about a range of events, using a self-report measure. As in the large-scale studies discussed here, administering such an inventory as a first step requires no physician time and may be more comfortable for both the physician and the patient (Green et al., 1997). Separate questions should be included for sexual traumas, physical traumas, serious accidents, serious illness, and combat. The traumatic event inventory would be followed up by questioning about symptoms of PTSD and then a consultation with or referral to mental health professionals, if needed (Breslau et al., 1999). The purpose of the first phase is to maximize the number of true cases of PTSD, while the second phase allows for reclassification of those who were wrongly classified as having the disorder. At all stages of assessment, the physician and medical staff should be sensitive to issues of privacy and confidentiality, which are especially salient when dealing with trauma. Training that addresses these issues, as well as how to ask follow-up questions and how best to interface with mental health, would be helpful.

Ideally, an initial screening for PTSD would be administered to all primary care patients, but in situations where this is not feasible, higher risk patients should be screened. Those patients (1) who were recently treated in the emergency room; (2) who have experienced major surgery, a difficult childbirth, or painful medical procedures; or (3) who the physician knows to be seriously or chronically ill would be clear targets for screening. In a discussion of mental health screening, Leon et al. (1995) strongly recommend assessing patients who are returning for follow-up care, rather than those coming for first visits. This is suggested because established patients and those with chronic medical problems are known to have higher rates of mental health disorder. From the perspective of PTSD assessment, such an approach also makes sense because the physician is more likely to have established a relationship of trust with a known patient, which may ease the inquiry process.

Even with a well-established physician–patient relationship, however, a patient may not be willing to accept a mental health referral. In such a case, Leskin et al. (1999) recommend that the physician offer education about the prevalence of trauma exposure, the normality of symptomatic reactions to trauma, the relationship of stress to health problems, and the benefits of mental health treatment. Written materials on PTSD can be provided so the patient can go over them at leisure. The physician should project an attitude of acceptance of the patient and comfort with the trauma material, and the patient should be assured that the referral will not interfere with the physician's continuing treatment of his or her physical health problems. If the patient continues to express reluctance to accept the referral, the physician can be supportive of the patient's right to decide but can continue to check in with the patient during later visits in order to "keep the door open" (Leskin et al., 1999).

Leskin and colleagues (1999) recommend that a PTSD assessment be a part of routine screening in primary care. They suggest using a brief initial questionnaire like Prins and colleagues' Primary Care PTSD Screen (PC-PTSD; Prins, Kimerling, Cameron, Oimette, & Shaw, 1999; see below for full description of this measure). Patients who report exposure to trauma or symptoms of PTSD would receive a more complete diagnostic evaluation, either a structured interview like the CAPS (Blake et al., 1995) or a self-report measure such as the Los Angeles Symptom Checklist (LASC; King, King, Leskin, & Foy, 1995) or the PTSD Checklist (PCL; Weathers, Litz, Huska, & Keane, 1991). Leskin et al. (1999) do not specify who would carry out this second step. If the results of the initial screen are not seen as sufficient to trigger a referral to a mental health professional, the physician or primary care staff could administer either of the two self-report measures to confirm the need for further treatment. However, the CAPS interview is complex and time-intensive, and it is unrealistic to expect a physician to be capable and sufficiently trained to administer a CAPS. Instead, we recommend that a positive screen for PTSD trigger a referral for a comprehensive confirmatory diagnostic assessment by a trained clinician.

PTSD Screening Measures for Use in Primary Care Settings

The Seven-Symptom Scale for PTSD (Breslau et al., 1999) is a brief screen that consists of five avoidance and numbing items and two hyperarousal items, selected from DSM-IV criteria (from the DIS/Composite International Diagnostic Interview PTSD section); it does not include a trauma probe. Avoidance/numbing is the least frequently met criterion for PTSD: few of those who report sufficient symptoms in the other two criterion groups meet this criterion. The diagnostic utility of items in this category led to their being the majority in the screening measure. A score of 4 or greater on the seven-symptom screening scale is indicative of PTSD. A validation study on a community sample of over 2,000 people compared the diagnosis of PTSD using the brief screen with that obtained from a full-length interview (the DIS/CIDI). With the cutoff score of 4, the measure had a sensitivity of 80%, a specificity of 97%, a positive predictive value of 71%, and a negative predictive value of 98%.

The PC-PTSD (Prins et al., 1999) is another brief measure that is appropriate for use in medical settings. This four-item screen was developed to be embedded in the omnibus PRIME-MD measure previously described. The questions reflect the major symptom clusters of PTSD, and the patient is assessed for current disorder. Like the seven-symptom screen, the PC-PTSD does not include a trauma probe. If a patient responds "yes" to two or more questions, more in-depth assessment of PTSD is warranted. A validation study was carried out on 59 randomly recruited veterans in primary care clinics. Diagnosis with the brief screen was compared to the results of the CAPS and PCL, given at a follow-up interview 2 to 4 weeks later. Internal consistency (alpha = .79) and test–retest reliability (r = .84) were both good. The screen had a sensitivity of 67%, a specificity of 91%, a positive predictive value of 60%, and a negative predictive value of 93%.

General Recommendations for PTSD Assessment in Primary Care

We offer the following recommendations with regard to assessing trauma and PTSD in the primary care setting:

1. Education of primary care providers to enhance their awareness of the subtle and explicit signs of trauma and PTSD.

2. Training in regard to what questions to ask of their patients and how to ask them sensitively and effectively.

3. Augmentation of existing mental health screening protocols to include PTSD. This would involve the addition of a few symptom questions to the self-report screening form, and the addition of a PTSD module to the structured interview portion of the two-step assessment procedure. Prins and colleagues have done this for the PRIME-MD, but the SDDS-PC and others would also benefit from such an addition.

4. Development of additional brief PTSD screening measures that can be utilized both as part of standard intake protocols and in such settings as emergency rooms and medical specialty clinics.

5. Use of the two-step assessment procedure described above as a part of routine screening of primary care patients. The setting and the context of the assessment will determine which measures should be used. During a regular medical appointment, where a patient's mental health status needs to be explored but there is no overt indication of trauma, an omnibus mental health screening protocol that includes a PTSD module could be used; currently, the PRIME-MD is the best choice. In situations and settings where trauma exposure is suspected but time prevents a comprehensive screening (e.g., the emergency room), the Breslau 7-item screen could be used for the first step, followed by the PCL for the more in-depth second step.

6. Detection of PTSD symptoms should result in a mental health referral, but only to a mental health professional who specializes or is experienced in treating PTSD.

7. Follow-up of symptomatic patients by the primary care physician is crucial. For those who accept a mental health referral, the physician should ask if they have made contact with the provider and should monitor their patients' progress to see if they experience a reduction in symptoms. For those who refuse the referral, the physician should inquire about the patient's symptoms during future appointments and continue to bring up the possibility of treatment, gauging the patient's readiness to engage in this process.

This last recommendation points to the usefulness of collaborative care within the primary care setting (Leskin et al., 1999; Strosahl, 1997). In such a model of care, physicians and behavioral health specialists work together with the patient to treat all aspects of the patient's health. Ideally, both providers are located within the primary care setting, so the patient can easily visit both, and they can readily consult with one another. Among recommendations for financial efficacy of assessment in the era of managed care concerns, Groth-Marnat (1999) suggests integrating treatment planning, monitoring progress, and evaluating outcome into the assessment process. A comprehensive team approach makes this goal possible, and it reduces the chance that traumatized individuals will "fall through the cracks" and fail to receive treatment for their PTSD.

ASSESSING AND MONITORING OUTCOME IN PTSD TREATMENT

The process of assessing and monitoring outcome is important to researchers and clinicians alike, as both are interested in the efficacy of their treatments for PTSD. However, the best way to measure outcome in patients with PTSD is not obvious. There are a number of possible indicators of change: symptom severity, diagnostic status, general mental health, level of comorbidity, quality of life, social functioning, physical health, and patient satisfaction are aspects of patient functioning that could serve as indicators of treatment success. In this section, we first list some general recommendations that have been made with regard to assessment and measurement of PTSD outcome. Next, we summarize the methods used to measure outcome in three recent cognitive-behavioral treatment outcome studies. Finally, we provide some specific suggestions that may be helpful for the scientist–practitioner who wishes to monitor outcome in therapy cases.

General Recommendations for Evaluating PTSD Treatment Outcome

Borkovec, Castonguay, and Newman (1997) make several suggestions with regard to conducting outcome measurement in PTSD. First, they recommend that, in addition to PTSD, all Axis I diagnoses that a patient carries be determined by diagnostic interviews given at all assessments. Second, the patient's degree of global impairment should be measured at every period; this includes the degree of interference with daily living in occupational, school, and social relationships and family functioning. Third, they stress the importance of studying long-term efficacy of treatment, and they suggest waiting a minimum of 1 year to perform a complete follow-up assessment, which should include information on any other kinds of treatment that the patient may have received in the interim.

Borkovec et al. (1997) also recommend examination of clinical and functional change. As defined by Jacobson and Truax (1991), this is the extent to which therapy moves someone outside the range of the dysfunctional population or within the range of the functional population. Statistically significant change indicates that the differences between treatment and control groups did not occur by chance, but it does not tell you if these differences are meaningful. When comparing the status of a patient before and after therapy, clinicians could use the reliable change index (Jacobson & Truax, 1991) to determine if the magnitude of a given change is statistically reliable. We also recommend that both patient and therapist rate the degree of global impairment. Composite outcome measures need to be developed (self-reports, behavioral performance, and clinical ratings) to better assess the significance of change (Borkovec et al., 1997), and this level of evaluation requires reliable norms for the measures used, for both PTSD groups and well-adjusted populations.

Evaluating patient satisfaction and its relation to cost and function is also important to consider in PTSD treatment studies (deGruy, 1996). These indicators are not usually examined, but they are worth considering by practitioners who have to function in the current managed care environment. Clinicians are faced with constraints in terms of number of sessions and types of treatment covered by patients' mental health plans. Researchers, too, should be aware of these constraints when they evaluate treatment efficacy.

Representative PTSD Treatment Outcome Studies

Three recent seminal PTSD treatment studies were examined to compare the state-of-the-art methods of measuring outcome (Foa et al., 1999; Marks, Lovell, Noshirvani, Livanou, & Thrasher, 1998; Tarrier et al., 1999). These three studies had several characteristics in common. They all measured PTSD severity and diagnostic status using state-of-the-art clinical interviews (e.g., the CAPS), and they evaluated comorbid depression and anxiety with self-report measures. Two of the three studies administered the entire SCID to assess a range of comorbid disorders. These measurements were obtained at pretreatment and at posttreatment follow-up, immediately posttreatment and over time. Although substance abuse was not measured during the treatment or follow-up portions of the studies, all reported screening out those individuals who were significant drug or alcohol users. Patients' general functional status was measured in all three studies. The researchers used a variety of change indicators (e.g., work functioning, social functioning, general mental health, and quality of life), and they examined markers of clinically significant change (e.g., effect sizes). End-state functioning was measured by improvement in symptom severity and diagnostic status after treatment, and the percentage of patients improved was calculated by examining scores on PTSD symptom clusters and general health measures.

On the negative side, the studies could have benefited from some measure of patient satisfaction: only Tarrier et al. (1999) examined the patient's view of treatment credibility, expectancy of benefit, and patient motivation. Treatment failures in their study viewed the therapy as less credible, were less motivated, and missed a significantly greater number of therapy sessions than those who improved, which highlights the importance of examining these factors and their effects on outcome. Only one study followed patients for as long as 1 year, even though this length of time is considered a minimum for determining long-term efficacy in the treatment of this chronic disorder (Borkovec et al., 1997). Although the number of measures used in the studies discussed in this section is typical for research protocols, it is impractical for clinicians who wish to track progress in their patients.

Recommendations for Monitoring PTSD Cases in Therapy

First, we recommend that clinicians conduct an initial screening evaluation of trauma history, treatment history, PTSD, and comorbid problems using the initial section of the SCID as a guide (session 1). The goal here is to screen for psychological and social problems, screen for lifespan trauma, and evaluate current resources and social context. The clinician can get an initial idea about whether PTSD is the primary problem and whether the person is appropriate for time-limited, problem-focused, cognitive-behavioral treatment, which requires considerable effort and compliance. If so, the clinician can begin to hypothesize about specific PTSD-related problems that may be the first target of intervention. An additional goal is to provide an open-ended format to allow patients to articulate their history and current status in their own way, which can reveal useful things about interpersonal and communication style and coping capacities. We feel that an open-ended format is also useful before structured interviews and tests are employed because it empowers patients and allows them to get a sense of the clinician as a person, which can be comforting.

The patient should be given paper-and-pencil questionnaires to fill out at the end of the meeting. These should include the BDI, BAI, SF-36 (Ware & Sherbourne, 1992), a screen for lifespan traumas, such as the initial section of the Evaluation of Lifetime Stressors (ELS; Krinsley et al., 1993), and the PCL. If possible, these tests should be scored before the second evaluation session and the results used to guide the next phase of the assessment. For example, specific SCID modules can be used to formally evaluate disorders suggested in the initial interview. In addition, reported traumas can be followed up to determine the presence of Criterion A for any number of events across the lifespan and to facilitate decision making about the index Criterion A event that is the referent for the PTSD evaluation. The majority of the second session should be devoted to administering the CAPS. During the interview, the clinician should take notes on factors that are relevant for a functional analysis of trauma-related behaviors. The CAPS is time-intensive and may need to be completed in the next meeting.

Before the third (or fourth) meeting, the clinician should have a working formulation of the patient's unique adaptation to trauma. The clinician should be able to determine the patient's appropriateness for problem-focused cognitive-behavioral interventions and to prioritize targets for intervention. The therapist should collaborate with the patient in coming up with a working plan and provide the patient with accurate expectations about the course of therapy. The modal PTSD case is very complex and requires a flexible, hierarchical approach to treatment (Flack et al., 1998). Usually, a period of psychoeducation and self-monitoring is followed by stress management (e.g., applied relaxation and stress inoculation training), which is followed by exposure therapy.

We recommend that patients self-monitor intrusive trauma-related emotional and cognitive responses daily. Patients should be instructed to write down where they were, what they were thinking about, the degree of negative affect they experienced using a global distress scale (0 to 100), and their coping response. We also recommend that patients fill out a PCL weekly (e.g., the night before they come to treatment). If a comorbid problem is salient, the patient should also fill out a weekly measure of that problem (e.g., the BDI, a measure of alcohol use). At the completion of treatment, the therapist should readminister the CAPS and the self-report questionnaires.

SUMMARY

In this chapter we provided the reader with an overview of the PTSD syndrome, a road map for the comprehensive clinical evaluation of traumatized adults, a rendering of the various measurement methods, a set of recommendations for evaluating trauma and PTSD in primary care, and recommendations for monitoring treatment process and outcomes. The PTSD assessment literature is currently at its apex in terms of methods of diagnosis and evaluating the severity of symptoms, which is particularly important when monitoring change. At present, the clinician can choose from a number of excellent measurement tools that can meet the objectives of any specific assessment context (e.g., screening, confirming a diagnosis). We wish to underscore, however, something emphasized in this chapter: the assessment of adults exposed to trauma is more complex than administering a reliable and valid diagnostic tool. We trust that we have provided some useful heuristic guidelines that can be used in treatment planning and treatment monitoring.

REFERENCES

American Psychiatric Association. (1994). *The diagnostic and statistical manual of mental disorders* (4th ed.). Washington, DC: Author.

American Psychological Association. (1994). *Psychology as a health care profession.* Washington, DC: Author.

Beck, A. T. (1988). *Beck Depression Inventory.* New York: Psychological Corporation.

Beck, A. T. (1990). *Beck Anxiety Inventory.* New York: Psychological Corporation.

Bernat, J. A., Ronfeldt, H. M., Calhoun, K. S., & Arias, I. (1998). Prevalence of traumatic events and peritraumatic predictors of posttraumatic stress symptoms in a nonclinical sample of college students. *Journal of Traumatic Stress, 11,* 645–664.

Blake, D. D. (1994). Rationale and development of the Clinician-Administered PTSD Scale. *PTSD Research Quarterly, 5,* 1–2.

Blake, D. D., Weathers, F. W., Nagy, L. M., Kaloupek, D. G., Gusman, F. D., Charney, D. S. & Keane, T. M. (1995). The development of a clinician-administered PTSD scale. *Journal of Traumatic Stress, 8,* 75–90.

Blake, D. D., Weathers, F. W., Nagy, L. M., Kaloupek. D. G., Klauminzer, G., Charney, D. S., & Keane, T. M. (1990). A clinician rating scale for assessing current and lifetime PTSD: The CAPS–1. *Behavior Therapist, 13,* 187–188.

Blanchard, E. B., & Buckley, T. C. (1999). Psychophysiological assessment of posttraumatic stress disorder. In P. A. Saigh & J. D. Bremner (Eds.), *Posttraumatic stress disorder: A comprehensive text* (pp. 248–266). Boston: Allyn & Bacon.

Blanchard, E. B., Gerardi, R. J., Kolb, L. C., & Barlow, D. H. (1986). The utility of the Anxiety Disorders Interview Schedule (ADIS) in the diagnosis of posttraumatic stress disorder (PTSD) in Vietnam veterans. *Behaviour Research and Therapy, 24,* 557–580.

Borkovec, T. D., Castonguay, L. G., & Newman, M. G. (1997). Measuring treatment outcome for posttraumatic stress disorder and social phobia: A review of current instruments and recommendations for future research. In H. H. Strupp, L. M. Horowitz, & M. J. Lambert (Eds.), *Measuring patient changes in mood, anxiety, and personality disorders: Toward a core battery* (pp. 117–154). Washington, DC: American Psychological Association.

Boudewyns, P. A., & Hyer, L. (1990). Physiological responses to combat memories and preliminary treatment outcome in Vietnam veteran PTSD patients treated with direct therapeutic exposure. *Behavior Therapy, 21,* 63–87.

Boudewyns, P. A., & Shipley, R. H. (1983). *Flooding and implosive therapy.* New York: Plenum Press.

Breslau, N., Davis, G. C., Andreski, P., & Peterson, E. (1991). Traumatic events and posttraumatic stress disorder in an urban population of young adults. *Archives of General Psychiatry, 48,* 216–222.

Breslau, N., Kessler, R. C., Chilcoat, H. D., Schultz, L. R., Davis, G. C., & Andreski, P. (1998). Trauma and posttraumatic stress disorder in the community. *Archives of General Psychiatry, 55,* 626–632.

Breslau, N., Peterson, E. L., Kessler, R. C., & Schultz, L. R. (1999). Short screening scale for DSM-IV posttraumatic stress disorder. *American Journal of Psychiatry, 156,* 908–911.

Briere, J. (1997). *Psychological assessment of adult posttraumatic states.* Washington, DC: American Psychological Association.

Briere, J., Elliott, D. M., Harris, K., & Cotman, A. (1995). Trauma Symptom Inventory: Psychometrics and association with childhood and adult trauma in clinical samples. *Journal of Interpersonal Violence, 10,* 387–401.

Broadhead, W. E., Leon, A. C., Weissman, M. M., Barrett, J. E., Blacklow, R. S., Gilbert, T. T.,

Keller, M. B., Olfson, M. & Higgins, E. S. (1995). Development and validation of the SDDS-PC screen for multiple mental disorders in primary care. *Archives of Family Medicine, 4*, 211–219.

Butcher, J. N., Dahlstrom, W. G., Graham, J. R., Tellegen, A., & Kaemmer, B. (1989). *Minnesota Multiphasic Personality Inventory (MMPI–2): Manual for administration and scoring.* Minneapolis: University of Minnesota Press.

Carlson, E. B. (1997). *Trauma assessments: A clinician's guide.* New York: Guilford Press.

Carroll, E. M., Rueger, D. B., Foy, D. W., & Donahoe, C. P. (1985). Vietnam combat veterans with posttraumatic stress disorder: Analysis of marital and cohabitating adjustment. *Journal of Abnormal Psychology, 94*, 329–337.

Centers for Disease Control, Vietnam Experience Study. (1988). Health status of Vietnam veterans: I. Psychosocial characteristics. *Journal of the American Medical Association, 259*, 2701–2707.

Chemtob, C., Roitblat, H., Hamada, R., Carlson, J., & Twentyman, C. (1988). A cognitive action theory of post-traumatic stress disorder. *Journal of Anxiety Disorders, 2*, 253–275.

Davidson, J., & Foa, E. (1991). Diagnostic issues in posttraumatic stress disorder: Considerations for the DSM-IV. *Journal of Abnormal Psychology, 100*, 346–355.

Davidson, J., Smith, R., & Kudler, H. (1989). Validity and reliability of the DSM-III criteria for posttraumatic stress disorder: Experience with a structured interview. *Journal of Nervous and Mental Disease, 177*, 336–341.

Davidson, L. M., & Baum, A. (1986). Chronic stress and posttraumatic stress disorders. *Journal of Consulting and Clinical Psychology, 54*, 303–308.

deGruy, F. V. (1996). Mental health care in the primary care setting. In M. S. Donaldson, K. D. Yordy, K. N. Lohr, & N. Vanselow (Eds.), *Primary care: America's health in a new era* (pp. 285–311). Washington, DC: National Academy Press.

Derogatis, L. R. (1983). *SCL-90-R: Administration, scoring, and procedures manual-II.* Towson, MD: Clinical Psychometric Research.

Derogatis, L. R. (1993). *Brief Symptom Inventory: Administration, scoring and procedures manual.* Minneapolis, MN: National Computer Systems.

Derogatis, L. R., Lipman, R. S., & Covi, S. (1973). SCL-90: An outpatient psychiatric rating scale—preliminary report. *Psychopharmacology Bulletin, 9*, 13–27.

Di Nardo, P., Brown, T. A., & Barlow, D. H. (1994). *Anxiety Disorders Interview Schedule for DSM-IV.* San Antonio, TX: Psychological Corporation.

Di Nardo, P. A., Moras, K., Barlow, D. H., Rapee, R. M., & Brown, T. A. (1993). Reliability of DSM-III-R anxiety disorder categories: Using the Anxiety Disorders Interview Schedule—Revised (ADIS-R). *Archives of General Psychiatry, 50*, 251–256.

Dollard, J., & Miller, N. E. (1950). *Personality and psychotherapy.* New York: McGraw-Hill.

Drossman, D. A., Leserman, J., Nachman, G., Li, Z., Gluck, H., Toomey, T. C., & Mitchell, M. (1990). Sexual and physical abuse in women with functional or organic gastrointestinal disorders. *Annals of Internal Medicine, 113*, 828–833.

Elliot, D., & Briere, J. (1992). Sexual abuse trauma among professional women: Validating the Trauma Symptom Checklist-40 (TSC–40). *Child Abuse and Neglect, 16*, 391–398.

Fairbank, J. A., & Keane, T. M. (1982). Flooding for combat-related stress disorders: Assessment of anxiety reduction across traumatic memories. *Behavior Therapy, 13*, 499–510.

Fairbank, J. A., McCaffrey R. J., & Keane, T. M. (1985). Psychometric detection of fabricated symptoms of posttraumatic stress disorder. *American Journal of Psychiatry, 142*, 501–503.

Fairbank, J. A., & Nicholson, R. A. (1987). Theoretical and empirical issues in the treatment of posttraumatic stress disorder in Vietnam veterans. *Journal of Clinical Psychology, 43*, 44–55.

Falsetti, S., Resnick, H., & Kilpatrick, D. (1993). The Modified PTSD Symptom Scale: A brief self-report measure for assessing post-traumatic stress disorder. *Journal of Traumatic Stress, 6*, 459–474.

Falsetti, S., Resnick, H., Kilpatrick, D., & Freedy, J. (1994). A review of the Potential Stressful Events Interview. *Behavior Therapist, 17*, 66–67.

Falsetti, S. A., Resnick, H. S., Resick, P. A., & Kilpatrick, D. G. (1993). The Modified PTSD Symptom Scale: A brief self-report measure of posttraumatic stress disorder. *The Behavior Therapist, 16*,161–162.

Fifer, S. K., Mathias, S. D., Patrick, D. L., Mazonson, P. D., Lubeck, D. P., & Buesching, D. P. (1994). Untreated anxiety among adult primary care patients in a health maintenance organization. *Archives of General Psychiatry, 51,* 740–750.

Finkelhor, D., Hotaling, G., Lewis, I. A., & Smith, C. (1990). Sexual abuse in a national survey of adult men and women: Prevalence, characteristics, and risk factors. *Child Abuse and Neglect, 14,* 19–28.

First, M. B., Spitzer, R. L., Gibbon, M., & Williams, J. B. W. (1996). *Structured Clinical Interview for Axis I and II DSM-IV Disorders—Patient Edition (SCID-IV/P)* New York: Biometrics Research Department, New York State Psychiatric Institute.

First, M. B., Spitzer, R. L., Gibbon, M., & Williams, J. B. W. (1997). *Structured Clinical Interview for Personality Disorders (SCID-II).* Washington, DC: American Psychiatric Press.

Flack, W. F., Litz, B. T., & Keane, T. M. (1998). Cognitive-behavioral treatment of combat-related PTSD: A flexible hierarchical approach. In V. M. Follette, J. I. Ruzek, & F. R. Abueg (Eds.), *Cognitive-behavioral therapies for trauma* (pp. 77–99). New York: Guilford Press.

Foa, E. B., Dancu, C. V., Hembree, E. A., Jaycox, L. H., Meadows, E. A., & Street, G. P. (1999). A comparison of exposure therapy, stress inoculation training, and their combination for reducing posttraumatic stress disorder in female assault victims. *Journal of Consulting and Clinical Psychology, 67,* 194–200.

Foa, E. B., Hearst-Ikeda, D., & Perry, K. J. (1995). Evaluation of a brief cognitive-behavioral program for the prevention of chronic PTSD in recent assault victims. *Journal of Consulting and Clinical Psychology, 63,* 948–955.

Foa, E., Riggs, D., Dancu, C., & Rothbaum, B. (1993). Reliability and validity of a brief instrument for assessing post-traumatic stress disorder. *Journal of Traumatic Stress, 6,* 459–474.

Foa, E. B., & Rothbaum, B. (1998). *Treating the trauma of rape.* New York: Guilford Press.

Foa, E. B., Steketee, G., & Rothbaum, B. O. (1989). Behavioral/cognitive conceptualizations of posttraumatic stress disorder. *Behavior Therapy, 20,* 155–176.

Ford, J. D., & Kidd, P. (1998). Early childhood trauma and disorders of extreme stress as predictors of treatment outcome with chronic posttraumatic stress disorder. *Journal of Traumatic Stress, 11,* 743–761.

Foy, D. W., Osato, S. S., Housecamp, B. M., & Neumann, D. A. (1992). Etiology of Post-traumatic Stress Disorder. In P. Saigh (Ed.), *Post-traumatic Stress Disorder: A behavioral approach to assessment and treatment* (pp. 50–84). Boston: Allyn & Bacon.

Freud, S., Ferenczi, S., Abraham, K., Simmel, E., & Jones, E. (1921). *Psychoanalysis and the war neurosis.* New York: International Psychoanalytic Press.

Friedman, M. J., & Schnurr, P. P. (1995). The relationship between trauma, post-traumatic stress disorder and physical health. In M. J. Friedman, D. S. Charney, & A. Y. Deutch (Eds.), *Neurobiological and clinical consequences of stress: From normal adaptation to post-traumatic stress disorder* (pp. 507–524). Philadelphia, PA: Lippincott-Raven.

Goodman, L. A., Corcoran, C., Turner, K., Yuan, N., & Green, B. L. (1998). Assessing traumatic event exposure: General issues and preliminary findings for the Stressful Life Events Screening Questionnaire. *Journal of Traumatic Stress, 11,* 521–542.

Green, B. L. (1991). Evaluating the effects of disasters. *Psychological Assessment, 3,* 538–546.

Green, B. L. (1993). Identifying survivors at risk: Trauma and stressors across events. In J. P. Wilson & B. Raphael (Eds.), *International handbook of traumatic stress syndromes* (pp. 135–144). New York: Plenum Press.

Green, B. L. (1996). Psychometric review of Trauma History Questionnaire. In B. H. Stamm (Ed.), *Measurement of stress, trauma, and adaptation.* Lutherville, MD: Sidran Press.

Green, B. L., Epstein, S. A., Krupnick, J. L., & Rowland, J. H. (1997). Trauma and medical illness: Assessing trauma-related disorders in medical settings. In J. P. Wilson & T. M. Keane (Eds.), *Assessing psychological trauma and PTSD* (pp. 160–191). New York: Guilford Press.

Gross, J. J., & Levenson, R. W. (1993). Emotional suppression: Physiology, self-report, and expressive behavior. *Journal of Personality and Social Psychology, 64,* 970–986.

Grossman, L. S., Willer, J. K., Stovall, J. G., McRae, S. G., Maxwell, S., & Nelson, R. (1997). Underdiagnosis of posttraumatic stress disorder and substance abuse disorders in hospitalized female veterans. *Psychiatric Services, 48,* 393–395.

Groth-Marnat, G. (1999). Financial efficacy of clinical assessment: Rational guidelines and issues for future research. *Journal of Clinical Psychology, 55,* 813–824.

Groth-Marnat, G., & Edkins, G. (1996). Professional psychologists in general health care settings: A review of the financial efficacy of direct treatment interventions. *Professional Psychology: Research and Practice, 27,* 161–174.

Hammarberg, M. (1992). Penn Inventory for Posttraumatic Stress Disorder: Psychometric properties. *Psychological Assessment: A Journal of Consulting and Clinical Psychology, 4,* 67–76.

Hankin, J. R., Steinwachs, D. M., Regier, D. A., Burns, B. J., Goldberg, I. D., & Hoeper, E. W. (1982). Use of general medical care services by persons with mental disorders. *Archives of General Psychiatry, 39,* 225–231.

Harvey, A., & Bryant, R. (1998). The relationship between acute stress disorder and posttraumatic stress disorder: A prospective evaluation of motor vehicle accident survivors. *Journal of Consulting and Clinical Psychology, 66,* 507–512.

Helzer, J. E., Robins, L. N., & McEvoy, L. (1987). Post-traumatic stress disorder in the general population. *New England Journal of Medicine, 317,* 1630–1634.

Herman, J. (1992a). *Trauma and recovery.* New York: Basic Books.

Herman, J. (1992b). Complex PTSD: A syndrome in survivors of prolonged and repeated trauma. *Journal of Traumatic Stress, 5,* 377–391.

Horowitz, M. J. (1986). *Stress response syndromes.* New York: Jason Aronson.

Horowitz, M. J., Wilner, N., & Alvarez, W. (1979). Impact of Event Scale: A measure of subjective stress. *Psychosomatic Medicine, 41,* 209–218.

Hyer, L., Fallon, J. H., Jr., Harrison, W. R., & Boudewyns, P. A. (1987). MMPI overreporting by Vietnam combat veterans. *Journal of Clinical Psychology, 43,* 79–83.

Jacobson, N. S., & Truax, P. (1991). Clinical significance: A statistical approach to defining meaningful change in therapy. *Journal of Consulting and Clinical Psychology, 59,* 12–19.

Jacobsen, P. W., Widows, M. R., Hann, D. M., Andrykowski, M. A., Kronish, L. E., & Fields, K. K. (1998). Posttraumatic stress disorder symptoms after bone marrow transplantation for breast cancer. *Psychosomatic Medicine, 60,* 366–371.

Janoff-Bulman, R. (1989). Assumptive worlds and the stress of traumatic events: Applications of the schema construct. *Social Cognition, 7,* 113–136.

Jordan, K. B., Marmar, C. R., Fairbank, J. A., Schlenger, W. E., Kulka, R. A., Hough, R. L., & Weiss, D. S. (1992). Problems in families of male Vietnam veterans with posttraumatic stress disorder. *Journal of Consulting and Clinical Psychology, 60,* 916–926.

Joukamaa, M., Lehtinen, V., & Karlsson, H. (1995). The ability of general practitioners to detect mental health disorders in primary health care. *Acta Psychiatrica Scandinavica, 91,* 52–56.

Keane, T. M. (1995). Guidelines for the forensic psychological assessment of posttraumatic stress disorder claimants. In R. Simon, *Posttraumatic stress disorder in litigation: Guidelines for forensic assessment* (pp. 99–115). Washington, DC: American Psychiatric Press.

Keane, T. M. (1997). Psychological and behavioral treatment of post-traumatic stress disorder. In P. Nathan & J. Gorman (Eds.), *A guide to treatments that work* (pp. 398–407). New York: Oxford University Press.

Keane, T. M., Caddell, J. M., & Taylor, K. L. (1988). Mississippi Scale for Combat-Related Posttraumatic Stress Disorder: Three studies in reliability and validity. *Journal of Consulting and Clinical Psychology, 56,* 85–90.

Keane, T. M., Fairbank, J. A., Caddell, J. M., Zimering, R. T., Taylor, K. L., & Mora, C. A. (1989). Clinical evaluation of a measure to assess combat exposure. *Psychological Assessment, 1,* 53–55.

Keane, T. M., Gerardi, R., Quinn, S., & Litz, B. T. (1992). Behavioral treatment of post-traumatic stress disorder. In S. M. Turner, K. S. Calhoun, & H. E. Adams (Eds.), *Handbook of Clinical Behavior Therapy* (2nd ed., pp. 87–98). New York: Wiley.

Keane, T. M., Kolb, L. C., Kaloupek, D. G., Orr, S. P., Blanchard, E. B., Thomas, R. G., Hsieh, F. Y., & Lavori, P. W. (1998). Utility of psychophysiological measurement in the diagnosis of posttraumatic stress disorder: Results from a Department of Veterans Affairs cooperative study. *Journal of Consulting and Clinical Psychology, 66,* 914–923.

Keane, T. M., Malloy, P. F., & Fairbank, J. A. (1984). Empirical development of an MMPI subscale for the assessment of combat-related posttraumatic stress disorder. *Journal of Consulting and Clinical Psychology, 52,* 888–891.

Keane, T. M., Scott, W. O., Chavoya, G. A., Lamparski, D. M., & Fairbank, J. A. (1985). Social support in Vietnam veterans with posttraumatic stress disorder: A comparative analysis. *Journal of Consulting and Clinical Psychology, 53,* 95–102.

Keane, T. M., Weathers, F. W., & Foa, E. B. (2000). Diagnosis and assessment. In E. B. Foa, T. M. Keane, & M. J. Friedman (Eds.), *Effective treatments for PTSD: Practice guidelines from the International Society for Traumatic Stress Studies.* New York: Guilford Press.

Keane, T. M., & Wolfe, J. (1990). Comorbidity in post-traumatic stress disorder: An analysis of community and clinical studies. *Journal of Applied Social Psychology, 20,* 1776–1788.

Keane, T. M., Zimering, R. T., & Caddell, J. M. (1985). A behavioral formulation of post-traumatic stress disorder in Vietnam veterans. *Behavior Therapist, 8,* 9–12.

Kessler, R. C., Andrews, G., Mroczek, D., Ustun, B., & Wittchen, H. U. (1998). The World Health Organization Composite International Diagnostic Interview—Short Form (CIDI-SF). *International Journal of Methods in Psychiatric Research, 7,* 171–185.

Kessler, R. C., Sonnega, A., Bromet, E., Hughes, M., & Nelson, C. B. (1995). Posttraumatic stress disorder in the National Comorbidity Survey. *Archives of General Psychiatry, 52,* 1048–1060.

Kilpatrick, D. G., Best, C. L., Veronen, L. J., Amick, A. E., Villeponteaux, L. A., & Ruff, G. A. (1985). Mental health correlates of criminal victimization: A random community survey. *Journal of Consulting and Clinical Psychology, 53,* 866–873.

Kilpatrick, D. G., Veronen, L. J., & Best, C. L. (1985). Factors predicting psychological distress among rape victims. In C. R. Figley (Ed.), *Trauma and its wake* (pp. 113–141). New York: Brunner/Mazel.

King, D. W., King, L. A., Foy, D. W., Keane, T. M., & Fairbank, J. A. (1999). Posttraumatic stress disorder in a national sample of female and male Vietnam veterans: Risk factors, war-zone stressors, and resilience-recovery variables. *Journal of Abnormal Psychology, 108,* 164–170.

King, D. W., King, L. A., Gudanowski, D. M., & Vreven, D. L. (1995). Alternative representations of war-zone stressors: Relationships to post-traumatic stress disorder in male and female Vietnam veterans. *Journal of Abnormal Psychology, 104,* 184–196.

King, L. A., & King, D. W. (1994). Latent structure of the Mississippi Scale for Combat-Related PTSD Post-traumatic Stress Disorder: Exploratory and higher-order confirmatory factor analyses. *Assessment, 1,* 275–291.

King, L. A., King, D. W., Leskin, G., & Foy, D. W. (1995). The Los Angeles Symptom Checklist: A self-report measure of posttraumatic stress disorder. *Assessment, 2,* 1–17.

Koopman, C., Classen, C., Cardena, E., & Spiegel, D. (1995). When disaster strikes, acute stress disorder may follow. *Journal of Traumatic Stress, 8,* 29–46.

Koss, M. P., Gidycz, C. A., & Wisniewski, N. (1987). The scope of rape: Incidence and prevalence of sexual aggression and victimization in a national sample of higher education students. *Journal of Consulting and Clinical Psychology, 55,* 162–170.

Krinsley, K. E., Weathers, F. W., Young, L. S., Vielhauer, M., Kimerling, R., & Newman, E. (1993). *Evaluation of lifetime stressors (ELS).* Boston, MA: National Center for PTSD.

Kubany, E. S., Leisen, M. B., Kaplan, A. S., Watson, S. B., Haynes, S. N., Owens, J. A., & Burns, K. (2000). Development and preliminary validation of a brief broad-spectrum measure of trauma exposure: The Traumatic Life Events Questionnaire. *Psychological Assessment, 12,* 210–224.

Kulka, R. A., Schlenger, W. E., Fairbank, J. A., Hough, R. L., Jordan, B. K., Marmar, C. R., & Weiss, D. S. (1988). *National Vietnam veterans readjustment study (NVVRS): Description, current status, and initial PTSD prevalence estimates.* Washington, DC: Veterans Administration.

Kulka, R. A., Schlenger, W. E., Fairbank, J. A., Hough, R. L., Jordan, B. K., Marmar, C. R., & Weiss, D. S. (1990). *Trauma and the Vietnam war generation: Report of the findings from the National Vietnam Veterans Readjustment Study.* New York: Brunner/Mazel.

Kulka, R. A., Schlenger, W. E., Fairbank, J. A., Jordan, B. K., Hough, R. L., Marmar, C. R., & Weiss, D. S. (1991). Assessment of post-traumatic stress disorder in the community: Prospects and pitfalls from recent studies of Vietnam veterans. *Psychological Assessment, 3,* 547–560.

Lang, P. (1979). A bio-informational theory of emotional imagery. *Psychophysiology, 16,* 495–512.

Lauterbach, D., & Vrana, S. (1996). Three studies on the reliability and validity of a self-report measure of posttraumatic stress disorder. *Assessment, 3,* 17–25.

Lebowitz, L., & Newman, E. (1996). The role of cognitive-affective themes in the assessment and treatment of trauma reactions. *Clinical Psychology and Psychotherapy, 3,* 196–207.

Leon, A. C., Olfson, M., Broadhead, W. E., Barrett, J. E., Blacklow, R. S., Keller, M. B., Higgins, E. S., & Weissman, M. W. (1995). Prevalence of mental disorders in primary care: Implications for screening. *Archives of Family Medicine, 4,* 857–861.

Leskin, G. A., Ruzek, J. I., Friedman, M. J., & Gusman, F. D. (1999). Effective clinical management of PTSD in primary care settings: Screening and treatment options. *Primary Care Psychiatry, 5,* 3–12.

Linehan, M. M. (1993). *Cognitive-behavioral treatment of borderline personality disorder.* New York: Guilford Press.

Litz, B. T., Blake, D., Gerardi, R., & Keane, T. M. (1990). Decision making guidelines for the use of direct therapeutic exposure in the treatment of Post-Traumatic Stress Disorder. *Behavior Therapist, 13,* 91–93.

Litz, B. T., & Keane, T. M. (1989). Information-processing in anxiety disorders: Application to the understanding of post-traumatic stress disorder. *Clinical Psychology Review. 9,* 243–257.

Litz, B. T., Keane, T. M., Fisher, L., Marx, B., & Monaco, V. (1992). Physical health complaints in combat-related post-traumatic stress disorder: A preliminary report. *Journal of Traumatic Stress, 5,* 131–141.

Litz, B. T., Orsillo, S. M., Kaloupek, D., & Weathers, F. (2000). Emotional-processing in posttraumatic stress disorder. *Journal of Abnormal Psychology, 109,* 26–39.

Litz, B. T., Penk, W. E., Gerardi, R., & Keane, T. M. (1992). Behavioral assessment of PTSD. In P. Saigh (Ed.), *Post-traumatic stress disorder: A behavioral approach to assessment and treatment* (pp. 50–84). New York: Pergamon Press.

Litz, B. T., & Weathers, F. (1994). The diagnosis and assessment of post-traumatic stress disorder in adults. In M. B. Williams & J. F. Sommer (Eds.), *The handbook of post-traumatic therapy* (pp. 20–37). Westport, CT: Greenwood Press.

Lyons, J., & Keane, T. M. (1989). Implosive therapy for the treatment of combat-related PTSD. *Journal of Traumatic Stress, 2,* 137–152.

Macklin, M. L., Metzger, L. J., Litz, B. T., McNally, R. J., Lasko, N. B., Orr, S. P., & Pitman, R. K. (1998). Lower precombat intelligence is a risk factor for posttraumatic stress disorder. *Journal of Consulting and Clinical Psychology, 66,* 323–326.

Marks, I., Lovell, K., Noshirvani, H., Livanou, M., & Thrasher, S. (1998). Treatment of posttraumatic stress disorder by exposure and/or cognitive restructuring: A controlled study. *Archives of General Psychiatry, 55,* 317–325.

Marks, J. N., Goldberg, D. P., & Hillier, V. F. (1979). Determinants of the ability of general practitioners to detect psychiatric illness. *Psychological Medicine, 9,* 337–353.

McCann, I. L., & Pearlman, L. A. (1990). *Psychological trauma and the adult survivor: Theory, therapy, and transformation.* New York: Brunner/Mazel.

McFarlane, A. C., Atchison, M., Rafalowicz, E., & Papay, P. (1994). Physical symptoms in post-traumatic stress disorder. *Journal of Psychosomatic Research, 38,* 715–726.

McNally, R. J. (1998). Experimental approaches to cognitive abnormality in posttraumatic stress disorder. *Clinical Psychology Review, 18,* 971–982.

Mechanic, D. (1997). Approaches for coordinating primary and specialty care for persons with mental illness. *General Hospital Psychiatry, 19,* 395–402.

Miller, B., & Farber, L. (1996). Delivery of mental health services in the changing health care system. *Professional Psychology: Research and Practice, 27,* 527–529.

Miller, M. W., Kaloupek, D. G., & Keane, T. M. (1999). Antisociality and physiological hyporesponsivity during exposure to trauma-related stimuli in patients with PTSD. *Psychophysiology, 36,* S81.

Myers, D. G. (1989). Mental health and disaster: Preventive approaches to intervention. In R. Gist & B. Lubin (Eds.), *Psychosocial aspects of disaster* (pp. 190–228). New York: Wiley.

Nezu, A., & Carnevale, G. (1987). Interpersonal problem solving and coping reactions of Vietnam veterans with posttraumatic stress disorder. *Journal of Abnormal Psychology, 96,* 155–157.

Norris, F. H. (1990). Screening for traumatic stress: A scale for use in the general population. *Journal of Applied Social Psychology, 20,* 1704–1718.

Norris, F. H. (1992). Epidemiology of trauma: Frequency and impact of different potentially traumatic events on different demographic groups. *Journal of Consulting and Clinical Psychology, 60,* 409–418.

Norris, F. H., & Perilla, J. L. (1996). The Revised Civilian Mississippi Scale for PTSD: Reliability, validity, and cross-language stability. *Journal of Traumatic Stress, 9,* 285–298.

Norris, F. H., & Uhl, G. A. (1993). Chronic stress as a mediator of acute stress: The case of Hurricane Hugo, *Journal of Applied Social Psychology, 23,* 1263–1284.

Olfson, M. (1991). Primary care patients who refuse specialized mental health services. *Archives of Internal Medicine, 151,* 129–132.

Orleans, C., George, L., Houpt, J., & Brodie, H. (1985). How primary care physicians treat psychiatric disorders: A national survey of family practitioners. *American Journal of Psychiatry, 142,* 52–57.

Orsillo, S. M., Weathers, F. W., Litz, B. T., Steinberg, H. R., Huska, J. A., & Keane, T. M. (1996). Current and lifetime psychiatric disorders among veterans with war zone-related posttraumatic stress disorder. *Journal of Nervous and Mental Disease, 184,* 307–313.

Pallak, M. S., Cummings, N. A., Dorken, H., & Henke, C. J. (1995). Effect of mental health treatment on medical costs. *Mind/Body Medicine, 1,* 7–12.

Pearse, W. H. (1994). The Commonwealth Fund Women's Health Survey: Selected results and comments. *Women's Health Issues, 4,* 38–47.

Pennebaker, J., Barger, S., & Tiebout, J. (1989). Disclosure of traumas and health among Holocaust survivors. *Psychosomatic Medicine, 51,* 577–589.

Prins, A., Kimerling, R., Cameron, R., Oimette, P., & Shaw, J. (1999). *The Primary Care PTSD Screen (PC-PTSD).* Unpublished measure, National Center for PTSD, Palo Alto, CA.

Resick, P., Calhoun, K., Atkeson, B., & Ellis, E. (1981). Social adjustment in victims of sexual assault. *Journal of Consulting and Clinical Psychology, 49,* 705–712.

Resnick, H. S., Falsetti, S. A., Kilpatrick, D. G., & Freedy, J. R. (1996). Assessment of rape and other civilian trauma-related PTSD: Emphasis on assessment of potentially traumatic events. In T. W. Miller (Ed.), *Theory and assessment of stressful life events* (pp. 235–271). Madison, CT: International Universities Press.

Resnick, H. S., Kilpatrick, D. G., Dansky, B. S., Saunders, B. E., & Best, C. L. (1993). Prevalence of civilian trauma and posttraumatic stress disorder in a representative national sample of women. *Journal of Consulting and Clinical Psychology, 61,* 984–991.

Resnick, H. S., Kilpatrick, D. G., & Lipovsky, J. A. (1991). Assessment of rape-related posttraumatic stress disorder: Stressor and symptom dimensions. *Psychological Assessment: A Journal of Consulting and Clinical Psychology, 3,* 561–572.

Robins, L. N., Cottler, L., Bucholz, K., & Compton, W. (1995). *Diagnostic Interview Schedule (DIS), Version IV.* St. Louis, MO: Washington University School of Medicine.

Robins, L. N., Helzer, J. E., Croughan, J., & Ratcliff, K. S. (1981). National Institute of Mental Health Diagnostic Interview Schedule: Its history, characteristics, and validity. *Archives of General Psychiatry, 38,* 318–389.

Rost, K., Smith, G. R., Matthews, D. B., & Guise, B. (1994). The deliberate misdiagnosis of major depression in primary care. *Archives of Family Medicine, 3,* 333–337.

Roth, S., Lebowitz, L., & DeRosa, R. R. (1997). Thematic assessment of posttraumatic stress reactions. In J. Wilson & T. Keane (Eds.), *Assessing psychological trauma and PTSD* (pp. 512–528). New York: Guilford Press.

Roth, S., Newman, E., Pelcovitz, D., van der Kolk, B., & Mandel, F. (1997). Complex PTSD in victims exposed to sexual and physical abuse: Results from the DSM-IV field trial for posttraumatic stress disorder. *Journal of Traumatic Stress, 10,* 539–555.

Rothbaum, B., Foa, E., Riggs, D., Murdock, T., & Walsh, W. (1992). A prospective examination of post-traumatic stress disorder in rape victims. *Journal of Traumatic Stress, 5,* 455–475.

Ruch, L. O., Gartrell, J. W., Ramelli, A., & Coyne, B. J. (1991). The clinical trauma assessment: Evaluating sexual assault victims in the emergency room. *Psychological Assessment: A Journal of Consulting and Clinical Psychology, 3,* 405–411.

Saunders, B. E., Arata, C. M., & Kilpatrick, D. G. (1990). Development of a crime-related post-traumatic stress disorder scale for women with Symptom-Checklist-90—Revised. *Journal of Traumatic Stress, 3,* 439–448.

Schlenger, W. E., Kulka,-R. A., Fairbank,-J. A., Hough, R. L., Jordan, K. B., Marmar, C. R., & Weiss, D. S. (1992). The prevalence of post-traumatic stress disorder in the Vietnam generation: A multimethod, multisource assessment of psychiatric disorder. *Journal of Traumatic Stress, 5,* 333–363.

Schnurr, P. P., Friedman, M. J., & Rosenberg, S. D. (1993). Preliminary MMPI scores as predictors of combat-related PTSD symptoms. *American Journal of Psychiatry, 150,* 479–483.

Shalev, A., Bleich, A., & Ursano, R. J. (1990). Posttraumatic stress disorders. In J. Lundeberg, & U. Otto (Eds.), *Wartime medical services: Second annual conference; Stockholm, Sweden, 25–29 June 1990: Proceedings* (pp. 364–478). Stockholm: Foersvarets Forskningsanstalt.

Shalev, A. Y., Orr, S. P., & Pitman, R. K. (1992). Psychophysiologic response during script-driven imagery as an outcome measure in posttraumatic stress disorder. *Journal of Clinical Psychiatry, 53,* 324–326.

Sierles, F. S., Chen, J., McFarland, R. E., & Taylor, M. A. (1983). Post-traumatic stress disorder and concurrent psychiatric illness. *American Journal of Psychiatry, 140,* 1177–1179.

Solomon, S. D., & Davidson, J. R. T. (1997). Trauma: Prevalence, impairment, service use, and cost. *Journal of Clinical Psychiatry, 58,* 5–11.

Solomon, Z., Mikulincer, M., & Avitzur, E. (1988). Coping, locus of control, social support, and combat-related posttraumatic stress disorder: A prospective study. *Journal of Personality and Social Psychology, 55,* 279–285.

Solomon, Z., Mikulincer, M., & Flum, H. (1988). Negative life events, coping responses, and combat-related psychopathology: A prospective study. *Journal of Abnormal Psychology, 97,* 302–307.

Somasundaram, D. J., & Sivayokan, S. (1994). War trauma in a civilian population. *British Journal of Psychiatry, 165,* 524–527.

Sparr, L. F., & Pitman, R. K. (1998). Forensic assessment of traumatized adults. In P. Saigh & J. Bremner (Eds.), *Posttraumatic stress disorder: A comprehensive text* (pp. 284–308). Boston: Allyn & Bacon.

Spitzer, R. L., Williams, J. B. W., Kroenke, K., Linzer, M., deGruy, F. V. III, Hahn, S. R., Brody, D., & Johnson, J. G. (1994). Utility of a new procedure for diagnosing mental disorders in primary care: The PRIME-MD 1000 study. *Journal of the American Medical Association, 272,* 1749–1756.

Steinert, Y., & Rosenberg, E. (1987). Psychosocial problems: What do patients want? What do physicians want to provide? *Family Medicine, 19,* 346–350.

Steketee, G., & Foa, E. B. (1987). Rape victims: Post-traumatic stress responses and their treatment: A review of the literature. *Journal of Anxiety Disorders, 1,* 69–86.

Strosahl, K. (1997). Building primary care behavioral health systems that work: A compass and a horizon. In N. A. Cummings, J. L. Cummings, & J. N. Johnson (Eds.), *Behavioral health in primary care: A guide for clinical integration* (pp. 37–58). Madison, CT: Psychosocial Press/International Universities Press.

Sutker, P., Uddo-Crane, M., & Allain, A. N. (1991). Clinical and research assessment of posttraumatic stress disorder: A conceptual overview. *Psychological Assessment, 3,* 520–530.

Tarrier, N., Pilgrim, H., Sommerfield, C., Faragher, B., Reynolds, M., Graham, E., & Barrowclough, C. (1999). A randomized trial of cognitive therapy and imaginal exposure in the treatment of chronic posttraumatic stress disorder. *Journal of Consulting and Clinical Psychology, 67,* 13–18.

Vasquez-Barquero, J. L., Garcia, J., Simon, J. A., Iglesias, C., Montejo, J., Herran, A., & Dunn, G. (1997). Mental health in primary care: An epidemiological study of morbidity and use of health resources. *British Journal of Psychiatry, 170,* 529–535.

Von Korff, M., & Meyers, L. (1987). The primary care physician and psychiatric services. *General Hospital Psychiatry, 9,* 235–240.

Vrana, S., & Lauterbach, D. (1994) Prevalence of traumatic events and post-traumatic psychological symptoms in a nonclinical sample of college students. *Journal of Traumatic Stress, 7,* 289–302.

Ware, J. E., & Sherbourne, C. D. (1992). The MOS 36-item short-form health survey (SF–36): I. Conceptual framework and item selection. *Medical Care, 30,* 473–483.

Watson, C. G. (1990). Psychometric post-traumatic stress disorder techniques: A review. *Psychological Assessment, 2,* 460–469.

Watson, C. G., Juba, M. P., & Anderson, P. E. (1989). Validities of five combat scales. *Psychological Assessment, 1,* 98–102.

Watson, C. G., Juba, M. P., Manifold, V., Kucala, T., & Anderson, P. E. D. (1991). The PTSD Interview: Rationale, description, reliability, and concurrent validity of a DSM-III based technique. *Journal of Clinical Psychology, 47,* 179–188.

Weathers, F. W. (1996). Psychometric review of War-Zone Related PTSD Scale of the SCL-90-R. *Measurement of stress, trauma, and adaptation.* Lutherville, MD: Sidran Press.

Weathers, F. W., Blake, D. D., Krinsley, K. K., Haddad, W. H., Huska, J. A., & Keane, T. M. (1992, November). *The Clinician-Administered PTSD Scale: Reliability and construct validity.* Paper presented at the annual meeting of the Association for Advancement of Behavior Therapy, Boston, MA.

Weathers, F. W., & Keane, T. M. (1999). Psychological assessment of traumatized adults. In P. Saigh & J. D. Bremner (Eds.), *Posttraumatic stress disorder: A comprehensive approach to research and treatment* (pp. 219–247). Boston, MA: Allyn & Bacon.

Weathers, F. W., Keane, T. M., King, L. A., & King, D. W. (1997). Psychometric theory in the development of posttraumatic stress disorder assessment tools. In J. P. Wilson & T. M. Keane (Eds.), *Assessing psychological trauma and PTSD* (pp. 98–138). New York: Guilford Press.

Weathers, F. W., & Litz, B. T. (1994). Psychometric properties of the Clinician Administered PTSD Scale. *PTSD Research Quarterly, 5,* 2–6.

Weathers, F. W., Litz, B. T., Herman, D., Huska, J., & Keane, T. M. (1993, October). *The PTSD Checklist (PCL): Reliability, validity, and diagnostic utility.* Paper presented at the meeting of the International Society for Traumatic Stress Studies, San Antonio, TX.

Weathers, F. W., Litz, B. T., Huska, J. A., & Keane, T. M. (1991). *The PTSD Checklist (PCL).* Boston: National Center for PTSD/Boston VA Medical Center.

Weathers, F. W., Litz, B. T., Keane, T. M., Herman, D. S., Steinberg, H. R., Huska, J. A., & Kraemer, H. C. (1996). The utility of the SCL-90 for the diagnosis of posttraumatic stress disorder. *Journal of Traumatic Stress, 9,* 111–128.

Weathers, F. W., Ruscio, A. M., & Keane, T. M. (1999). Psychometric properties of nine scoring rules for the Clinician Administered Posttraumatic Stress Disorder Scale. *Psychological Assessment, 11,* 124–133.

Weaver, T. L., & Clum, G. A. (1993). Early family environments and traumatic experiences associated with borderline personality disorder. *Journal of Consulting and Clinical Psychology, 61,* 1068–1075.

Weiss, D. S., & Marmar, C. R. (1997). The Impact of Event Scale—Revised. In J. P. Wilson & T. M. Keane (Eds.), *Assessing psychological trauma and PTSD* (pp. 399–411). New York: Guilford Press.

Weiss, D. S., Marmar, C. R., Metzler, T. J., & Ronfeldt, H. M. (1995). Predicting symptomatic distress in emergency services personnel. *Journal of Consulting and Clinical Psychology, 63,* 361–368.

Weissman, M. M., Olfson, M., Leon, A. C., Broadhead, E., Gilbert, T. T., Higgins, E. S., Barrett, J. E., Blacklow, R. S., Keller, M. B., & Hoven, C. (1995). Brief diagnostic interviews (SDDS-PC) for multiple mental disorders in primary care: A pilot study. *Archives of Family Medicine, 4,* 220–227.

Wilson, J. P., & Keane, T. M. (Eds.). (1997). *Assessing psychological trauma and PTSD.* New York: Guilford Press.

Zatzick, D. F., Marmar, C. R., Weiss, D. S. Browner, W. S., Metzler, T. J., Golding, J. M., Stewart, A., Schlenger, W. E., & Wells, K. B. (1997). Posttraumatic stress disorder and functioning and quality of life outcomes in a nationally representative sample of male Vietnam veterans. *American Journal of Psychiatry, 154,* 1690–1695.

Zimmerman, M., & Mattia, J. I. (1999). Is posttraumatic stress disorder underdiagnosed in routine clinical settings? *Journal of Nervous and Mental Disease, 187,* 420–428.

8

Depression

David J. A. Dozois
Keith S. Dobson

Although the term "depression" is often used in the vernacular to refer to a transient and relatively mild negative mood state (i.e., dysphoria), clinical depression is a debilitating and pernicious cluster of symptoms that may persist for a period of weeks, months, or even years. This disorder is associated with significant cognitive, emotional, behavioral, somatic, and social impairments (American Psychiatric Association, 1994).

This chapter focuses on the assessment of major depression. As described in the current nomenclature, the *Diagnostic and Statistical Manual of Mental Disorders* (DSM-IV; American Psychiatric Association, 1994), major depressive disorder (MDD) is a heterogeneous syndrome that is characterized by either depressed mood or markedly diminished interest or pleasure in most activities. Additional symptoms listed in the DSM-IV include worthlessness or excessive guilt, suicidal ideation, attempted suicide or recurrent thoughts of death, psychomotor retardation or agitation, insomnia or hypersomnia, weight loss or weight gain, impaired concentration, indecisiveness or difficulty thinking, and loss of energy or fatigue. The diagnostic criteria for MDD require that a minimum of five out of nine symptoms be present and cause notable distress or impairment nearly every day for a period of at least 2 weeks. At least one of these symptoms must be either depressed mood or anhedonia.

Notwithstanding what is often the time-limited duration of a major depressive episode, the course of MDD appears to be chronic and recurrent across the lifespan. Clinically significant first-onset depression among never-depressed individuals is seemingly quite rare and is usually preceded by a series of subthreshold episodes (Coyne, Pepper, & Flynn, 1999; Horwath, Johnson, Klerman, & Weissman, 1992). For the vast majority of persons who experience major depressive episodes, the disorder is also recurrent. Between 50% and 85% of depressed patients experience multiple subsequent episodes (Coyne et al., 1999).

Despite the fact that only one in three depressed individuals seek formal treatment (Greenberg, Stiglin, Finkelstein, & Berndt, 1993), MDD is actually one of the most common presenting complaints encountered by mental health professionals (Zheng et al., 1997). The current prevalence rate is nearly 5%, and the lifetime prevalence rate is approximately 17% (Blazer, Kessler, McGonagle, & Swartz, 1994; Kessler et al., 1994). Women are approximately twice as likely as men to suffer from depression.

This chapter presents an empirical review of the various instruments that are available for the assessment of depression and provides practical assessment recommendations for clinicians. Even though we emphasize depression, most of our review and discussion is equally relevant to the assessment of dysthymia. We begin by describing some of the most commonly used instruments and reviewing their strengths and limitations. Following this review, we discuss a number of practical strategies for the assessment of depression; address the necessary integration among assessment, treatment planning, and outcome evaluation; and briefly highlight some of the issues and strategies for assessing depression in managed care and primary care settings.

AN EMPIRICAL EVALUATION OF ASSESSMENT MEASURES FOR DEPRESSION

Although assessment instruments may be categorized in a number of different ways, one broad distinction is between diagnostic and symptom severity measures. Another main discrimination among assessment instruments pertains to whether the evaluation information derives from the clinician or the patient. We have divided our review of assessment instruments according to this basic typology. We begin by examining clinician-determined and self-report indexes of diagnostic criteria and then evaluate clinician and self-ratings of symptom severity. A range of assessment methods are reviewed, and their defining features and their psychometric properties are described. Without reliable and valid assessment instruments and techniques, it would be extremely difficult to accurately assess the symptoms and severity of depression, determine targets for intervention, or evaluate treatment efficacy (Katz, Shaw, Vallis, & Kaiser, 1995).

Structured Diagnostic Interviews

Chapter 1 (Summerfeldt & Antony) in this volume reviews structured interviews in greater detail. Rather than reiterating these issues, we present briefly two of the most well known structured interviews used to date and discuss their appropriateness for the assessment of depression.

Structured Clinical Interview for DSM-IV Axis I Disorders (SCID-I)

The SCID-I (First, Gibbon, Spitzer, & Williams, 1996a; First, Spitzer, Gibbon, & Williams, 1997) is a semistructured interview that covers the spectrum of DSM-IV Axis I clinical syndromes. This instrument was designed to increase the reliability of diagnoses and improve differential diagnosis of mental health professionals who are already trained in conducting unstructured clinical interviews. There are two main versions of the SCID that focus on Axis I conditions. The clinician version includes diagnoses that are seen most frequently in clinical practice (i.e., mood disorders, psychotic disorders, substance use disorders, and anxiety disorders). This version is shorter than the research version that, in addition, covers somatoform disorders, eating disorders and adjustment disorders and includes course and severity specifiers. Each version permits the assessment of both current and lifetime mood disorders.

Before beginning the interview proper, individuals using the research version of the SCID administer 12 screening questions that are used to determine which modules of the SCID require further assessment. The SCID begins with an overview of the patient's presenting complaints and history. The interviewer then proceeds through the various required diagnostic modules until the interview is complete. Administration time typically ranges between 45 and 90 minutes. In our experience, the average interview usually takes under an hour to administer with depressed patients. However, the SCID may be more time-consuming, depending on the number of coexisting disorders present and the interviewee's general response style. The SCID includes numerous open-ended questions, as well as a skip structure that allows the interviewer to proceed through alternate diagnostic decision-trees, contingent upon the patients' responses (First, Gibbon, Spitzer, & Williams, 1996b). For each item, the interviewer makes a judgment about whether the symptom or criterion is present, absent, or subthreshold and whether adequate information is available with which to rate the item. Clinicians and researchers are also encouraged to use all available sources of information in making their ratings (e.g., referral notes, medical records, observations of significant others).

Reliability studies of diagnostic instruments are generally conducted by comparing the agreement among raters and calculating the kappa coefficient. This statistic allows one to assess the degree of concordance between ratings, controlling for chance levels of agreement. Kappa values $\geq$ .85 indicate excellent agreement between raters; .84 to .70 suggest good agreement; .69 to .40 denote marginally acceptable agreement; and coefficients < .40 suggest poor agreement. Because the SCID for DSM-IV is relatively new, there are few reliability data available specifically on this measure. However, a number of studies that have evaluated the earlier versions of the SCID (e.g., for DSM-III-R) suggest that several nosological categories yield moderate to excellent interrater reliability. Kappa coefficients range from .72 to .92 for general mood disorders and from .64 to .93 for major depression (Riskind, Beck, Berchick, Brown, & Steer, 1987; Segal, Hersen, & Van Hasselt, 1994; Skre, Onstad, Torgersen, & Kringlen, 1991; Spitzer, Williams, & Gibbon, & First, 1992; Williams et al., 1992). Williams et al. (1992) found acceptable to good agreement for mood disorders (kappa coefficients were .40, .64, and .84 for dysthymia, major depression, and bipolar disorder, respectively). Although poorer interrater agreement was obtained in nonpatient samples, this finding is not too surprising, given the relatively restricted range of scores on such research participants.

Because the SCID is derived from DSM-IV, its validity depends to a large extent on the validity of the DSM nosological system. Validity studies have indicated that the convergence between SCID-generated and clinician-rated diagnoses is somewhat lower than its interrater reliability (Dunner & Tay, 1993; Fennig, Craig, Lavelle, Kovasznay, & Bromet, 1994; Steiner, Tebes, Sledge, & Walker, 1995); however, there is no completely objective and infallible "gold standard" for psychiatric diagnosis available.

Schedule for Affective Disorders and Schizophrenia (SADS)

The SADS (Endicott & Spitzer, 1978; Spitzer & Endicott, 1975) represents one of the earliest attempts to reduce information variance and thus enhance the reliability of psychiatric assessment. This semistructured interview includes criteria on eight scales for differential diagnoses of mood disorders, schizophrenia, and a limited number of anxiety disorders. The SADS is designed to be administered in two parts. The first section emphasizes current symptomatology, while the second focuses on past episodes. The SADS predates the introduction, in DSM-III, of explicit diagnostic criteria for evaluating psychopathology; as such, diagnoses are made using the Research Diagnostic Criteria (Spitzer, Endicott, & Robins, 1978).

The SADS was developed for use by clinicians who are trained in psychiatric interviewing and psychopathology. The interviewer proceeds through specific questions and follow-up prompts to arrive at diagnoses, using a decision-tree model of diagnosis. Items are rated according to whether they are present or absent. Interviewers may also indicate that insufficient information was available to make such a determination. In addition to employing a dichotomous scoring format, some items are rated using Likert-type scales. There are four scales that assess various aspects of depression: depressed mood and cognition, neurovegetative features of depression, suicidal ideation, and associated features. A fifth scale assesses manic symptoms. The SADS also provides criteria for classifying 10 subtypes of major depressive disorder. To enhance diagnostic accuracy, clinicians and researchers are prompted to consult ancillary information from a range of sources (e.g., medical records, family).

This instrument has demonstrated high interrater reliability, especially for mood disorders. Matarazzo (1983) for instance, reported that the average weighted kappa coefficients across major diagnostic categories ranged from .75 to .95. Spitzer et al. (1978) and Simon, Endicott, and Nee (1987) reported kappas of .90 and .99, respectively, for major depressive disorder (MDD). The stability of lifetime major depressive episodes is more difficult to establish and may be suspect. Validity studies suggest that the SADS correlates in the expected directions with independent measures of depression, anxiety, and thought disorder (Johnson, Magaro, & Stern, 1986).

A 45-item form of the SADS (the SADS-C) allows clinicians to assess changes in a patient's clinical presentation over a period of a week or longer. The SADS-C takes approximately 20 minutes to complete (Altshuler, Post, & Fedio, 1991) and appears to be reliable, valid, and sensitive to treatment change (Basco, Krebaum, & Rush, 1997; Johnson et al., 1986).

Probably the greatest liability of the full SADS is its length. Administration time generally ranges between 90 and 120 minutes, which makes its use in clinical settings cumbersome and unlikely. Both this instrument and the SCID are also prohibitive in terms of their training requirements. In addition to being familiar with clinical interviewing and psychopathology, SADS and SCID training may involve several weeks. One of strengths of the SADS, however, is in making fine discriminations among different subtypes of mood disorder and schizophrenia. Both the SADS and the SCID are recommended for use in research studies, where diagnostic precision is often required.

Self-Administered Diagnostic Instruments

Inventory to Diagnose Depression (IDD)

The IDD (Zimmerman, Coryell, Corenthal, & Wilson, 1986) is a 22-item self-rating scale that was designed specifically for the diagnosis of MDD. Each item is rated on a 5-point scale, ranging from 0 (no disturbance) to 4 (severe), with a score of 2 or greater denoting the presence of a symptom. The time frame for the evaluation of the presence of a symptom is 1 week. A diagnostically meaningful feature of this instrument is that respondents are also asked to indicate the duration of each reported symptom (i.e., whether it has lasted more or less than 2 weeks). Twenty items are required to diagnose MDD; the remaining two items (anxiety and somatic complaints) are used to calculate the severity of the episode at its most acute point in time. This scale closely follows DSM-III criteria. However, since the changes between DSM-III and DSM-IV have not been substantial for major depression, the IDD likely remains applicable. The reliability of this scale appears to be good. Zimmerman et al. (1986) reported a split-half reliability of .93 and an alpha coefficient of .92. The item–total correlations were significant and ranged from .15 to .84. Test–retest reliability over a 2-day period was .98. In a college sample, Goldston, O'Hara, and Schartz (1990) found test–retest coefficients of .92 over 2 days and .56 over 2 weeks.

The IDD correlates significantly with related depression scales. Correlations with the Beck Depression Inventory (BDI; Beck, Steer, & Brown, 1996), the Hamilton Rating Scale for Depression (HRSD; Hamilton, 1960, 1967), and the Carroll Rating Scale for Depression (CRSD; Carroll, Feinberg, Smouse, Rawson, & Greden, 1981) were .87, .80, and .81, respectively. The IDD also appears to discriminate adequately among different levels of depressive severity and corresponds well to diagnoses based on the SCID (Sakado, Sato, Uehara, Sato, & Kameda, 1996; Uehara, Sato, Sakado, & Kameda, 1997), the SADS (Zimmerman et al., 1986), and the Diagnostic Interview Schedule (DIS; Zimmerman & Coryell, 1987, 1994). However, the IDD does occasionally identify individuals with anxiety disorders as having MDD (Sakado et al., 1996; Uehara et al., 1997), although this problem is not unique to this instrument (e.g., Haaga, McDermut, & Ahrens, 1993). Regardless of its fairly good diagnostic efficiency when compared to diagnoses derived from structured interviews, the IDD is not recommended to be used as the sole diagnostic tool. Rather, this instrument is intended to supplement more detailed diagnostic interviews.

Clinician Ratings of Symptomatology

There are over nine clinician-rating scales of depression (Nezu, Ronan, Meadows, & McClure, 2000). In this section we review the Hamilton Rating Scale for Depression and the Brief Psychiatric Rating Scale, as these instruments are the most well known, they are used extensively, and they have high research and clinical utility (Nezu et al., 2000).

Hamilton Rating Scale for Depression (HRSD)

The HRSD (Hamilton, 1960, 1967) is the most frequently used clinician-rating instrument of depressive severity. This 21-item scale was initially developed for use as an index of severity in individuals who already had been diagnosed with clinical depression. It has been used frequently in clinical trials, especially psychopharmacological outcome research.

The HRSD appears to be a valuable instrument for assessing depressive severity in both psychotherapy and pharmacotherapy outcome studies and in clinical outcome evaluation. Unfortunately, there are a number of versions of the HRSD (17-item, 21-item, 24-item, and 27-item versions), and investigators have not consistently specified which version was used in their studies. These factors have made comparison of the scale's psychometric properties difficult. If summary scores are presented, it is important for clinicians and researchers to report clearly which version of the HRSD they are using.

The original scale consisted of 21 items, only 17 of which were formally scored. Nine items were scored on a scale that ranged from 0 to 4, whereas eight items were scored from 0 to 2, with frequency and intensity of symptoms equally weighted (Basco et al., 1997). The remaining items (diurnal variation, depersonalization, obsessions/compulsions, and paranoia) were not used to calculate the severity of depression. Total scores range from 0 to 52, with scores between 7 and 17 reflecting mild depression, scores between 18 and 24 indicating moderate severity, and scores of 25 or higher signifying severe depression. Administration of the HRSD takes approximately 30 minutes, and the format involves an open-ended interview.

The HRSD focuses primarily on behavioral and somatic symptoms of depression and assesses symptoms such as early, middle, and late insomnia; psychomotor retardation; agitation; anxiety; loss of appetite and weight loss; and muscular aches and pains. In another version of this scale, three cognitive items (helplessness, hopelessness, worthlessness) were added.

This instrument appears to be reliable and sensitive to treatment change. Interrater agreement often exceeds .84 (Hedlund & Vieweg, 1979). Bech, Bolwig, Kramp, and Rafaelsen (1979) found that the item–total correlations ranged between –.02 and .81, suggesting that the homogeneity of the scale is moderate. In a sample of medical patients, Schwab, Bialow, and Holzer (1967) found item–total correlations that ranged from .45 to .78.

The correlation between the HRSD and other self-report measures of depressive symptomatology (Katz et al., 1995) and clinical ratings (Knesevich, Biggs, Clayton, & Ziegler, 1977) has been reported to be between .60 and .98. These findings lend support to the convergent validity of the HRSD; however, the concurrent validity of the HRSD has become more difficult to determine, largely because this instrument has become the measure to which others are compared. As such, it is difficult to know whether discrepancies with other instruments reflect poor psychometric properties of the HRSD or the instrument being compared (Rabkin & Klein, 1987).

There are fewer data available on the discriminant validity of the HRSD. The data that are available suggest that the HRSD differentiates well between psychiatric and nonpsychiatric persons, although specificity among patient groups is poorer. For example, the HRSD does not appear to clearly distinguish between depression and anxiety. This lack of specificity is likely due to the fact that the HRSD includes items explicitly related to anxiety.

The factorial validity of the HRSD has been supported in a number of studies. Generally, two reliable factors are extracted (Katz et al., 1995; Rabkin & Klein, 1987). One factor seems to represent general severity of depression, while the other constitutes a bipolar factor that ranges from retardation to agitation (Hedlund & Vieweg, 1979). In a sample of 370 patients who met Research Diagnostic Criteria for MDD, Gibbons, Clark, and Kupfer (1993) found that the HRSD measured five distinct factors, with only one of these (global depressive severity) being well defined and interpretable. The authors concluded that the total HRSD score may be a weaker index of depressive severity than is the factor score.

The HRSD appears to be a reliable instrument with well-documented research and clinical utility. Some of the limitations of the HRSD include (1) the emphasis on somatic items to the relative exclusion of mood and cognitive symptoms of depression; (2) the lack of data on its discriminant validity, and the fact that some items are confounded with other disorders (e.g., pain, anxiety); (3) differential item weightings (e.g., some items are scored 0 to 4 and others 0 to 2); and (4) a time frame that is incongruent with that in DSM-IV (i.e., a focus on the past week rather than the past 2 weeks). Despite its weaknesses, this measure continues to represent the state-of-the-art in terms of being an instrument to which others are compared. Most clinical research trials (e.g., Elkin et al., 1989) use the HRSD as a principal outcome measure. A revised version of the HRSD has recently been developed (see Nezu et al., 2000). Time will tell about the clinical and research utility of this revised measure of depression severity.

Brief Psychiatric Rating Scale (BPRS)

The BPRS (Overall & Gorman, 1962) was designed both to provide comprehensive coverage of the primary symptoms of a number of psychiatric conditions and to assess treatment change. Although the scale was initially intended for use with psychiatric inpatients (Rabkin & Klein, 1987), it has become one of the most frequently employed clinician-rating instruments for assessing symptom severity in schizophrenia and mood disorders (Faustman & Overall, 1999). To date, more than 1,900 studies have used this scale.

The BPRS is a clinician-rating scale that consists of 18 symptom constructs (e.g., somatic complaints; depressed mood; feelings of guilt, hostility, grandiosity). Depressed mood is rated on the basis of both expressed symptoms and behavioral observations. For example, verbalized pessimism, sadness, hopelessness, and discouragement are used to make a rating on this item. Crying and other methods of communicating one's mood state are also taken into account, but vegetative complaints (e.g., psychomotor retardation) are rated elsewhere on this scale. The original BPRS consisted of 16 constructs that were derived from other rating scales. Two items were later added to increase the classification rates (Faustman & Overall, 1999), and an expanded 24-item BPRS has also been developed recently (Dingemans, Linszen, Lenior, & Smeets, 1995). Symptom constructs are scored on 7-point Likert-type scales, ranging from 1 (not present) to 7 (extremely severe). Six of the items are rated on the basis of the patient's behavior as observed during the interview (e.g., mannerisms, motor retardation), and the remaining 12 are rated based primarily on the content of the interview. The BPRS is scored by summing the 18 items.

This instrument was developed to be used by trained professionals in conjunction with an informal clinical interview (Faustman & Overall, 1999). Thus, although there are sample questions available for assessing each construct (Rhoades & Overall, 1988) there are no mandatory questions for this scale. The data required to make the appropriate ratings may be collected in approximately 10 minutes during a 20- to 30-minute routine clinical interview. The BPRS lacks normative information, but Faustman and Overall (1999) suggested that this lack is because it was not developed for the purpose of making clinical decisions but for assessing treatment-related changes. Several studies have reported high interrater reliability (e.g., .85; Hedlund & Vieweg, 1980). In addition, a number of studies that have evaluated the validity of the BPRS indicate that it provides an accurate assessment of various symptoms, is sensitive to symptom changes, and correlates highly with other clinical scales (for a review, see Faustman & Overall, 1999). Unfortunately, most of this research has been conducted with individuals diagnosed with schizophrenia.

The main limitation of the BPRS for specifically assessing depression is that fewer than half of the items are especially relevant to depression, while the others are related to thought disorder (e.g., disorientation, hallucinations, grandiosity) (Rabkin & Klein, 1987). One advantage of the BPRS is that it allows for the rapid and reliable assessment of a number of clinical symptoms and syndromes. Most clinicians interested in specifically assessing depression will likely want to use the HRSD or its revision, but the BPRS permits a broader picture of psychopathology and may be helpful in assessing the severity of comorbid conditions and complaints.

Self-Report Measures of Symptomatology

Approximately 25 self-report measures of the severity of depression have been identified in the literature. Of these questionnaires, 17 were specifically developed to measure depressive symptoms, mood, and/or severity in adults populations, whereas 8 were created for use with special populations (e.g., depression in schizophrenia, depression in children, depression in primary care settings) (Nezu et al., 2000). Nezu et al. (2000) rated each available measure of depression in terms of both its clinical and research utility. A rating of "high" was assigned to instruments that were frequently and meaningfully used in research or practice. Self-report questionnaires were rated of "limited" value if they were either not frequently used in clinical settings or were prohibitive in terms of the cost or time required. A rating of "limited" was designated for research utility if, in the opinion of the editors, there was insufficient empirical data related to the instrument. Table 8.1 highlights the adult-focused self-report instruments that were rated positively in terms of *both* research and clinical utility (see Nezu et al., 2000, for a more detailed review).

Notwithstanding the number of self-report measures of depressed mood and symptoms, only a few have achieved widespread acceptance and use. As such, we review here

TABLE 8.1. Self-Report Assessment Instruments with High Clinical and High Research Utility

Instrument	No. of items	Format	Time needed (minutes)	User fee?	Reference
Beck Depression Inventory–II	21	4-point	5–10	Yes	Beck, Steer, & Brown (1996)
Carroll Rating Scale for Depression—Revised	61	Yes/no	5–10	Yes	Carroll (1998)
Depression Anxiety Stress Scales	42	4-point	10–20	Yes	Lovibond & Lovibond (1995)
Depression Questionnaire	24	Yes/no	20	No	Sanavio et al. (1988)
Hamilton Depression Inventory[a]	23	3- and 4-point	10–15	Yes	Kobak & Reynolds (1999)
Hopelessness Depression Symptom Questionnaire	32	4-point	10	Yes	Metalsky & Joiner (1997)
Inventory of Depressive Symptomatology[b]	30	4-point	30–45	No	Rush, Gullion et al. (1996)
IPAT Depression Scale	36	3-point	10–20	Yes	Krug & Laughlin (1976)
Multiscore Depression Inventory for Adolescents and Adults	118	True/false	20–25	Yes	Berndt (1986)
Positive and Negative Affect Scales	20	5-point	5	Yes	Watson et al. (1988)
Primary Care Evaluation of Mental Disorders (PRIME-MD)	26	Yes/no	5–10	No	Spitzer et al. (1993)
Profile of Mood States	65	5-point	3–5	Yes	McNair et al. (1992)
Revised HRSD Self-Report Problem Inventory	76	True/false	10–20	Yes	Warren (1994)
Reynolds Depression Screening Inventory[a]	19	Varies	5–10	Yes	Reynold & Kobak (1998)
State–Trait Depression Adjective Checklist	34	Yes/no	3	Yes	Lubin (1994)
Zung Self-Rating Depression Scale	20	4-point	5	No	Zung (1965)

Note. Adapted from Nezu, Ronan, Meadows, and McClure (2000). Copyright 2000 by Kluwer Academic/Plenum Publishers. Adapted by permission.
[a]These instruments were rated high on clinical utility, but their research utility is presently unknown, although promising.
[b]This instrument is also available in a clinician-rated form.

four of the most commonly cited self-report measures of depression: the Beck Depression Inventory–II (BDI-II), the Zung Self-Rating Depression Scale (ZSDS), the Carroll Rating Scale for Depression (CRSD), and the Center for Epidemiological Studies Depression Scale (CES-D).

Beck Depression Inventory–II (BDI-II)

The BDI-II (Beck, Steer, & Brown, 1996) is a 21-item questionnaire that is presented in a multiple-choice format. Each item is scored 0 to 3 in terms of intensity, with total scores ranging from 0 to 63. Both the BDI-II and its predecessor (Beck, Ward, Mendelson, Mock, & Erbaugh, 1961; Beck, Rush, Shaw, & Emery, 1979; Beck, Steer, & Brown, 1996) were designed to measure the presence and severity of depressive symptomatology, in both normal populations and psychiatrically diagnosed patients (Beck, Steer, & Garbin, 1988; Steer, Clark, Beck, & Ranieri, 1998). This instrument has been accepted as one of the better self-report measures of depression and has been employed extensively in both research and practice. In fact, the BDI consistently falls within the "top 10" of the most frequently used psychological tests (Camara, Nathan, & Puente, 2000).

The original BDI has demonstrated adequate internal consistency, test–retest reliability, construct validity, and factorial validity (see Beck et al., 1988 for a review). As a result of problems noted with its content validity (e.g., the BDI measured only decreases in appetite, weight, and sleep rather than reversed vegetative symptoms; its coverage included only six of nine DSM-IV diagnostic criteria), a number of changes were made to the BDI to make it more congruent with DSM nosology. There were 23 item changes in total (4 items were deleted, the wording of 17 response options was altered, and 2 items were moved to another location in the new inventory). The BDI-II also differs from its predecessor in that the time frame was extended from 1 week to 2 weeks, consistent with the diagnostic criteria for depression in DSM-IV (see Beck, Steer, Ball, & Ranieri, 1996). Although this instrument is not intended as a diagnostic tool and never should be used as such, the BDI-II now covers all of the DSM-IV symptom criteria.

The BDI-II may be completed in 5 to 10 minutes. The following cutoff scores were recommended in the manual: 0 to 13, "minimal depression"; 14 to 19, mild depression; 20 to 28, "moderate depression"; and, 29 to 63, "severe depression." Because the BDI-II is frequently used to study vulnerability to depression in analogue samples, it is worth noting that slightly different cutoffs have been recommended for undergraduate samples (see Dozois, Dobson, & Ahnberg, 1998).

Internal consistency (coefficient alpha) of the BDI ranges from .73 to .95, and test–retest reliability has been reported to be above .90 (Beck et al., 1988).The BDI-II also has demonstrated high internal consistency (alpha = .91–.93 among college students; alpha = .92 among outpatients) (Beck, Steer, & Brown, 1996; Dozois et al., 1998; Steer, Kumar, Ranieri, & Beck, 1998. One-week test–retest reliability of the BDI-II is .93 (Beck, Steer, & Brown, 1996). The convergent validity of the BDI-II is supported by significant correlations with other indices of depression, including a correlation of .93 with the earlier version of this instrument. The BDI-II correlates .71 with the HRSD (Beck, Steer, & Brown, 1996). This instrument is also more highly associated with the Depression subscale of the Symptom Check List-90—Revised (.89) than the Anxiety subscale of the same instrument (.71) (Steer, Ball, Ranieri, & Beck, 1997). One of the criticisms of the BDI-II that probably generalizes to all depression instruments (see Gotlib & Cane, 1989) is that this instrument does not discriminate adequately between depression and anxiety.

Earlier factor-analytic studies of the BDI revealed that a three-factor solution (Negative AttitudesToward Self, Performance Impairment, Somatic Disturbance) was most frequently identified in the literature (Beck et al., 1988). However, a stable factor solution was not consistently found across studies and samples, as the number of factors extracted in various studies ranged anywhere from 1 to 7 (see Beck et al., 1988). Studies thus far conducted seem to indicate that stronger factor structure exists for the BDI-II (Beck, Steer, & Brown, 1996; Dozois et al., 1998; Steer, Ball, Ranieri, & Beck, 1999; Steer, Clark et al., 1998). Across psychiatric and nonpsychiatric samples, two main factors appear to emerge consistently. One of these factors refers to cognitive symptoms, and the other refers to somatic and affective components of depression.

Many of the limitations of the BDI appear to have been resolved with the 1996 revision. The BDI-II has numerous strengths that make it an excellent choice for both research and practice. These strengths include the BDI-II's consistency with DSM-IV criteria, its strong psychometric properties, the ease of use and administration, its sensitivity to treatment change, and its large empirical database with which to compare results.

Zung Self-Rating Depression Scale (ZSDS)

The ZSDS (Zung, 1965) is a 20-item self-report measure of depressive symptomatology. This instrument was designed to provide a quantitative assessment of the various affective (2 items—crying, feeling downhearted), somatic (8 items; e.g., retardation, tachycardia), and psychological (10 items; e.g., irritability, dissatisfaction) components of depression. Respondents are instructed to rate each item in terms of how much of the time each statement describes them during the past number of days. The anchors provided for each item are "a little," "some," "a good part," and "most of the time." Each item is scored on a 4-point scale, for a total possible score of 80. Of the 20 items, 10 are reverse keyed and scored, in that a negative answer indicates the presence of a symptom (e.g., "Morning is when I feel best"). The remaining items are symptomatically positive (e.g., "I feel downhearted and blue"). Administration time is approximately 10 to 15 minutes.

Scoring involves summing the total of the 20 items. A depression index (obtained score divided by the total possible score) may also be generated. This index may range between .25 and 1.00. The following cutoff scores are recommended for interpretation of the summary scores: less than 50, normal; 50 to 59, mild depression; 60 to 69, moderate to marked depression; 70 or greater, severe depression. A cutoff score of 50 results in a correct classification rate of 88% (sensitivity = 88%; specificity = 88%) (Basco et al., 1997). Most people with depression achieve scores between 50 and 69.

Surprisingly, given its long history of clinical and research use, few data exist to address the reliability of this instrument. The internal consistency of the ZSDS appears to be adequate with a split-half (odd/even) reliability of .94 (Gabrys & Peters, 1985). Internal consistency is also high, with a coefficient alpha of .79 to .88 (Gabrys & Peters, 1985; Knight, Waal-Manning, & Spears, 1983). The ZSDS correlates moderately with other depression instruments, including the BDI, the HRSD, the Geriatric Depression Scale, and the Centre for Epidemiological Studies—Depression Scale (described below) (Dunn & Sacco, 1989; Faravelli, Albanesi, & Poli, 1986; Plutchik & van Praag, 1987; Schotte, Maes, Cluydts, & Cosyns, 1996). In contrast to the strong convergent validity of the ZSDS, its discriminant validity is more suspect. Although the ZSDS appears to distinguish between depressed and nonpsychiatric individuals (Gabrys & Peters, 1985), it is less able to differentiate between depression and anxiety (e.g., Schotte et al., 1996) or between different severity levels of the depressive syndrome (Rabkin & Klein, 1987).

Factor-analytic studies of the ZSDS have identified between one and seven factors. The factor scores do not, however, appear to provide incremental utility over the ZSDS total score (Rabkin & Klein, 1987). Schotte and associates (1996) have recently questioned the construct validity of the ZSDS. These researchers challenged empirically the assumption that positively and negatively worded items tap the same construct. In a sample of 338 depressed patients, Schotte et al. found that the reverse scoring on the ZSDS resulted in an inflation of average item scores. In addition, the effects of phrasing items in this manner strongly influenced the resultant factor structure of the ZSDS. Most symptom-negative and symptom-positive items loaded on separate factors. Although these findings are not unique to the ZSDS, they cast doubt on its construct validity as a measure of depressive symptoms. In other words, the factor structure may, at least in part, represent a semantic differential (i.e., positive vs. negative) rather than assessing mood and psychomotor components of depression.

Despite its popularity, a number of authors have suggested that the ZSDS may not be the most appropriate instrument for assessing depressive severity or treatment change (Altshuler et al., 1991; Basco et al., 1997; Gotlib & Cane, 1989). We agree with this general conclusion. Among the most cogent criticisms are its limited usefulness at discriminating between levels of depression (e.g., depressed inpatients, moderately depressed day hospital patients, less severe outpatients), its dubious construct validity, and the paucity of psychometric information. Given its classification rates, it is possible that the ZSDS may be useful for screening depression. It may also be used in conjunction with a more psychometrically sound instrument such as the BDI-II. Although high correlations have been found between the ZSDS and the BDI (Plutchik & van Praag, 1987), these instruments may each provide complementary information. For instance, the BDI-II focuses on the intensity of depressive symptoms, while the ZSDS emphasizes their frequency.

Carroll Rating Scale for Depression (CRSD)

The CRSD (Carroll, Feinberg, Smouse, Rawson, & Greden, 1981) is a 52-item self-report measure of the severity of depressive symptoms. The items are primarily behavioral and somatic in content. At least two and up to four items assess each of the following constructs: depression, guilt, suicide, initial insomnia, middle insomnia, delayed insomnia, work and interests, retardation, agitation, psychological anxiety, somatic anxiety, gastrointestinal, general somatic, libido, hypochondriasis, loss of insight, and loss of weight. Each item is presented in a "yes"/"no" self-descriptive format (e.g., "I get hardly anything done lately"), and respondents are instructed to rate their symptoms based on how they felt over the previous few days. Items are rated dichotomously, either present or absent, with total scores ranging from 0 to 52. Twelve of the 52 items are reverse-scored to control for acquiescent response styles. This instrument takes approximately 20 minutes to complete. Scores greater than 10 are suggestive of clinically significant depression.

One objective in the development of the CRSD was to minimize the discrepancies among clinician ratings and self-report scores. This instrument was specifically designed to correspond to the HRSD. Carroll et al. (1981) found moderate correlations between each item on the CRSD and the parallel HRSD item (median $r = .60$; range $= -.06$ to .73). This correlation matrix indicated that there is only modest correspondence between these two measures at the individual item level. However, the CRSD and the HRSD total scores correlated at .80. Thus, depending on one's assessment needs, the CRSD may be used to supplement the HRSD.

Internal consistency estimates (split-half reliability) are .87 for odd/even item comparisons and .97 for first/last items. Item–total correlations range between .05 and .78 (median $= .55$). Convergent validity of the CRSD is supported by studies showing that its total scores correlate significantly with other conceptually similar indices (e.g., correlations with the HRSD ranged from .66 to .85; and with the BDI they were .86) (Carroll et al., 1981). The CRSD is able to accurately classify the severity of depression in low to moderately severe depression; however, as depression intensifies, it tends to overestimate depressive severity (Katz et al., 1995; Shaver & Brennan, 1991).

One advantage of the CRSD is that because its items are similar to the HRSD, it may permit a more direct comparison between clinician and patient ratings. With 52 items, it is somewhat longer and more complex to score than other self-report measures of the severity of depression. More recently, a self-report version of the HRSD has been developed; it serves the same purpose as the CRSD and exhibits excellent psychometric properties (see Kobak & Reynolds, 1999). The CRSD itself has also recently been revised and now includes 61 items (see Nezu et al., 2000, for review).

Center for Epidemiological Studies Depression Scale (CES-D)

The CES-D (Radloff, 1977) is a brief self-report measure that was developed specifically for the identification of depression in the general community. The CES-D items were derived from previously established instruments, including the BDI, the ZSDS, and the Minnesota Multiphasic Personality Inventory (MMPI; Hathaway & McKinley, 1983). This instrument consists of 20 items that measure the frequency of depressive symptomatology. Respondents rate, on a 4-point (0 to 3) scale, how often they experienced each symptom over the past week, from "rarely" (i.e., less than once per day) to "most of the time" (i.e., 5 to 7 days). Total scores may range from 0 to 60, with 16 being the recommended cutoff characteristic of significant depressive symptomatology. In contrast to the other self-report measures described here, which tend to have more comprehensive assessment of different depressive symptoms, the emphasis of the CES-D is on depressed mood (Radloff, 1977).

The reliability and validity of the CES-D appear to be good. Radloff (1977) reported a coefficient alpha of .90 and .85 for patients and nonpatients, respectively. Test–retest reliability over 6 months was .54 (Radloff, 1977). Similar findings have been reported in older (Lewinsohn, Seeley, Roberts, & Allen, 1997) and younger (Roberts, Andrews, Lewinsohn, & Hops, 1990) populations. The CES-D has been found to correlate significantly with other indices of depressive symptomatology, which indicates that its convergent validity is acceptable. The construct validity of the CES-D is also supported by its consistent factor structure. Four factors generally emerge in factor analyses of the CES-D: dysphoria, well-being, somatic complaints and interpersonal difficulties (Radloff, 1977; Hertzog, Van Alstine, Usala, Hultsch, & Dixon, 1990; Knight, Williams, McGee, & Olaman, 1997; Zich, Attkisson, & Greenfield, 1990). The well-being or positive affect factor, however, may be related to the fact that some of the items are positively worded.

Given that a main purpose of the CES-D was to screen for depression, a number of investigators have also examined its operating characteristics, including sensitivity (the ability of the instrument to correctly detect individuals with the disorder), specificity (the ability of the instrument to correctly identify individuals without the disorder), and positive predictive power (the number of individuals identified by the test as depressed who are diagnosed as depressed). The CES-D has good sensitivity, but its specificity and positive predictive value are unsatisfactory. Several studies have found that the CES-D overestimates the prevalence of depression with the threshold set at a score of 16 (Fechner-Bates, Coyne, & Schwenk, 1994; Santor & Coyne, 1997; Santor, Zuroff, Ramsey, Cervantes, & Palacios, 1995). Fechner-Bates et al. (1994) found that one-fifth of individuals who were diagnosed as depressed according to the SCID were not so identified by the CES-D. In addition, 72% of individuals with elevated scores on the CES-D did not meet diagnostic criteria. Because the purpose of the CES-D is to provide an initial screen of depressive symptoms that can later be monitored more closely, this low sensitivity and poor positive predictive power may not pose too much of a problem. Screening instruments are intended to maximize sensitivity so that "true positives" (i.e., individuals who actually meet diagnostic criteria) will not be missed. However, clinicians should be aware that this instrument produces a large number of "false positives" (i.e., individuals who are identified as meeting criteria, when in fact they do not) and may wish to adjust the cutoff scores to optimally correspond to the base rate of depression in their setting.

One limitation of the CES-D is that its items do not cover all of the DSM-IV criteria. Zimmerman & Coryell (1994) also noted that several of the CES-D items (e.g., "I felt fearful" and "People were unfriendly") do not coincide with the diagnostic criteria for MDD, which reduces its specificity for clinical depression. Another limitation is that at least two of the CES-D items ("I had crying spells" and "I talked less than usual") contain possible gender bias (Stommel et al., 1993). Finally, the recommended cutoff score results in an overestimation of depression. Notwithstanding these liabilities, the CES-D remains a popular instrument.

Collateral Areas of Assessment

Although space limits prohibit a description all of the collateral areas of assessment in depression, it is important to point out that many other measures than those discussed here are available. All these instruments assess related aspects of depression, including interpersonal processes and relatedness, social support, coping styles, life events, degree of functional impairment, and readiness for change. We have identified three main instruments that are particularly useful for assessment using cognitive-behavioral approaches.

Beck Hopelessness Scale (BHS)

The presence of suicidal ideation and suicide risk is an important factor to consider with depressed samples. The BHS (Beck & Steer, 1988) is a 20-item ("true"/"false") self-report scale that measures the degree to which an individual is pessimistic about his or her future. Scores range from 0 (no hopelessness) to 20 (extreme hopelessness). To control for acquiescent response styles, 11 items are positively keyed and 9 items are negatively keyed. Administration time is approximately 5 minutes.

Empirical research supports a strong positive relationship between BHS scores and indices of suicidal ideation and intent, as well as between scores on this instrument and depression (Canon et al., 1999). This instrument has high internal consistency (coefficient alphas range from .84 to .93) (Hill, Gallagher, Thompson, & Ishida, 1988). Test–retest reliability over a period of 1 and 6 weeks has been reported to be .69 and .66, respectively. This instrument also demonstrates excellent content, concurrent, discriminative, and construct validity. For example, the BHS is positively related to dysfunctional cognition, poor problem-solving skills, and greater severity of depression, and it is believed to be the best single predictor of present suicide risk (Canon et al., 1999).

Dysfunctional Attitude Scale (DAS)

The DAS (Weissman & Beck, 1978) was designed to measure the "silent assumptions"—dysfunctional cognitions and maladaptive beliefs—that depressed individuals tend to exhibit. This instrument consists of 40 statements that reflect measures of conditional worth (e.g., "It is impossible for me to be happy unless I have the respect and admiration of those around me") that are scored using a 1 (totally agree) to 7 (totally disagree) Likert-type scale. Some items are reverse-scored.

Norms exist for both student samples and clinically depressed patients (Beck, Brown, Steer, & Weissman, 1991). Coefficient alphas range from .88 to .97, and a 6-week test–retest reliability coefficient of .73 has been reported. The DAS correlates moderately with the BDI ($r = .41$), and several studies attest to its ability to differentiate reliably between depressed and nondepressed groups. Factor-analytic studies have generally revealed two main factors that reflect beliefs surrounding affiliative and achievement needs. This measure also appears to be sensitive to changes in depressed mood via psychotherapy.

Automatic Thoughts Questionnaires

The Automatic Thoughts Questionnaire—Negative ATQ-N (Hollon & Kendall, 1980) is a 30-item questionnaire that assesses the frequency of automatic negative thoughts. Each item is rated on a 5-point scale (1, "not at all," to 5, "all the time"). This instrument has excellent psychometric properties (e.g., coefficient alpha = .96) and has been shown to differentiate significantly between depressed and nondepressed groups.

In addition to being associated with a preponderance of negative thinking, depression is also frequently characterized by a deficit in positive thinking. This lack of positive thinking appears to be specific to depression (Dozois & Dobson, 2001). Thus, the assessment of positive cognition may also be important as an outcome measure. The Automatic Thoughts Questionnaire—Positive (ATQ-P; Ingram & Wisnicki, 1988) is a 30-item (1 to 5) questionnaire that assesses the frequency of automatic positive self-statements. Like the ATQ-N, this instrument has strong psychometric properties (Ingram, Kendall, Siegle, Guarino, & McLaughlin, 1995). The ATQ-P is the most widely used measure of positive cognition in studies of depression (Ingram, Slater, Atkinson, & Scott, 1990).

PRACTICAL RECOMMENDATIONS FOR THE ASSESSMENT OF DEPRESSION

Beyond being familiar with the various available quantitative instruments, there are a number of practical issues that a practitioner needs to consider in the assessment of depression. We begin by focusing on various aspects of the clinical interview, including the clinician's demeanor, important variables to assess during the interview, behavioral observations, and differential diagnosis. Following this overview, we discuss some ways to optimize one's assessment strategies, provide a sample assessment battery, and highlight some of the more complicated factors related to the assessment and diagnosis of depression.

The Clinical Interview

Much of the information necessary for the assessment of depression results from the clinical interview. Aside from a solid background in psychopathology and adequate training in interviewing skills, several basic considerations are particularly pertinent to evaluating depressed patients. First, it is important to set the stage. Patients feel more comfortable and are more willing to discuss their problems if they have a clear understanding of what they will be doing and what is required of them throughout the assessment phase. Depressed individuals tend to be particularly sensitive to being interrupted, so warning them of this possibility early in the interview and providing a rationale will help reduce the possible negative impact. For example, the clinician can state that certain information is required in a limited amount of time to understand the patient's problems, determine what is wrong, and generate a optimal treatment options.

An interviewer's style will obviously vary, depending on his or her own personal preferences and personality, as well as on the patient's current state (e.g., agitated versus tearful). Regardless of one's style, it is important to make the patient feel relaxed and to allow him or her sufficient time to reflect on and respond to the interviewer's questions. Severely depressed patients may experience psychomotor retardation as a symptom of depression, so it is particularly important for the interviewer not to rush the interview process with this type of patient. After explaining the assessment process, it is often helpful to begin the interview by asking the patient to explain in his or her own words the presenting complaints and what the experience of depression has been like for him or her. Throughout the assessment interview, it is also beneficial to check on the accuracy of the patient's report. Depressed individuals frequently exhibit negative biases (e.g., Beck et al., 1979) that may influence the clinician's appraisal of the degree of impairment and distress that is present. Consequently, it is important to conduct a thorough functional analysis of the patient's daily routines to obtain a clear idea of the amount of actual impairment that is evident. The clinician should focus on specific details of a patient's symptomatology, such as its frequency, duration, and intensity. This information is also useful after treatment is initiated to assess therapeutic efficacy.

A number of salient variables and areas of functioning should be evaluated during the initial assessment interview. The main variables that need to be assessed are the major systems that are affected in major depression (i.e., affective, cognitive, behavioral, somatic, social). It is important to gain a clear understanding of the severity of each symptom domain. Quantitative evaluation of this information will best come from the psychometric instruments reviewed; however, it is helpful to obtain qualitative descriptions of the symptoms from the patient's life. For instance, it is not enough to simply ask whether the patient has experienced loss of interest. A more lucid picture of symptom severity and functional impairment would stem from ascertaining what kinds of things a patient used to be interested in and has now lost interest in. Similarly, the assessment of anhedonia should be conducted using a number of related questions: "What kinds of things do you like to do when you are not working?" "Do you have any hobbies or activities that you enjoy?" "Do you enjoy reading or watching television?" "Have you been able to get out of the house and socialize?" "Do you enjoy socializing?" The same general rule applies to the assessment of each of the symptom criteria (see Shea, 1988). In addition to assessing each diagnostic criterion in a variety of ways, it is also useful to be aware of the colloquial variants that patients use to describe their symptoms (Murphy, Monson, Laird, Sobol, & Leighton, 2000). Patients may also describe their experiences and symptoms in vague or idiosyncratic ways, and it is the clinician's responsibility to translate these descriptions into the language of our current nosological system. For some of the more externally apparent symptoms (e.g., psychomotor retardation, concentration difficulties), it is often useful to determine whether other individuals had noticed them as well. With the patient's consent, briefly interviewing a significant other can provide important corroborative information and clarify ambiguity regarding symptom severity and functional impairment.

A depressed patient may perceive his or her impediments to be far worse than others might perceive them to be (see Katz et al., 1995). Procuring a detailed review of a patient's symptoms and presenting complaints not only helps in making appropriate diagnoses and treatment recommendations, it also conveys messages that the interviewer is interested in the patient and knowledgeable about the symptoms and difficulties that he or she is experiencing. Other areas worthy of thorough assessment are the frequency of depressive episodes and the number of past episodes. This information is particularly meaningful because the duration of an episode and the number of previous episodes relate to the speed of recovery (Rush et al., 1993) and to the risk of subsequent relapse (Soloman et al., 2000). However, the clinician should be suspect of this information, as unintentional memory biases may occur. Bromet, Dunn, Connell, Dew, and Schulberg (1986), for instance, found that even when patients were reliable reporters about most details of their disorder, they were frequently inconsistent about the age of first episode, the duration of the longest episode, and the past number of episodes. One way in which the clinician may reduce symptom reporting biases is to ensure that the patient understands which time frame is being referred to. When reviewing the DSM-IV criteria for a major depressive episode, for example, it is helpful to periodically remind the patient that you are referring to the presence and intensity of symptoms over the past 2 weeks. The reliability and validity of information about past episodes may also be enhanced by providing contextual cues to a patient's memory, such as relating the onset of symptoms to certain dates or special occasions or holidays (Shea, 1988).

Past treatments and their effectiveness, medical history, factors maintaining depression, and the patient's motivation for change are also essential variables to consider during the assessment interview. It is important to assess previous treatments, including hospitalizations, outpatient psychotherapy, medications, previous ECT, current treatment, past diagnoses, and self-help groups or products that may or may not have been useful. This information can be extremely valuable to help identify resources for change and overcome future treatment obstacles. Similarly, a detailed review of a patient's family history provides valuable clues as to diagnosis and what treatment(s) might be successful with a particular patient. It is also helpful to assess an individual's strengths (coping that has previously worked, social support, etc.) to capitalize on these forces in treatment.

The potential for suicide and a review of other areas of psychopathology (e.g., alcohol and drug abuse history) should also be addressed. Because completed suicide has such a low base rate of occurrence, assessing risk is extremely difficult. On the other hand, it is not sufficient to simply ask a patient if he or she is suicidal, although open and frank questioning is effective. Clinicians also need to be cognizant of potential risk factors (e.g., hopelessness, impulsivity, substance abuse, having a mental disorder, physical illness—especially if it results in pain, disfigurement, loss of mobility, social isolation, etc.) (Shea, 1988) and more immediate suicide indicators (e.g., specific plan, time frame, means). A recent survey of 220 psychologists revealed eight critical risk factors for suicide (Peruzzi & Bongar, 1999). These variables included the medical gravity of previous attempts, a history of suicide attempts, acute ideation, seeing death as attractive, a family history of suicide, current alcohol abuse, and recent loss. Several other factors (e.g., depressive turmoil, cognitive rigidity, and loneliness) were rated as moderately important to the prediction of suicide risk. Psychometric instruments such as the Beck Hopelessness Scale may also be beneficial for documenting risk. However, the clinician should be aware that these instruments necessarily yield a high number of false positives. Given the low base rate for completion of suicide, the clinician is sometimes required to rely on his or her own intuition and experience rather than on actuarial data. Therefore a "mental factor-analysis" of risk factors, self-report scores, and the results of direct questioning is often necessary. Because hopelessness and the risk of suicide are part of the nature of depression, clinicians working in this area are strongly recommended to be familiar with local laws and procedures regarding involuntary hospitalization.

In addition to obtaining content-oriented information, it is also important for clinicians to be aware of some of the behavioral indices of depression that may be evident during the assessment process. In particular, it is important for clinicians to attend to the patient's appearance, movements, and mannerisms. Research has shown that depressed individuals make less eye contact; demonstrate slower speech; and exhibit fewer hand, head, and body movements during conversation than nonpsychiatric controls (e.g., Schelde, 1998). Depressed persons also tend to show decreased social interaction and increased self-occupation. Many of these behaviors have also been shown to improve with remission. Schelde (1998) found that increased social interest and initiative, smiles, raised eyebrows, nods, and laughter were associated with recovery.

When a patient complains of depression, it is important for the clinician to examine the possibility of other psychiatric and medical conditions. Depression is frequently associated with dysthymia, cyclothymia, anxiety disorders, personality disorders (e.g., borderline, dependent, and histrionic personality disorders), various medical conditions (e.g., hypothyroidism, myocardial infarct, and stroke), substance abuse, and adjustment disorders (see Stefanis & Stefanis, 1999). Assessing various comorbid conditions has important implications for diagnosis and for treatment planning. For example, depressive individuals frequently abuse substances, and a clinician needs to be aware of this potential obstacle to ensure that it does not undermine the treatment of depression. It is also important to distinguish major depression from an adjustment disorder with depressed mood, and both of these from uncomplicated bereavement. All three of these problems share symptoms of depression. Clinicians should also evaluate the possibility of past or current mania during the intake assessment and monitor this periodically over the course of treatment and follow-up. Simon et al. (1987) found that 2% to 3% of patients switch from unipolar to bipolar disorder. When the interview focuses on the negative aspects of the patient's experience, it becomes quite easy for clinicians to neglect to assess for mania.

The optimal strategy to accurately diagnose depression and to make differential diagnoses is through the use of structured interviews. However, if time does not permit the use of, for instance, the SCID, then the clinician may opt to conduct a clinical interview. This interview could be followed by specific relevant modules from a structured interview and then from clinician-rating scales and self-report measures that are most pertinent to the patient's presenting complaint(s).

Choosing Optimal Assessment Strategies

In addition to the clinical interview, an accurate assessment of depression requires a thorough review of specific symptoms using multiple strategies for assessment (i.e., structured and unstructured interviews, clinician ratings, and self-report inventories), and ideally these are obtained from multiple perspectives (e.g., patient, significant others, clinician, employer). Table 8.2 presents a sample assessment battery that may be used throughout the various stages of assessment. In addition to assessing depressive symptoms and diagnostic criteria (DSM-IV inclusion criteria), it is also crucial to rule out other variables (DSM-IV exclusion criteria). For instance, it is critical to ensure that a comprehensive enough physical evaluation is conducted to rule out depression that may be due to substances or a general medical condition. A investigation of the patient's family, social, and occupational history is also valuable, not simply to ensure that the patient's depression causes significant impairment but also to develop targets for intervention and strategies for generalizing treatment change.

The reliability of diagnostic interviews is enhanced with the use of structured clinical interviews (Groth-Marnat, 1999; Zimmerman & Mattia, 1999). Although the SADS was at one time the most frequently utilized structured interview, the SCID now seems to have generated at least as much research. As our earlier review suggests, both the SCID and the SADS exhibit excellent reliability and validity in the assessment of mood disorders, and either instrument is appropriate to use, depending on one's clinical and research needs. These

TABLE 8.2. Sample Assessment Battery for Depression

Session	Recommended instruments
Initial assessment	*Symptoms/diagnosis* Structured Clinical Interview for DSM-IV Axis I Disorders (SCID) Hamilton Rating Scale for Depression (HRSD) Beck Depression Inventory–II (BDI-II) Hopelessness Scale (HS) *Theory-specific measures* Automatic Thoughts Questionnaire—Negative (ATQ-N) Automatic Thoughts Questionnaire—Positive (ATQ-P) Dysfunctional Attitude Scale (DAS)
Weekly assessment (acute phase)	BDI-II, ATQ-N, ATQ-P, DAS, HS
Monthly assessment	HRSD, BDI-II, HS
Assessment at each session (continuance/maintenance phase)	BDI-II
Discharge assessment	SCID, HRSD, BDI-II, ATQ-N, ATQ-P, DAS, HS
Follow-up assessment	BDI-II, HS

structured interviews are also helpful as guides to the types of treatment-related questions that need to be asked and the diagnostic criteria that should be covered. The main disadvantages of these instruments is that they are time-consuming to administer, require extensive training, and do not cover many of the areas needed to formulate a coherent treatment plan (e.g., motivation for change, social supports). Another disadvantage that has frequently been cited regarding all of the structured interviews is the potential loss of rapport relative to clinical interviews (see Groth-Marnat, 1999). However, loss of rapport has certainly not been our experience with the SCID, especially with increased familiarity with and use of the instrument. Although there are few data to directly address this issue, one exception is an investigation by Scarvalone et al. (1996), who found that participants' distress decreased rather than increased during a structured SCID interview. In this study, however, there was no adequate control condition to rule out extraneous factors (e.g., the passage of time), and the researchers did not contrast the effects of a SCID interview with those of another, less-structured method.

Although training is time-consuming, we encourage clinicians to become familiar with either the SCID or the SADS, as these are the best methods for diagnosing mood disorders. In our opinion, the SCID is preferred over the SADS because it is a more comprehensive structured diagnostic interview, it requires less time to administer, it has a clinician version available, and it is most congruent with DSM-IV criteria.

Clinician rating scales and self-report instruments also provide important strategies to describe patients and to index the severity of their symptoms. These scales may be used in treatment, both to identify which problem areas to target in therapy and to measure change after treatment. The most used clinician-rating scale for depression is the HRSD, and among these measures we recommend its routine use in clinical practice. One advantage with using a well-established measure such as the HRSD is that clinicians may more easily integrate the findings from their practice with the literature on psychotherapy outcomes. Another benefit of using a clinician-rating scale is to provide an index of disability and recovery using a different method than self-report.

Self-report measures of depressive severity vary in terms of their psychometric properties and their coverage of the core symptoms of depressive symptomatology (Faravelli et al., 1986). They also differ in terms of their primary content focus. The BDI-II is consistent with DSM-IV criteria, but it is more focused on cognitive symptoms than other measures; the CES-D was designed to have more of an affective component; the ZSDS focuses more on somatic and affective symptoms; and the CRSD tends to be more behavioral and somatic in emphasis. As noted previously, these scales also differ in their format. Despite these format and content differences, self-report measures of depression correlate quite highly with one another. For example, Plutchik and van Praag (1987) found high correlations among the BDI, the CES-D, and the Zung ($r = .87$ to $.89$). In addition, by regressing one scale onto another, these authors demonstrated that it was possible to estimate one depression score quite accurately by having knowledge of another self-report depression score. Given these similarities among self-report indices of depressive severity, there are no simple rules for choosing which scale(s) to use. Different scales yield slightly different information about a patient's presenting problems. Thus, clinicians should consider an instrument's psychometric properties, content, and operating characteristics and should choose an instrument based on the purpose of assessment and the specific content (e.g., cognitive, affective, somatic) or format (multiple-choice versus "yes"/"no") required. For example, in elderly or more severely impaired samples, multiple-choice questionnaires may be too cumbersome and thus result in a lower response rate. In such instances, a clinician may opt to use a less complicated or less time-consuming assessment strategy such as the CRSD (which has a "yes"/"no" format) or one of the abbreviated instruments we describe in a subsequent section of this chapter.

We recommend the BDI-II for the assessment of depressive severity and the evaluation of psychotherapy outcome. The BDI-II is most congruent with the criteria in DSM-IV; it has excellent psychometric properties, and it emphasizes cognitive and attitudinal symptoms more than do the other popular self-report measures. The BDI-II now covers all 9 symptoms of depression listed in DSM-IV and includes questions of reversed vegetative symptoms. The BDI-II is also the most frequently used self-report measure of depression, a fact that permits greater comparability of clinical results to the literature. The CRSD, ZSRD, and CES-D each focus on slightly different themes and include items that are not directly related to diagnostic criteria, features that have the unintended effect of decreasing overall specificity. In addition, the CES-D and Zung need to be updated to accommodate to changes made with DSM-IV.

There are several limitations of relying on self-report, both in general and in the specific instance of depression. In addition to their vulnerability to misinterpretation and response biases, self-reports are not well suited for individuals who have difficulty with reality testing, have a thought disorder, or have such severe symptoms that they are unable to concentrate. Therefore, self-report instruments should not be the only assessment measures used, but should instead be used to supplement other assessment techniques.

Clinician ratings and self-report scales correlate only moderately, suggesting that different perspectives may yield different information about a depressed individual (Plutchik & van Praag, 1987). There is a tendency for self-report indices to show rightward asymmetry (in that patients judge their own symptoms as being more severe than clinicians judge them to be), while clinician-rating scales lean more toward leftward asymmetry (Faravelli et al., 1986). Part of the reason for this discrepancy is that patients do not have a normative database on which to compare their symptoms. Self-report measures are thus ideal for the assessment of one's internal state, while clinician ratings and other-report indices are better for assessing behavioral symptoms and interpersonal styles. Combining instruments appears to produce a greater amount of information than would otherwise be possible (Faravelli et al., 1986; Plutchik & van Praag, 1987). Moreover, by using a few different measures, clinicians can increase the reliability and convergent validity of their assessment results and can cross-validate their findings (Kellner, 1994).

A number of factors complicate the assessment of depression. For example, it is necessary to consider a unique set of variables when assessing depression in the elderly (Lewinsohn et al., 1997) or in different ethnic groups. Three of the most common complications entail psychiatric comorbidity, medical comorbidity, and the overlap of depression with dementia.

Comorbidity

Depression tends to co-occur with most Axis I disorders. Particularly high rates of comorbidity have been noted between depression and schizophrenia, substance abuse, anxiety disorders, and eating disorders (Maser, Weise, & Gwirtsman, 1995). In most instances, self-report measures of depression do not differentiate among these patient groups. This lack of specificity is particularly true with measures of depression and anxiety (Dobson, 1985). Although a review of strategies for differential diagnosis extends beyond the scope of this chapter, one general recommendation is for clinicians to increase the reliability of diagnosing comorbid conditions by using structured diagnostic interviews. Zimmerman and Mattia (1999) found that clinicians were more likely to diagnose comorbid conditions using structured rather than unstructured interviews (e.g., roughly 33% using the SCID, compared to fewer than 10% otherwise). Proper recognition of comorbidity also assists with deriving a solid case formulation and predicting treatment outcome. For instance, depending on the severity of the disorders in question, one would treat an individual with comorbid depression and panic differently than an individual with pure depression. Comorbidity generally predicts a poorer treatment response for patients with depression and is also associated with greater psychosocial impairment.

Medical Comorbidity

Another complication involved in assessing depressive symptoms and severity is that of medical comorbidity. Many patients who seek treatment for depression in medical facilities present with vague somatic complaints including dizziness, bodily pains, sleep disturbance, muscle tension, fatigue, lack of appetite, and gastrointestinal disturbances (the "masking" somatic complaints; see Stefanis & Stefanis, 1999). Consequently, many of these patients are misdiagnosed as having a medical condition when none is present. Patients who present with somatic complaints tend to be elderly or poorly educated, to feel ashamed to admit to psychological difficulties, to have poor psychological insight, and to be reluctant or unable to express emotions verbally.

Adding to this complexity is the fact that depression is frequently comorbid with a diverse array of medical conditions. There is a high prevalence of depression in individuals with Parkinson's disease, multiple sclerosis, temporal lobe epilepsy, Alzheimer's disease, cardiovascular illnesses, cancer, endocrine disorders (e.g., hypothyroidism, hyperthyroidism, Cushing's syndrome), and metabolic disturbances (e.g., Addison's disease, diabetes mellitus) (Kaplan, Sadock, & Grebb, 1994; Stefanis & Stefanis, 1999; Stevens, Merikangas, & Merikangas, 1995). When a nonpsychiatric condition causes a mood disorder, the DSM-IV diagnosis is not MDD, but mood disorder due to a general medical condition (American Psychiatric Association, 1994). It is also possible that a medical condition exacerbates a depression that would exist in any event. In this case, the diagnosis would be MDD and the medical condition would be listed on Axis III of DSM-IV.

The overlap of depressive symptoms and physical conditions is high and may result in an overestimation of depression in such populations. This overlap may make the determination of treatment efficacy for depression in these populations very difficult. For example, treating a patient who is diagnosed with both MDD and Parkinson's disease will not likely result in many changes in the neurovegetative symptoms of depression. Further, scores on self-report indices may be inflated, indicating that the severity of depression continues to warrant treatment. In attempting to differentiate between depression and medical complaints, a number of researchers have suggested using questionnaires that focus less on the somatic aspects of depression. Cognitive and affective items may be the best indicators of depression and symptom change in such populations.

Depression and Dementia

Finally, it is important to differentiate between the pseudodementia in depression and the dementia that is related to a disease process (e.g., Alzheimer's). Although making this distinction can be very difficult, some key differences may be noticed. For example, in depression the cognitive symptoms typically have a sudden onset, and symptoms such as self-reproach and inappropriate guilt are usually also apparent. In depression, recent memory is affected more than remote memory, and depressed individuals can usually be trained to remember. These features are not true in dementia. Moreover, in depression cognitive difficulties frequently show a pattern of diurnal variation that is not seen in dementia. Finally, depressed patients with cognitive difficulties tend to give up rather than attempt to answer difficult questions, whereas demented individuals often confabulate (Kaplan et al., 1994).

Unfortunately, there is no phenotypical marker for depression. Thus, a combination of several assessment approaches is the most useful, both diagnostically and in terms of case conceptualization and treatment planning (see Table 8.2). Understandably, many clinicians may not have the available time to conduct such thorough assessments. In such cases, we recommend choosing at least two approaches to try to obtain convergent evidence about the initial complaints and the outcome of treatment. There are also some simple, time effective ways to assess problem areas and define concrete treatment goals operationally (e.g., via specific functional analysis). We therefore discuss strategies to integrate assessment with the development of treatment plans and outcome evaluation.

INTEGRATING ASSESSMENT, TREATMENT PLANNING, AND OUTCOME EVALUATION

We begin this section by discussing how assessment data may be used to develop a coherent case conceptualization, to identify targets for intervention, and to propose an appropriate plan for treatment. Following this brief overview, we focus our attention on the continued importance of assessment throughout the course of treatment and illustrate how data may be used to monitor and enhance treatment efficacy. Finally, we review tactics for the evaluation of treatment outcome and the assessment of the risk of relapse and recurrence. A case example is used to highlight several of the points we raise in this discussion.

An Overview of Empirically Supported Treatments for Depression

Ideally, one's assessment results should signify which overall treatment plan is most appropriate. Although the guidelines for the treatment of depression continue to evolve, and some of the following recommendations will likely change over time, antidepressant medication is typically recommended when the episode of depression is severe, recurrent, or chronic. Medication is also preferred if there is psychosis, if there is a family history of depression, or if there is a previous positive response to medication. Psychotherapy is generally recommended when the episode is less severe or chronic; nonpsychotic; when there is a prior positive response to psychotherapy; and when medication is contraindicated or unacceptable to the patient. Combined treatment is advocated for more severe and chronic depression and when there is a partial response to either single treatment modality (Rush et al., 1993). A number of these guidelines have been challenged in recent years. For example, based on results from the National Institute of Mental Health Treatment of Depression Collaborative Research Program (Elkin et al., 1989), but inconsistent with more recent data (see Hollon, DeRubeis, & Evans, 1996), many clinicians have held on to the belief that medication is necessary to alleviate severe depression. Contrary to this opinion, Hollon et al. (1996) reviewed a number of studies that attest to the efficacy of cognitive therapy for severe depression. In addition, cognitive therapy has also demonstrated a more powerful prophylactic effect (approximately half the rate of relapse) than antidepressants. As another example, researchers have attempted to find specific subtypes of depression in the hope that differential treatment efficacy might be shown. It is commonly understood, for instance, that melancholic depression is more amenable to pharmacological intervention. However, attempts at subtyping depression, save the unipolar/bipolar distinction, have not been very reliable or successful in predicting treatment responsivity. Also, the literature is inconsistent as to whether psychotherapy or pharmacotherapy, or their combination, is best for individuals with melancholic features (see Jarrett, 1995).

There is similar confusion regarding "differential therapeutics" for depression (Groth-

Marnat, 1999). The past few years have witnessed dramatic growth of the movement toward identifying and disseminating empirically supported psychosocial treatments (Chambless et al., 1996). The therapies that have achieved the status of empirically supported for depression include cognitive therapy, behavioral therapy, and interpersonal psychotherapy (DeRubeis & Crits-Christoph, 1998). However, there is a lack of clarity in the literature as to which of these therapies is most appropriate for a given client (Beutler, Goodrich, Fisher, & Williams, 1999). Despite the limitations of assessment for determining which specific treatment modalities are most appropriate for a given client, assessment data are crucial for case conceptualization and treatment planning, as well as for monitoring and evaluating the effects of treatment. Consistent case assessment may also assist with the development of databases to make determinations about which patient characteristics are associated with optimal response to various treatments.

Using Assessment Methods to Derive a Solid Case Formulation and Treatment Plan

To adequately formulate a case and generate a strategy for intervention, it is important to make appropriate diagnoses, to have a clear understanding of the range of the patient's presenting problems and their severity, and to prioritize this problem list (see Persons, 1989; Persons & Davidson, 2001). The structured interviews and symptom severity measures described earlier in this chapter are important instruments for case conceptualization and treatment planning for depression. Other instruments that tap specific areas of functioning (e.g., readiness for change, social support, coping styles) may also assist in the quantification and understanding of a patient's problems and strengths (Maruish, 1999).

Obtaining an accurate diagnosis is an obvious important step in treatment planning. This step is especially crucial when depression is comorbid with other psychiatric conditions. Depending on the nature of the comorbidity, for instance, the clinician may choose to target either the depression or the comorbid disorder as the first line of attack. If the comorbid diagnosis involves substance dependence, the clinician will need to treat this problem before interventions for depression will be successful. Concurrent obsessive–compulsive disorder or an eating disorder are also important to treat prior to the introduction of depression-specific interventions. In the case of comorbid generalized anxiety disorder, it is typically recommended that the depression is treated first (see Rush et al., 1993). Diagnosis alone is not usually sufficient for establishing a focused treatment plan (Moras, 1997). Symptom-specific psychometric instruments such as the BDI-II are beneficial supplements for treatment planning. For example, it is sometimes difficult to know which disorder to treat initially if a depressed person presents with a comorbid condition of panic disorder. In this instance, researchers generally recommend treating the disorder that is primary (i.e., most severe or longstanding) (Rush et al., 1993).

For example, one of our patients presented with comorbid depression and panic disorder with agoraphobia. After administering various symptom severity measures of both depression and anxiety, it was clear that his depression was not particularly severe relative to his panic. Based on these results, treatment began by focusing on the cognitive-behavioral treatment of panic disorder, with the hope that the patient's depression would dissipate as his anxiety reduced and his coping skills improved. In contrast, psychometric indices used with another patient suggested that her panic and depression were both very severe. When depression is very severe, one must question whether the patient would have the energy and motivation to comply with the demanding interoceptive and in vivo exposure tasks required to treat panic disorder. Symptom severity measures provide this valuable information, and in this case supported the need to treat the patient's depression before undertaking treatment of her panic disorder. Based on cases such as these, we advocate for the integration of self-report data with other information acquired from a comprehensive assessment protocol.

Providing the patient with specific feedback about his or her test results and presenting a case formulation that incorporates these results helps educate patients about their difficulties and how they might be alleviated. Patients also have the opportunity through this feedback process to clarify any issues that have been inadequately or incorrectly assessed, or to simply confirm the assessment results. This information is also beneficial because it increases the probability that patients will adopt the therapeutic rationale. For example, during the initial assessment interview, one patient stated that her depression was completely biological and that therapy would not likely assist her. Rather than wasting valuable time trying to persuade this patient that depression is a heterogeneous disorder with multiple causes, her belief was approached as a hypothesis that could be tested with assessment data. By conducting a timeline analysis of her experience with depression, it became evident that her depression was tied to a number of significant psychosocial stressors. In addition, the administration of the DAS, ATQ-P, and ATQ-N helped the patient realize that her cognition was maladaptive and likely contributing to her depression. Finally, having patients list very concrete and operationalized goals also provides accessory data to self-report indices that helps to ascertain the effects of treatment and its generalizability.

Assessment throughout the Process of Treatment

The line between assessment and treatment is often blurry, as there is a dynamic interplay between the two (Groth-Marnat, 1999). Assessment obviously influences treatment because it provides a means of identifying problems, understanding their severity, recognizing important patient characteristics, and prioritizing strategies for intervention. Assessment has also been shown to have a therapeutic benefit in its own right, whether derived from feedback of personality inventory scores (Meyer et al., 1998) or structured interviews (Scarvalone et al., 1996). Indeed, several research studies attest to the value of ongoing assessment throughout the process of treatment (see Meyer et al., 1998). In this section, we present a general approach to repeated assessment and highlight some of its advantages.

Once problem areas have been identified and the approach to treatment has been determined, it is important to choose which instruments to use on an ongoing basis. In making this decision, there is an obvious need to balance the costs of time and other resources with the benefit of the information accrued. It is also important for clinicians to choose instruments that are reliable, easy to administer and understand, and sensitive to change. We encourage clinicians to choose at least one symptom-based measure and to augment this measure with one or more theoretically applicable instrument. By choosing both types of measures, clinicians are more able to monitor the effects of a given intervention both on outcome and on variables that are purported to be causally related to depression.

It is important to first establish a baseline index on various scores and then have patients complete the questionnaires most pertinent to the focus of therapy. Although there are no data that directly address when to measure, we suggest monitoring scores on selected instruments each session, which in most cases is roughly equivalent to once a week (also see Maruish, 1999). It is crucial to protect test security. One strategy that is often useful is to have patients complete and score the questionnaires in the waiting room or before arriving for their session. At the beginning of the therapy session, they can simply report their scores to the therapist, who then records them in a log (H. Westra, personal communication, May 1999). In this way, the clinician and patient are immediately cognizant of how the patient is doing, and there is an ongoing record of treatment change, without requiring valuable therapeutic time. After six to eight sessions, it is often helpful to more formally review treatment progress with the patient, to ensure that therapy is producing the desired effects. Although such procedures do use therapy time, using measures other than self-report (e.g., the HRSD) can provide convergent evidence regarding treatment change and any discrepancies between self- and observer-report can be addressed. Depending on one's approach to treatment, collecting data using behavioral assessment strategies (e.g., daily logs of behavior and cognition) can also provide useful information to guide the process of treatment (see Beck et al., 1979).

There are a number of advantages to monitoring change over time:

1. The clinician is able to determine whether or not his/her approach is effective. The therapist can monitor problems, determine their cause (e.g., poor administration of treatment, faulty case conceptualization, low patient motivation or compliance) and address these issues early in the course of treatment (e.g., altering one's approach to therapy, reconceptualizing the case, confronting the patient).
2. Collecting data throughout the treatment phase often encourages patients. It relays the message that the therapist is confident in his or her ability to help patients overcome their problems and that the therapist is credible and respects accountability. It also conveys a powerful message to the patient that the therapist and patient are both there to get a job done.
3. Data can be used to show patients who may not feel like they are making significant progress (e.g., disqualifying the positives) that they are indeed taking steps toward recovery.
4. Test data can be used to examine the stability of the treatment response (e.g., to ensure that a patient's change does not simply reflect a flight into health).
5. This information provides a clear indication of when treatment is successful and can be safely concluded, or if early termination and referral are required (Mash & Hunsley, 1993).
6. The data gathered can be tabulated across different cases and can provide an opportunity for therapists to evaluate their own efficacy with different types of diagnoses and genders or based on other patient characteristics.

Evaluating Treatment Outcome

One of the most common uses of assessment is to evaluate the outcome of treatment. The collection of objective data provides crucial information to the therapist and third-party payers about what has or has not worked with a given patient. Outcome data also provide critical information for a patient regarding his or her improvement. Such information may cultivate a greater sense of confidence and self-efficacy in a patient's ability to manage subsequent stressors autonomously; it provides a realistic picture of where he or she is functioning psychologically; and it depicts how far a patient has progressed. Outcome data may also imply when further treatment may be necessary (Maruish, 1999). There is little consensus as to which measures of outcome are optimal for the evaluation of treatments for depression. Although attempts have been made to identify a core battery of outcome measures for depression (Moras, 1997), a singular standardized assessment package does not appear to be practical, especially given the heterogeneous nature of this disorder and the multiple perspectives on outcome. The three most popular outcome measures for depression are the BDI, the HRSD, and the ZSDS. The HRSD tends to provide a larger indication of change than does the BDI or the ZSDS. It is possible that the HRSD overestimates the magnitude of clinical improvement, that the BDI and ZSRS underestimate improvement, or that the "truth" lies somewhere in between (Lambert & Lambert, 1999).

Horowitz, Nelson, and Person (1997) argue, as do many others, that the use of self-report as the principal outcome procedure is fraught with problems. Patients are not always accurate in reporting their level of distress. For instance, patients may respond to demand characteristics and underreport their difficulties during or at the end of treatment in order to please a therapist. Patient satisfaction surveys also have low correlations with patient problem change variables (e.g., Pekarik & Guidry, 1999). Alternatively, therapists may not always be accurate judges of a patient's distress, in part because distress is a subjective phenomenon and because a therapist is motivated to perceive treatment as effective. The fact that these outcomes may yield slightly different sets of results suggests that researchers and clinicians should utilize more than one symptom-focused instrument to determine treatment outcome.

This chapter has focused primarily on symptom-based measures of depression. Although diagnostic interviews and clinician-rating scales use a different method of data collection and capture a slightly discrete vantage point, they nonetheless rely heavily on a patient's self-report. Behavioral measures of depression (e.g., recall of negative events, organization of negative adjectives, selective attention to negative content) have not yet become commonplace in clinical practice, but we anticipate that these techniques will be used more frequently in the future, attendant to the growth in popularity of cognitive-behavioral treatments of depression. These assessment strategies not only surmount many of the problems associated with self-report measures, but many are also quick and easy to administer and provide accessory data about the cognitive variables related to a patient's index episode of depression. Most of these techniques have not yet been validated for use in routine clinical practice, but there exist several potentially useful behavioral indices of change (see Horowitz et al., 1997, for review).

Another important consideration in the assessment of treatment outcome is that improvement is undeniably in the "eye of the beholder" (Maruish, 1999). Which criterion of improvement is recognized varies according to which perspective is regarded. Patients are typically interested in changes in subjective distress and symptomatology; families usually want to see improvement in well-being, as well as interpersonal and occupational functioning; therapists are most attentive to the reduction of symptoms or other characteristics related to psychopathology; employers are most concerned with how quickly a patient can get back to work and reassume productivity; and managed care companies and health policy makers are invested in rapid recovery and cost-containment (Docherty & Streeter, 1996; Dorwart, 1996; Moras, 1997). As such, several additional areas may need to be assessed, including patient satisfaction, coping strategies, social support, interpersonal functioning, occupational functioning, quality of life, and cost-effectiveness (for elaboration see Basco et al., 1997; Moras, 1997).

Adding to the complexity of outcome assessment for depression is the fact that different symptoms and problems related to depression may change at different rates. For example, reductions in hopelessness may be evident prior to changes in vegetative symptoms (Kobak & Reynolds, 1999). As well, a clinician will typically find that subjective distress changes prior to a decrease in other symptoms of depression, and that symptom reduction will be found before improved functioning becomes evident (Howard, Lueger, & Kolden, 1997). Given these nuances and complexities, it is important to ensure that outcome assessment is multidimensional. It is also important that the clinician carefully select instruments that will provide the best data not only for the patient but also for addressing the demands of external agents. In choosing outcome measures, the clinician will want to ensure that the instruments considered are relevant to the population of interest, convenient (in terms of cost, ease of use, and time), of high psychometric quality, intelligible to nonprofessionals, and compatible with theory and practice (Moras, 1997; Newman, Ciarlo,

& Carpenter, 1999). Operationally defined treatment goals, generated during the initial assessment interview, are also viable measures of outcome that can supplement psychometric instruments and address other areas of functioning without accruing additional costs.

Keeping adequate assessment data will support demonstrated efficacy of treatment and also will help determine average response–dose curves, expected rates of change, and factors involved in change. Clinicians also need to be aware of the base rates for recovery from depression and to use this information to ensure that a patient's change is reliable and clinically significant (see Doctor, 1999; Maruish, 1999). This information may be invaluable for addressing the queries of managed care companies, providing appropriate informed consent to future patients, justifying therapeutic choices and actions, supporting one's professional image, and "managing" one's relationship with managed care companies.

Using Assessment Strategies to Assist in the Prevention of Relapse or Recurrence

Assessment data collected over the course of therapy can also be used to ensure that the patient is equipped enough to maintain his or her gains and prevent relapse or future recurrence. Based on her data from cognitive therapy outcome trials (Jarrett et al., 1999), Jarrett suggested that additional treatment may be indicated to prevent relapse when a patient's HRSD (17-item) score is over 6 (mild or above) during the last 6 weeks of the acute phase of cognitive therapy (R. B. Jarrett, personal communication, January 11, 2000). Extended treatment may also be important for depressed patients who have experienced multiple previous episodes, as their risk for relapse is particularly high. The probability of experiencing a subsequent episode following a first-onset episode of depression is approximately 50%. This figure increases to 75% after the second episode, and to 90% after the third episode (Craighead, Craighead, & Brosse, 1999).

The prediction and prevention of relapse in depression will undoubtedly be an important direction for future research. Over the past decade, researchers have demonstrated that, although successfully treated depressives no longer differ from nonpsychiatric controls on self-report indices of depressive severity or dysfunctional attitudes, they may remain cognitively vulnerable to depression. This vulnerability becomes evident in former depressives once core negative beliefs have become activated through the use of cognitive or emotional priming. Priming methodologies may be employed to temporarily access latent negative cognition and thereby assess a patient's risk of relapse (see Segal, 1997). As a prophylactic strategy, the therapist may then help the patient work through his or her cognitions and anticipated future challenges, which will serve to solidify the strategies and skills learned in therapy and increase their generalizability.

Case Example

Sarah was a 50-year-old divorced woman with a history of major depressive episodes dating back almost 25 years. The onset of her most recent difficulties began approximately 2 years ago, when she experienced considerable stress at her place of employment. Sarah had been out of work since that time, and she claimed that this episode was the most severe in terms of both intensity and duration. Although her mood had improved since being stabilized on antidepressant medication, she continued to exhibit significant depressive symptomatology and reported that her thinking was extremely negative. Sarah believed that her negative thinking stemmed from her upbringing and from an emotionally abusive marriage. After 15 years, Sarah terminated the relationship and had been living alone for the past 9 years. She completed her educational requirements and passed her entry examination to become a certified accountant. She was working in an accounting firm until her most recent exacerbation of depressive symptoms.

Following an unstructured clinical interview, Sarah was administered the mood disorders module of the SCID-I. This semistructured interview indicated that she met diagnostic criteria for MDD. Sarah also completed a number of questionnaires that measured self-reported depressive severity (BDI-II), automatic thoughts (ATQ-P, ATQ-N), and distorted beliefs (DAS). Her BDI-II score indicated that the intensity of her depressive symptoms was in the low end of the severe range. Many of her self-derogatory thoughts and beliefs focused on themes of perfectionism, self-loathing, and a high need for social approval as a means of validating her self-worth. This maladaptive pattern of thinking appeared to have developed during childhood and was exacerbated during her marriage. The stress she experienced, due to a verbally abusive employer during her last job, seemed to have activated core beliefs that she was worthless and ineffectual.

The clinical interview indicated that Sarah had developed a number of maladaptive behavioral patterns (e.g., frequently sleeping in late) and that her depression was in the severe range. As such, the initial course of therapy focused on behavioral activation in order to help Sarah increase the number of pleasure- and task-oriented activities in her life and ultimately improve her energy, interest, and mood to prepare her for subsequent cognitive work (see Beck et al., 1979). Weekly self-report ratings of mood and cognition revealed that these tasks had a fairly quick and positive impact on her mood and energy. Given her scores on the cognitive indices, therapy focused on cognitive restructuring, with particular emphasis on themes of perfectionism, need for social approval, and extreme negativity about self. Much of this work was conducted using the Daily Record of Dysfunctional Thoughts (see Beck et al., 1979; Greenberger & Padesky, 1995). Once Sarah had improved symptomatically according to the BDI-II, the SCID mood disorders module was readministered. The results of the SCID concurred with the BDI-II and indicated that Sarah no longer met diagnostic criteria for MDD. Consequently, therapy began to emphasize strategies for maintaining gains and preventing relapse. Data were collected weekly until the end of treatment.

This case example illustrates a number of important points. First, the data from the initial intake assessment were used to formulate a case conceptualization and treatment plan. For example, Sarah's scores on the cognitively based questionnaires provided important data about the severity and frequency of her distorted thinking. Examination of the factor scores and individual items from these questionnaires also suggested a number of themes that were important to address in therapy. These data also were used to supplement the unstructured interview. We know from this interview, for instance, that Sarah developed a number of negative beliefs about herself, likely from past abusive interpersonal and occupational relationships, the latter of which triggered her most recent depressive episode. The BDI-II also provided important information about the severity of Sarah's depressive symptomatology and presented an initial baseline against which to evaluate the effect of treatment.

A second important point demonstrated in this example is the value of ongoing assessment. The weekly collection of cognitive- and symptom-based measures facilitated Sarah's understanding of the important link between these two variables and reinforced her confidence in the cognitive model. As shown in Figure 8.1, when Sarah's cognition shifted, so did her symptoms. Another advantage of ongoing assessment was that it allowed the therapist to gauge how treatment was progressing. In this case, the data indicated that Sarah's BDI-II scores were improving as sessions continued. If, however, the data had suggested that Sarah's scores were not changing as quickly as should be the case, the therapist would be cognizant of this fact early on in treatment, and appropriate remedial steps could be taken.

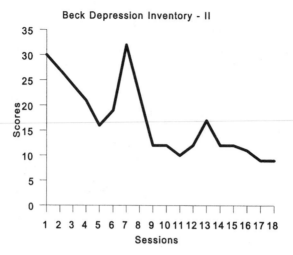

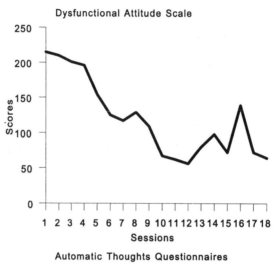

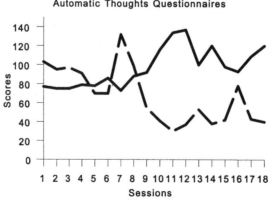

FIGURE 8.1. Case example: Assessment throughout the course of treatment.

Depressed individuals frequently distort information in a negatively biased fashion. These biases also tend to manifest themselves in the patient's view of treatment response. After the fourth session, for instance, Sarah questioned the extent to which therapy was helping her overcome her depression. Having weekly data on her symptoms helped Sarah recognize that, although her depression was not completely alleviated, she was clearly on the way to remission. In fact, within four sessions her BDI-II score had improved by 10 points. Assuming the same rate of change, it would have been possible to draw a regression line and estimate the number of sessions needed for complete remission. By using theory-specific measures, the efficacy of treatment was also enhanced. One factor that appears to be specific to depression is low positive affect or cognition (Dozois & Dobson, 2001). During the course of Sarah's treatment it became apparent that while her negative thinking was diminishing, her positive thinking had not yet shifted. Specific techniques then were implemented to help Sarah fend off negative cognition and to begin to increase self-reinforcement, acceptance, and enjoyment. As shown in Figure 8.1, the frequency of positive cognitions began to increase after the seventh session.

A third main point raised in this case example is that the outcome data indicated not only that the treatment was effective but also when therapy might be terminated. After session 10, Sarah no longer met criteria for MDD according to the SCID; however, her BDI-II scores were still in the mild range of severity. Jarrett recommends that therapy should continue past the acute stage when scores are in the mild range of severity or there is a history of recurrent depression, and because both of these risk factors were present in the current case, treatment continued in order to prevent relapse. Specific strategies for relapse prevention were also highlighted during these remaining sessions. Sessions 14 to 18 indicated that Sarah's BDI-II scores remained fairly stable and were in the minimal range of severity. Treatment continued on for a few more weeks to consolidate gains, review the cognitive tactics she had learned, and address termination issues.

ASSESSING DEPRESSION IN MANAGED CARE AND PRIMARY CARE SETTINGS

The proliferation of managed care organizations in the United States has resulted in an emphasis on cost containment in health care delivery. Concomitantly, the value of psychological assessment has been challenged (Eisman et al., 2000). Third-party payers and policy-makers continue to question whether psychological assessment is cost-effective. Fortunately, there are data to support the notion that psychological assessment is beneficial and leads to improved prediction (i.e., of functional behavior, health care utilization, mental health outcomes, and response to treatment), more effective clinical decision making (Kubiszyn et al., 2000), and better treatment planning (Ben-Porath, 1997; Meyer et al., 1998). The drawback of managed care is that the measures chosen and the manner in which assessment and treatment are conducted have become dictated equally, if not more, by fiscal restraint rather than quality of care. Conversely, the demand for greater accountability in health care is a positive consequence of managed care as mental health services have increasingly become empirically based. It is now imperative that clinicians conduct sophisticated and comprehensive assessment to respond to external pressures and to maximize quality of care.

As illustrated previously, psychological assessment provides a means to identify a patient's needs, make effective treatment recommendations, and monitor progress and outcome. It is important to remember that treatment outcome may be defined very differently, depending on which perspective of the "consumer" is being considered. Although many of the instruments reviewed in this chapter are suitable for managed care settings because of their psychometric properties, sensitivity to change, and brevity, the clinician may wish to supplement these tools with other indices of change.

Many of the measures described here are too time-consuming to be of practical use in some settings. In primary care settings, for example, the typical physician visit lasts less than 15 minutes and the average number of presenting complaints is six (Williams et al., 1999). Clearly, there is little time in such settings to devote to the assessment of emotional problems. Although effective screening tools in health care settings (Zich et al., 1990), instruments such as the BDI and the CES-D may be too lengthy for common usage in primary care. Consequently, a number of abridged measures have been developed to screen for depression in primary care settings.

Another reason for the development of depression screeners is that, despite a high prevalence of depression in primary care (30% to 50%) (Santorius et al., 1993), there is poor recognition of mood disorders among primary care physicians. Fewer than half the individuals with clinically significant depression are detected (Katon & Von Korff, 1990; Klinkman & Okkes, 1998). Both patient and clinician factors appear to contribute to the lack of recognition and misdiagnosis of depression in primary care. Patient factors include (1) differences of severity in symptom presentation across psychiatric, general medical practice, and community settings (Katon & Von Korff, 1990); (2) comorbidity between medical and mental health problems; and (3) the failure of patients to report or discuss emotional problems. Cape and McCulloch (1999) surveyed 83 patients who scored high on a measure of psychological distress. Only 23% of these patients mentioned emotional difficulties in consultation with their family practitioner. Many patients neglected to discuss their problems because they believed that their doctor did not have enough time or was not interested, that there was little their general practitioner could do about their emotional problems, that they might waste physician's time, or that their symptoms were not all that debilitating. Clinician-related variables noted for the underdiagnosis of depression in primary care include (1) many physicians are not well versed in the DSM-IV criteria for MDD; (2) most physicians lack sufficient time to screen for depression; (3) it is possible that some physicians overestimate their ability to diagnose depression (e.g., clinical hermeneutics error); and (4) some physicians underestimate the importance of formal diagnosis (Main, Lutz, Barrett, Matthew, & Miller, 1993; Williams et al., 1999). In addition to the obvious solution of increasing the recognition of MDD by being aware of these issues, physicians may benefit from using brief screening instruments. A number of studies have documented that the use of screening instruments increases the identification of MDD by physicians (e.g., Schade, Jones, & Wittlin, 1998).

The main brief screening instruments available for primary care settings are presented in Table 8.3. We recognize that there are other measures available that we have not included. For example, Melchoir, Huba, Brown, and Reback (1993) presented 4-item and 8-item versions of the CES-D. Although these screeners may be effective, the operating characteristics described in this study were calculated by comparing the shortened versions of the CES-D to the full 20-item instrument rather than to diagnostic status. Thus, the figures these authors presented are most likely inflated estimates. As another example, Weissman and her colleagues (1998) developed a computerized measure that screens MDD in fewer than 4 minutes. This instrument appears to be very promising for use in primary care; however, it is not presented in this chapter because it also screens for a number of other disorders. Also, the requirement of computerized assessment will likely limit the use of this strategy in many settings. Thus, the list of scales presented in Table 8.3 is meant to be illustrative rather than exhaustive.

When considering which specific screening instruments to use, it is important to consider their psychometric properties, performance characteristics (e.g., specificity and sensitivity), cost in terms of direct resources and time, and acceptability to the patient. It is also

TABLE 8.3. Screening Instruments for Depression in Primary Care Settings

Instrument	No. of items	Item content	Sensitivity (%)	Specificity (%)	PPP (%)	NPP (%)	AUC	Reference
BDI-PC (Primary Care)	7	Sadness, anhedonia, suicidal thoughts/wishes, pessimism, past failure, self-dislike, self-critical	82–97	82–99	—	—	.92	Beck et al. (1997); Steer et al. (1999)
BDI, Short Form	13	Sadness, pessimism, failure, dissatisfied, guilt, self-dislike, suicidal, withdrawal, indecisive, self-image, work inhibition, fatigue, weight/appetite loss	79	77	18–27	97–98	—	Beck & Beck (1972); Volk et al. (1993)
Brief Screen for Depression	4	Hopelessness/sadness; relaxed past 2 days; difficulty initiating/completing tasks; satisfied with ability to conduct day-to-day activities	94	69	—	—	—	Hakstian & McLean (1989)
CES-D (5-item)	5	Could not shake off blues; felt depressed; hopeful; fearful; sleep difficulties	80	80	26	98	.87	Lewinsohn et al. (1997)
CES-D (9-item)	9	Bothered; could not shake off blues; concentration; felt depressed; everything was an effort; sleep difficulties; enjoyed life; sad	78	80	46	94	—	Santor & Coyne (1997)
DIS Depressive Disorder Screener	2	Sad, blue or depressed; loss of pleasure	83–94	90–92	17–24	99	—	Rost et al. (1993)
Mental Health Screen–5	5	Downhearted and blue; nervous person; felt calm and peace; happy person; down in the dumps	—	—	—	—	.89	Berwick et al. (1991)
RAND-3	3	Felt depressed; sad, blue, depressed or anhedonia (past year); sad (2 years)	81	95	33	99	—	Kemper & Babonis (1992); Rost et al. (1993)

Note. PPP, positive predictive power; NPP, negative predictive power (see Finn & Kamphuis, 1995, for elaboration of these terms); AUC, area under the receiver operating curve, where the sensitivity of an instrument is plotted against 1 minus its specificity; when the AUC equals .50, no predictive information is provided about a diagnosis; a perfect test (distinguishing accurately between all depressed and nondepressed individuals) has an AUC of 1.00 (see Lewinsohn et al., 1997, for clarification); DIS, Diagnostic Interview Schedule; —, not reported.

289

important to weigh the costs and benefits of false positives and false negatives. False positives can lead to unnecessary and costly diagnostic testing and therapeutic interventions. Conversely, false negatives may result in treatment being delayed until a patient's symptoms are significantly worse. Treatment delay may have detrimental effects on patients' well-being and day-to-day functioning (Feldman, 1990), and even their eventual treatment, as longer episodes of depression are more difficult to treat effectively (Rush et al., 1993).

Screening instruments typically yield too many false positives, but they serve the important function of the alerting practitioners to think of conditions they might otherwise miss (Barrett, 1990). In addition, research has demonstrated that even when individuals are classified as being "false positive" for MDD, they usually have other psychiatric problems that warrant treatment (Leon et al., 1997; Leon et al., 1999). It is important to recognize that a screening is just that: it merely indicates whether further investigation is warranted. The responsibility rests with the clinician to decide how to proceed with a positive test.

Visual inspection of Table 8.3 reveals that the operating characteristics (i.e., sensitivity, specificity, positive predictive power, negative predictive power, and receiver operating curves) are quite similar across instruments, despite the fact that the number of items per measure ranges from 2 to 13. It is worth noting that the content of items is also generally quite similar across measures. Perhaps not surprisingly when one considers the criteria in DSM-IV, the two most important questions to ask patients appear to be some variant of "Do you often feel sad, depressed, or blue?" and "Have you lost interest in things you typically cared about or enjoyed?"

For a number of reasons[1] the majority of depressed individuals are seen by their primary care physicians rather than by mental health specialists (Attkisson & Zich, 1990). Primary care physicians are therefore in a unique and strategic position to detect depression and either treat it or refer a patient to mental health. Although screening for depression in primary care is controversial, research supports the idea that it is possible to detect depression, that screening instruments outperform clinical impressions in recognition, and that very brief instruments perform about as well as longer screening measures (Schade et al., 1998). Even single-item questions may be effective in detecting the majority of depressed individuals (Berwick et al., 1991; Mahoney et al., 1994). Thus, rather than the number of items per se, the crucial issue appears to be whether or not screening instruments are used. We encourage clinicians to screen their patients routinely in order to improve recognition of depression in their clinic population and to convey the messages that emotional problems are worth discussing and that effective treatments are available.

SUMMARY AND CONCLUSIONS

We have reviewed some of the main measures and techniques for assessing major depressive disorder and discussed several practical strategies for the assessment of this debilitating disorder. Also we have highlighted the important link between assessment, treatment planning, and outcome assessment, and we have reviewed issues and instruments for use in primary care settings. Several observations are noteworthy from this review. Before discussing these observations, it is important to restate that many of the issues considered in this chapter also apply to the assessment of dysthymia.

---

[1]Individuals with depression may be reluctant to acknowledge their mental health problems or may not even be cognizant of them. Increased vegetative signs, which are associated with increased medical visits, may be perceived by patients as symptoms of physical illness (Attkisson & Zich, 1990). There are also financial constraints (e.g., limitations of health insurance coverage) that limit the number of persons seen by mental health (Zich et al., 1990).

Recently, there has been considerable discussion (e.g., Moras, 1997; Rabkin & Klein, 1987) about the use of a core battery of strategies and instruments for the assessment of depression. It is extremely unlikely that such a battery would be adopted by all clinicians and psychotherapy outcome researchers because different theoretical orientations emphasize different outcome and process measures for depression. Notwithstanding the sheer number of clinician-rating and self-report instruments for measuring depression and their various strengths and weaknesses, we recommend that clinicians adopt a select few of the most used and validated tests to use for research and practice. These instruments can easily be supplemented with theory-specific indices. We have suggested that the SCID, the HRSD, and the BDI-II remain the instruments of choice for depression. When these measures are combined with other assessment approaches and theory-specific measures over time, the assessment of the depressive symptoms, severity, course, and outcome is maximized.

We have also highlighted the importance of (1) choosing reliable and valid measures, (2) weighing specificity and sensitivity, (3) being aware of the base rates of improvement, (4) using measures to provide convergent evidence to clinical conclusions and decision making, and (5) utilizing assessment throughout the entire process for a host of important reasons, including treatment outcome, and both process and management issues. There are so many excellent instruments available with which to derive accurate diagnoses, understand symptom severity, conduct case formulation, monitor the effects of treatment, determine outcome, examine the utility and scientific validity of the therapeutic techniques, and predict and prevent relapse that it is no longer justified not to measure.

We are not advocating that the development of assessment instruments in depression should cease. Although we think that comparative assessment of the wide range of self-report and interview-based severity and diagnostic instruments is an important next step in evaluating assessment procedures, we believe that one outcome of such an assessment would be the need for more definitive, and more generally accepted, measures. As noted in this discussion, although we recommend the regular use of the BDI-II and the HRSD, each of these measures has its limitations and strengths. We maintain that it is likely possible to generate more theory-neutral assessment methods that optimize psychometric test characteristics without sacrificing concurrent validity with other measures of depression, divergent validity with other constructs (e.g., anxiety), and sensitivity to change. Certainly, much more needs to be known about the correspondence between depression assessment and other related processes in depression (e.g., behavior change, cognitive features of depression, neurovegetative symptoms). Researchers are therefore enjoined to continue their inquiry into the optimal assessment strategies in the area of assessment.

ACKNOWLEDGMENTS

During the preparation of this chapter, David J. A. Dozois was supported by a research grant from the Ontario Mental Health Foundation, and Keith S. Dobson was assisted by a grant from the Alberta Heritage Foundation for Medical Research. This support is gratefully acknowledged.

REFERENCES

Altshuler, L. L., Post, R. M., & Fedio, P. (1991). Assessment of affective variables in clinical trials. In E. Mohr & P. Brouwers (Eds.), *Handbook of clinical trials: The neurobehavioral approach* (pp. 141–164). Amsterdam: Swets & Zeitlinger.

American Psychiatric Association. (1994). *Diagnostic and statistical manual of mental disorders* (4th ed.). Washington, DC: Author.

Attkisson, C. C., & Zich, J. M. (1990). Depression screening in primary care: Clinical needs and research challenges. In C. C. Attkisson & J. M. Zich (Eds.), *Depression in primary care: Screening and detection* (pp. 3–11). New York: Routledge.

Barrett, J. (1990). Issues of criterion validity for screening measures for depressive disorders in primary care. In C. C. Attkisson & J. M. Zich (Eds.), *Depression in primary care: Screening and detection* (pp. 27–42). New York: Routledge.

Basco, M. R., Krebaum, S. R., & Rush, A. J. (1997). Outcome measures of depression. In H. H. Strupp, L. M. Horowitz, & M. J. Lambert (Eds.), *Measuring patient changes in mood, anxiety, and personality disorders: Toward a core battery* (pp. 191–245). Washington, DC: American Psychological Association.

Bech, P., Bolwig, T., Kramp, P., & Rafaelsen, O. (1979). The Bech–Rafaelsen Mania Scale and the Hamilton Depression Scale. *Acta Psychiatrica Scandinavica, 59,* 420–430.

Beck, A. T., & Beck, R. W. (1972). Screening depressed patients in family practice: A rapid technique. *Postgraduate Medicine, 52,* 81–85.

Beck, A. T., Brown, G., Steer, R. A., & Weissman, A. N. (1991). Factor analysis of the Dysfunctional Attitude Scale in a clinical population. *Psychological Assessment, 31,* 478–483.

Beck, A. T., Guth, D., Steer, R. A., & Ball, R. (1997). Screening for major depression disorders in medical inpatients with the Beck Depression Inventory for primary care. *Behaviour Research and Therapy, 35,* 785–791.

Beck, A. T., Rush, A. J., Shaw, B. F., & Emery, G. (1979). *Cognitive therapy of depression.* New York: Guilford Press.

Beck, A. T., & Steer, R. A. (1988). *Beck hopelessness scale.* San Antonio, TX: Psychological Corporation.

Beck, A. T., Steer, R. A., Ball, R., & Ranieri, W. F. (1996). Comparison of the Beck Depression Inventories–IA and –II in psychiatric outpatients. *Journal of Personality Assessment, 67,* 588–597.

Beck, A. T., Steer, R. A., & Brown, G. K. (1996). *Beck Depression Inventory Manual* (2nd ed.). San Antonio, TX: Psychological Corporation.

Beck, A. T., Steer, R. A., & Garbin, M. G. (1988). Psychometric properties of the Beck Depression Inventory: Twenty-five years of evaluation. *Clinical Psychology Review, 8,* 77–100.

Beck, A. T., Ward, C. H., Mendelson, M., Mock, J., & Erbaugh, J. (1961). An inventory for measuring depression. *Archives of General Psychiatry, 5,* 53–63.

Ben-Porath, Y. S. (1997). Use of personality assessment instruments in empirically guided treatment planning. *Psychological Assessment, 9,* 361–367.

Berndt, D. J. (1986). *Multiscore Depression Inventory (MDI) manual.* Los Angeles: Western Psychological Services.

Berwick, D. M., Murphy, J. M., Goldman, P. A., Ware, J. E., Barsky, A. J., & Weinstein, M. C. (1991). Performance of a five-item mental health screening test. *Medical Care, 29,* 169–176.

Beutler, L. E., Goodrich, G., Fisher, D., & Williams, O. B. (1999). Use of psychological tests/instruments for treatment planning. In M. E. Maruish (Ed.), *The use of psychological testing for treatment planning and outcomes assessment* (2nd ed., pp. 81–113). Mahwah, NJ: Erlbaum.

Blazer, D. G., Kessler, R. C., McGonagle, K. A., & Swartz, M. S. (1994). The prevalence and distribution of major depression in a national community sample: The national comorbidity survey. *American Journal of Psychiatry, 151,* 979–986.

Bromet, E. J., Dunn, L. O., Connell, M. M., Dew, M. A., & Schulberg, H. C. (1986). Long-term reliability of diagnosing lifetime major depression in a community sample. *Archives of General Psychiatry, 43,* 435–440.

Camara, W. J., Nathan, J. S., & Puente, A. E. (2000). Psychological testing usage: Implications in professional psychology. *Professional Psychology: Research and Practice, 31,* 141–154.

Canon, B., Mulroy, R., Otto, M. W., Rosenbaum, J. F., Fava, M., & Nierenberg, A. A. (1999). Dysfunctional attitudes and poor problem solving skills predict hopelessness in major depression. *Journal of Affective Disorders, 55,* 45–49.

Cape, J., & McCulloch, Y. (1999). Patients' reasons for not presenting emotional problems in general practice consultations. *British Journal of General Practice, 49,* 875–879.

Carroll, B. J. (1998). *Carroll Depression Scales—Revised (CDS-R): Technical manual.* Toronto: Multi-Health Systems.

Carroll, B. J., Feinberg, M., Smouse, P. E., Rawson, S. G., & Greden, J. F. (1981). The Carroll Rating Scale for Depression: I. Development, reliability, and validation. *British Journal of Psychiatry, 138,* 194–200.

Chambless, D. L., Sanderson, W. C., Shoham, V., Johnson, S. B., Pope, K. S., Crits-Christoph, P., Baker, M., Johnson, B., Woody, S. R., Sue, S., Beutler, L., Williams, D. A., & McCurry, S. (1996). An update on empirically validated therapies. *Clinical Psychologist, 49,* 5–18.

Coyne, J. C., Pepper, C. M., & Flynn, H. (1999). Significance of prior episodes of depression in two patient populations. *Journal of Consulting and Clinical Psychology, 67,* 76–81.

Craighead, W. E., Craighead, L. W., & Brosse, A. L. (1999, May). *Prevention of relapse and recurrence of major depressive disorder.* Paper presented at the meeting of the Canadian Psychological Association, Halifax, Nova Scotia.

DeRubeis, R. J., & Crits-Christoph, P. (1998). Empirically supported individual and group psychological treatments for adult mental disorders. *Journal of Consulting and Clinical Psychology, 66,* 37–52.

Dingemans, P. M., Linszen, D. H., Lenior, M. E., & Smeets, R. M. (1995). Component structure of the expanded Brief Psychiatric Rating Scale (BPRS-E). *Psychopharmacology, 122,* 263–267.

Dobson, K. S. (1985). An analysis of anxiety and depression scales. *Journal of Personality Assessment, 49,* 522–527.

Docherty, J. P., & Streeter, M. J. (1996). Measuring outcomes. In L. I. Sederer & B. Dicket (Eds.), *Outcome assessment in clinical practice* (pp. 8–18). Baltimore: Williams & Wilkins.

Doctor, J. N. (1999). Recovery after treatment and sensitivity to base rate. *Journal of Consulting and Clinical Psychology, 67,* 219–227.

Dorwart, R. A. (1996). Outcomes management strategies in mental health: Application and implications for clinical practice. In L. I. Sederer & B. Dicket (Eds.), *Outcome assessment in clinical practice* (pp. 45–54). Baltimore: Williams & Wilkins.

Dozois, D. J. A., & Dobson, K. S. (2001). Information processing and cognitive organization in unipolar depression: Specificity and comorbidity issues. *Journal of Abnormal Psychology, 110,* 236–246.

Dozois, D. J. A., Dobson, K. S., & Ahnberg, J. L. (1998). A psychometric evaluation of the Beck Depression Inventory–II. *Psychological Assessment, 10,* 83–89.

Dunn, V. K., & Sacco, W. P. (1989). Psychometric evaluation of the Geriatric Depression Scale and the Zung Self-rating Depression Scale using an elderly community sample. *Psychology and Aging, 4,* 125–126.

Dunner, D. L., & Tay, L. K. (1993). Diagnostic reliability of the history of hypomania in bipolar II patients and patients with major depression. *Comprehensive Psychiatry, 34,* 303–307.

Eisman, E. J., Finn, S. E., Kay, G. G., Meyer, G. J., Dies, R. R., Eyde, L. D., Kubiszyn, T. W., & Moreland, K. L. (2000). Problems and limitations in using psychological assessment in the contemporary health care delivery system. *Professional Psychology: Research and Practice, 31,* 131–140.

Elkin, I., Shea, M. T., Watkins, J. T., Imber, S. D., Sotsky, S. M., Collins, J. F., Glass, D. R., Pilkonis, P. A., Leber, W. R., Docherty, J. P., Fiester, S. J., & Parloff, M. B. (1989). National Institute of Mental Health Treatment of Depression Collaborative Research Program: General effectiveness of treatments. *Archives of General Psychiatry, 46,* 971–982.

Endicott, J., & Spitzer, R. L. (1978). A diagnostic interview: The Schedule for Affective Disorders and Schizophrenia. *Archives of General Psychiatry, 35,* 837–844.

Faravelli, C., Albanesi, G., & Poli, E. (1986). Assessment of depression: A comparison of rating scales. *Journal of Affective Disorders, 11,* 245–253.

Faustman, W. O., & Overall, J. E. (1999). Brief Psychiatric Rating Scale. In M. E. Maruish (Ed.), *The use of psychological testing for treatment planning and outcomes assessment* (2nd ed., pp. 791–830). Mahwah, NJ: Erlbaum.

Fechner-Bates, S., Coyne, J. C., & Schwenk, T. L. (1994). The relationship of self-reported distress to depressive disorders and other psychopathology. *Journal of Consulting and Clinical Psychology, 62,* 550–559.

Feldman, W. (1990). How serious are the adverse effects of screening? *Journal of General Internal Medicine, 5*(Suppl.), S50–S53.

Fennig, S., Craig, T., Lavelle, J., Kovasznay, B., & Bromet, E. J. (1994). Best-estimate versus structured interview-based diagnosis in first-admission psychosis. *Comprehensive Psychiatry, 35,* 341–348.

Finn, S. E., & Kamphuis, J. H. (1995). What the clinician needs to know about base rates. In J. N. Butcher (Ed.), *Clinical personality assessment: Practical approaches* (pp. 224–235). Oxford: Oxford University Press.

First, M. B., Gibbon, M., Spitzer, R. L., & Williams, J. B. W. (1996a). *Structured Clinical Interview for DSM-IV Axis I Disorders - Research Version* (SCID-I, Version 2.0, February, 1996, Final version). New York: Biometrics Research.

First, M. B., Gibbon, M., Spitzer, R. L., & Williams, J. B. W. (1996b). *User's guide for the Structured Clinical Interview for DSM-IV Axis I Disorders—Research Version (SCID-I, Version 2.0, February, 1996, Final version).* New York: Biometrics Research.

First, M. B., Spitzer, R. L., Gibbon, M., & Williams, J. B. W. (1997). *Structured Clinical Interview for DSM-IV Axis I Disorders—Clinician Version (SCID-CV).* Washington, DC: American Psychiatric Press.

Gabrys J. B., & Peters, K. (1985). Reliability, discriminant and predictive validity of the Zung Self-rating Depression Scale. *Psychological Reports, 57,* 1091–1096.

Gibbons, R. D., Clark, D. C., & Kupfer, D. J. (1993). Exactly what does the Hamilton Depression Rating Scale measure? *Journal of Psychiatric Research, 27,* 259–273.

Goldston, D. B., O'Hara, M. W., & Schartz, H. A. (1990). Reliability, validity, and preliminary normative data for the Inventory to Diagnose Depression in a college population. *Psychological Assessment, 2,* 212–215.

Gotlib, I. H., & Cane, D. B. (1989). Self-report assessment of depression and anxiety. In P. C. Kendall & D. Watson (Eds.), *Anxiety and depression: Distinctive and overlapping features. Personality, psychopathology, and psychotherapy* (pp. 131–169). San Diego, CA: Academic Press.

Greenberg, P. E., Stiglin, L. E., Finkelstein, S. N., & Berndt, E. R. (1993). Depression: A neglected major illness. *Journal of Clinical Psychiatry, 54,* 419–424.

Greenberger, D., & Padesky, C. A. (1995). *Mind over mood: A cognitive therapy treatment manual for clients.* New York: Guilford Press.

Groth-Marnat, G. (1999). *Handbook of psychological assessment* (3rd ed.). New York: Wiley.

Haaga, D. A. F., McDermut, W., & Ahrens, A. H. (1993). Discriminant validity of the Inventory to Diagnose Depression. *Journal of Personality Assessment, 60,* 285–289.

Hakstian, A. R., & McLean, P. D. (1989). Brief screen for depression. *Psychological Assessment, 1,* 139–141.

Hamilton, M. (1960). A rating scale for depression. *Journal of Neurology, Neurosurgery and Psychiatry, 23,* 56–62.

Hamilton, M. (1967). Development of a rating scale for primary depressive illness. *British Journal of Social and Clinical Psychology, 6,* 278–296.

Hathaway, S. R., & McKinley, J. C. (1983). *The Minnesota Multiphasic Personality Inventory manual.* New York: Psychological Corporation.

Hedlund, J. L., & Vieweg, B. W. (1979). The Hamilton Rating Scale for Depression: A comprehensive review. *Journal of Operational Psychiatry, 10,* 149–162.

Hedlund, J. L., & Vieweg, B. W. (1980). The Brief Psychiatric Rating Scale (BPRS): A comprehensive review. *Journal of Operational Psychiatry, 11,* 48–65.

Hertzog, C., Van Alstine, J., Usala, P. D., Hultsch, D. F., & Dixon, R. (1990). Measurement properties of the Center for Epidemiological Studies Depression Scale (CES-D) in older populations. *Psychological Assessment, 2,* 64–72.

Hill, R. D., Gallagher, D., Thompson, L. W., & Ishida, T. (1988). Hopelessness as a measure of suicidal intent in the depressed elderly. *Psychology and Aging, 3,* 230–232.

Hollon, S. D., DeRubeis, R. J., & Evans, M. D. (1996). Cognitive therapy in the treatment and prevention of depression. In P. M. Salkovskis (Ed.), *Frontiers of cognitive therapy* (pp. 293–317). New York: Guilford Press.

Hollon, S. D., & Kendall, P. C. (1980). Cognitive self-statements in depression: Development of an automatic thoughts questionnaire. *Cognitive Therapy and Research, 4,* 383–395.

Horowitz, L. M., Nelson, K. L., & Person, E. A. (1997). Using empirical research findings to develop a behavioral measure of depression: A proposed direction for future research. In H. H. Strupp, L. M. Horowitz, & M. J. Lambert (Eds.), *Measuring patient changes in mood, anxiety, and personality disorders: Toward a core battery* (pp. 339–368). Washington, DC: American Psychological Association.

Horwath, E., Johnson, J., Klerman, G. L., & Weissman, M. (1992). Depressive symptoms as relative and attributable risk factors for first-onset major depression. *Archives of General Psychiatry, 49,* 817–823.

Howard, K. I., Lueger, R. J., & Kolden, G. G. (1997). Measuring progress and outcome in the treatment of affective disorders. In H. H. Strupp, L. M. Horowitz, & M. J. Lambert (Eds.), *Measuring patient changes in mood, anxiety, and personality disorders: Toward a core battery* (pp. 263–281). Washington, DC: American Psychological Association.

Ingram, R. E., Kendall, P. C., Siegle, G., Guarino, J., & McLaughlin, S. C. (1995). Psychometric properties of the Positive Automatic Thoughts Questionnaire. *Psychological Assessment, 7,* 495–507.

Ingram, R. E., Slater, M. A., Atkinson, J. H., & Scott, W. (1990). Positive automatic cognition in major affective disorder. *Psychological Assessment, 2,* 209–211.

Ingram, R. E., & Wisnicki, K. S. (1988). Assessment of positive automatic cognition. *Journal of Consulting and Clinical Psychology, 56,* 898–902.

Jarrett, R. B. (1995). Comparing and combining short-term psychotherapy and pharmacotherapy for depression. In E. E. Beckham & W. R. Leber (Eds.), *Handbook of depression* (2nd ed., pp. 435–464). New York: Guilford Press.

Jarrett, R. B., Kraft, D., Doyle, J., Foster, B., Eaves, G., & Silver, P. (1999, November). Does continuation phase cognitive therapy reduce relapse? In D. Kraft (Chair), *Improving the long-term well-being of depressed patients by predicting and preventing relapse.* Symposium conducted at the 33rd meeting of the Association for Advancement of Behavior Therapy, Toronto, Ontario.

Johnson, M. H., Magaro, P. A., & Stern, S. L. (1986). Use of the SADS-C as a diagnostic and symptom severity measure. *Journal of Consulting and Clinical Psychology, 54,* 546–551.

Kaplan, H. I., Sadock, B. J., & Grebb, J. A. (1994). *Synopsis of psychiatry* (7th ed.). Baltimore: Williams & Wilkins.

Katon, W., & Von Korff, M. (1990). Caseness criteria for major depression: The primary care clinicians and the psychiatric epidemiologist. In C. C. Attkisson & J. M. Zich (Eds.), *Depression in primary care: Screening and detection* (pp. 43–62). New York: Routledge.

Katz, R., Shaw, B. F., Vallis, T. M., & Kaiser, A. S. (1995). The assessment of severity and symptom patterns in depression. In E. E. Beckham & W. R. Leber (Eds.), *Handbook of depression* (2nd ed., pp. 61–85). New York: Guilford Press.

Kellner, R. (1994). The measurement of depression and anxiety. In J. A. den Boer & J. M. Ad Sitsen (Eds.), *Handbook of depression and anxiety: A biological approach* (pp. 133–158). New York: Marcel Dekker.

Kemper, K. J., & Babonis, T. R. (1992). Screening for maternal depression in pediatric clinics. *Journal of Diseases of Children, 146,* 876–878.

Kessler, R. C., McGonagle, K. A., Zhao, S., Nelson, C. B., Hughes, M., Eshleman, S., Wittchen, H., & Kendler, K. S. (1994). Lifetime and 12-month prevalence of DSM-III-R psychiatric disorders in the United States: Results from the National Comorbidity Survey. *Archives of General Psychiatry, 51,* 8–19.

Klinkman, M. S., & Okkes, I. (1998). Mental health problems in primary care. *Journal of Family Practice, 47,* 379–384.

Knesevich, J. W., Biggs, J. T., Clayton, P. J., & Ziegler, V. E. (1977). Validity of the Hamilton Rating Scale for Depression. *British Journal of Psychiatry, 131,* 49–52.

Knight, R. G., Waal-Manning, H. J., & Spears, G. F. (1983). Some norms and reliability data for the State–Trait Anxiety Inventory and the Zung Self-Rating Depression Scale. *British Journal of Clinical Psychology, 22,* 245–249.

Knight, R. G., Williams, S., McGee, R., & Olaman, S. (1997). Psychometric properties of the Center for Epidemiologic Studies Depression Scale (CES-D) in a sample of women in middle life. *Behaviour Research and Therapy, 35,* 373–380.

Kobak, K. A., & Reynolds, W. M. (1999). Hamilton Depression Inventory. In M. E. Maruish (Ed.), *The use of psychological testing for treatment planning and outcomes assessment* (2nd ed., pp. 935–969). Mahwah, NJ: Erlbaum.

Krug, S. E., & Laughlin, J. E. (1976). *Handbook for the IPAT Depression Scale.* Champaign, IL: Institute for Personality and Ability Testing.

Kubuszyn, T. W., Meyer, G. J., Finn, S. E., Eyde, L. D., Kay, G. G., Moreland, K. L., Dies, R. R., & Eisman, E. J. (2000). Empirical support for psychological assessment in clinical health care settings. *Professional Psychology: Research and Practice, 31,* 119–130.

Lambert, M. J., & Lambert, J. M. (1999). Use of psychological tests for assessing treatment outcome. In M. E. Maruish (Ed.), *The use of psychological testing for treatment planning and outcomes assessment* (2nd ed., pp. 115–151). Mahwah, NJ: Erlbaum.

Leon, A. C., Portera, L., Olfson, M., Kathol, R., Farber, L., & Sheehan, D. V. (1999). Diagnostic errors of primary care screens for depression and panic disorder. *International Journal of Psychiatry in Medicine, 29,* 1–11.

Leon, A. C., Portera, L., Olfson, M., Weissman, M. M., Kathol, R. G., Farber, L., Sheehan, D. V., & Pleil, A. M. (1997). False positive results: A challenge for psychiatric screening in primary care. *American Journal of Psychiatry, 154,* 1462–1464.

Lewinsohn, P. M., Seeley, J. R., Roberts, R. E., & Allen, N. B. (1997). Center for Epidemiologic Studies Depression Scale (CES-D) as a screening instrument for depression among community-residing older adults. *Psychology and Aging, 12,* 277–287.

Lovibond, S. H., & Lovibond, P. F. (1995). *Manual for the Depression Anxiety Stress Scales.* Sydney: Psychology Foundation of Australia.

Lubin, B. (1994). *State–Trait Depression Adjective Checklists: Professional manual.* Odessa, FL: Psychological Assessment Resources.

Mahoney, J., Drinka, T. J. K., Abler, R., Gunter-Hunt, G., Matthews, C., Gravenstein, S., & Carnes, M. (1994). Screening for depression: Single question versus GDS. *Journal of the American Geriatric Society, 42,* 1006–1008.

Main, D. S., Lutz, L. J., Barrett, J. E., Matthew, J., & Miller, R. S. (1993). The role of primary care clinical attitudes, beliefs, and training in the diagnosis and treatment of depression. *Archives of Family Medicine, 2,* 1061–1066.

Maruish, M. E. (1999). Introduction. In M. E. Maruish (Ed.), *The use of psychological testing for treatment planning and outcomes assessment* (2nd ed., pp. 1–39). Mahwah, NJ: Erlbaum.

Maser, J. D., Weise, R., & Gwirtsman, H. (1995). Depression and its boundaries with selected Axis I disorders. In E. E. Beckham & W. R. Leber (Eds.), *Handbook of depression* (2nd ed., pp. 86–106). New York: Guilford Press.

Mash, E. J., & Hunsley, J. (1993). Assessment considerations in the identification of failing psychotherapy: Bringing the negatives out of the darkroom. *Psychological Assessment, 5,* 292–301.

Matarazzo, J. D. (1983). The reliability of psychiatric and psychological diagnosis. *Clinical Psychology Review, 3,* 103–145.

McNair, D. M., Lorr, M., & Droppleman, L. F. (1992). *EdITS manual for the Profile of Mood States.* San Diego, CA: EdITS.

Melchior, L. A., Huba, G. J., Brown, V. B., & Reback, C. J. (1993). A short depression index for women. *Educational and Psychological Measurement, 53,* 1117–1125.

Metalsky, G. I., & Joiner, T. E. (1997). The Hopelessness Depression Symptom Questionnaire. *Cognitive Therapy and Research, 21,* 359–384.

Meyer, G. J., Finn, S. E., Eyde, L. D., Kay, G. G., Kubiszyn, T. W., Moreland, K. L., Eisman, E. J., & Dies, R. R. (1998). *Benefits and costs of psychological assessment in healthcare delivery: Report of the Board of professional affairs psychological assessment work group, Part 1.* Washington, DC: American Psychological Association.

Moras, K. (1997). Toward a core battery for treatment efficacy research on mood disorders. In H. H. Strupp, L. M. Horowitz, & M. J. Lambert (Eds.), *Measuring patient changes in mood, anxiety, and personality disorders: Toward a core battery* (pp. 301–338). Washington, DC: American Psychological Association.

Murphy, J. M., Monson, R. R., Laird, N. M., Sobol, A. M., & Leighton, A. H. (2000). A comparison of diagnostic interviews for depression in the Stirling County study. *Archives of General Psychiatry, 57,* 230–236.

Newman, F. L., Ciarlo, J. A., & Carpenter, D. (1999). Guidelines for selecting psychological instruments for treatment planning and outcome assessment. In M. E. Maruish (Ed.), *The use of psychological testing for treatment planning and outcomes assessment* (2nd ed., pp. 153–170). Mahwah, NJ: Erlbaum.

Nezu, A. M., Ronan, G. F., Meadows, E. A., & McClure, K. S. (2000). *Clinical assessment series: Vol. 1. Practitioner's guide to empirically-based measures of depression.* New York: Kluwer/Plenum.

Overall, J. E., & Gorman, D. R. (1962). The Brief Psychiatric Rating Scale. *Psychological Reports, 10,* 799–812.

Pekarik, G., & Guidry, L. L. (1999). Relationship of satisfaction to symptom change, follow-up adjustment, and clinical significance in private practice. *Professional Psychology: Research and Practice, 30,* 474–478.

Persons, J. B. (1989). Cognitive therapy in practice: A case formulation approach. New York: Norton.

Persons, J. B., & Davidson, J. (2001). Cognitive-behavioral case formulation. In K. S. Dobson (Ed.), *Handbook of cognitive-behavioral therapies* (2nd ed., pp. 86–110). New York: Guilford Press.

Peruzzi, N., & Bongar, B. (1999). Assessing risk for completed suicide in patients with major depression: Psychologists' views of critical factors. *Professional Psychology, Research and Practice, 30,* 576–580.

Plutchik, R., & van Praag, H. M. (1987). Interconvertability of five self-report measures of depression. *Psychiatry Research, 22,* 243–256.

Rabkin, J. G., & Klein, D. F. (1987). The clinical measurement of depressive disorders. In A. J. Marsella & R. M. A. Hirschfeld (Eds.), *The measurement of depression* (pp. 30–83). New York: Guilford Press.

Radloff, L. S. (1977). The CES-D Scale: A self-report depression scale for research in the general population. *Applied Psychological Measurement, 1,* 385–401.

Reynold, W. M., & Kobak, K. A. (1998). *Reynolds Depression Screening Inventory: Professional manual.* Odessa, FL: Psychological Assessment Resources.

Rhoades, H. M., & Overall, J. E. (1988). The semi-structured BPRS interview and rating guide. *Psychopharmacology Bulletin, 24,* 101–104.

Riskind, J. H., Beck, A. T., Berchick, R. J., Brown, G., & Steer, R. A. (1987). Reliability of DSM-III diagnoses for major depression and generalized anxiety disorder using the Structured Clinical Interview for DSM-III. *Archives of General Psychiatry, 44,* 817–820.

Roberts, R. E., Andrews, J. A., Lewinsohn, P. M., & Hops, H. (1990). Assessment of depression in adolescents using the Center for Epidemiologic Studies Depression Scale. *Psychological Assessment, 2,* 122–128.

Rost, K., Burnam, A., & Smith, G. R. (1993). Development of screeners for depressive disorders and substance disorder history. *Medical Care, 31,* 189–200.

Rush, A. J., Golden, W. E., Hall, G. W., Herrera, M., Houston, A., Kathol, R. G., Katon, W., Hatchett, C. L., Petty, F., Schulberg, H. C., Smith, G. R., & Stuart, G. (1993). *Depression in primary care: Vol. 2. Treatment of major depression: Clinical practice guideline, Number 5* (AHCPR Publication No. 93-0551). Rockville, MD: U.S. Department of Health and Human Services, Public Health Service, Agency for Health Care Policy and Research.

Rush, A. J., Gullion, C. M., Basco, M. R., Jarrett, R. B., & Trivedi, M. H. (1996). The Inventory of Depressive Symptomatology (IDS): Psychometric properties. *Psychological Medicine, 26,* 477–486.

Sakado, K., Sato, T., Uehara, T., Sato, S., & Kameda, K. (1996). Discriminant validity of the Inventory to Diagnose Depression, lifetime version. *Acta Psychiatrica Scandinavia, 93,* 257–260.

Sanavio, E., Bertolotti, G., Michielin, P., Vidotto, G., & Zotti, A. M. (1988). CBA–2.0 Cognitive behavioral assessment: Scale primarie. Manuale. Florence, Italy: Organizzazioni Speciali.

Santor, D. A., & Coyne, J. C. (1997). Shortening the CES-D to improve its ability to detect case of depression. *Psychological Assessment, 9,* 233–243.

Santor, D. A., Zuroff, D. C., Ramsay, J. O., Cervantes, P., & Palacios, J. (1995). Examining scale discriminability in the BDI and CES-D as a function of depressive severity. *Psychological Assessment, 7,* 131–139.

Santorius, N., Üstün, T. B., Costa e Silva, J., Goldberg, D., Lecrubier, Y., Ormel, J., Von Kroff, M., & Wittchen, H. (1993). An international study of psychological problems in primary care: Preliminary report from the World Health Organization Collaborative Project on "Psychological Problems in General Health Care." *Archives of General Psychiatry, 50,* 819–824.

Scarvalone, P. A., Cloitre, M., Spielman, L. A., Jacobsberg, L., Fishman, B., & Perry, S. W. (1996). Distress reduction during the Structured Clinical Interview for DSM-III-R. *Psychiatry Research, 59,* 245–249.

Schade, C. P., Jones, E. R. Jr., & Wittlin, B. J. (1998). A ten-year review of the validity and clinical utility of depression screening. *Psychiatric Services, 49,* 55–61.

Schelde, J. T. M. (1998). Major depression: Behavioral parameters of depression and recovery. *Journal of Nervous and Mental Disease, 186,* 141–149.

Schotte, C. K. W., Maes, M., Cluydts, R., & Cosyns, P. (1996). Effects of affective-semantic mode of item presentation in balanced self-report scales: Biased construct validity of the Zung Self-Rating Depression Scale. *Psychological Medicine, 26,* 1161–1168.

Schwab, J. J., Bialow, M. R., & Holzer, C. E. (1967). A comparison of two rating scales for depression. *Journal of Clinical Psychology, 23,* 94–96.

Segal, D. L., Hersen, M., & Van Hasselt, V. B. (1994). Reliability of the structured clinical interview for DSM-III-R: An evaluative review. *Comprehensive Psychiatry, 35,* 316–327.

Segal, Z. V. (1997). Implications of priming for measures of change following psychological and pharmacological treatments. In H. H. Strupp, L. M. Horowitz, & M. J. Lambert (Eds.), *Measuring patient changes in mood, anxiety, and personality disorders: Toward a core battery* (pp. 81–99). Washington, DC: American Psychological Association.

Shaver, P. R., & Brennan, K. A. (1991). Measures of depression and loneliness. In J. P. Robinson, P. R. Shaver, & L. S. Wrightsman (Eds.), *Measures of personality and social psychological attitudes* (Vol. 1, pp. 195–289). San Diego, CA: Academic Press.

Shea, S. C. (1988). *Psychiatric interviewing: The art of understanding.* Philadelphia: Harcourt Brace.

Simon, R., Endicott, J., & Nee, J. (1987). Intake diagnoses: How representative? *Comprehensive Psychiatry, 28,* 389–396.

Skre, I., Onstad, S., Torgersen, S., & Kringlen, E. (1991). High interrater reliability for the Structured Clinical Interview for DSM-III-R Axis I (SCID-I). *Acta Psychiatrica Scandinavica, 84,* 167–173.

Solomon, D. A., Kellerm M. B., Leon, A. C., Mueller, T. I., Lavori, P. W., Shea, T., Coryell, W., Warshaw, M., Turvey, C., Maser, J. D., & Endicott, J. E. (2000). Multiple recurrences of major depressive disorder. *American Journal of Psychiatry, 157,* 229–233.

Spitzer, R. L., & Endicott, J. (1975). *The Schedule for Affective Disorders and Schizophrenia (SADS).* New York: Biometrics Research Division, New York State Psychiatric Institute.

Spitzer, R. L., Endicott, J., & Robins, E. (1978). Research Diagnostic Criteria. *Archives of General Psychiatry, 35,* 733–782.

Spitzer, R. L., Williams, J. B. W., Gibbon, M., & First, M. B. (1992). The Structured Clinical Interview for DSM-III-R (SCID): I. History, rationale, and description. *Archives of General Psychiatry, 49,* 624–629.

Spitzer, R. L., Williams, J. B. W., Kronenke, K., Linzer, M., deGruy III, F. V., Hahn, S. R., & Brody, D. (1993). *PRIME-MD: Clinician evaluation guide.* New York: Pfizer.

Steer, R. A., Ball, R., Ranieri, W. F., & Beck, A. T. (1997). Further evidence for the construct validity of the Beck Depression Inventory–II with psychiatric outpatients. *Psychological Reports, 80,* 443–446.

Steer, R. A., Ball, R., Ranieri, W. F., & Beck, A. T. (1999). Dimensions of the Beck Depression Inventory–II in clinically depressed outpatients. *Journal of Clinical Psychology, 55,* 117–128.

Steer, R. A., Clark, D. A., Beck, A. T., & Ranieri, W. F. (1998). Common and specific dimensions of self-reported anxiety and depression: The BDI-II versus the BDI-IA. *Behaviour Research and Therapy, 37,* 183–190.

Steer, R. A., Kumar, G., Ranieri, W. F., & Beck, A. T. (1998). Use of the Beck Depression Inventory–

II with adolescent psychiatric outpatients. *Journal of Psychopathology and Behavioral Assessment, 20,* 127–137.

Stefanis, C. N., & Stefanis, N. C. (1999). Diagnosis of depressive disorders: A review. In M. Maj & N. Sartorius (Eds.), *Depressive disorders* (pp. 1–51). New York: Wiley.

Steiner, J. L., Tebes, J. K., Sledge, W. H., & Walker, M. L. (1995). A comparison of the Structured Clinical Interview for DSM-III-R and clinical diagnoses. *Journal of Nervous and Mental Disease, 183,* 365–369.

Stevens, D. E., Merikangas, K. R., & Merikangas, J. R. (1995). Comorbidity of depression and other medical conditions. In E. E. Beckham & W. R. Leber (Eds.), *Handbook of depression* (2nd ed., pp. 147–199). New York: Guilford Press.

Stommel, M., Given, B. A., Given, C. W., Kalaian, H. A., Schulz, R., & McCorkle, R. (1993). Gender bias in the measurement properties of the Center for Epidemiologic Studies Depression Scale (CES-D). *Psychiatry Research, 49,* 239–250.

Uehara, T., Sato, T., Sakado, K., & Kameda, K. (1997). Discriminant validity of the Inventory to Diagnose Depression between patients with major depression and pure anxiety disorders. *Psychiatry Research, 71,* 57–61.

Volk, R. J., Pace, T. M., & Parchman, M. L. (1993). Screening for depression in primary care patients: Dimensionality of the short form of the Beck Depression Inventory. *Psychological Assessment, 5,* 173–181.

Warren, W. L. (1994). *Revised Hamilton Rating Scale for Depression (RHRSD): Manual.* Los Angeles: Western Psychological Services.

Watson, D., Clark, L. A., & Tellegen, A. (1988). Development and validation of brief measures of positive and negative affect: The PANAS scales. *Journal of Personality and Social Psychology, 54,* 1063–1070.

Weissman, A. N., & Beck, A. T. (1978). *Development and validation of the Dysfunctional Attitude Scale: A preliminary investigation.* Paper presented at the annual meeting of the Association for Advancement of Behavior Therapy, Chicago.

Weissman, M. M., Broadhead, W. E., Olfson, M., Sheehan, D. V., Hoven, C., Conolly, P., Fireman, B. H., Farber, L., Blacklow, R. S., Higgins, E. S., & Leon, A. C. (1998). A diagnostic aid for detecting (DSM-IV) mental disorders in primary care. *General Hospital Psychiatry, 20,* 1–11.

Williams, J. B. W., Gibbon, M., First, M. B., Spitzer, R. L., Davies, M., Borus, J., Howes, M. J., Kane, J., Pope, H. G., Rounsaville, B., & Wittchen, H. (1992). The Structured Clinical Interview for DSM-III-R (SCID): II. Multisite test–retest reliability. *Archives of General Psychiatry, 49,* 630–636.

Williams, J. W., Rost, K., Dietrich, A. J., Ciotti, M. C., Zyzanski, S. J., & Cornell, J. (1999). Primary care physicians' approach to depressive disorders. *Archives of Family Medicine, 8,* 58–67.

Zheng, D., Macera, C. A., Croft, J. B., Giles, W. H., Davis, D., & Scott, W. K. (1997). Major depression and all-cause mortality among white adults in the United States. *Annals of Epidemiology, 7,* 213–218.

Zich, J. M., Attkisson, C. C., & Greenfield, T. K. (1990). Screening for depression in primary care clinics: The CES-D and the BDI. *International Journal of Psychiatry in Medicine, 20,* 259–277.

Zimmerman, M., & Coryell, W. (1987). The Inventory to Diagnose Depression (IDD): A self-report scale to diagnose major depressive disorder. *Journal of Consulting and Clinical Psychology, 55,* 55–59.

Zimmerman, M., & Coryell, W. (1994). Screening for major depressive disorder in the community: A comparison of measures. *Psychological Assessment, 6,* 71–74.

Zimmerman, M., Coryell, W., Corenthal, C., & Wilson, S. (1986). A self-report scale to diagnose major depressive disorder. *Archives of General Psychiatry, 43,* 1076–1081.

Zimmerman, M., & Mattia, J. I. (1999). Psychiatric diagnosis in clinical practice: Is comorbidity being missed? *Comprehensive Psychiatry, 40,* 182–191.

Zung, W. W. K. (1965). A self-rating depression scale. *Archives of General Psychology, 12,* 63–70.

9

Obesity and Eating Disorders

Linda W. Craighead

Eating and weight concerns encompass a range of problems that include medical concerns and psychological issues; frequently they involve complex interactions between psychological distress and changes in weight. It is useful to conceptualize this range of problems as consisting of the four categories that appear at the top of Table 9.1 (i.e., obesity, binge-eating disorder, bulimia nervosa, and anorexia nervosa). Only three of these categories are psychiatric diagnostic entities (i.e., eating disorders); obesity (by itself) is considered a medical problem. Although these four categories do not form a true continuum, the categories closest to each other in Table 9.1 have the most in common. Thus, in most cases, diagnostic difficulties revolve around making meaningful distinctions between the adjacent categories.

Incidence rates are highest for the category of obesity, with about one-third of adults (in the United States) being at least 20% over ideal weight. Rates are higher among women than among men and higher among African Americans and Mexican Americans than among Caucasians. The greatest increase in the incidence of obesity occurs in the early 20s to early 30s, but weight typically increases gradually over time (Williamson, 1995). Rates for full diagnostic-level eating disorders (EDs) are much lower. Binge-eating disorder (BED) is estimated to occur in about 4% of community samples (equally among males and females), but it has been found in as many as 30% of individuals (primarily women) seeking weight loss treatment (Spitzer et al., 1992). Among adolescent and young adult females, rates of bulimia nervosa (BN) range from 1% to 3%, (with the purging type being more common than the nonpurging type) and rates of anorexia nervosa (AN) range from 0.5% to 1% (with about half being the restricting type). Among males, rates are substantially lower for both BN and AN and are estimated at less than 10% of diagnosed cases (American Psychiatric Association, 1994). Approximately 6% to 10% of young women demonstrate significantly disordered eating patterns that don't quite meet the criteria for the specific types of EDs. Since all weight and eating concerns are more common among women, I will use female pronouns throughout the chapter. Very little research is available to guide the clinician in adapting treatment for males.

The criteria required by DSM-IV for the specific types of EDs are indicated in Table 9.1 by an [a]. Other (nonrequired) characteristics are also provided in the table to underscore

TABLE 9.1. Characteristics of Obesity and Eating Disorders

Domain	Obesity	Binge-eating disorder	Bulimia nervosa		Anorexia nervosa	
			Nonpurging	Purging	Binge/purge	Restricting
Physiological	Overweight by medical standard	Normal to overweight	Mildly overweight to underweight		Amenorrhea (three cycles; in postmenarcheal females)[a] Weight < 85% of normal (BMI < 17.5)[a]	
Eating-related behaviors	Overeating	Objective bingeing (loss of control) (two times a week for 6 months)[a]	Objective bingeing (loss of control) (two times a week for 3 months)[a]		Bingeing[a]	No bingeing[a]
		No inappropriate compensatory behavior[a]	Nonpurging compensatory behavior[a] (two times a week for 3 months)	Purging[a]	Purging[a]	Nonpurging compensatory behavior (fasting, exercise)[a]
Eating-related affect	Not as prominent	Distress over binge eating and weight[a]	Distress over weight, binge/purge, or fear of weight gain		Intense fear of weight gain[a]	
Eating-related cognitions	Not as prominent	Overconcern with weight and shape	Overconcern with weight and shape[a]		Body image disturbance or denial of low weight as a medical problem[a]	
Other psychiatric problems	Not as frequent	Frequent: depression; anxiety disorders; substance abuse; personality disorders (borderline, hysterical, and avoidant); history of sexual abuse				

[a]Diagnostic criteria from DSM-IV (American Psychiatric Association, 1994).

the commonalities among the categories. As noted in the table, the experience of recurrent binge eating, defined by loss of control (the feeling that one cannot control what or how much one is eating, or behavioral indicators of impaired control), is the primary distinction between obesity and BED. In addition, the binges must cause distress, must be objectively large (defined as eating in a discrete period of time, usually fewer than 2 hours, an amount definitely larger than most people would eat under similar circumstances), and must be characterized by at least three of the following: eating more rapidly than normal; eating until feeling uncomfortably full; eating large amounts when not physically hungry; eating alone because of being embarrassed by the large amounts; and feeling disgusted with oneself, depressed, or very guilty after overeating. The more overweight an individual is, the more likely he or she is to meet criteria for BED or to resemble individuals with BED, even if the person does not experience the sense of losing control. Within the BED category, the less overweight the individual is, the more similar the person is to individuals with BN. Such individuals typically demonstrate some efforts to compensate (dieting and exercise), but their behaviors are not clearly "inappropriate." Within the BN category, individuals who are higher weight are more similar to individuals with BED (having larger or more frequent binges), whereas those who are underweight are more similar to individuals with AN (having longer or more frequent periods of severe restriction and smaller or less frequent binges).

The clinician's first diagnostic decision is to establish the appropriate general category. The second decision is to determine whether the severity (the frequency and/or duration criteria) is such that a full diagnosis can be given. Importantly, the severity criteria are relatively arbitrary and have been questioned by many researchers. DSM-IV does provide a diagnosis, eating disorder not otherwise specified (EDNOS; 307.50), which can be used for any pattern of disturbed eating that does not meet the specific criteria for AN or BN but warrants intervention because it is distressing or impairing. In fact, the criteria for a diagnosis of BED are still provisional, so such individuals are currently diagnosed as having EDNOS. DSM-IV provides five examples to illustrate additional symptom patterns that warrant a diagnosis of EDNOS: females meeting all criteria for AN except amenorrhea; significant weight loss and all criteria for AN except weight remains in the normal range; all criteria for BN except frequency or duration is less than required; regular use of inappropriate compensatory behaviors after small amounts of food; and repeatedly chewing and spitting out, but not swallowing, large amounts of food.

Assessment of individuals with disordered eating patterns often involves a medical evaluation. In that case, actual weight and height and presence or absence of amenorrhea are assessed as part of the physical exam. Detailed information regarding medical assessment (and treatments) associated with eating disorders is found in Andersen (1992); this chapter focuses on psychological assessment of eating disorders.

The initial psychological assessment typically includes an interview that focuses on history of symptoms and prior treatment, retrospective reports of specific eating and compensatory behaviors, and, when appropriate, assessment of comorbid conditions. Self-report measures may be administered to obtain more detailed information on relevant constructs; such measures provide quantitative indicators of the severity of behavioral, cognitive, and affective variables that are useful for monitoring progress and documenting outcome of treatment. Self-monitoring may be used to supplement information gathered during the initial assessment, but it is most often used as a component of treatment where it serves to facilitate functional analyses of problem behaviors.

The specific assessment instruments most commonly used with eating problems are described in the next section of this chapter and are organized by type of assessment. Most of the measures described here have adequate psychometric data available, but some additional measures, most of which are still in development, have been included because they appear to have potential clinical utility. For more detailed psychometric information on many of the measures described herein, see Allison (1995); many of the actual measures are reprinted in Allison's appendices. The second part of this chapter discusses how assessment can be used to answer specific questions relevant to making treatment decisions.

ASSESSMENT INSTRUMENTS

Weight

Assessment of degree of obesity or underweight is complicated if one needs an exact measurement of body fat (see discussion in Wardle, 1995). However, for clinical purposes, the *body mass index* (BMI = kg body weight/height in m^2) is generally adequate (see discussion in Hannan, Wrate, Cowen, & Freeman, 1995). A BMI of 18 or below is considered underweight; below 17 is considered to confer some health risk. A normal BMI is 19 to 24. A BMI of 25 or above is considered "overweight." Above a BMI of 27, some medical risk due to weight alone is present. A BMI over 30 is considered "obese," and the health risks increase as weights go higher. BMI charts indicating these ranges can be useful in terms of discussing current and ideal weight with clients. Many clients have focused so exclusively on "magic" numbers (e.g. "I can't be over 110 pounds"), that they do not think in terms of what is a reasonable range. Most clients do not realize how much BMI is related to height. Although no chart will convince a client to accept a certain weight, it can be useful in helping the client to make the distinction between being "fat" and being "normal" with a strong preference to be "thin–normal" or even "very thin" (what I call "model-thin"). We have calculated BMI for a number of models and TV stars for whom height and weight have been published. Several TV stars have been publicly noted for recent weight losses; they had typically been in the thin–normal range (BMI = 19–20), but had dropped down to the 17 to 18 range. Virtually all professional models are in the 16 to 17 range; note that 17.5 is the BMI given as a guide for meeting criteria for AN. It is also useful to point out to clients that weight is only one criteria for AN. A broad range of eating patterns may be clinically significant and can be diagnosed as EDNOS if distress or interference is present (e.g., excessive preoccupation, avoidance behaviors, or failure to carry out major life responsibilities).

It should be noted that BMI only approximates the percentage of body fat. Skinfold measurements of body fat tend to be more accurate than BMI, but the tester needs to be well trained in the technique. Otherwise, skinfold estimates are not very reliable, and they are especially poor for the very lean or very overweight. Body-fat scales, which are based on bioelectrical impedance, can be a practical alternative. This method sends a weak current through the body; the current travels more slowly through fat (which contains less water) than through muscle, providing an estimate of body fat. Such scales need to be recalibrated often and can be inaccurate if the person is dehydrated or overhydrated, but no special training is needed to operate them. Either method may be useful in a particular case, for example a female athlete, and may help a highly fit client understand that her weight will be higher than a less fit individual. For assessing medical risk, the waist–hip ratio is a useful index; ratios greater than 1 indicate excessive abdominal fat. Central fat (more common in men) appears to confer greater health risk than peripheral fat (more common in women) (Bjorntorp, 1988).

Most important, the client's desired weight should be considered in the context of her own (and her family's) weight history. This information is likely to be most helpful in efforts to differentiate between an "ideal" weight for a person her height and a "reasonable" weight goal for her as a unique individual. It is also useful to determine the extent to which a client's feelings about her weight are related to having family members with significant weight problems or significant others who held excessively thin ideals or were overly weight conscious.

History of Symptoms

A life chart (see Apple, 1999) is a useful way to obtain an overview of the client's eating symptoms and weight history, as well as to establish relationships between the onset and exacerbation of symptoms over time and other important events in the client's life. Generating such a life chart is the purpose of the initial, assessment stage of interpersonal therapy (IPT; see Weissman, Markowitz, & Klerman, 2000). In IPT, the chart takes between three and five sessions to complete and is an essential component in providing the rationale and basis for treatment. Four areas are traced chronologically from the client's earliest memories to the present: significant life events, mood and self-esteem, interpersonal relationships, and changes in weight (onset and changes in compensatory behaviors are assessed as well, if relevant). Past treatments should also be noted. When the life chart is done as part of IPT, it includes a detailed discussion of current relationships (number, type, quality, and degree of reciprocity), which helps identify the primary interpersonal problem that will be the focus of treatment. However, a brief life chart can be done in a single assessment interview or can be given to the client to complete out of session. This linear representation over time can be very useful for understanding eating problems because they often present as a chronic concern with weight and specific symptoms having a widely fluctuating course over time.

It is useful to note whether individuals report that binge eating or dieting occurred first. Both sequences are reported in BN and BED, with binge eating first being more common in BED than in BN. Haiman and Devlin (1999) reported that individuals with BN who binged first resemble individuals with BED more closely than do those who dieted first. They report higher weight, higher shape and weight concern, and lower age of onset of binge eating.

Diagnostic Interviews

Eating Disorder Examination, 12th Edition (EDE)

The EDE (Fairburn & Cooper, 1993) is the most widely used semistructured interview for eating disorders. It was designed to measure psychological constructs and specific eating patterns and behaviors, as well as to provide a means to generate specific diagnoses. It has been used primarily with late adolescents and adults. Bryant-Waugh, Taylor, and Lask (1996) reported that a slightly modified version was appropriate to use with children ages 7 to 14. The interview begins with providing a calendar to orient the participant to the time periods for which questions will be asked. The calendar indicates the specific 28 days prior to the interview and, in addition, specifies the dates that mark the 2 prior months. The participant is asked to mark any significant events that occurred during the past 28 days and may use her personal calendar for reference. The purpose of the calendar is simply to improve recall for the time period in question; specific eating episodes are not marked on the calendar. Most questions refer to the past 28 days; however, frequency questions are asked about the preceding months as needed to determine certain diagnoses. The interview provides specific questions (i.e., probes) that must be asked and suggests additional prompts; the interviewer is free to ask further questions as needed to clarify the participant's responses. About 30 questions cover various eating and weight concerns, and responses are rated by the interviewer on a scale of 1 to 6. In addition, the specifics of the participant's eating pattern are determined (i.e., number of meals and snacks eaten). The frequencies of specific compensatory behaviors and of each of three types of overeating are obtained. First, the interviewer describes the three different types of overeating and asks for recent examples of episodes. The interviewer decides, based on the examples provided, whether these episodes meet the "large amount" criterion. Average frequency is asked for each type of episode.

Objective Binge Episode (OBE). For an OBE, the amount eaten must be "large" (guidelines suggest three or more times a normal portion), and "loss of control" must be reported. Number of calories is not used to decide if a binge is objectively large; however, it is useful to note that several self-monitoring studies give average caloric values of reported binges. Rosen, Leitenberg, Fischer, and Khazam (1986) reported that binge episodes reported by individuals with BN averaged 1,459 calories (range = 45 to 5,138) whereas nonbinge episodes averaged 321 calories (range = 10 to 1,652). Notably, 65% of the "binge" episodes were actually within the range of the nonbinge episodes. Rossiter, Agras, and McCann (1991) reported a lower average, about 600 calories per binge, among individuals with BED. Initially, Fairburn (1987) had recommended 1,000 calories as a guide for determining if an episode was "large." However, given the variability that has been reported, it is recommended that the amount be evaluated as "large" primarily in terms of the context in which it occurs.

Subjective Binge Episode (SBE). An SBE is defined as any amount eaten that is less than "large" but is viewed by the individual as excessive and is accompanied by a sense of "loss of control." Thus, a SBE might consist of a single candy bar (a normal portion size), or it might be two pieces of pie (larger than a normal portion but less than an OBE).

Objective Overeating (OOE). OOE is used to refer to amounts eaten that are clearly "large" but for which no loss of control is reported. Eldredge and Agras (1996) reported on six individuals who presented for weight loss treatment and met all the criteria for BED, except that they did not endorse the sense of loss of control. These six individuals did not differ from subjects who met all the criteria for BED, except that they were, on average, currently heavier and had higher "highest ever weights." The authors suggested that such individuals may have formerly experienced loss of control but had "burned out" and given up efforts to control eating. Future research will need to determine if it is useful to consider such individuals as different from people who meet all the criteria for BED. In our weight control programs, participants who do not experience loss of control (therefore no true "binges") are encouraged to use the terms "large versus moderate overeating episodes" in order to differentiate the times they become clearly overfull from more "normative" overeating. In treatment, we find it useful to identify the larger overeating episodes as most problematic and to target them first during treatment.

The EDE is the only measure that allows for separate reporting of objective and subjective binge episodes. Thus, in evaluating research findings, it is important to determine what measure of binges is being used and how (or if) a binge is defined for the respondent. Most self-report measures do not clearly define a binge or "large" amounts of food. Without clear guidelines, results across studies can be highly variable. Some investigators consider the distinction between OBEs and SBEs to be both fairly unreliable and not useful. However, further research may be able to suggest particular modifications of treatment that would be more useful for one type of binge than another.

In addition to the specific frequencies of compensatory behaviors and eating episodes, the EDE provides four subscale scores: Restraint, Eating Concern, Shape Concern, and Weight Concern. These scores can be summed to provide an overall severity measure. Norms for various groups are provided in Fairburn and Cooper (1993); the available data on discriminant and concurrent validity, internal consistency, interrater reliability, and sensitivity to change are also summarized. These are all judged to be adequate to good.

The EDE allows the interviewer to ask many specific and sensitive questions that might otherwise feel more intrusive in a first interview. Thus, this semistructured interview is an excellent way to cover a lot of ground in a relatively short amount of time. However, it does not ask about past symptoms or previous treatment, so it would need to be supplemented with additional questions if used as an initial assessment. The clear standards for definitions of "large" make diagnoses of BN and BED quite reliable. For clinical purposes, however, the distinction between OBEs and SBEs may be less critical because degree of distress is typically related to the feeling of being out of control. The EDE requires some expertise to administer, and considerable training is needed to obtain adequate interrater reliability. The EDE was initially developed to assess BN, but it is now used for AN and BED as well. Some of the questions are marked as inappropriate for use when the participant is clearly overweight.

Clinical Eating Disorder Rating Instrument (CEDRI)

The CEDRI (Palmer, Christie, Cordle, Davies, & Kendrick, 1987) asks about 31 symptoms, which are rated on the basis of the past 4 weeks. This semistructured interview can be used both as an initial assessment and to measure change in symptoms. Questions and probes are provided and may be supplemented by the clinician in order to facilitate making ratings. The interview is not set up specifically to tie symptom ratings to diagnostic criteria. The initial report indicated adequate reliability, and a more recent report (Palmer, Robertson, Cain, & Black, 1996) found differences between anorexic, bulimic, and dieting women, thus supporting its validity.

Interview for the Diagnosis of Eating Disorders–IV (IDED)

This semistructured interview was developed by Williamson (1990) to focus specifically on assessing the symptoms needed to make clear diagnoses, and it has been revised to conform to DSM-IV (Kutlesic, Williamson, Gleaves, Barbin, & Murphy-Eberenz, 1998). Twenty symptoms are rated on a 5-point scale; ratings are designed to determine the presence or absence of diagnostic criteria. It does not ask about some of the other eating concerns that are assessed in the EDE. However, the IDED asks for demographic information, eating disorder history, and individual and family psychiatric history. It is designed to be used as a complete initial assessment tool. It includes a diagnostic checklist to assist in making differential diagnoses for the major disorders, as well as for subthreshold diagnoses and specific types of EDNOS. Psychometric data are summarized in Kutlesic et al. (1998) and indicate moderate to high interrater reliability, internal consistency, content validity, and convergent and discriminant validity. No studies have directly compared the EDE and the IDED. The IDED is easier to administer and score, but it provides less detailed information in certain areas.

Structured Interview for Anorexic and Bulimic Disorders for Expert Ratings (SIAB-EX)

The SIAB-EX (Fichter et al., 1998) has 61 items rated on a 5-point scale. Factor analysis indicated six factors: Body Image and Slimness Ideal; General Psychopathology; Sexuality and Social Integration; Bulimic Symptoms; Measures to Counteract Weight Gain, Fasting, and Substance Abuse; and Atypical Binges. The interview is designed to provide current and lifetime diagnoses; these diagnoses may be derived using a computer algorithm. Fitchter and his colleagues report adequate interrater reliability and internal consistency for the most recent revision of the interview.

Self-Report Questionnaires

Symptom Measures

Table 9.2 briefly describes the most frequently used eating symptom self-report questionnaires. Some are useful as screening devices, but most are used to provide an index of change during treatment. The primary use of the measure is indicated in the table with an asterisk; the number of items, any subscales, and a brief summary of the psychometric data available for the measure are also indicated. A few measures are able to provide a tentative initial diagnosis, but, as noted earlier, it is highly recommended that semistructured interviews be used to establish reliable diagnoses. Due to the overlap among the eating disorders in terms of attitudes, cognitions, and associated problems, self-report measures typically do not differentiate reliably among diagnostic groups. In addition, although most measures do ask about eating behaviors, the questions are usually too general. The measures may not clarify what is considered a binge, establish amounts of food eaten, or clearly document symptom frequencies. In using any of these questionnaires, the clinician is cautioned to look

TABLE 9.2. Descriptive and Psychometric Data for Disordered Eating Symptom Self-Report Measures

Measure	Length	Eating-related scales	Body Image Scales	Noneating Scales	Psychometric data available
Binge Eating Scale (BES)	16 items Multiple choice RL: 5th grade	Total score CC = 20			Norms IC (good) CV *Severity index
Bulimia Test—Revised (BULIT-R)	36 items Multiple choice RL: 11th grade	28 items used for total score CC = 102			Norms IC (.97) TRT (.95) CV *Severity index
Bulimic Investigatory Test (BITE)	33 items Format varied RL: 4th grade	Symptom and severity subscales CC = 25 (total score)			Norms IC (.62–.96) TRT (.86) CV *Severity index
Eating Attitudes Test (EAT-26)	26 items 6-point ratings RL: 5th grade	Dietary restraint Bulimia and food preoccupation Oral control CC = 20 (total score)			Norms IC (.8 –.9) TRT (.84) CV FA *Severity index
Eating Disorders Examination Questionnaire (EDE-Q)	36 items Format of ratings considered difficult for client use	Restraint Eating concern Binge/purge (frequencies)	Shape concern Weight concern		Items (but not frequency counts) correlate well with EDE interview *Severity index
Eating Disorders Inventory (EDI; EDI-2)	EDI (64 items) EDI-2 (91 items) 6-point ratings RL: 5th grade	Drive for thinness Bulimia	Body dissatisfaction	Ineffectiveness Perfectionism Interpersonal distrust Interoceptive awareness Maturity fears EDI-2: Ascetism Impulse regulation Social insecurity	Norms IC (.6–.9, except ascetism) TRT (.4–.9) CV FA *Comprehensive outcome measure

(continued)

307

TABLE 9.2. *(continued)*

Measure	Length	Eating-related scales	Body Image Scales	Noneating Scales	Psychometric data available
Eating Symptoms Inventory (ESI)	17 items Multiple choice RL: 7th grade	Total score			Norms IC (.76) CV Sensitivity (.71) Specificity (.81) *Screen
Eating Questionnaire—Revised (EQ-R)	15 items Multiple choice RL: 7th grade	Total score			Norms IC (.87) TRT (.9) CV *BN symptom checklist
Multifactorial Assessment of Eating Disorders Symptoms (MAEDS)	56 items 7 point ratings	Restrictive eating Binge eating Purgative behavior Forbidden foods	Fear of fatness	Negative affect	Norms IC (.8–9) TRT (.8–9) CV FA *Comprehensive outcome measure
Stirling Eating Disorder Scales (SEDS)	80 items	Anorexic behavior Anorexic cognitions Bulimic behavior Bulimic cognitions		Perceived external control Assertiveness Low self-esteem Self-directed hostility/guilt	Norms IC TRT CV *Comprehensive outcome measure
Questionnaire on Eating and Weight Patterns—Revised (QEWP-R)	28 items Format varied RL: 5th grade	Total score			IC (.79) Kappa (.6) with interview version *Tentative diagnosis for BED and BN
Weight Loss Behavior Scale (WLBS)	35 items 5 point rating RL: 5th grade	Concern with dieting and weight Overeating Avoidance of fattening foods and sweets Emotional eating		Exercise	Norms IC (.7) TRT (.78) CV FA *Treatment outcome for weight loss programs

Note. Asterisk (*) indicates primary use of this instrument. RL, reading level; CC, clinical cutoff; IC, internal consistency; TRT, test–retest reliability; CV, concurrent validity; FA, factor analyzed.

carefully at the items to ensure that the needed information is assessed. For example, an item on a scale might say, "I think about vomiting" rather than ask how frequently one vomits after eating.

The Eating Attitudes Test (EAT-26; Garner & Garfinkel, 1979; Garner, Olmsted, Bohr, & Garfinkel, 1982) was designed as a brief screen to identify individuals with eating disorders (primarily BN and AN) in college or community samples. The test differentiates between AN, BN, BED, and nonclinical controls, but it does not differentiate between AN and BN. The clinical cutoff will yield a fair number of false positives in term of individuals meeting full criteria for an ED diagnosis, but it is unlikely to miss many individuals with eating disorders unless the person intentionally misrepresents herself. A children's version (ChEAT), more suitable for screening in middle school, is also available (Smolak & Levine, 1994). The Eating Symptoms Inventory (ESI; Whitaker et al., 1989) and the Setting Conditions for Anorexia Nervosa Scale (SCANS; Slade & Dewey, 1986) are also appropriate screens for high school populations; they also do not differentiate between AN and BN.

The Eating Disorders Inventory (EDI: Garner, Olmsted, & Polivy, 1983; EDI-2: Garner, 1991) is the most widely used general symptom measure. A total EDI score is frequently used as an outcome measure in studies of AN. The Bulimia scale includes both binge eating and purging questions. Psychometric properties of all of the scales except Maturity Fears and Ascetism appear to be adequate. Joiner and Heatherton (1998) confirmed the factor structure of five of the subscales in a nonclinical population.

The Stirling Eating Disorder Scales (SEDS; Williams et al., 1994) are less widely used but offer certain advantages. The SEDS is the only self-report measure that has separate scales (both for dietary behavior and for cognitions) to differentiate between AN and BN. The four, non-eating-specific scales do not differentiate between AN and BN.

The Multifactorial Assessment of Eating Disorders Symptoms (MAEDS; Anderson, Williamson, Duchmann, Gleaves, & Barbin, 1999) was designed specifically to focus on variables that can be manipulated in treatment and to serve as a single measure of treatment outcome that is shorter and easier to use than are batteries of separate measures. Factor analyses confirmed the six factors, but failed to support a seventh factor, which attempted to assess resistance and denial. As noted later in this chapter, efforts to assess resistance and denial have not been very successful. Evidence of criterion validity is also reported (Martin, Williamson, & Thaw, 2000) indicating that different diagnostic groups show the expected patterns among the subscales.

The Eating Disorders Examination Questionnaire (EDE-Q; Fairburn & Beglin, 1994) is a self-report version of the EDE (described earlier). Several questions are marked to be excluded if the individual is overweight, so it can be used for BED. Specific symptom frequencies are reported and scores are generated for the same four subscales as for the EDE. Some of the items are rated in terms of number of days, out of the past 28, and some individuals report finding this format difficult to use. A number of the items correlate highly with the interview version, but, most notably, binge eating frequency does not. This is to be expected because the amount of food constituting a binge is simply described as "what most people would regard as unusually large" and loss of control is not defined further. Thus, although it may be efficient to use the self-report version to obtain subscale scores (one has to worry less about rater reliability), the determination of frequency of different types of eating episodes is more reliable with the interview. Loeb, Pike, Walsh, and Wilson (1994) suggest that the EDE-Q be used to track change over time once clients have been instructed about the nature and size of binges.

The remaining assessment measures are more specific to particular eating problems. Three were designed specifically to assess BN symptoms, but they do not differentiate BN from AN groups: the Bulimia Test (BULIT; Smith & Thelen, 1984; BULIT-R; Thelen,

Farmer, Wonderlich, & Smith, 1991), the Bulimic Investigatory Test (BITE; Henderson & Freeman, 1987) and the Eating Questionnaire—Revised (EQ-R; Williamson, Davis, Bennett, Goreczny, & Gleaves, 1989). The Binge Eating Scale (BES; Gormally, Black, Daston, & Rardin, 1982) is the most appropriate severity index for BED. It does include one question on which the individual can endorse "I sometimes have to induce vomiting to relieve my stuffed feeling;" however, it does not ask about other compensatory behaviors. The Questionnaire on Eating and Weight Patterns-Revised (QEWP-R; Spitzer et al., 1992) is the most appropriate to use as a screen for BED among participants in a weight control program. The Weight Loss Behavior Scale (WLBS; Smith, Williamson, Womble, Johnson, & Burke, 2000) is a new measure that is designed to serve as a comprehensive treatment outcome measure for weight loss programs.

Self-Reports Relevant to Specific Eating Behaviors

Three measures include some assessment of dietary restraint, the degree to which individuals are attempting to diet, and whether they are successful. These measures were designed to be used with general or obese populations, and they indicate levels of dieting or binge eating but are not designed to assess clinical levels of symptoms. The Restraint Scale—Revised (Herman & Polivy, 1980; Polivy, Herman, & Howard, 1988) is a very brief (10-item) index. The total score has been used extensively and predicts counterregulatory eating in laboratory settings. The authors describe the scale as reflecting a pattern of unsuccessful dieting (i.e., individuals who attempt to restrain and periodically lose control). The scale has two distinct factors. The concern with dieting factor shows considerable overlap with the cognitive restraint factors of the two questionnaires described next. The weight fluctuation factor taps a unique construct that is not assessed in the other questionnaires.

The Three Factor Eating Questionnaire (TFEQ; Stunkard & Messick, 1985, 1988) is more comprehensive than the Restraint Scale. It has 51 items and includes cognitive restraint, disinhibition, and hunger subscales. The latter two factors have been found to be moderately correlated in general populations. Marcus, Wing, and Lamparski (1985) found that those two factors correlated with binge eating severity among obese women, and Lowe and Caputo (1991) reported that all three factors were associated with binge eating. Westenhoefer, Stunkard, and Pudel (1999) attempted to improve the cognitive restraint scale by adding additional items and dividing it into two scales to reflect flexible/appropriate versus rigid/maladaptive approaches to controlling eating. However, the two scales are highly correlated ($r = .77$), and both are positively correlated with disordered eating symptoms.

The Dutch Eating Behavior Questionnaire (DEBQ; van Strien, Frijters, Staveren, Defares, & Deurenberg, 1986) is a 33-item measure with subscales for dietary restraint, external eating, and emotional eating. The latter two correlate highly with the disinhibition and hunger scales on the TFEQ. Gorman and Allison (1995) reviewed the high overlap among the restraint scales in the three measures just discussed. They concluded that the TFEQ and DEBQ restraint scales assess the more successful aspects of dieting behavior, while the Restraint Scale—Revised assesses the consequences of chronic, unsuccessful dieting. In addition, the DEBQ scale appears to assess more purely "cognitive" restraint (i.e., intentions to restrict), whereas the TFEQ scale assesses both the cognitive and the more behavioral (overt) aspects of restraint. Because the concept of restraint appears to have several components, it is not surprising that current evidence does not present a clear picture of its relationship to various disordered eating patterns. Thus, continued research is needed to clarify this construct and to develop measures that are clinically useful.

The Emotional Eating Scale (EES; Arnow, Kenardy, & Agras, 1995) is similar to the DEBQ emotional eating subscale. The participant rates the extent to which each of the specified feeling states lead her to feel an urge to eat. Internal consistency is good. Given the importance accorded to binge eating that is triggered by emotions, either of these measures can be used to quickly assess the degree to which emotional eating is likely to be a problem for a particular client.

Three scales assess aspects of cravings for food. The Craving Questionnaire (Weingarten & Elston, 1991) asks the respondent to indicate which foods have been craved, how frequently cravings occur, and several other questions (e.g., how much of the time the person eats the craved food). Interestingly, one-third of the women surveyed in that study reported cravings were related to their menstrual cycle. The Hill, Weaver, and Blundell (1991) craving questions assess frequency and strength of cravings. Their results suggest that both hunger and negative moods precipitate food cravings. The most recent measure attempts to capture the multidimensional nature of cravings and provides both a state and a trait version (Cepeda-Benito, Gleaves, Williams & Eroth, 2000). Schlundt, Virts, Sbrocco, Pope-Cordle, and Hill (1993) found that people with high and low levels of cravings could be differentiated: craving was highly related to moods and cognitions. However, in a general sample (Weingarten & Elston, 1991), there were no differences in cravings between women who were and were not on a diet. Thus, the role of dieting in creating cravings is not clear. Current evidence does not indicate whether greater cravings are associated with poorer response to treatment, but this idea would be worth further investigation.

In the Forbidden Food Survey (see Schlundt & Johnson, 1990), the respondent rates how she would feel about herself after eating specified foods. A total score on the 45-item scale can be used as a summary measure of fear of forbidden foods. The scale has not yet been used to evaluate response to treatment, but it could be useful in both generating hierarchies and evaluating the effectiveness of gradual exposure to feared foods, which is often part of treatment for AN and BN.

An Eating Hedonics Questionnaire (Mitchell et al., 1999) has been recently developed to assess the cognitions and feelings associated with binge eating. The authors report that individuals with BED differ from those with BN in that they are more likely to enjoy the sensations associated with binge eating and to report more relaxation and less physical discomfort. Understanding the apparent positive function of binges in BED may be useful in tailoring treatment for that group.

Hagan, Whitworth, and Moss (1999) recently reported on the development of a measure to assess the occurrence of what are labeled semistarvation behaviors (e.g., bizarre mixing of foods, deception, eating soiled or discarded foods). College students who reported high levels of binge eating also reported significant frequencies of some peculiar eating habits and some drastic measures to resist binges. This scale may be clinically useful since individuals may be unlikely to report these atypical behaviors unless they are specifically asked to do so.

Self-Reports Specific to Cognitions

Cognitions and attitudes are assessed to some degree in all the symptom measures reviewed earlier, but several specific measures are also available. Mizes and Christiano (1995) provide a detailed review of the various self-report and alternative assessment methodologies (e.g., thought sampling) that have been developed to assess cognitions. These authors concluded that (1) there was little evidence to suggest that the alternative methods yielded more valid or more sensitive data and (2) self-report measures were briefer and easier to score. Thus, only the more commonly used self-reports are described here.

The Mizes Anorectic Cognitions Questionnaire (MAC; Mizes & Klesges, 1989) is probably the best established measure. It has 33 Likert-type items. Factor analyses supported the existence of three factors (assessing perception of weight and eating as the basis of approval from others; beliefs that rigid self-control is fundamental to self-worth; and rigidity of weight and eating regulation efforts). The scale has been revised, and several reports (Kettlewell, Mizes, & Wasylyshyn, 1992; Mizes, 1988, 1990, 1991, 1992) provide extensive evidence of its reliability, internal consistency, validity (correlations with in vivo cognitive measures and symptom severity measures), sensitivity, and discrimination between eating disorder and other comparison groups.

The Bulimic Thoughts Questionnaire (Phelan, 1987) assesses three factors (self-schema, self-efficacy, and salient beliefs). It consists of 20 thoughts derived from the thought diaries of a bulimic sample (10 worded positively and 10 worded negatively). The thoughts are rated on the basis of how often the individual has such thoughts (1, not at all, to 5, all the time). Bulimic women score higher than do nonbulimic women. The author reports that bulimics typically score above 25 on the sum of the negative thoughts and below 25 on the sum of the positive thoughts; greater discrepancy between the scores indicates greater severity. Scores decreased significantly after short-term cognitive-behavioral therapy. Normal-weight, nonbulimic women usually show the opposite patterns, scoring above 25 on the positive scale and below 25 on the negative scale. Overweight, non-bingeing women tend to score between 20 and 30 on both scales.

The Modified Distressing Thoughts Questionnaire (MDTQ; Clark, Feldman & Channon, 1989) was designed to assess dimensions of thoughts other than frequency: emotional intensity (degree of sadness and worry generated by the thought), difficulty of removing the thought, guilt generated by the thought, and degree of belief in the thought. Adequate internal consistency and temporal reliability were reported. Some evidence of external validity was demonstrated by the differential relationship of the different types of thoughts (depressive vs. weight-related) to measures of dysphoria and eating disturbance. Bulimic individuals scored higher than anorexic individuals (who scored higher than normal controls) on all six dimensions for the weight-related thoughts. In the anorexic sample, weight-related thoughts were uniquely associated with the level of eating disturbance; it was not clear why this relationship did not hold for bulimics. The MDTQ format for assessing degree of preoccupation with eating and weight thoughts and degree of distress associated with the thoughts is well suited for most ED populations. BN and BED clients typically report significant preoccupation and distress about their thoughts. The MDTQ asks questions about six specific weight-related thoughts; however, the response format can easily be applied to a wider range of thoughts, or the questions can be asked about an individual client's ideosyncratic thoughts. In our research, we obtain an overall estimate of the extent of preoccupation by asking the MDTQ questions about two general categories of thoughts: thoughts about food (e.g., what you are going to eat, what you have eaten, what you want to eat) and thoughts about weight and shape (e.g., how you look and what you weigh).

Although it is a semistructured interview rather than a self-report, the *Yale–Brown–Cornell Eating Disorder Scale* (YBC-EDS; Mazure, Halmi, Sunday, Romano, & Einhorn, 1994) is discussed here because it is relevant to the assessment of eating-disordered cognitions. This interview is a modification of one designed to assess general obsessive–compulsive symptoms. It provides the most comprehensive assessment of eating-related preoccupations, as well as eating-related rituals and body-checking rituals. Participants are asked to describe any preoccupations and rituals they have. To assist them, an extensive checklist of possibilities is provided (organized according to content). Each preoccupation or ritual is rated according to various dimensions, such as severity, ego-syntonicity, time consumed, distress, and interference with functioning. Since the interview is quite time-intensive, it has primarily been used for research purposes. However, it might be worthwhile for some clients (particularly those with severe AN) as they might fail to spontaneously bring up preoccupations and rituals because of the eating disorder's predominately ego-syntonic nature.

Numerous investigators (see Cooper, 1997) have suggested the need to investigate the role of more general, underlying maladaptive core beliefs rather than focusing on specific, eating-related automatic thoughts. Schemas have been considered particularly important for understanding individuals with personality disorders and to partly explain those individual's relatively poorer response to traditional cognitive-behavioral therapy (CBT). Although many individuals with EDs respond well to short-term CBT, it is possible that those who do not are characterized by these more entrenched, unconditional, negative core beliefs. If this is correct, better assessment of these generalized beliefs may help predict who will not respond to treatment, as well as to improve treatment. At the present time, only two studies have looked at such beliefs. Both studies used Young's Schema Questionnaire (YSQ; Young, 1994). This 205-item self-report questionnaire provides a score for 16 different core beliefs. Each item is rated on a 6-point scale from "completely untrue of me" to "describes me perfectly." Waller, Ohanian, and Meyer (2000) compared three bulimic groups (bulimic–anorexic, bulimic, binge eaters); Leung, Waller, and Thomas (1999) included a restricting anorexic group. Both studies found that women with EDs had more unhealthy core beliefs than did normal comparison groups. The overall strength of beliefs did not generally differ between the clinical groups. This assessment tool is quite time-consuming, but a shorter version is now available (Young & Klosko, 1993) that may be useful.

Self-efficacy (i.e., beliefs about how well one is likely to handle eating in certain situations) is another cognitive feature that is relevant to eating disorders. The Dieter's Inventory of Eating Temptations (DIET; Schlundt & Zimering, 1988) presents 30 problem situations and provides a "competent" response; the subject indicates what percentage of the time they would make that response (e.g., "What percent of the time would you turn down a second helping?"). The measure discriminated well between overweight and normal weight subjects, was modestly related to community persons' reported ability to lose and maintain weight loss, and added modestly to the prediction of 1-year weight loss following treatment. Five subscales are reported: emotional eating, exercise, craving sweets, overeating, and food preparation. The Situation-Based Dieting Self-Efficacy Scale (SDS; Stotland, Zuroff, & Roy, 1991) has respondents rate 25 specific situations in terms of their confidence that they could stick to their diet in the situation. The authors' results indicate that the measure taps into something different from dietary restraint, but the implications for treatment are not clear since it has not been used in outcome research. The Situational Appetite Measure (SAM; Stanton, Garcia, & Green, 1990) presents 30 somewhat more general descriptions of problem situations than the two previously described measures (e.g., "when I am watching television") in five domains: relaxation, food present, hunger, reward, and negative feelings. The respondent rates both the strength of urges to eat in the situation and self-efficacy (the degree to which they could control their eating in that situation).

A very similar and correlated measure is the Eating Self-Efficacy Scale (ESES; Glynn & Ruderman, 1986), a 25-item scale in which individuals rate how difficult it is to control overeating in general situations (e.g., after work or school). Factor analysis confirmed two factors, one consisting of eating in response to various types of negative affect and one consisting of eating in response to various "socially acceptable circumstances." Improved total scores after a behavioral weight loss program were reported by these authors. Also reported were improved scores for the negative affect situations scale after CBT for BED (Allen & Craighead, 1999). The Self-Efficacy Questionnaire (SEQ; Schneider, O'Leary, & Agras, 1987), with 56 items representing seven domains, is designed more specifically to rate areas that are relevant to recovery from bulimia. The authors reported it was sensitive to changes in vomiting frequency following treatment.

Bruch's "ineffectiveness" construct has been considered important for understanding the core pathology of anorexia, but assessments of self-esteem or ineffectiveness have generally not differentiated between anorexics and psychiatric controls. Bers and Quinlan (1992) reported on an Interests and Abilities Questionnaire that was developed specifically to assess perceived-competence deficits (PCD, or discrepancy between one's interest in various activities and perceived abilities). This measure differentiated hospitalized anorexics from both normal controls and hospitalized psychiatric controls; anorexics reported low abilities (as did the psychiatric controls) but high levels of interest (as did the controls but not the psychiatric controls). Anorexics reported large discrepancies between what they wanted to do and what they felt they did well, whereas normal controls reported very little discrepancy. For anorexics, dieting was the only activity in which they experienced no perceived deficit in competence (i.e., they rate it as high importance and high ability). Several other measures of self-esteem and depression were included in the study, but only the self-criticism factor of the Depressive Experiences Questionnaire (Blatt, D'Afflitti, & Quinlan, 1976) also discriminated between the groups. No comparisons to other ED groups were made, so it is unclear whether this finding is unique to anorexia. This measure may prove useful in pointing out specific areas that ED patients feel are important but in which they do not measure up to their high standards.

Another cognitive measure with the potential to influence the type of treatment offered has recently been reported. Hohlstein, Smith, and Atlas (1998) reported on the development of the following two measures, which were based on expectancy theory. The 34-item Eating Expectancy Inventory (EEI) includes five subscales that reflect the person's beliefs that eating will help manage negative affect, alleviate boredom, enhance cognitive competence, be useful as a reward, or lead to feeling out of control. The 44-item Thinness and Restricting Expectancy Inventory had only one clear factor, which assessed beliefs about the positive consequences of being thin/restricting (i.e., overgeneralized self-improvement). These two scales point to a potentially useful distinction between bulimics and anorexics. Both groups expect positive consequences from being thin, but only bulimics expect negative reinforcement from eating. Anorexics expect significantly less positive reinforcement from eating than do bulimics or controls. If these results prove reliable, such a measure might be useful in tailoring cognitive treatments specifically to address maladaptive beliefs about the functions of eating for a particular client or type of ED.

Body Image Assessment

Body image problems can be assessed in a number of ways. The most commonly used self-report measures provide a general index of body dissatisfaction (e.g., the Body Dissatisfaction subscale of the EDI and the Body Shape Questionnaire (Cooper, Taylor, Cooper, & Fairburn, 1987). The EDE interview and the EDE-Q also have specific weight and shape concern subscales. Thompson (1995) describes additional measures that more specifically tap into the affective, cognitive, or behavioral components of negative body image. Self-reports (as well as *in vivo* behavioral avoidance tests) of avoidance of body-image-related situations have also been developed. Rosen (1996) provides a comprehensive review of body image intervention, pointing out that current ED treatments often fail to address this important topic directly. Rosen, Reiter, and Orosan (1995) reported on the use of the Body Dysmorphic Disorder Examination with eating disorder patients. This semistructured interview could be useful in assessing individuals with very severe body image disturbance, but it is not necessary in most cases.

In addition to questionnaire measures, various types of figure drawings have been used as a way to more clearly quantify perceived discrepancy from ideal body shape. Subjects select the figure that best represents their current body shape and the one that represents their "ideal." Additional information can be gathered, such as what a "reasonable/maintainable" body shape for the respondent might be, or what shape the respondent thinks other groups (e.g., males) would select as ideal. Williamson and his colleagues have reported on several versions of this assessment that are appropriate for different groups: normal or underweight women (Williamson et al., 1989), moderately to severely overweight persons (Williamson et al., 2000), and male and female children and preadolescents (Veron-Guidry & Williamson, 1996). Notably, in their administrations, the silhouettes are on separate cards, which are presented to the subject in random order for each question asked. This is likely helpful in reducing response biases that might be elicited when the figures are presented in ascending size order, as is done in most self-report versions (e.g., Stunkard, Sorenson, & Schulsinger, 1983 shows nine figures all on one page in ascending size). However, those measures are more efficient for larger scale uses such as screenings. Altabe and Thompson (1992) compared two different types of body image measures and found that the figural drawings were better predictors of eating disturbance than were perceptual estimation measures. The latter have generally failed to demonstrate clinical utility.

The Psychosocial Risk Factors Questionnaire (PRFQ; Whisenhunt, Williamson, Netemeyer, & Womble, 2000) assesses constructs that are related to body image, but it was designed specifically as a brief inventory (18 items rated on a 7-point scale from "strongly disagree" to "strongly agree") to assess *risk* for eating disorders. It has four scales (Social Pressure for Thinness, Media Pressure for Thinness, Concern for Physical Appearance, and Perception of Physical Appearance), which assess constructs that are considered important in sociocultural models of the etiology of eating disorders. The scales have been shown to correlate with ED symptoms, but additional work is needed to determine if the measure is useful and cost-effective for identifying at-risk individuals. The authors report adequate reliability and validity.

Self-Reports for Relevant Personality Traits

Clinical reports have frequently noted that perfectionism is associated with eating disorders, particularly AN. The EDI Perfectionism subscale is most commonly used to assess this construct. Szabo and Terre Blanche (1997) reported that the Perfectionism subscale was the only one that did not show significant improvement at discharge from treatment for a sample with AN. This result supports previous findings regarding the enduring quality of trait perfectionism. Mitzman, Slade, and Dewey (1994) have developed a Neurotic Perfectionism Questionnaire, specifically for use with EDs, that discriminates between normal controls and ED patients. Satisfactory internal consistency and validity were reported.

Slade and Dewey (1986) developed a 40-item screening instrument (SCANS) based on a functional analytic model of AN. That model hypothesizes that perfectionism and general dissatisfaction are the major setting conditions that predispose an individual toward having a high need for bodily control (including weight control). The measure was designed to assess constructs that could be detected before the onset of overt symptoms, so it does not include specific symptom questions. Because its purpose is not as obvious, it may be a more acceptable and effective screen for young, high-risk populations. Factor analyses indicated five scales: perfectionism, general dissatisfaction, social and personal anxiety, adolescent problems, and need for weight control. A combination of scores on the first two constructs provided the best discrimination between ED patients and controls.

Bulik, Sullivan, Carter, McIntosh, and Joyce (1999) included the Temperament and Character Inventory in a treatment study (CBT for BN) and reported that the self-directedness scale predicted a positive short-term response to this treatment, independent of the baseline frequency of binge eating. Thus, this scale may be useful in identifying individuals for whom self-help or less intensive forms of therapy might be adequate.

Fahy and Eisler (1993) reported using the Impulsivity Questionnaire in a sample of ED patients. Patients with BN had higher scores (and reported more impulsive behaviors in an interview) than did those with AN. Individuals with BN who reported low impulsiveness demonstrated a more rapid response to treatment; however, by follow-up there were no differences between groups. This scale may also prove useful in identifying individuals for whom less intensive therapy might be adequate.

Motivation to Change

Assessing motivation to change has been a relatively recent focus in the eating disorder literature, despite the clinical consensus that denial and resistance to treatment are commonly encountered (particularly in the treatment of AN). Early work, primarily based on clinician ratings, did not prove particularly helpful, at least in terms of predicting response to treatment. However, recent measures are more promising. The Goldberg Anorectic Attitude Scale (Goldberg et al., 1980) includes a four-item "denial of illness" factor that was shown to correlate negatively with weight gain in the hospital and positively with body size overestimation and staff ratings of anorexic behavior. However, the factor was not related to *clinician* ratings of denial (Casper, Halmi, Goldberg, Eckert, & Davis, 1979; Eckert, Goldberg, Halmi, Caster, & Davis, 1981; Goldberg et al., 1980; Steinhausen, 1986). On the Concerns about Change Scale (Vitousek, Watson, & Wilson, 1998), anorexics scored higher than bulimics, agoraphobics, and specific phobics on four subscales that were related to resistance to change. Engel and Wilms (1986) compared patient and therapist ratings on 15 aspects of motivation and found that therapists considered the patients less motivated than they viewed themselves, both at the beginning and at the end of treatment. Sunday, Halmi, and Einhorn (1995) confirmed that restricting anorexics were less likely to wish to change their preoccupations/rituals than were purging anorexics or bulimics.

In summary, the little empirical work currently available on the constructs of denial and motivation to change certainly support clinical intuition about the importance of these variables, but the research makes it clear that there is no one construct that can be easily assessed. Findings appear to differ considerably, depending on the specific measure that is used. Therefore, researchers and clinicians will need to be clearer about which aspect of this construct they are attempting to assess. At a minimum, the following dimensions need to be considered: degree of insight or denial of problems or motivation for treatment (typically as rated by a clinician), expectancies of treatment, fears and concerns about changing, perceived benefits of symptoms, self-reported desire to change, attempts to change, and actual ability to change (treatment response). Anorexics, and to some degree bulimics, have high levels of concern about the prospect of losing the perceived benefits of their predominately ego-syntonic symptoms. Ambivalence about change will likely interfere with responsiveness to treatment recommendations and thus needs to be assessed and addressed directly.

The most recent work in this area has been the adaptation of measures developed within the "transtheoretical" model of change, which was developed in the area of addictions. This model describes four different stages of readiness to change: precontemplation, contemplation, action, and maintenance. Readiness to change has proven to be useful in predicting treatment outcome and treatment dropout (Prochaska & Norcross, 1994; Smith, Subich, & Kalodner, 1995) in substance abuse treatment. However, initial work applying the construct to eating problems was less successful (Blake, Turnbull, &

Treasure, 1997; Stanton, Rebert, & Zinn, 1986). The most recent development, the Readiness and Motivation Interview (RMI; Geller & Drab, 1999), appears to be more promising because it is designed specifically to address the multidimensional nature of the symptoms of eating disorders. In eating disorders, individuals are generally more willing to make changes in bingeing behaviors than they are in restricting behaviors or in the importance of weight and shape. The RMI also uses a semistructured interview (rather than self-report) format, which the authors consider critical in helping the participant articulate her feelings more clearly. The interview was designed to be used in conjunction with the EDE (described earlier). The motivation questions are asked for each symptom cluster (Cognitive/Affective, Restriction, Bingeing, and Compensatory Behaviors) after the severity ratings have been made for that cluster. The interviewer asks to what extent that symptom is experienced as a problem by the client and then makes three ratings indicating the extent to which the individual identifies herself as being in each stage of change: for instance, precontemplation (25%), contemplation (50%), and action (25%) (action and maintenance are not considered to be separate stages). The ratings must sum to 100%. If the individual is in the action stage at all, a rating is also given to indicate the degree to which she is doing this for herself versus others (e.g., 50% internality). Subscale scores can be summed to provide overall ratings for each of the three stages of change and for internality. Geller, Cockell, and Drab (2001) reported on the psychometric properties of the RMI in a sample of women with anorexia. High interrater reliability (over 90%) and acceptable internal consistency were reported. RMI scores correlated with questionnaire readiness scores and psychiatric distress, and they were predictive of two (analogue) behavioral measures of change. Discriminant validity was demonstrated by the lack of correlation with BMI, a measure of desirable responding, and a measure of symptom severity. Readiness is hypothesized to be independent of symptom severity. The authors note that, in this study, the assessors assured clients that their responses would not be shared with those making treatment decisions, and this was likely significant in terms of obtaining candid responses. This notion would need careful consideration when the RMI is used in a clinical context. The authors suggest that different types of treatment should be made available to individuals, depending on their readiness to change, rather than excluding individuals from treatment who are in the earlier stages. By clearly identifying those symptoms the person is most willing to change, Geller and Drab (1999) suggest that initial stages of treatment may be better tailored to the specific individual. They note that "treatment programmes may at times attempt to bring about change in individuals who are not yet ready to change . . . this mismatch . . . may cause a well-intentioned therapy to deteriorate into an entrenched battle between therapist and client over food and weight" (p. 260). Clinton (1996) found that lack of congruence between patients' and therapists' expectations of treatment was related to treatment dropout. Thus, appropriate matching of stage of change to type of intervention might reduce dropout, improve initial engagement and treatment outcome, and reduce recidivism. Howver, the RMI has not yet been evaluated in outcome studies. Treasure et al. (1999) used a 24-item self-report measure of stage of change and found it did predict initial (4-week) response to treatment and development of a therapeutic alliance in a sample of women with BN. It did not predict dropout during that initial phase. It may be that assessing readiness will be even more useful with women with AN, as they are generally less distressed about their symptoms and are more often brought to treatment by concerned others.

Less has been done to assess readiness for weight control programs. Pendleton et al. (1998) reported on the development of a Diet Readiness Test, which had adequate internal consistency but failed to predict changes in a clinical population during treatment.

Self-Monitoring

Self-monitoring measures that assess nutrient intake and/or various aspects of eating behavior are commonly used as part of behavioral treatment programs. Such records provide the most clinically useful data in terms of conducting functional analyses of eating behaviors. However, as an initial assessment device, self-monitoring is time-intensive (for the subject) and provides such a small sample of behavior (perhaps 1 to 2 weeks) that it is not particularly useful in terms of establishing diagnoses. Eating behavior, particularly binge eating, is known to be highly variable over time and very responsive to environmental contexts. Thus, a minimum of 4 weeks is generally recommended as necessary to have a valid estimate of the frequency of binge eating. Thus, retrospective self-report (as in the EDE) is more practical as an initial assessment tool. In addition, most behaviors show an initial, reactive effect from self-monitoring. Asking a client who has just presented for treatment to do a week of self-monitoring is not likely to produce a valid indicator of her typical eating patterns.

A variety of instructions and forms for the self-monitoring of food intake have been used. Such data are more often utilized as process measures to demonstrate change during treatment than as pre–post measures. Williamson (1990) has reported some support for the predictive and concurrent validity of his form of self-monitoring; each eating episode is rated on a separate form that includes the specific amounts and types of food eaten, as well as information about antecedents and consequences of eating. Caloric and nutrient data (e.g., percentage of fat) can be generated from food records, although that is a time-intensive procedure. However, evaluating changes in dietary patterns may be quite useful in weight loss treatments.

Appetite ratings are the focus of self-monitoring records developed by Craighead and Allen (1995). Subjects rate each eating episode, indicating on a scale of 1 (very hungry) to 7 (very full) where they were before and after eating. These ratings are used to determine the number of "hunger violations" (when the individual's rating is below 2.5 before eating) and "satiety violations" (when the individual's rating is above 5.5 after eating). In addition, the person's feelings about the eating episode are rated as positive, negative, or "out of control." Also, for any satiety violation, the subject circles which of five hypothesized problematic patterns had been invoked: getting too hungry before eating, eating when not hungry because food was available, eating in response to emotions, not attending to moderate satiety cues, or giving up control after overeating (or eating "forbidden" food). These ratings are utilized during treatment to identify which patterns need to be the focus of intervention. Such assessments may be particularly useful in BED, as initial findings suggest a broader range of patterns is associated with this disorder, whereas excessive dietary restriction is hypothesized to be the primary factor driving binges associated with AN and BN.

Self-monitoring may be a useful way to ask very specific research questions about the eating behaviors of various diagnostic groups, as well as to tailor treatment to the individual. For example, if an individual reports that she does a lot of emotional eating, self-monitoring may confirm this or may point out that many of her overeating episodes are due to responding to food that is available. Those episodes may not have been as salient to her as the emotion-cued episodes, but they may be contributing as much, if not more, to her weight problem.

Family Functioning

Family variables can be important, particularly for adolescents (or others) who live with their families. However, few measures of family attitudes or interactions have been reported in ED studies. Van Furth et al. (1996) used the Camberwell Family Interview to obtain measures from each parent on "expressed emotion" (EE); this included five ratings (critical comments, hostility, emotional overinvolvement, warmth, and positive remarks). Although overall levels of EE were quite low in that sample and did not differ between parents, the mothers' critical comments were shown to be a substantial predictor of outcome both at posttest and at follow-up; EE was a better predictor than were a number of standard clinical variables, including severity of illness. However, this interview-based measure is time-consuming and requires trained raters, so it is not easily used in a clinical situation. Furthermore, parents of individuals with EDs demonstrate relatively low levels of critical comments and emotional overinvolvement, compared to several other disorders (see Hodes, Dare, Dodge, & Eisler, 1999), so it is unclear how useful assessment of family variables will prove to be. Using a self-report measure of family functioning (Family Relations Scale), Szabo, Goldin, and Le Grange (1999) found families across types of EDs to be quite similar.

LINKING ASSESSMENT WITH TREATMENT

Reliability, specificity, and validity are the primary criteria for evaluating the utility of assessments. Valid assessment is essential to the research process as the utility of the findings rests on appropriate assessment of whatever construct is being evaluated. Many of the measures presented earlier have been widely used in research studies and serve research purposes quite well. However, choosing assessments for clinical purposes must take into account additional factors such as the practical issues of cost and time requirements, both for the client (e.g., satisfaction with treatment or dropout) and the clinician (e.g., level of training needed to give the assessment). Ideally, clinical assessment serves three purposes:

1. Initially—to provide specific diagnostic and descriptive information to help with treatment planning.
2. Ongoing—to monitor progress so that other treatment options may be considered if progress is not being made.
3. At termination or during follow-up—to document outcomes for funding and accountability and, potentially, to identify early relapse and facilitate reinstating an appropriate intervention.

However, the realities of clinical practice may limit the implementation of assessment-based recommendations for treatment: financial resources must be considered; some options (partial hospitalization, specialized inpatient units, etc.) may not be accessible; and available clinicians may not be trained in certain approaches. In the following discussion we present the major questions that might be asked during an assessment and make some recommendations based, whenever possible, on empirical findings.

Screenings

Adolescent and young adult females (ages 13 to 24) are clearly the highest risk group for AN and BN and, ideally, should be assessed briefly on a yearly basis. The relative ease of conducting screenings for girls in school compared to the relatively poor treatment response, expense of treatment, and mortality associated with AN makes a compelling argument for screening adolescent girls for EDs despite the low base rate of AN. Although eating disorders also affect males and can emerge later in life, regular screening of those populations would likely not be cost-effective. However, individuals seeking treatment for weight control should be screened for BED since the base rate is very high in that population. Black and Wilson (1996) also suggest screening women in substance abuse treatments due to high rates of comorbid eating problems in that population. Garner, Rosen, and Barry (1998) describe the use of screenings appropriate for athletes, another at-risk group.

The primary target symptoms of a screening should be consistent with the different ages at which individuals are at highest risk of the various disorders. The mean age of onset of anorexia is 17, but bimodal peaks at ages 14 and 18 are reported (DSM-IV; American Psychiatric Association, 1994) suggesting that stressors associated with the transition to high school and to college may precipitate the onset of acute illness. The onset of BN is most commonly between the ages of 17 and 18. The onset of objective binge eating (subclinical levels of BED) is most often in the late teens or early 20s, even though most individuals do not meet the frequency criteria for a full diagnosis until later. Fortunately, the problematic attitudes (i.e., primarily negative body image and overconcern with weight or shape) that are characteristic of girls at greatest risk can usually be identified well before the onset of clinically significant symptoms (e.g., inappropriate weight loss or compensatory behaviors).

Screenings are best used to identify the top 20% of girls, i.e., those reporting the highest eating and weight concerns. "Normative" discontent with weight or shape is quite prevalent and is not an adequate indication of risk for EDs. Brief screening at entry to high school and college would be ideal in terms of identifying individuals at risk who could then be monitored more closely or could be targeted for early intervention. Hsu (1996) reviewed a number of epidemiology studies that support the conclusion that false negatives are quite uncommon. Essentially all clinical and subclinical cases identified through interviews (as well as extensive case finding) came from individuals whose self-report identified them as high or moderate risk, with none coming from the low-risk group. Rathner and Messner (1993) used two symptom self-report measures and measured actual weight; they commented specifically on the added benefit of obtaining *actual* weight. Early detection of eating symptoms is considered important because long intervals between the initial development of symptoms and the beginning of treatment are hypothesized to be associated with poorer treatment response. However, a recent review of AN treatment by Schoemaker (1997) concluded that methodological concerns and the paucity of studies make it difficult to adequately evaluate that hypothesis.

Early detection for BN and BED can be done on the basis of self-report alone; however, monitoring measured weight and assessing significant other's reports of eating habits enhances early detection for anorexia. The ego-syntonic nature of AN means that, at early stages, the client is highly motivated to hide her symptoms and is generally not motivated for treatment. Vandereycken (1992) reported on the use of an Anorectic Behavior Observation Scale that was developed for parents' reports; a cutoff score of 19 yielded excellent sensitivity and specificity. Powers and Powers (1984) noted that only 20% of their cases of anorexia were underweight before the onset of the problem; 50% were normal weight, and 30% were overweight. Thus, underweight girls do not necessarily have the greatest risk for developing AN, but if they also report negative body attitudes and overconcern, close monitoring is warranted; when the individual is already underweight, weight loss can more quickly get to medically dangerous levels. Powers (1996) reported a case study that illustrated how monitoring an adolescent's weight on a growth chart enabled her to identify when the girl's relative percentage of normal weight dropped; this happened before there was any *actual weight loss* since she was growing taller.

Noticeable weight loss that occurs over a fairly short period of time is a risk marker even in normal and overweight girls. Unusual initial success in losing weight (whether due to intentional dieting, illness, or other reasons) can trigger the acute onset of AN or BN.

The substantial weight loss may convince the girl that she can restrict successfully, spurring her on to even more severe restriction in order to achieve a very thin ideal, or it may lead to extreme fears of regaining the weight just lost, triggering compensatory behaviors. The initial effects of being thinner (e.g., internal satisfaction, others' reactions) are generally so extremely positive that, having experienced these, an individual may develop extreme fears of regaining weight and become willing to resort to compensatory behaviors to quell those fears. Untested beliefs about how easily one regains weight can drive unneeded restrictive efforts. The restriction may lead to binge eating and purging, or the individual may start to compensate when she eats even a small amount of "forbidden" foods. At least 30% of individuals starting out as restricting AN eventually develop binge eating and/or purging (Strober, Freeman, & Morrell, 1997).

Several self-report indicators that have been shown to confer risk include feeling out of control while eating, negative body image despite normal weight status (a very thin ideal weight), high perfectionism, perceived competence deficits (ineffectiveness or dissatisfaction), overconcern with weight and shape as the basis for self-evaluation, maladaptive approaches to dieting (skipping meals, use of rigid food rules, and very low calorie/fat limits), and reports of being teased about weight (see Leon, Keel, Klump, & Fulkerson, 1997). Although the EAT-26 has been the most commonly used screen, other, even briefer screens are available. Powers (1996) describes seven brief questions that a health professional can incorporate into a routine visit or physical. Freund, Boss, Handleman, and Dell (1999) used just two questions: "Do you eat in secret?" and "Are you satisfied with your weight?" In our screenings of college women, we ask, "Are you more concerned about your weight and shape than your peers?" That seems to work well for identifying women with clinical or subclinical BN (or various forms of EDNOS), but less well in identifying currently successful high restrictors. Whether one should use a brief, less obvious screen or a well-validated instrument (such as the EAT-26), which asks specific questions about symptoms, depends on the population being assessed.

Girls and young women identified in screenings as at-risk, who are also objectively overweight and distressed by their weight, need to be provided options for instruction in healthy dieting practices. If not assisted, many turn to unhealthy, quick weight loss schemes as popularized in the media. The use of maladaptive (rigid) dieting strategies is associated with the development of binge eating, which, over time, is associated with further weight gain. Given that cognitive behavioral interventions are quite effective in reducing binge eating and stabilizing weight, and that no treatments are very effective in promoting substantial, long-term weight loss, it is of utmost priority to prevent mildly overweight adolescent girls and college women from becoming obese. Programs also need to focus on improving body image since the majority of these individuals are unlikely to achieve the thin ideals that they hold. Stabilization (or modest weight loss) and acceptance of a weight that can be maintained by eating normally would be the goals for such programs. For those individuals who are still growing, weight stabilization alone will lead to lower BMI over time.

Adolescents identified as at-risk by their attitudes who are normal or only slightly underweight warrant at least monitoring of weight. Weight loss of any significant amount in this developmental stage is not "normal"; adolescents normally gain weight as they get taller. BN is more difficult than AN for others to detect since weight loss is often minimal or nonexistent. Parents, teachers, dentists, and physicians need to be educated about other possible signs of eating disorders (e.g., dental problems, swollen [salivary] glands, excessive use of mouthwash, changes in health of hair or skin, secretive eating, failure to eat normal meals with family and friends, excessively rigid restrictions on type of food, frequenting the bathroom after eating, fainting). Parents need to be educated about not responding in an overcontrolling, intrusive manner yet not colluding in denial of a problem. Once a young woman has been identified by a significant other as at risk, an interview with a sympathetic, trained person is the best way to ask further about current efforts to diet and possible use of compensatory behaviors (these may still be denied). The Motivational Interviewing stance (described earlier) is likely to promote getting the most accurate information. Such an interview can serve as the basis for a treatment referral, or it may just initiate some contemplation about the potential negative aspects of the individual's current behaviors. Body-image therapy (see Cash, 1996; Franko, 1998) is most appropriate for high-risk girls and women who do not yet display inappropriate binge eating or compensatory behaviors. Such interventions have been shown to reduce negative body image and, as such, best address the core issue for those who are not overweight. Girls who report any level of purging warrant early intervention. Cost-effective groups, or brief interventions incorporating self-help strategies, are effective for many individuals at this early point. Intervention also identifies those individuals who do not respond and who need more intensive intervention.

It is important to note here that primary prevention programs that target unselected populations have demonstrated little success. Although knowledge levels are generally shown to increase, there is little evidence that attitudes change and even less that problematic behaviors change or that EDs are prevented by primary prevention efforts. In at least one case (Mann, Nolen-Hoeksema, Huang, & Burgard, 1997), such a program appears to have exacerbated weight and shape concerns. Those investigators hypothesized that the program may "normalize" eating concerns or may even educate girls about maladaptive dieting strategies. Secondary prevention programs (for those with some level of symptoms already) may turn out to be a better alternative for EDs. Schwitzer, Bergholz, Dore, and Salimi (1998) describe a multiple-level model of intervention that is particularly appropriate for a college setting.

We are currently evaluating group CBT with appetite monitoring for individuals with early-stage BED (Elder & Craighead, 2000) because we were concerned about encouraging food monitoring in early-stage clients. Although there are currently no data to substantiate this concern, clinical reports suggest that food monitoring may exacerbate cognitive preoccupations with food. We find that early-stage binge eaters are more accepting of appetite monitoring than food monitoring. Further work is needed to confirm our hypothesis that a combination of appetite monitoring and body-image work will provide a noniatrogenic way to encourage behavior change (reduce binge and overeating) and to address the core cognitive concerns of early stage binge eaters.

Initial Assessment Questions

• *Does this person have a diagnosable disorder and what treatment is recommended?* As noted earlier, symptom self-report measures are not sufficiently accurate or specific to generate clinical diagnoses for EDs. Other standard assessments, such as the Minnesota Multiphasic Personality Inventory (MMPI-2), also do not distinguish between the diagnostic subtypes of EDs (see Pryor & Wiederman, 1996). In addition to the major subtypes, there are a wide variety of presentations that may be diagnosed as EDNOS. EDNOS currently includes subsyndromal cases (not meeting criteria for frequency or duration of AN or BN) and BED. As noted earlier, it is unclear if loss of control is important for obese clients meeting all other criteria for BED. Mizes and Sloan (1998) describe another common EDNOS subgroup; these individuals resemble BED in being overweight, but resemble BN in reporting some purging.

Clinical interviews are needed to establish reliable and accurate diagnoses. Clear information about size and frequency of binges is needed to establish BN and BED diagnoses, and sensitive probing is needed to elicit accurate information about compensatory behaviors and fears of weight gain. Individuals will be differentially motivated to over- or under-report what they are eating, depending on their motivation to get help. Although clinicians can obtain the appropriate information to make a diagnosis in an unstructured interview, a semistructured interview is recommended for several reasons. Even a well-trained clinician can become sidetracked by the client's distress in the moment or by a very involved history. Information needed to make the diagnosis may be missed. Letting the client know that you will be asking a structured series of questions can make it a little easier to stay on track, and to redirect a client who is providing too much detail or to probe a reticent client who is less willing to bring up the more upsetting aspects of the problem. The client is often reassured when the clinician asks knowledgeable questions about atypical behaviors/attitudes and may then be more forthcoming. In a semistructured interview, the clinician ensures that all the important information is obtained and that his or her notes will always be in the same format; this makes it easier to find information later (to write up a report) than to retrieve information from a set of unstructured notes. In particular, when the assessor is not going to be the treating clinician (as is often the case in clinics), a structured assessment may be more comfortable for the client. Any of the interviews discussed earlier are adequate, but those designed to serve as a complete interview (including obtaining an adequate history) and those with clear decision trees for making diagnoses may be better if the interviewers are less experienced or do not have specific training.

A number of treatment options have been developed within the experimental-clinical tradition. These include behavioral treatments to restore weight in anorexia nervosa, cognitive behavior therapy, family therapy, interpersonal psychotherapy, pharmacological treatments, and integrative treatments. For recent reviews of effective treatments for eating disorders, see the American Psychiatric Association practice guidelines (American Psychiatric Association, 2000) or Garner and Garfinkel (1997).

Treatments for AN have been the most difficult to evaluate due to the low base rates and practical problems that limit the use of random assignment and make it difficult to standardize length of treatment. Also, by their nature, inpatient programs are generally multicomponent interventions, making it difficult to draw firm conclusions about different aspects of treatment. Behavioral programs focused on weight restoration, cognitive-behavioral therapy, and family therapy have received the most support, but few comparative studies have been done. Dare, Eisler, Russell, and Szmukler (1990) reported family therapy was more effective than individual, supportive psychotherapy for AN patients with early onset and short duration of the disorder. No differences were found for subjects with later onset or duration more than 3 years or for those with BN. For both BN and BED, CBT has been the most extensively evaluated treatment and has the most support in terms of rapid initial symptom reduction. In one study, clients with BED who did not respond to CBT did not appear to do better when they were switched to IPT (Agras et al., 1995). Lengthening the standard course of CBT was shown to improve outcome for BED nonresponders (Eldredge et al., 1997). Antidepressants are commonly used with all the EDs. Despite these generally effective treatment options, substantial subsets of clients do not respond or are only partial responders. Thus, research continues to explore modifications and alternatives to current treatments. For discussions of stepped-care models and integrative treatment models, see Wilson (1999) and Garner and Needleman (1997).

• *To what extent is the client motivated for treatment at this point?* The RMI, described earlier, appears to be the best way to assess readiness for treatment. Asking the motivational change questions about each symptom separately (e.g., bingeing, purging, restricting) seems particularly important for EDs. The RMI was designed for use with the EDE, but the questions could easily be adapted for use with other interviews. As the authors note, the most honest information is likely to be revealed when the client does not think that her responses will affect being accepted for treatment. If the interview suggests the client is not ready for an active treatment (typically CBT), yet not in medical danger (e.g., very low weight), other options may be recommended. Some clients may be willing to accept a referral for IPT. IPT does not require that the client be willing to start directly making changes in her eating behavior. Agras, Wilson, Fairburn, and Walsh (1999) reported no client characteristics that predicted differential response to CBT compared to IPT treatment. Thus, client preference (or therapist expertise) may be a reasonable basis for choosing one approach over the other. One can use the Life Chart (described earlier) to determine if onset of or fluctuations in eating symptoms are clearly related to interpersonal events. Apple (1999) described the successful application of IPT for a case of BN in which that model seemed to fit the case particularly well.

If the client is not motivated for standard CBT, another option is motivational enhancement therapy (MET), which is based on the principles of stages of change (Miller, 1985; Schmidt & Treasure, 1997). Such therapy is focused on increasing dissonance and moving the client forward with respect to stages of change. As the client becomes ready for more active techniques, they are introduced. The model assumes that clients may shift back and forth in terms of readiness to change. Whenever the clinician detects resistance to more active techniques, he or she returns to the basic motivational interviewing stance. MET utilizes CBT interventions in its active phases. Further investigation is needed to determine the effectiveness of this approach or how it can best be combined with other interventions. MET may turn out to be particularly applicable to AN as ambivalence about change is often quite apparent with respect to restricting symptoms. Vitousek et al. (1998) describe a number of strategies to reduce resistance and discuss specifically how the Socratic method appears to be quite well suited to dealing with those issues.

• *Is the client willing to self-monitor?* Even if a client appears ready to take direct action to make changes, some are resistant to a fundamental aspect of CBT—food monitoring. Wilson and Vitousek (1999) discuss how best to present self-monitoring and describe ways to reduce resistance to self-monitoring. They point out that although fairly good compliance is reported in research studies, clinicians often report problems with compliance. Poor compliance appears to be one of the reasons that therapists choose not to use CBT. We recommend asking clients directly about their past experiences with self-monitoring. Clients are typically asked to do 1 or 2 weeks of baseline monitoring. The client's response helps clarify whether she sees monitoring as useful or if it is likely to be difficult to sustain for a long period. CBT can be modified to use appetite instead of food monitoring (Craighead & Allen, 1995); this approach is more acceptable to some clients. Negative reactions to food monitoring are often related to the shame experienced in recording large binges; some clients who need more feedback about food type become more receptive to adding food monitoring to their appetite monitoring once their binges are smaller. Negative reactions to food monitoring can also be related to philosophical issues. For such clients, the rationale for appetite monitoring may be better accepted. However, many clients have found food monitoring very helpful in the past and find that recording intake of specific foods provides a welcome structure that helps them inhibit impulsive eating. The type of self-monitoring used may turn out to be less important than the fact that careful attention is focused on the structure of eating. Involving the client in the decision about type of monitoring, and being willing to individualize that monitoring, is likely to enhance compliance with either food or appetite monitoring.

• *For clients who are binge eating only, is the client willing to focus on reducing binge eating before addressing weight loss? Is the client interested in a nondieting intervention?* CBT (for BN or BED) asks the client to focus first on stopping binge eating before attempting weight loss directly. This recommendation is based on results reported in Agras, Telch,

Arnow, Eldredge, and Marnell (1997) for BED participants who received CBT followed by a modified behavioral weight loss program. Participants who stopped binge eating completely during the first phase were more successful in subsequently losing (and maintaining) weight than were those who continued binge eating. Early studies had suggested that BED clients might do more poorly (or be more likely to relapse) in standard behavioral weight loss programs than non-bingeing obese. Only one study (Marcus, Wing, & Fairburn, 1995) has directly compared CBT to a primarily behavioral weight loss (BWL) program for the treatment of BED. At the end of active treatment, both interventions were equally effective for reducing binge eating, but individuals who received BWL had lost a moderate amount of weight whereas those in CBT had not. At follow-up, those receiving BWL did not increase the frequency of binges but they did regain some (about half) of the weight lost. Although their total loss remained below that of the CBT group, it was quite modest by follow-up. Only additional follow-up will indicate whether the experience of regaining some weight undermines the longer-term effectiveness of BWL and whether those clients are more likely to relapse with respect to their binge eating. One important note about this study is that all treatment was provided individually, rather than in a group format. Individualized behavioral weight loss treatment is likely to be better able to adapt to the special needs of a BED client than are group weight loss treatments, which include many obese individuals who do not binge. Thus, for overweight BED clients, standard weight loss interventions are not contraindicated, but treatment may need to be individualized and relapse prevention may need to be emphasized. Future studies will help determine the optimal combination of CBT and BWL strategies.

CBT with appetite monitoring is designed to focus on reducing both binge and overeating episodes from the beginning of treatment. Appetite monitoring is used first to set (internal) limits on amounts and establish moderate fullness cues as a functional signal to stop eating. Only when that boundary is firmly in place is the client to consider altering the types of foods eaten to achieve lower calorie and lower fat intake. Monitoring of satiety (e.g., moderate fullness) is continued to prevent the tendency to increase amounts to compensate for not feeling very satisfied (either physically or psychologically) when calories or fat are restricted. Substituting higher volume, lower fat foods is only effective for weight loss if a person does not increase amounts. Restricting the type of food eaten often feels "depriving" even when the calorie amount is normal. This deprived feeling can be a particularly potent trigger for individuals with a history of binge eating. Thus, we recommend assessing feelings of deprivation throughout treatment so treatment can be modified if needed.

Some individuals who binge eat may accept, or may even prefer, a nondieting intervention. Preliminary reports suggest that such interventions can reduce binge eating and moderate the negative body image, low self-esteem, anxiety, and depression that often accompany obesity (Goodrick, Poston, Kimball, Reeves, & Foreyt, 1998).

• *Does the client have other mental health problems that might influence the choice of and/or the expected length of treatment?* Knowledge of comorbid Axis I and Axis II conditions is useful when treating any psychiatric disorder, as the literature is fairly clear that the presence of comorbid disorders is generally associated with poorer response to treatment (see discussion in Reich & Vasile, 1993). Margolis, Spencer, DePaulo, and Simpson (1994) document the very high rate of multiple diagnoses found among ED inpatient populations. Telch and Stice (1998) found that women with BED had higher rates of Axis I and Axis II disorders than did community controls. A full semistructured interview (described in other chapters) is certainly warranted, but when that is not possible there are several specific concerns that at least should be assessed through a briefer informal interview or through self-report.

The most common Axis I complication in the treatment of eating problems is affective disorder (see also Wonderlich & Mitchell, 1997). A history of mood disorder is common in all types of EDs. Bulik, Sullivan, Carter, and Joyce (1996) reported that 75% of subjects with BN in a treatment study had a current mood disorder and 45% of those reported that the mood disorder came before the eating disorder. Having a current mood disorder was associated with greater body image disturbance and lower general levels of functioning. Using a cluster analysis, Stice and Agras (1999) reported that 62% of bulimic women were designated a pure dietary subtype, while 38% were designated a mixed dietary–depressive subtype. The latter reported more eating and weight-related obsessions, social maladjustment, and personality disorders and had poorer treatment response. North and Gowers (1999) found the presence of depression in AN was associated with more abnormal cognitions on the EDI, but depression was not associated with poorer treatment outcome. Over half of patients with BED have a history of depression. Furthermore, depression does not correlate with degree of obesity, so the depression is unlikely to be due to the obesity alone.

Many clients with EDs who present for psychosocial treatment will have already tried medications; therefore, information about medication use should always be part of the history that is taken. Some will be currently taking antidepressants. If these clients are still reporting depressive symptoms, or report their depression has improved but that the medication has had minimal effects on eating, it is important to determine whether they have had an adequate trial of medications. Investigators report occasionally seeing significant reductions in binge eating when clients have gone to larger doses or switched to other antidepressants. The effect of medication alone on eating behaviors is generally similar to the effects of CBT alone, with 30% to 40% of patients reporting complete abstinence from binge eating (see Agras, 1998). Clear advantages of combining medication with therapy have not yet been demonstrated convincingly. Some evidence suggests that with BN, CBT prevents the relapse that is typically seen when medication is stopped and, with BED, medication may enhance weight loss when it is added to CBT.

If a client who presents for psychosocial treatment is not currently on medication, a decision must be made about whether to try medication. In most cases of BN, the client's depression will remit with improvements in the eating symptoms, suggesting that the depression was secondary to the eating disorder and did not necessarily warrant being treated directly. No studies are available to indicate whether those individuals who report depression before the onset of eating symptoms are more likely to need medication. However, Freeman (1998) notes that the small group (perhaps 10% to 15% of those with BN) who report clear melancholic symptoms (e.g., early morning wakening, retardation, poor concentration) appear to benefit the most from medication. Agras (1998) reviewed the data on antidepressants for AN, finding that these medications do not enhance weight restoration, but they may improve weight maintenance over follow-up periods.

Antidepressants appear to act in a way that is incompatible with the goals of CBT for BN. Rossiter et al. (1991) indicate antidepressants work by (temporarily) reducing hunger levels, allowing clients to restrict food intake more successfully (thus reducing the need to purge). This would explain why relapse is such a problem after medication is stopped. In contrast, clients who are successfully treated with CBT report normalized food intake. However, for BED, the addition of medication is less likely to compromise the effects of CBT as those individuals are not typically overrestricting food at the start of treatment. Agras et al. (1994) found that the addition of antidepressants to CBT for BED did not further reduce binges, but it did facilitate weight loss. Our experience is that adding medication has been most helpful for individuals with BED who report substantial fatigue and anhedonia or long-term dysthymic symptoms. Medication often energizes such clients, which promotes compliance with exercise and facilitates the development of incompatible alternative behaviors that are needed to replace emotional eating.

Medication would be compatible with IPT for either BN or BED, but no studies are available to assess whether the combination enhances the effects of IPT. However, it seems likely that the early effects of medication on symptoms might compensate for the IPT's initially weaker effect on eating symptoms. However, this hypothesis needs further evaluation. At this point, medication might best be reserved for individuals who show severe depressive symptoms or for those choosing IPT. A trial of medication may also be warranted for those individuals who do not respond well to a reasonable course of CBT or for BED clients who fail to lose weight once binges are stopped.

Anxiety disorders are also a common comorbid condition for EDs. Bulik et al. (1996) reported that 64% of BN clients in a clinical trial had a comorbid anxiety disorder and, of these, 92% reported that the anxiety disorder had an earlier onset than did the eating disorder. Anxiety disorders were also related to having a history of AN. We noted earlier that assessing for food or eating-related obsessions and rituals is more likely to be useful in cases of AN than in the other EDs. The YBC-EDS interview format can be used to assess both food-related and non-food-related obsessions and rituals. No evidence has been presented to suggest that standard ED treatment is less effective or should be modified when anxiety disorders are present. Craighead and Aibel (2000) describe some of the specific ways in which anxiety may relate to eating concerns and how these issues may be addressed in treatment. If medication would be warranted for anxiety symptoms, antidepressant medication is generally recommended. Thus, the previous discussion regarding their use is relevant. Beumont et al. (1997) reported that antidepressant medication enhanced the effectiveness of nutritional counseling for EDs, specifically for reducing eating and weight concerns, as well as restraint in food intake. However, those who had received antidepressants demonstrated greater relapse during follow-up, so the benefits did not continue after medication was stopped. Future research needs to better evaluate the specific effect of antidepressants on cognitive preoccupations and comorbid anxiety symptoms.

Standard CBT for EDs already includes a strong emphasis on cognitive restructuring, which is a primary component of CBT for many anxiety disorders. Other CBT anxiety techniques would be compatible with the model of treatment if they needed to be incorporated for a particular client. We frequently recommend relaxation training or meditation as alternative ways to create a shift in mood state and consciousness, which is often one of the functions that binges perform.

Substance abuse is the third most common complicating Axis I disorder and is particularly common with BN. Bulik et al. (1996) reported that 48% of BN clients in a clinical trial also had alcohol dependence. Welch and Fairburn (1996) found that rates of alcohol and drug use in BN were higher than among normal controls but were not different from psychiatric controls. However, they concluded that designating an "impulsive" subtype of BN was not useful. Wilson (1993) concluded that there was no evidence to support the conceptualization of binge eating as an "addictive" behavior, and no evidence has been presented to indicate that treatments based on a 12-step addiction model are effective for binge eating. Wilson does recommend that severe substance abuse be treated first, before eating symptoms are addressed. Substance use is a frequent trigger for binge eating, so it is likely to be difficult to make progress with binge eating until those problems are addressed. In addition, severe substance abuse should take priority in that it is likely to have even more negative effects on the client's overall functioning than do disordered eating patterns. However, if the substance abuse is not severe, there is no evidence to suggest that such clients will not respond to standard CBT for the eating disorder. However, Keel, Mitchell, Miller, Davis, and Crow (1999) reported that a history of substance abuse was associated with a poorer long-term (10-year) outcome for BN.

Axis II comorbidity may also be relevant in terms of selecting treatment options.

Semistructured interviews are a more accurate, but more time-consuming, way to make an Axis II diagnosis. The Personality Disorders Questionnaire (Hyler & Reider, 1987) is a self-report measure of Axis II pathology that has been used in several studies of EDs. Raymond, Mussell, Mitchell, de Zwann, and Crosby (1995) found that self-report appeared to be associated with overreporting of symptoms compared to an interview. However, if the clinician simply wants to note possible Axis II pathology for treatment consideration, overreporting is less problematic. Borderline personality disorder (BPD) is the most common Axis II diagnosis for individuals with EDs. Waller (1997) found that BPD was associated with greater severity of eating symptoms and a higher likelihood of dropout from treatment for BN clients. Linehan's Dialectical Behavior Therapy (DBT) for BPD has recently been adapted for use with BED (Telch, 1997; Wiser & Telch, 1999). Other investigators (Marcus, Blocher, Levine, & Sebastiani, 1999) have reported promising pilot work using DBT with a mixed group of chronic, treatment-resistant ED patients, many of whom had borderline features such as self-harm behaviors and dissociative episodes. Thus, although definitive recommendations cannot be made, clinicians might consider DBT for clients with borderline features who are not responding well to the standard treatments.

One additional area that may warrant assessment is a history of sexual abuse. Sexual abuse has been shown to be a general risk factor for psychiatric problems rather than one specific to EDs. However, a history of abuse is quite common among clients with EDs, and a client may not disclose this unless specifically asked. Even when asked, clients may initially deny abuse or may downplay its relevance to their problems. There are no data to suggest that initial treatment focused on the ED is contraindicated or that it should be modified. However, if treatment is not going well, the possibility of sexual abuse should be among those issues that a clinician considers when evaluating the appropriateness of the current treatment. Kearney-Cooke and Striegel-Moore (1996) describe several ways in which sexual abuse may relate to eating problems and illustrate possible ways to incorporate specific techniques to address abuse issues when treating EDs.

During-Treatment Question

- *What are the functions of the binge eating, the purging or the restriction?* In order to individualize treatment for clients with binge eating, it is useful to assess the triggers for and functions of specific binge episodes. Cognitive-behavioral models of BN and BED hypothesize that binges may be triggered by the hunger (or cravings) associated with excessively restricting intake (i.e., skipping meals, fasting, avoiding forbidden foods), and that binges may serve as a reliable (and overly relied upon) means of regulating affect. However, binge patterns vary considerably among individuals, and the functions served by binge eating when it initially developed may not be the primary factors that are maintaining the pattern at a later point in time. A number of self-report measures (described earlier) can be used to alert a clinician to a client's problematic eating patterns. Such measures provide general indicators of emotional eating, ease of disinhibition, eating when not hungry, skipping meals, and other nonadaptive behaviors. However, ongoing assessment during treatment provides more specific information to assist the clinician in setting priorities and choosing appropriate strategies to use during treatment. Clients can be asked to write out a functional analysis for a given binge (or binge/purge) episode, indicating the more remote antecedents, the immediate trigger, and the consequences. These analyses can be written informally or on Problem Analysis Forms found in Linehan (1993).

Self-monitoring forms can also be adapted to provide ongoing measures of the most commonly encountered patterns. The BED/BN model provided by Craighead (2000) identifies maladaptive cycles: emotional eating, eating in response to food available rather than hunger, getting too hungry or restricting type of food, ignoring satiety clues, "what the heck" eating, and planned binges. On the appetite monitoring forms provided, each time the client goes past moderate satiety (over 5.5 on the appetite scale) she indicates which cycle(s) were involved. This information is used to tailor the treatment to the client's specific problems. These self-monitoring records are also helpful in responding to shifts in patterns that occur over the course of treatment. For example, getting too hungry is an initially frequent trigger. This problem responds well to the structured meal pattern. At that point, the role of emotions or the preference for the full feeling may become more salient. Clients differ considerably in terms of which cycles are most resistant to change.

Most clients endorse the idea that they do "emotional eating." However, having to identify emotional eating when it is happening highlights the specific type of emotion that triggers the problem eating (e.g., boredom rather than procrastination), and often points out how even a minor shift in affect can trigger emotional eating once it is an established mode of comforting oneself. CBT utilizes many strategies (e.g., problem solving, pleasurable alternative activities, and cognitive restructuring) to address emotional eating. If a specific emotional problem (e.g., stress at work or a relationship problem) is identified and it is presenting an obstacle to further progress on the eating issues, the focus of treatment may need to shift. If this is needed, I recommend maintaining the focus on eating behavior (i.e., continuing the appetite monitoring to increase awareness of cues), but designating substantial time to the non-eating problem until it is no longer creating such interference. Maintaining the eating focus is generally reassuring to the client that her eating concerns are not being minimized.

Maintaining a dual focus on eating and "other" problems is also a useful way to help a client whose dichotomous thinking style leads her to alternating periods of focusing on one or the other. We emphasize "both-and" thinking (an alternative to "either-or" thinking; see Linehan, 1993) in our stance that one can continue to work on eating patterns while dealing with other concerns. A consistent focus on eating is particularly needed for overweight clients. If clients alternate between periods of intense focus on dieting and periods of ignoring the problem, they are likely to experience a yo-yo pattern of weight loss and weight regain, which is distressing and undermines the client's sense of self-efficacy. With BN/AN clients, a dual focus can be difficult to maintain. The therapist, or the client, may feel that the most urgent problem (e.g., low weight or compensatory behaviors) is not being adequately addressed. However, if a client is not making progress in eating behaviors, continuing to focus on eating may collude with the client's desire to avoid dealing with other difficult issues. In that case, the therapist may do better to switch entirely to a treatment such as IPT, being absolutely clear about why the purging or low weight is no longer the focus of treatment.

It is often useful to distinguish between planned binges and unplanned binges. Unplanned binges are more often due to ignoring fullness. The individual loses awareness or more deliberately "checks out" once she starts eating, or she may focus only on the pleasant taste sensations, thereby avoiding awareness of the increasing fullness sensations. Upon realizing that she has overeaten, even if only slightly, she may experience the abstinence violation effect ("what the heck" response). Thus, intervention for unplanned binges is most effective when focused on appetite awareness and on cognitive restructuring to deal with the dichotomous thinking that is the basis for the "what the heck" response. Planned binges, in contrast, are more closely connected to situations in which restricted foods are readily available or the binge serves a clear affect regulation function. In some cases, the binge is experienced more as an entrenched habit, almost a ritual. The client does not necessarily experience negative affect at the time but feels compelled to binge when in a certain situation or at a certain time, usually when privacy is available. Stimulus control, as well as exposure and response prevention strategies, are most useful in breaking well-established patterns. Techniques drawn from Linehan (1993) that increase distress tolerance can be useful for addressing the distress experienced when the client tries to break a long-standing binge pattern.

Clinicians are advised to ask about any experiences of dissociation that may be associated with binges since the client may not volunteer them. Current self-report measures do not assess such experiences very well. We also advise assessing the role of sleep as it relates to binges. Sleeping may serve an escape function (i.e., avoiding the aversive feelings of being fat or overfull), or the binge may serve as a way to get to sleep, which may be difficult for the client. We have had cases (usually in sleep-deprived college students) in which planned afternoon naps (or meditation) successfully replaced a pattern of planned binges. A relaxation tape (or similar aid) can be used to provide structure if needed.

Careful functional analyses sometimes reveal idiosyncratic functions of binge eating or purging that the client has only somewhat recognized. In one case, vomiting (initiated with ipecac) was serving partially as a self-treatment for migraine headaches for which the client had refused to take appropriate medication. Addressing her concerns and convincing her to utilize appropriate medications eliminated one of her binge/purge triggers.

Appetite monitoring forms allow one to assess emotional feelings about what was eaten, as well as fullness sensations. This is particularly useful in the treatment of BN as the therapist can see (for each episode) whether purging is being triggered by objective overeating, by thinking negatively about the type of food eaten, or by both. Some clients find purges following "small" amounts of forbidden foods easier to give up first. Purges that are driven by fixed ideas that eating any amount of certain foods is bad are best addressed with cognitive restructuring. Other clients do better working first on eliminating large amounts (i.e., ignoring fullness) as a trigger to purge. As with binges, if purges seem to be more like well-established rituals, they may respond best to exposure techniques. While the literature on exposure and vomit prevention does not show strong support for its routine use, further work is needed to determine whether there may be a subset of clients for whom it is useful.

Functional analyses may also serve to identify more general social and lifestyle problems that need to be addressed. Many clients have social anxiety/avoidance that limits their ability to find effective alternatives to eating. Also, significant others may be sabotaging the client's efforts to make lifestyle changes. The client may live a life dominated by "shoulds." Marlatt and Gordon (1985) discuss how such a lifestyle renders individuals generally vulnerable to addictive behaviors.

End-of-Treatment Question

• *Is the client ready to terminate?* Few data are available to serve as a guide for making recommendations about the use of assessment as a way to decide when to end treatment, particularly in the treatment of AN. In research studies, a fixed amount of therapy is usually provided. In clinical practice, the client typically decides when she has made adequate progress and is ready to stop. Detailed follow-ups from clinical trials make clear that, even when the average effects indicate that treatment gains are well maintained, some individuals improve over the course of follow-up whereas others relapse. The chronic, fluctuating course of EDs makes it difficult to know when the client would benefit from working alone on her concerns and when continued treatment is necessary. Cost-effectiveness clearly favors less intensive approaches, but not enough work on this issue has been done to provide specific, empirically supported recommendations.

With IPT, much of the improvement in target behaviors does not manifest itself until the follow-up period. Thus, a prescribed length of IPT treatment is recommended. With CBT, it may be more important to continue until the specific target behaviors (i.e., binge eating and compensatory behaviors) are essentially eliminated. In a study of CBT for BN, complete abstinence from purging by the end of treatment was associated with better maintenance (Maddocks, Kaplan, Woodside, Langdon, & Piran, 1992). Also, participants who had experienced only partial reduction in the target behaviors did not experience as much improvement on broader measures such as self-esteem and depression. It may be that abstinence from binge eating (and purging) is necessary to enhance self-efficacy more generally, or perhaps it is only at the point of abstinence that one no longer labels oneself as having an eating disorder. In CBT for BED, individuals who stopped binge eating lost more weight in a subsequent weight loss intervention than did those who just reduced the frequency of binge eating (Agras et al., 1997).

Few data are available to address the issue of whether residual problems render an individual more prone to relapse. However, once target behaviors have been essentially eliminated, the clinician would do well to assess for the presence and strength of any residual urges (to binge or purge). A standard self-report measure, which includes questions about urges, could be used, or the client could be asked to self-monitor urges for a few weeks. A self-efficacy measure might also be a useful way to assess the client's readiness to continue on her own. Before termination, the clinician should also reassess the client's maladaptive beliefs about dieting, excessive fears of weight gain, or unrealistic body image. Normalization of these types of cognitions has been associated with better maintenance of treatment gains in studies on BN (Fairburn, Marcus, & Wilson, 1993). Although interventions that target body image directly may be warranted, one would not expect to completely eliminate weight and shape concerns given the "normative" discontent that characterizes non-eating-disordered women. Norms on measures of weight concern could provide useful comparison information.

SUMMARY

Assessment measures that are commonly used in the diagnosis and treatment of disordered eating are described. Clinical interviews are recommended to provide a valid diagnosis, to obtain a weight history, and to explore the client's perceptions and beliefs about her current and ideal weights. A primary difficulty in diagnosis is the subjective nature of the definition of binge episodes. To reliably differentiate objective binges from subjective binges, a trained evaluator is needed. Once a client understands the specific definitions of binge episodes, self-reports may be adequate for measuring change in binge frequency over time. Due to the variable nature of bingeing and compensatory behaviors, a period of 4 weeks is recommended to provide reasonable estimates of binge frequency.

Numerous self-reports have been developed to assess the various symptoms of eating disorders, and many have demonstrated adequate psychometric properties. The types of self-reports described in this chapter include general symptom measures, disorder-specific symptom measures, eating behavior measures, body-image measures, cognitive measures, and measures of related personality characteristics. Self-monitoring is another important assessment tool that is discussed.

Specific assessment questions related to treatment issues are discussed. High-risk groups that warrant screening are easily identified; thus, screening is recommended despite low base rates of EDs. Early intervention in AN and the prevention of obesity (due to binge eating) are high priorities due to the morbidity associated with AN and the lack of effective treatments for obesity. Assessment can be used to inform the choice of initial treatment strategies. Assessing the client's motivation to change is a new area of investigation that may lead to better matching of clients to particular treatments; it may also serve as a way to continue to work with clients who are not responding to active treatments.

Assessment of comorbid psychiatric conditions is particularly recommended for inpatient populations and may be useful for choosing treatments and understanding why treatment may not be effective in some cases. The most important issues to consider are current and past mood disorders, anxiety and substance abuse disorders, borderline personality traits, and a history of sexual abuse.

Ongoing assessment of the primary target behaviors (weight, binge eating, and compensatory behaviors) provides feedback about the effects of treatment and indicates when the client may be ready to consider termination. Once primary target behaviors have improved, reassessment of residual problems (particularly negative body image) that may maintain the person at greater risk of relapse is recommended. Interventions that directly target body image and related avoidance behaviors have been developed and may prove to reduce risk of relapse.

REFERENCES

Agras, W. S. (1998). Treatment of eating disorders. In A. F. Schatzberg & C. B. Nemeroff (Eds.), *The American Psychiatric Press textbook of psychopharmacology* (2nd ed., pp. 869–900). Washington, DC: American Psychiatric Press.

Agras, W. S., Telch, C. F., Arnow, B., Eldredge, K., Ketzer, M. J., Henderson, J., & Marnell, M. (1995). Does interpersonal therapy help patients with binge eating disorder who fail to respond to cognitive-behavioral therapy? *Journal of Consulting and Clinical Psychology, 63,* 356–360.

Agras, W. S., Telch, C. F., Arnow, B., Eldredge, K., & Marnell, M. (1997). One-year follow-up of cognitive-behavioral therapy for obese individuals with binge eating disorder. *Journal of Consulting and Clinical Psychology, 65,* 343–347.

Agras, W. S., Telch, C. F., Arnow, B., Eldredge, K., Wilfley, D. E., Raeburn, S. D., Henderson, J., & Marnell, M. (1994). Weight loss, cognitive-behavioral, and desipramine treatments in binge eating disorder: An additive design. *Behavior Therapy, 25,* 225–238.

Agras, W. S., Wilson, G. T., Fairburn, C. G., & Walsh, B. T. (1999, November). *Cognitive behavior therapy versus interpersonal psychotherapy in the treatment of bulimia nervosa.* Paper presented at the meeting of the Association for Advancement of Behavior Therapy, Toronto, Ontario.

Allen, H. N., & Craighead, L. W. (1999). Appetite monitoring in the treatment of binge eating disorder. *Behavior Therapy, 30,* 253–272.

Allison, D. B. (Ed.). (1995). *Handbook of assessment methods for eating behaviors and weight-related problems.* Thousand Oaks, CA: Sage.

Altabe, M., & Thompson, J. K. (1992). Size estimation versus figural ratings of body image disturbance: Relation to body dissatisfaction and eating dysfunction. *International Journal of Eating Disorders, 11,* 397–402.

American Psychiatric Association. (1994). *Diagnostic and statistical manual of mental disorders* (4th ed.). Washington, DC: Author.

American Psychiatric Association (2000). *Practice guideline for the treatment of patients With eating disorders,* second edition. Washington, DC: Author.

Andersen, A. E. (1992). Medical complications of eating disorders. In J. Yager & H. E. Gwirtsman (Eds.), *Special problems in managing eating disorders* (pp. 119–144). Washington, DC: American Psychiatric Press.

Anderson, D. A., Williamson, D. A., Duchmann, E. G., Gleaves, D. H., & Barbin, J. M. (1999). Development and validation of a multifactorial treatment outcome measure for eating disorders. *Assessment, 6,* 7–20.

Apple, R. F. (1999). Interpersonal therapy for bulimia nervosa. *Journal of Clinical Psychology, 55,* 715–725.

Arnow, B., Kenardy, J., & Agras, W. S. (1995). The Emotional Eating Scale: The development of a measure to assess coping with negative affect by eating. *International Journal of Eating Disorders, 18,* 79–90.

Bers, S. A., & Quinlan, D. M. (1992). Perceived-competence deficit in anorexia nervosa. *Journal of Abnormal Psychology, 101,* 423–431.

Beumont, P. J., Russell, J. D., Touyz, S. W., Buckley, C., Lowinger, K., Talbot, P., & Johnson, G. F. (1997). Intensive nutritional counseling in bulimia nervosa: A role for supplementation with fluoxetine? *Australian and New Zealand Journal of Psychiatry, 31,* 514–524.

Bjorntorp, P. (1988). Therapeutic indications in obesity. *Lakartidningen, 85,* 3551–3553.

Black, C. M., & Wilson, G. T. (1996). Assessment of eating disorders: Interview versus questionnaire. *International Journal of Eating Disorders, 20,* 43–50.

Blake, W., Turnbull, S., & Treasure, J. (1997). Stages and processes of change in eating disorders: Implications for therapy. *Clinical Psychology and Psychotherapy, 4,* 186–191.

Blatt, S. J., D'Afflitti, J. P., & Quinlan, D. M. (1976). Experiences of depression in normal young adults. *Journal of Abnormal Psychology, 85,* 383–389.

Bryant-Waugh, R. J. C. P. J., Taylor, C. L., & Lask, B. D. (1996). The use of the Eating Disorder Examination with children: A pilot study. *International Journal of Eating Disorders, 19,* 391–397.

Bulik, C. M., Sullivan, P. F., Carter, F. A., & Joyce, P. R. (1996). Lifetime anxiety disorders in women with bulimia nervosa. *Comprehensive Psychiatry, 37,* 368–374.

Bulik, C. M., Sullivan, P. F., Carter, F. A., McIntosh, V. V., & Joyce, P. R. (1999). Predictors of rapid and sustained response to cognitive-behavioral therapy for bulimia nervosa. *International Journal of Eating Disorders, 26,* 137–144.

Cash, T. F. (1996). The treatment of body image disturbance. In J. K. Thompson (Ed.), *Body image, eating disorders and obesity: An integrative guide for assessment and treatment* (pp. 83–108). Washington, DC: American Psychological Association.

Casper, R. C., Halmi, K. A., Goldberg, S. C., Eckert, E. D., & Davis, J. M. (1979). Disturbances in body image estimation as related to other characteristics and outcome in anorexia nervosa. *British Journal of Psychiatry, 134,* 60–66.

Cepeda-Benito, A., Gleaves, D. H., Williams, T. L., & Erath, S. A. (2000). The development and validation of the State and Trait Food-Cravings Questionnaires. *Behavior Therapy, 31,* 151–173.

Clark, D. A., Feldman, J., & Channon, S. (1989). Dysfunctional thinking in anorexia and bulimia nervosa. *Cognitive Therapy and Research, 13,* 377–387.

Clinton, D. N. (1996). Why do eating disorder patients drop out? *Psychotherapy and Psychosomatics, 65,* 29–35.

Cooper, M. (1997). Bias in interpretation of ambiguous scenarios in eating disorders. *Behaviour Research and Therapy, 35,* 619–626.

Cooper, P. J., Taylor, M. J., Cooper, Z., & Fairburn, C. G. (1987). The development and validation of the Body Shape Questionnaire. *International Journal of Eating Disorders, 6,* 485–494.

Craighead, L. W. (2000). *Eating with your appetite.* Unpublished manual.

Craighead, L. W., & Aibel, C. (2000). The role of anxiety in weight management. In D. E. Mostofsky & D. H. Barlow (Eds.), *The management of stress and anxiety in medical disorders* (pp. 346–360). Needham Heights, MA: Allyn & Bacon.

Craighead, L. W., & Allen, H. N. (1995). Appetite awareness training: A cognitive behavioral intervention for binge eating. *Cognitive and Behavioral Practice, 2,* 249–270.

Dare, C., Eisler, I., Russell, G. F., & Szmukler, G. I. (1990). The clinical and theoretical impact of a controlled trial of family therapy in anorexia nervosa. *Journal of Marital and Family Therapy, 16,* 39–57.

Eckert, E. D., Goldberg, S. C., Halmi, K. A., Caster, R. C., & Davis, J. M. (1981). Depression in anorexia nervosa. *Psychosomatic Medicine, 11,* 115–122.

Elder, K., & Craighead, L. W. (2000). *Early intervention with subclinical BED.* Unpublished manuscript.

Eldredge, K. L., & Agras, W. S. (1996). Burned out binge eaters: A preliminary investigation. *International Journal of Eating Disorders, 19,* 411–414.

Eldredge, K. L., Agras, W. S., Arnow, B., Telch, C. F., Bell, S., Castonguay, L., & Marnell, M. (1997). The effects of extending cognitive-behavioral therapy for binge eating disorder among initial treatment nonresponders. *International Journal of Eating Disorders, 21,* 347–352.

Engel, K., & Wilms, H. (1986). Therapy motivation in anorexia nervosa: Theory and first empirical results. *Psychotherapy and Psychosomatics, 46,* 161–170.

Fahy, T. A., & Eisler, I. (1993). Impulsivity and eating disorders. *British Journal of Psychiatry, 162,* 193–197.

Fairburn, C. G. (1987). The definition of bulimia nervosa: Guidelines for clinicians and research workers. *Annals of Behavioral Medicine, 9,* 307.

Fairburn, C. G., & Beglin, S. J. (1994). Assessment of eating disorders: Interview or self-report questionnaire? *International Journal of Eating Disorders, 16,* 363–370.

Fairburn, C. G., & Cooper, Z. (1993). The Eating Disorders Examination (12th ed.). In C. G. Fairburn & G. T. Wilson (Eds.), *Binge eating: Nature, assessment, and treatment* (pp. 317–360). New York: Guilford Press.

Fairburn, C. G., Marcus, M. D., & Wilson, G. T. (1993). Cognitive-behavioral therapy for binge eating and bulimia nervosa: A comprehensive treatment manual. In C. G. Fairburn & G. T. Wilson (Eds.), *Binge eating: Nature, assessment, and treatment* (pp. 361–404). New York: Guilford Press.

Fichter, M. M., Elton, M., Engel, K., Meyer, A., Poutska, F., Mall, J., & von der Heydte, S. (1998). The Structured Interview for Anorexia and Bulimia Nervosa (SIAB): Development and characteristics of a (semi-) standardized instrument. In M. M. Fichter (Ed.), *Bulimia nervosa: Basic research, diagnosis, and therapy* (pp. 57–70). Chichester, UK: Wiley.

Franko, D. L. (1998). Secondary prevention of eating disorders in college women at risk. *Eating Disorders: The Journal of Treatment and Prevention, 6,* 29–40.

Freeman, C. (1998). Drug treatment for bulimia nervosa. *Neuropsychobiology, 37,* 72–79.

Freund, K. M., Boss, R. D., Handleman, E. K., & Dell, S. A. (1999). Secret patterns: Validation of a screening tool to detect bulimia. *Journal of Women's Health and Gender-Based Medicine, 8,* 1281–1284.

Garner, D. M. (1991). *Eating Disorders Inventory–2.* Odessa, FL: Psychological Assessment Resources.

Garner, D. M., & Garfinkel, P. E. (1979). The Eating Attitudes Test: An index of the symptoms of anorexia nervosa. *Psychological Medicine, 9,* 273–279.

Garner, D. M., & Garfinkel. P.E. (Eds.). (1997). *Handbook of treatment for eating disorders* (2nd ed.). New York: Guilford Press.

Garner, D. M., & Needleman, L. D. (1997). Sequencing and integration of treatments. In D. M. Garner & P. E. Garfinkel (Eds.), *Handbook of treatment for eating disorders* (2nd ed., pp. 50–63). New York: Guilford Press.

Garner, D. M., Olmsted, M., Bohr, Y., & Garfinkel, P. E. (1982). The Eating Attitudes Test: Psychometric features and clinical correlates. *Psychological Medicine, 12,* 871–878.

Garner, D. M., Olmsted, M., & Polivy, J. (1983). Development and validation of a multidimensional Eating Disorder Inventory for anorexia nervosa and bulimia. *International Journal of Eating Disorders, 2,* 15–34.

Garner, D. M., Rosen, L. W., & Barry, D. (1998). Eating disorders among athletes: Research and recommendations. *Child and Adolescent Psychiatric Clinics of North America, 7,* 839–857.

Geller, J., Cockell, S. J., & Drab, D. L. (2001). Assessing readiness to change in anorexia nervosa: The psychometric properties of the Readiness and Motivation Interview. *Psychological Assessment, 13*(2), 189–198.

Geller, J., & Drab, D. L. (1999). The Readiness and Motivation Interview: A symptom-specific measure of readiness for change in the eating disorders. *European Eating Disorders Review, 7,* 259–278.

Glynn, S. M., & Ruderman, A. J. (1986). The development and validation of an Eating Self-Efficacy Scale. *Cognitive Therapy and Research, 10,* 403–420.

Goldberg, S. C., Halmi, K. A., Eckert, E. D., Casper, R. C., Davis, J. M., & Roper, M. (1980). Attitudinal dimensions in anorexia nervosa. *Journal of Psychiatric Research, 15,* 239–251.

Goodrick, G. K., Poston, W. S., Kimball, K. T., Reeves, R. S., & Foreyt, J. P. (1998). Nondieting versus dieting treatment for overweight binge-eating women. *Journal of Consulting and Clinical Psychology, 66*, 363–368.

Gormally, J., Black, S., Daston, S., & Rardin, D. (1982). The assessment of binge eating severity among obese persons. *Addictive Behaviors, 7*, 47–55.

Gorman, B. S., & Allison, D. B. (1995). Measures of restrained eating. In D. B. Allison (Ed.), *Handbook of assessment methods for eating behaviors and weight-related problems: Measures, theory, and research*, pp.149–184. Thousand Oaks, CA: Sage.

Hagan, M. M., Whitworth, R. H., & Moss, D. E. (1999). Semistarvation-associated eating behaviors among college binge eaters: A preliminary description and assessment scale. *Behavioral Medicine, 25*, 125–133.

Haiman, C., & Devlin, M. J. (1999). Binge eating before the onset of dieting: A distinct subgroup of bulimia nervosa? *International Journal of Eating Disorders, 25*, 151–157.

Hannan, W. J., Wrate, R. M., Cowen, S. J., & Freeman, C. P. L. (1995). Body mass index as an estimate of body fat. *International Journal of Eating Disorders, 18*, 91–97.

Henderson, M., & Freeman, C. P. L. (1987). A self-rating scale for bulimia: The BITE. *British Journal of Psychiatry, 150*, 18–24.

Herman, C. P., & Polivy, J. (1980). Restrained eating. In A. J. Stunkard (Ed.), *Obesity* (pp. 208–225). Philadelphia: Saunders.

Hill, A. J., Weaver, C. F., & Blundell, J. E. (1991). Food craving, dietary restraint, and mood. *Appetite, 17*, 187–197.

Hodes, M., Dare, C., Dodge, E., & Eisler, I. (1999). The assessment of expression emotion in a standardized family interview. *Journal of Child Psychology and Psychiatry and Allied Disciplines, 40*, 617–625.

Hohlstein, L. A., Smith, G. T., & Atas, J. G. (1998). An application of expectancy theory to eating disorders: Development and validation of measures of eating and dieting expectencies. *Psychological Assessment, 10*, 49–58.

Hsu, L. K. (1996). Epidemiology of the eating disorders. *Psychiatric Clinics of North Amercia, 19*, 681–700.

Hyler, S. E., & Reider, R. O. (1987). *PDQ-R: Personality Diagnostic Questionnaire—Revised*. New York: New York State Psychiatric Institute.

Joiner, T. E., & Heatherton, T. F. (1998). First- and second-order factor structure of five subscales of the Eating Disorders Inventory. *International Journal of Eating Disorders, 23*, 189–198.

Kearney-Cooke, A., & Striegel-Moore, R. H. (1996). Treatment of childhood sexual abuse in anorexia nervosa and bulimia nervosa: A feminist psychodynamic approach. In M. F. Schwartz & L. Cohn (Eds.), *Sexual abuse and eating disorders* (pp. 155–175). New York: Brunner/Mazel.

Keel, P. K., Mitchell, J. E., Miller, K. B., Davis, T. L., & Crow, S. J. (1999). Long-term outcome of bulimia nervosa. *Archives of General Psychiatry, 56*, 63–69.

Kettlewell, P. W., Mizes, J. S., & Wasylyshyn, N. A. (1992). A cognitive-behavioral group treatment of bulimia. *Behavior Therapy, 23*, 657–670.

Kutlesic, V., Williamson, D. A., Gleaves, D. H., Barbin, J. M., & Murphy-Eberenz, K. P. (1998). The Interview for the Diagnosis of Eating Disorders—IV. Application to DSM-IV diagnostic criteria. *Psychological Assessment, 10*, 41–48.

Leon, G. R., Keel, P. K., Klump, K. L., & Fulkerson, J. A. (1997). The future of risk factor research in understanding the etiology of eating disorders. *Psychopharmacology Bulletin, 33*, 405–412.

Leung, N., Waller, G., & Thomas, G. (1999). Core beliefs in anorexic and bulimic women. *Journal of Nervous and Mental Disease, 187*, 736–741.

Linehan, M. M. (1993). *Skills training manual for treating borderline personality disorder*. New York: Guilford Press.

Loeb, K. L., Pike, K. M., Walsh, B. T., & Wilson, G. T. (1994). Assessment of diagnostic features of bulimia nervosa: Interview versus self-report format. *International Journal of Eating Disorders, 16*, 75–81.

Lowe, M. R., & Caputo, G. C. (1991). Binge eating in obesity: Toward the specification of predictors. *International Journal of Eating Disorders, 10*, 49–55.

Maddocks, S. E., Kaplan, A. S., Woodside, D. B., Langdon, L., & Piran, N. (1992). Two year followup of bulimia nervosa: The importance of abstinence as the criterion of outcome. *International Journal of Eating Disorders, 12,* 133–141.

Mann, T., Nolen-Hoeksema, S., Huang, K., & Burgard, D. (1997). Are two interventions worse than none? Joint primary and secondary prevention of eating disorders in college females. *Health Psychology, 16,* 215–225.

Marcus, J. D., Blocher, M. E., Levine, M., & Sebastiani, L. (1999, November). *DBT in the treatment of eating disorders.* Workshop presented at the meeting of the Association for the Advancement of Behavior Therapy, Toronto, Ontario.

Marcus, M. D., Wing, R. R., & Fairburn, C. G. (1995). Cognitive treatment of binge eating versus behavioral weight control in the treatment of binge eating disorder. *Annals of Behavioral Medicine, 17,* S090.

Marcus, M. D., Wing, R. R., & Lamparski, D. M. (1985). Binge eating and dietary restraint in obese patients. *Addictive Behaviors, 10,* 163–168.

Margolis, R. L., Spencer, W., DePaulo, J. R., & Simpson, S. G. (1994). Psychiatric comorbidity in subgroups of eating-disordered inpatients. *Eating Disorders: The Journal of Treatment and Prevention, 2,* 231–236.

Marlatt, G. A., & Gordon, J. R. (Eds.). (1985). *Relapse prevention: Maintenance strategies in the treatment of addictive behaviors.* New York: Guilford Press.

Martin, C. K., Williamson, D. A., & Thaw, J. M. (2000). *Criterion validity of the multiaxial assessment of eating disorders symptoms.* Unpublished manuscript, Louisiana State University.

Mazure, C. M., Halmi, K. A., Sunday, S. R., Romano, S. J., & Einhorn, A. M. (1994). The Yale–Brown–Cornell Eating Disorder Scale: Development, use, reliability and validity. *Journal of Psychiatric Research, 28,* 425–445.

Miller, W. R. (1985). Motivation for treatment: A review with special emphasis on alcoholism. *Psychological Bulletin, 98,* 84–107.

Mitchell, J. E., Mussell, M. P., Peterson, C. B., Crow, S., Wonderlich, S. A., Crosby, R. D., Davis, T., & Weller, C. (1999). Hedonics of binge eating in women with bulimia nervosa and binge eating disorder. *International Journal of Eating Disorders, 26,* 165–170.

Mitzman, S. F., Slade, P., & Dewey, M. E. (1994). Preliminary development of a questionnaire designed to measure neurotic perfectionism in the eating disorders. *Journal of Clinical Psychology, 50,* 516–522.

Mizes, J. S. (1988). Personality characteristics of bulimic and non-eating-disordered female controls: A cognitive behavioral perspective. *International Journal of Eating Disorders, 7,* 541–550.

Mizes, J. S. (1990). Criterion-related validity of the Anorectic Cognitions Questionnaire. *Addictive Behaviors, 15,* 153–163.

Mizes, J. S. (1991). Construct validity and factor stability of the Anorectic Cognitions Questionnaire. *Addictive Behaviors, 16,* 89–93.

Mizes, J. S. (1992). Validity of the Mizes Anorectic Cognitions Scale: A comparison between anorectics, bulimics, and psychiatric controls. *Addictive Behaviors, 17,* 283–289.

Mizes, J. S., & Christiano, B. A. (1995). Assessment of cognitive variables relevant to cognitive behavioral perspectives on anorexia nervosa and bulimia nervosa. *Behaviour Research and Therapy, 33,* 95–105.

Mizes, J. S., & Klesges, R. C. (1989). Validity, reliability, and factor structure of the Anorectic Cognitions Questionnaire. *Addictive Behaviors, 14,* 589–594.

Mizes, J. S., & Sloan, D. M. (1998). An empirical analysis of eating disorder, not otherwise specified: Preliminary support for a distinct subgroup. *International Journal of Eating Disorders, 23,* 233–242.

North, C., & Gowers, S. (1999). Anorexia nervosa, psychopathology, and outcome. *International Journal of Eating Disorders, 26,* 386–391.

Palmer, R., Christie, M., Cordle, C., Davies, D., & Kendrick, J. (1987). The clinical eating disorder rating instrument (CEDRI): A preliminary investigation. *International Journal of Eating Disorders, 6,* 9–16.

Palmer, R., Robertson, D., Cain, M., & Black, S. (1996). The clinical eating disorders rating instrument (CEDRI): A validation study. *European Eating Disorders Review, 4*, 149–156.

Pendleton, V. R., Poston, W. S. II, Goodrick, G. K., Willems, E. P., Swank, P. R., Kimball, K. T., & Foreyt, J. P. (1998). The predictive validity of the Diet Readiness Test in a clinical population. *International Journal of Eating Disorders, 24*, 363–369.

Phelan, P. W. (1987). Cognitive correlates of bulimia: The Bulimic Thoughts Questionnaire. *International Journal of Eating Disorders, 6*, 593–607.

Polivy, J., Herman, P. H., & Howard, K. I. (1988). Restraint scale: Assessment of dieting. In M. Hersen & A. S. Bellack (Eds.), *Dictionary of behavioral assessment techniques* (pp. 377–380). New York: Pergamon.

Powers, P. S. (1996). Initial assessment and early treatment options for anorexia nervosa and bulimia nervosa. *Psychiatric Clinics of North America, 19*, 639–655.

Powers, P. S., & Powers, H. P. (1984). Inpatient treatment of anorexia nervosa. *Psychosomatics, 25*, 512–527.

Prochaska, J. O., & Norcross, J. C. (1994). *Systems of psychotherapy: A transtheoretical analysis.* Pacific Grove, CA: Brooks Cole.

Pryor, T., & Wiederman, M. W. (1996). Use of the MMPI–2 in the outpatient assessment of women with anorexia nervosa or bulimia nervosa. *Journal of Personality Assessment, 66*, 363–373.

Rathner, G., & Messner, K. (1993). Detection of eating disorders in a small rural town: An epidemiological study. *Psychological Medicine, 23*, 175–184.

Raymond, N. C., Mussell, M. P., Mitchell, J. E., de Zwaan, M., & Crosby, R. D. (1995). An age-matched comparison of subjects with binge eating disorder and bulimia nervosa. *International Journal of Eating Disorders, 18*, 135–143.

Reich, J. H., & Vasile, R. G. (1993). Effect of personality disorders on the treatment outcome of Axis I conditions: An update. *Journal of Nervous and Mental Disease, 181*, 475–484.

Rosen, J. C. (1996). Body image assessment and treatment in controlled studies of eating disorders. *International Journal of Eating Disorders, 20*, 331–343.

Rosen, J. C., Leitenberg, H., Fischer, C., & Khazam, C. (1986). Binge eating episodes in bulimia nervosa: The amount and type of food consumed. *International Journal of Eating Disorders, 9*, 255–267.

Rosen, J. C., Reiter, J., & Orosan, P. (1995). Assessment of body image in eating disorders with the Body Dysmorphic Disorder Examination. *Behaviour Research and Therapy, 33*, 77–84.

Rossiter, E. M., Agras, W. S., & McCann, U. D. (1991). Are antidepressants appetite suppressants in bulimia nervosa? *European Journal of Psychiatry, 5*, 224–231.

Schlundt, D. G., & Johnson, G. F. (1990). *Eating disorders: Assessment and treatment.* Boston: Allyn & Bacon.

Schlundt, D. G., Virts, K. L., Sbrocco, T., Pope-Cordle, J., & Hill, J. O. (1993). A sequential behavioral analysis of craving sweets in obese women. *Addictive Behaviors, 18*, 67–80.

Schlundt, D. G., & Zimering, R. T. (1988). The Dieter's Inventory of Eating Temptations: A measure of weight control competence. *Addictive Behaviors, 13*, 151–164.

Schmidt, U., & Treasure, J. (1997). *Clinician's guide to getting better bit(e) by bit(e): A survival kit for sufferers of bulimia nervosa and binge eating disorders.* Hove, UK: Psychology Press.

Schneider, J. A., O'Leary, A., & Agras, W. S. (1987). The role of perceived self-efficacy in recovery from bulimia: A preliminary examination. *Behaviour Research and Therapy, 25*, 429–432.

Schoemaker, C. (1997). Does early intervention improve the prognosis in anorexia nervosa? A systematic review of the treatment-outcome literature. *International Journal of Eating Disorders, 21*, 1–15.

Schwitzer, A. M., Bergholz, K., Dore, T., & Salimi, L. (1998). Eating disorders among college women: Prevention, education, and treatment responses. *Journal of American College Health, 46*, 199–207.

Slade, P. D., & Dewey, M. E. (1986). Development and preliminary validation of SCANS: A screening instrument for identifying individuals at risk of developing anorexia and bulimia nervosa. *International Journal of Eating Disorders, 5*, 517–538.

Smith, C. F., Williamson, D. A., Womble, L. G., Johnson, J., & Burke, L. E. (2000). Psychometric development of a multidimensional measure of weight-related attitudes and behaviors. *Eating and Weight Disorders, 5,* 73–89.

Smith, K. J., Subich, L. M., & Kalodner, C. (1995). The transtheoretical model's stages and processes of change and their relation to premature termination. *Journal of Counseling Psychology, 42,* 34–39.

Smith, M. C., & Thelen, M. H. (1984). Development and validation of a test for bulimia nervosa. *Journal of Consulting and Clinical Psychology, 52,* 863–872.

Smolak, L., & Levine, M. (1994). Psychometric properties of the Children's Eating Attitudes Test. *International Journal of Eating Disorders, 16,* 275–282.

Spitzer, R. L., Devlin, M., Walsch, B. T., Hasin, K. D., Wing, R. R., Marcus, M. D., Stunkard, A., Wadden, T., Yanovski, S., Agras, W. S., Mitchell, J. E., & Nonas, C. (1992). Binge eating disorder: A multisite field trial of the diagnostic criteria. *International Journal of Eating Disorders, 11,* 191–203.

Stanton, A. L., Garcia, M. E., & Green, S. B. (1990). Development and validation of the situational appetite measures. *Addictive Behaviors, 15,* 461–472.

Stanton, A. L., Rebert, W. M., & Zinn, L. M. (1986). Self-change in bulimia: A preliminary study. *International Journal of Eating Disorders, 5,* 917–924.

Steinhausen, H. C. (1986). Attitudinal dimensions in adolescent anorexic patients: An analysis of the Goldberg Anorectic Attitude Scale. *Journal of Psychiatric Research, 20,* 83–87.

Stice, E., & Agras, W. S. (1999). Subtyping bulimic women along dietary restraint and negative affect dimensions. *Journal of Consulting and Clinical Psychology, 67,* 460–469.

Stotland, S., Zuroff, D. C., & Roy, M. (1991). Situational dieting self-efficacy and short-term regulation of eating. *Appetite, 17,* 81–9.

Strober, M., Freeman, R., & Morrell, W. (1997). The long-term course of severe anorexia nervosa in adolescents: Survival analysis of recovery, relapse, and outcome predictors over 10–15 years in a prospective study. *International Journal of Eating Disorders, 22,* 339–360.

Stunkard, A., & Messick, S. (1985). The Three-Factor Eating Questionnaire to measure dietary restraint, disinhibition, and hunger. *Journal of Psychosomatic Research, 29,* 71–83.

Stunkard, A. J., & Messick, S. (1988). *The eating inventory.* San Antonio, TX: Psychological Corporation.

Stunkard, A., Sorenson, T., & Schlusinger, F. (1983). Use of the Danish Adoption Register for the study of obesity and thinness. In S. Kety, L. P. Rowland, R. L. Sidman, & S. W. Matthysse (Eds.), *The genetics of neurological and psychiatric disorders* (pp. 115–120). New York: Raven.

Sunday, S. R., Halmi, K. A., & Einhorn, A. (1995). The Yale–Brown–Cornell Eating Disorder Scale: A new scale to assess eating disorders symptomatology. *International Journal of Eating Disorders, 18,* 237–245.

Szabo, C. P., Goldin, J., & Le Grange, D. (1999). Application of the Family Relations Scale to a sample of anorexics, bulimics, and nonpsychiatric controls: A preliminary study. *European Eating Disorders Review, 7,* 37–46.

Szabo, C. P., & Terre Blanche, M. J. (1997). Perfectionism in anorexia nervosa [letter; comment]. *American Journal of Psychiatry, 154,* 132.

Telch, C. F. (1997). Skills training treatment for adaptive affect regulation in a woman with binge-eating disorder. *International Journal of Eating Disorders, 22,* 77–81.

Telch, C. F., & Stice, E. (1998). Psychiatric comorbidity in women with binge eating disorder: Prevalence rates from a non-treatment-seeking sample. *Journal of Consulting and Clinical Psychology, 66,* 768–776.

Thelen, M. H., Farmer, J., Wonderlich, S., & Smith, M. C. (1991). A revision of the Bulimia Test: BULIT-R. *Psychological Assessment, 3,* 119–124.

Thompson, J. K. (1995). Assessment of Body Image. In D. B. Allison (Ed.), *Handbook of assessment methods for eating behaviors and weight-related problems* (pp. 119–148). Thousand Oaks, CA: Sage.

Treasure, J. L., Katzman, M., Schmidt, U., Troop, N., Todd, G., & de Silva, P. (1999). Engagement and outcome in the treatment of bulimia nervosa: First phase of sequential design comparing motivation enhancement therapy and cognitive behavioural therapy. *Behaviour Research and Therapy, 37,* 405–418.

Vandereycken, W. (1992). Validity and reliability of the Anorectic Behavior Observation Scale for parents. *Acta Psychiatrica Scandinavica, 85,* 163–166.

van Furth, E. F., van Strien, D. C., Martina, L. M. L., van Son, M. J. M., Hendrickx, J. J. P., & van Engeland, H. (1996). Expressed emotion and the prediction of outcome in adolescent eating disorders. *International Journal of Eating Disorders, 20,* 19–31.

van Strien, T., Frijters, J. E. R., Staveren, W. A., Defares, P. B., & Deurenberg, P. (1986). The predictive validity of the Dutch restrained eating questionnaire. *International Journal of Eating Disorders, 5,* 747–755.

Veron-Guidry, S., & Williamson, D. A. (1996). Development of a body image assessment procedure for children and preadolescents. *International Journal of Eating Disorders, 20,* 287–293.

Vitousek, K., Watson, S., & Wilson, G. T. (1998). Enhancing motivation for change in treatment-resistant eating disorders. *Clinical Psychology Review, 18,* 391–420.

Waller, D., Ohanian, V., & Meyer, C.O.S. (2000). Cognitive content among bulimic women: The role of core beliefs. *International Journal of Eating Disorders, 28,* 235–241.

Waller, G. (1997). Drop-out and failure to engage in individual outpatient cognitive behavior therapy for bulimic disorders. *International Journal of Eating Disorders, 22,* 35–41.

Wardle, J. (1995). The assessment of obesity: Theoretical background and practical advice. *Behaviour Research and Therapy, 33,* 107–117.

Weingarten, H. P., & Elston, D. (1991). Food cravings in a college population. *Appetite, 17,* 167–175.

Weissman, M. M., Markowitz, J. C., & Klerman, G. L. (2000). *Comprehensive guide to interpersonal psychotherapy.* New York: Basic Books.

Welch, S. L., & Fairburn, C. G. (1996). Impulsivity or comorbidity in bulimia nervosa: A controlled study of deliberate self-harm and alcohol and drug misuse in a community sample. *British Journal of Psychiatry, 169,* 451–458.

Westenhoefer, J., Stunkard, A. J., & Pudel, V. (1999). Validation of the flexible and rigid control dimensions of dietary restraint. *International Journal of Eating Disorders, 26,* 53–64.

Whisenhunt, B. L., Williamson, D. A., Netemeyer, R. G., & Womble, L. G. (2000). Reliability and validity of the psychosocial risk factors questionnaire (PRFQ). *Eating and Weight Disorders, 5,* 1–6.

Whitaker, A., Davies, M., Shaffter, D., Johnson, J., Abrams, S., Walsh, B. T., & Kalikow, K. (1989). The struggle to be thin: A survey of anorexic and bulimic symptoms in a non-referred adolescent population. *Psychological Medicine, 19,* 143–163.

Williams, G. J., Power, K. G., Miller, H. R., Freeman, C. P., Yellowless, A., Dowds, T., Walker, M., & Parry-Jones, W. (1994). Development and validation of the Stirling Eating Disorder Scales. *International Journal of Eating Disorders, 16,* 35–43.

Williamson, D. A. (1990). *Assessment of eating disorders.* New York: Pergamon.

Williamson, D. A., Davis, C. J., Bennett, S. M., Goreczny, A. J., & Gleaves, D. H. (1989). Development of a simple procedure for assessing body image disturbances. *Behavioral Assessment, 11,* 433–446.

Williamson, D. A., Womble, L. G., Zucker, N. L., Reas, D. L., White, M. A., Blouin, D. C., & Greenway, F. (2000). Body image assessment for obesity (BIA-O): Development of a new procedure. *International Journal of Obesity, 24,* 1326–1332.

Williamson, D. F. (1995). Prevalence and demographics of obesity. In K. D. Brownell & C. G. Fairburn (Eds.), *Eating disorders and obesity: A comprehensive handbook* (pp. 391–395). New York: Guilford Press.

Wilson, G. T. (1993). Binge eating and addictive disorders. In C. G. Fairburn & G. T. Wilson (Eds.), *Binge eating: Nature, assessment and treatment* (pp. 97–120). New York: Guilford Press.

Wilson, G. T. (1999). Cognitive behavior therapy for eating disorders: Progress and problems. *Behaviour Research and Therapy, 37,* S79–S95.

Wilson, G. T., & Vitousek, K. M. (1999). Self-monitoring in the assessment of eating disorders. *Psychological Assessment, 11*, 480–489.

Wiser, S., & Telch, C. F. (1999). Dialectical behavior therapy for Binge-Eating Disorder. *Journal of Clinical Psychology, 55*, 755–768.

Wonderlich, S. A., & Mitchell, J. E. (1997). Eating disorders and comorbidity: empirical, conceptual, and clinical implications. *Psychopharmacology Bulletin, 33*, 381–390.

Young, J. E. (1994). *Cognitive therapy for personality disorders: A schema-focused approach* (2nd ed.). Sarasota, FL: Professional Resource Press.

Young, J. E., & Klosko, J. S. (1993). *Reinventing your life*. New York: Penguin Books.

10

Couple Distress

Douglas K. Snyder
Brian V. Abbott

OVERVIEW OF PARTNER RELATIONAL PROBLEMS

The fourth edition of the *Diagnostic and Statistical Manual of Mental Disorders* (DSM-IV; American Psychiatric Association, 1994) defines a "partner relational problem" (the closest DSM-IV comes to legitimizing couple-based interventions) as a pattern of interaction that is characterized by negative or distorted communication, or "noncommunication (e.g., withdrawal)"; it is associated with clinically significant impairment in individual or relationship functioning or the development of symptoms in one or both partners. The acknowledgment of relational problems as a "frequent focus of clinical attention" but their separation from other emotional and behavioral disorders comprises only a marginal improvement over earlier versions of DSM that all but ignored the interpersonal context of distressed lives.

What are the limitations to this conceptualization of partner relational problems? First is an almost exclusive emphasis on the etiological role of communication in the impairment of functioning or development of symptoms in one or both partners. Although group comparisons document differences in communication between clinic and community couples (Heyman, 2001), and "communication problems" comprise the most frequent presenting complaint of couples (Geiss & O'Leary, 1981), evidence that communication differences precede rather than follow from relationship distress is weak or nonexistent. Moreover, recent research with community samples indicates that some forms of "negative" communication predict better rather than worse relationship outcomes longitudinally (Gottman, 1993). In addition, positive changes in relationship satisfaction after couple therapy correspond only weakly or nonsignificantly with actual changes in communication behavior (Jacobson, Schmaling, & Holtzworth-Munroe, 1987; Sayers, Baucom, Sher, Weiss, & Heyman, 1991). Even the distinction between communication and "noncommunication" seems flawed, in that most couple and family theorists would argue that all behavior (including withdrawal) is communicative (Fraenkel, 1997).

Also lacking in the DSM-IV conceptualization of partner relational problems is recognition of "nonsymptomatic" deficiencies that couples often present as a focus of concern, including those that detract from optimal individual or relationship well-being. These include deficits in security, closeness, shared values, trust, joy, love, and similar positive emotions that individuals typically pursue in their intimate relationships. Not all such deficits reflect communication difficulties, nor do they necessarily culminate in "clinically significant" impaired functioning or emotional and behavioral symptoms as traditionally conceived; yet frequently these deficits are experienced as significant concerns that may culminate in partners' disillusion or dissolution of the relationship.

The most positive features of DSM's conceptualization of partner relational problems are its emphasis on the interactions between partners and its recognition that relational problems are frequently associated with individual symptoms in one or both partners. The prevalence of partner relational problems (which we will refer to more simply as "couple distress") and their comorbidity with other individual disorders are described in this chapter.

The Prevalence of Couple Distress

The most visible and discrete indicator for the prevalence of couple distress continues to be the high rate of divorce among married couples. Estimates of divorce among first marriages in the United States range from 50% to 67% (Martin & Bumpass, 1989); half of these divorces occur in the first 7 years. Divorce rates for second marriages are either comparable or about 10% higher. Only the rate of increase in divorce over the past 50 years appears to be slowing.

Some have argued that a significant percentage of marriages reflect stable but unsatisfactory relationships (Lederer & Jackson, 1968). Indeed, it is not unreasonable to presume that most marriages experience periods of significant turmoil that place them at risk for dissolution or symptom development (e.g., depression or anxiety) in one or both partners at some point in their lifespan. Only one-third of married persons report being "very happy" with their marriage, down from more than one-half 25 years ago. In a recent national survey, the most frequently cited causes of acute emotional distress were relationship problems, including divorce, separation, and other marital strains (Swindle, Heller, Pescosolido, & Kikuzawa, 2000).

Even these findings from national surveys may underestimate the prevalence of couple distress due to design flaws and susceptibility to response biases in the instrumentation (Stuart, 1980). On a standardized measure of relationship distress, the Global Distress (GDS) scale of the Marital Satisfaction Inventory—Revised (MSI-R; Snyder, 1997), half of community respondents report at least moderate dissatisfaction with their marriage, and 15% indicate extensive distress. About 37% of men aged 50 to 59 and 20% of women aged 40 to 49 report having had an affair at least once during their marriage (Laumann, Gagnon, Michael, & Michaels, 1994). It does not come as a surprise, then, that more people seek therapy for marital problems than for any other type of problem (Veroff, Kulka, & Douvan, 1981).

Linkage of Couple Distress to Disruption of Individual Well-Being

The linkage of relationship distress to disruption of individual emotional and physical well-being has achieved increasing documentation. In a recent analysis of responses from 2,538 married persons in the National Comorbidity Survey, Whisman (1999) found that greater marital dissatisfaction was associated with 7 of 12 specific disorders for women (with the largest associations obtained for posttraumatic stress disorder, dysthymia, and major depression) and with 3 of 13 specific disorders for men (dysthymia, major depression, and alcohol dependence). Earlier reviews have similarly substantiated the linkage of marital dissatisfaction with the onset, course, and treatment of adult psychiatric disorders (cf. Halford

& Bouma, 1997). Empirical support has been garnered for the effectiveness of couple-based interventions for a variety of emotional and behavioral disorders, including depression, anxiety, alcohol abuse, and physical aggression (for reviews, see Baucom, Shoham, Mueser, Daiuto, & Stickle, 1998; Christensen & Heavey, 1999).

Just as compelling is evidence that links marital functioning to physical health. Marital dissolution is associated with significant immunosuppression (Kiecolt-Glaser, Malarkey, Cacioppo, & Glaser, 1994), increased risk of physical illness and mortality from diseases (Burman & Margolin, 1992), and decreased longevity (Friedman, Tucker, Schwartz, & Tomilson, 1995). An unhappy marriage increases a person's risk of physical illness by 35% and shortens the expected lifespan by 4 years. A recent study indicated that maritally distressed partners have twice the risk of their nondistressed counterparts in developing Type II diabetes (Gaskill, Williams, Stern, & Hazuda, 2000).

Nor are the effects of couple distress confined to the adult partners. More than 1 million children have experienced parental divorce each year since 1970 (Wallerstein, Lewis, & Blakeslee, 2000). Gottman (1999) cites evidence indicating that "marital distress, conflict, and disruption are associated with a wide range of deleterious effects on children, including depression, withdrawal, poor social competence, health problems, poor academic performance, a variety of conduct-related difficulties, and markedly decreased longevity" (p. 4).

In brief, couple relationship distress has a markedly high prevalence; has a strong linkage to emotional, behavioral, and health problems in the adult partners and their offspring; and comprises the most frequent primary or secondary concern among individuals who seek assistance from mental health professionals.

Organization of This Chapter

The remainder of this chapter has four sections. First, we present a comprehensive conceptual model for directing and organizing assessment strategies and findings relevant to couples. Thinking about domains and levels of a couple's relationship and understanding *what* to assess necessarily precede consideration of any specific assessment techniques or evaluation tactics. Second, we offer both general clinical guidelines and specific strategies for *how* to assess couples that follow from our conceptual model. We initially emphasize idiographic techniques and the clinician as a measurement instrument, and only then turn to standardized measures that provide a nomothetic basis for evaluating couples in clinical or research settings. Third, we briefly summarize findings regarding the effectiveness of couple therapy and present a model for integrating findings and interventions from diverse theoretical perspectives. We relate this integrative intervention model to the comprehensive assessment strategy outlined earlier. The importance of integrating couple assessment with treatment planning and evaluation is illustrated with a clinical case example of a couple struggling to recover from an extramarital affair. Finally, we offer recommendations for screening for relationship distress in primary care facilities and documenting couples' functioning before and after treatment in managed care settings.

A CONCEPTUAL MODEL FOR ASSESSING COUPLES

There is little that is not relevant to assessing couples! Most obvious is the need to assess the dyadic behaviors, quality of affect, and patterning of expectancies and related cognitions that define the couple's relationship. Relationship constructs emerge, in part, from the interaction of individual characteristics that both partners bring to their exchanges. At a broader level, a couple's relationship influences and is influenced by persons outside the dyad, and these include children, families of origin, and social or community support or stressors. Although, theoretically, comprehensive assessment of individuals entails evaluation across a similar breadth of domains and levels of the psychosocial ecological system, the interpersonal context of presenting concerns is rarely as compelling as with couples and families.

The Conceptual Model

Snyder and colleagues (Heffer & Snyder, 1998; Snyder, Cavell, Heffer, & Mangrum, 1995; Snyder, Cozzi, Grich, & Luebbert, 2001) have proposed a comprehensive model for directing and organizing assessment strategies for couples and families (see Figure 10.1). The model proposes five construct domains: cognitive, affective, behavioral and control, structural/developmental, and communication and interpersonal. Constructs relevant to each of these domains can be assessed at each of the multiple levels that make up the psychosocial system in which the couple or family functions. The model posits five distinct levels of this system: individuals, dyads, the nuclear family, the extended family and related social systems, and the community and cultural systems. Each of the five target domains may be assessed with varying degrees of relevance and specificity across each of the five system levels, using both formal and informal assessment approaches to self-report and observational techniques. Our model emphasizes the fluid nature of individual and system functioning by linking structural with developmental processes. It also presumes that individual members of a couple or family recursively influence, and are influenced by, the broader social system.

Constructs across Domains and Levels

Table 10.1 provides a modest sampling of specific constructs relevant to each domain at each system level. Our intent in this table is not to attempt a comprehensive list of all constructs relevant to individual, couple, or broader systemic functioning but, instead, to offer a way of thinking about how specific constructs map onto different domains of functioning and generalize across individual, couple or family, and broader system levels.

For example, important constructs within the cognitive domain at the individual level include general cognitive resources that underlie the ability to understand and apply concepts and the capacity for self-reflection and insight. A second cognitive dimension involves each individual's self-view, including self-efficacy and the extent to which individuals regard themselves as contributing to their own distress and able to effect change. Cognitive constructs at the dyadic level emphasize views toward the relationship and include (1) assumptions the individual makes about how this relationship or relationships in general function, (2) standards for how a relationship or members of a relationship ought to function, (3) selective attention to relationship events congruent with existing belief systems, (4) expectancies regarding the course and impact of their own and others' behaviors in a relationship, and (5) attributions regarding the causes for relationship events (Baucom, Epstein, Sayers, & Sher, 1989). Similar to standards at the dyadic level are values at the family level, and norms or mores at the cultural level. For example, families differ in the extent to which they espouse intellectual and aesthetic endeavors, recreational activity, religious or moral pursuits, personal achievement, and independence.

Persons vary in their general range of affective intensity and the extent to which affect persists across time and situations. Affective dimensions of cohesion, expressiveness, satisfaction, and commitment have all been identified in the dyadic relationship literature. Indeed, relationship satisfaction is the most widely investigated dimension of intimate dyads. Recent literature has begun to address the constructs of acceptance and forgiveness in relationships—that is, the ability to suspend the hurt or anger associated with relationship con-

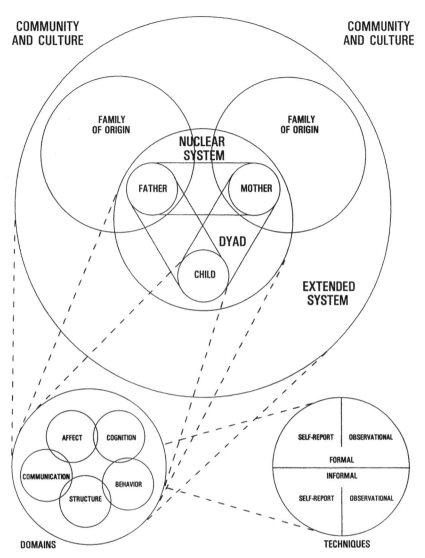

FIGURE 10.1. Conceptual model for assessing couples from a systems perspective. The model presents five system levels: individuals, dyads, the nuclear family, the extended family system, and the community and cultural systems. Each system level may be assessed across five overlapping domains: cognitive, affective, behavioral, structural/developmental, and communication and interpersonal. Information across domains may be gathered using multiple assessment strategies, including both formal and informal self-report and observational techniques. From Snyder, Cavell, Heffer, and Mangrum (1995). Copyright 1995 by the American Psychological Association. Reprinted by permission.

flicts (Gordon, Baucom, & Snyder, 2000; Jacobson & Christensen, 1996). Affective constructs have been described in the family literature as well. For example, families often convey a collective mood that varies along dimensions of optimism, contentment, anger, worry, guilt, or despair. High levels of emotional connectedness and social support at the extended family and community levels provide a vital resource for couples. An important focus of assessment involves the extent to which family members have balanced developmental tasks of differentiating from extended systems while retaining the ability to draw on the support functions of those systems.

TABLE 10.1. Sample Assessment Constructs across Domains and Levels of Couple and Family Functioning

Domain	Individual	Dyad (couple, parent–child)	Nuclear family system	Extended system (family of origin, friends)	Culture/community
Cognitive	Intelligence; memory functions; thought content; thought quality; analytic skills; cognitive distortions; schemas; capacity for self-reflection and insight.	Cognitions regarding self and other in relationship; expectancies; attributions; attentional biases; shared understanding of the relationship.	Shared or co-constructed meanings within the system; family ideology or paradigm; thought sequences between members contributing to family functioning.	Intergenerational patterns of thinking and believing; co-constructed meaning shared by therapist and family or other significant friends or family.	Prevailing societal and cultural beliefs and attitudes; ways of thinking associated with particular religious or ethnic groups that are germane to the family or individual.
Affective	Mood; affective range, intensity, and valence; emotional lability.	Predominant emotional themes or patterns in the relationship; cohesion; range of emotional expression; commitment and satisfaction in the relationship; acceptance and forgiveness.	Family emotional themes of fear, shame, guilt, or rejection; system properties of cohesion or emotional disaffection; emotional atmosphere in the home.	Emotional themes and patterns in extended system; intergenerational emotional legacies; patterns of fusion or differentiation across generations.	Prevailing emotional sentiment in the community, culture, and society; cultural norms and mores regarding the expression of emotion.
Behavioral/ control	Capacity for self-control; impulsivity; aggressiveness; capacity to defer gratification. Overall energy and drive.	Recursive behavioral sequences displayed in the relationship; behavioral repertoire; reinforcement contingencies; strategies used to control other's behavior.	Repetitive behavioral patterns or sequences used to influence family structure and power.	Behavioral patterns displayed by the extended system (significant friends, family of origin, therapist) used to influence the structure and behaviors of the extended system.	Cultural norms and mores of behavior; behaviors prescribed or proscribed by the larger society.

Interpersonal/ communication	Characteristic ways of communicating and interacting across relationships or personality (e.g. shy, gregarious, narcissistic, dependent, controlling, avoidant).	Quality and frequency of the dyad's communication; speaking and listening skills; how couples share information, express feelings, and resolve conflict.	Information flow in the family system; paradoxical messages; family system boundaries, hierarchy, and organization; how the family system uses information regarding its own functioning.	Degree to which information is shared with and received from significant others outside the nuclear family system or dyad; has implications about the relative permeability of boundaries and the degree to which the family or couple is receptive to outside influences.	Information that is communicated to the family or individual by the community or culture in which they live; how the family or individual communicates their needs and mobilizes resources.
Structural/ developmental	All aspects of physiological and psychosocial development; personal history that influences current functioning; intrapersonal consistency of cognitions, affect, and behavior.	History of the relationship and how it has evolved over time; congruence of partners' cognitions, affect, and behavior.	Changes in the family system over time; current stage in the family life cycle; congruence in needs, beliefs, and behaviors across family members.	Developmental changes across generations; significant historical events influencing current system functioning (e.g. death, illness, divorce, abuse).	The cultural and political history of the society in which the family or individual lives; current political and economic changes; congruence of the individual's or couple's values with those of the larger community.

347

In assessing behavior and control at an individual level, capacity for self-control reflects the extent to which partners can defer self-gratification for the sake of the other or for their relationship. At the dyadic level, the means by which partners struggle to influence each other and the models adopted for decision making (e.g., unilateral versus collaborative) are key dimensions in a couple's relationship. Couples may use different decision-making models across different domains of family life or across different subsystems within the family; thus, assessment should differentiate between typical decision-making strategies and their variability across situations. Also central to behavioral control at the dyadic level is the management of conflict and aggression. Extended systems at the family or community level exert influence or control to the degree that they make the availability of desired resources contingent on one or more family members' behavior. Couples frequently experience conflict when partners differ in their perception or tolerance of control that is exerted by others outside their own relationship.

As noted earlier, communication difficulties rank first among the reasons couples give for entering marital therapy. Most frequently studied among dyads is the ability to resolve conflicts and negotiate mutually acceptable solutions. Although communication typically is viewed as involving two or more persons, consistency in a person's relational style across diverse topics and situations with others points to an important individual source of communication behaviors. Communication may be direct or indirect, deliberate or haphazard, constructive or destructive. Similar to individuals and dyads, conflict resolution behaviors and the expression of both positive and negative feelings emerge as important components of communication at the family system level as well. Critical to couples' functioning are the means by which partners attempt to negotiate conflict resolution with elements of the extended family and their strategies for securing social support and mobilizing community resources.

Structural considerations include intrapersonal consistency across cognitive, affective, and behavioral dimensions (e.g., Does the individual behave in a manner congruent with his beliefs and feelings?), as well as interpersonal congruence or discrepancies between partners along these same dimensions. Also relevant are critical events in the partners' developmental histories and in the course of their relationship. Both the likelihood of specific conflicts and their interpretation and impact may vary, not only as a function of partners' ages but also as a function of the stage or duration of the relationship. Changes in a couple's interactions often reflect the modification of norms, roles, and other characteristics as their relationship adapts or fails to adapt to new challenges over time.

How one approaches the task of assessing couples across the domains and levels of functioning defined by this conceptual model will vary according to purposes of the evaluation, resources of time and instrumentation, willingness of partners to participate in various assessment tasks, and theoretical orientation of the clinician. In the section that follows, we offer general guidelines and strategies for how to assess couples, bearing in mind that decisions regarding the specific process and the content of the assessment must be tailored to the unique needs of each couple and the objectives of the evaluation.

GUIDELINES AND STRATEGIES FOR ASSESSING COUPLES

General Considerations

Separating assessment from treatment creates a false dichotomy. The process of couple therapy requires continuous assessment of moment-to-moment fluctuations in affect and cognitions within sessions, as well as sustained progress toward behavior change and resolution of presenting problems between and across sessions. Continuous assessment allows the therapist to evaluate the appropriateness of current treatment strategies and suggests changes in either the content or the modality of interventions. Similarly, assessment directed exclusively at information gathering in the absence of therapeutic benefit fails to advance the couple's conceptual understanding and motivation toward resolving relationship difficulties, and it may heighten resistance and impede subsequent treatment progress. Assessment should be therapeutic in and of itself. Therapeutic assessment (Finn & Tonsager, 1997) requires collaborating with the couple in framing relevant questions, reviewing test findings, generating a tentative formulation regarding factors contributing to relationship difficulties, establishing initial treatment goals, and deciding on therapeutic strategies.

Stuart (1980) asserted that therapeutic assessment can be achieved "only if the language of assessment is specific, intelligible, and acceptable to the couple; if the assessment broadens the partners' perspectives to include awareness of their own roles in shaping their interaction; and if the data collected are positive and strength-oriented" (p. 70). Similarly, Jacobson and Margolin (1979) noted that "the most desirable goal of an initial interview is not to gather assessment information but rather to set the stage for therapeutic change by building positive expectancies and trust in the couple, and by actually providing them with some benefits" (p. 51). An initial or primary emphasis on identifying presenting problems can magnify partners' defensiveness, antagonisms, and hopelessness.

Thus, techniques of couple assessment—whether they emphasize informal or structured self-report or observational methods—should complement one another in serving dual purposes of generating information and helping the couple construct a more optimistic formulation of their current difficulties, how they came about, and how they can be remediated (L'Abate, 1994). These dual goals are facilitated when the therapist conveys confidence and enthusiasm, allows partners an equal opportunity to be heard, establishes a safe environment and sets appropriate limits on negative exchanges, and provides a constructive model of empathic listening.

The Clinical Interview

The clinical interview remains the most important tool in couple assessment (L'Abate & Bagarozzi, 1993). Various formats for organizing and conducting an initial assessment interview with couples have been proposed (cf., Baucom & Epstein, 1990; Gottman, 1999; Jacobson & Margolin, 1979; Karpel, 1994; L'Abate, 1994; Stuart, 1980). For example, Karpel (1994) suggested a four-part evaluation that includes an initial meeting with the couple together, followed by separate sessions with each partner individually and then an additional joint meeting with the couple. Although this format potentially permits greater exploration of relationship and individual concerns, it has several potential drawbacks. The length of this assessment may not be feasible in many managed-care environments that limit the number of treatment sessions. Couples in crisis may also become discouraged if the pacing of assessment requires several weeks before initial interventions are undertaken to reduce immediate distress. Finally, individual assessment sessions for some couples may elicit unilateral disclosure of secrets, engender imbalances in the therapist's alliance with each partner or partners' fears of such imbalances, and subsequently detract from a collaborative therapeutic alliance.

We prefer an extended initial assessment interview that lasts about 2 hours in which the following goals are stated at the outset:

1. Getting to know each partner as an individual separate from the marriage
2. Understanding the structure and organization of the marriage

3. Learning about current relationship difficulties, their development, and previous efforts to address them

4. Reaching an informed decision together about whether to proceed with couple therapy and, if so, discussing respective expectations.

Getting to Know the Individuals

Each partner should be interviewed in turn to obtain information about their age, education, current occupation if working outside the home, and employment history. To what extent does the individual's work contribute to his or her stress or sense of well-being? Information is also obtained regarding physical health and both current and previous medical and psychological treatment. If previously in therapy, what were the primary issues addressed at that time? What worked well in that treatment, what worked less well, and how do previous experiences in therapy influence the individual's hopes, fears, or expectations about pursuing couple therapy now?

Also reviewed briefly are the structure and history of the family of origin and any previous marriages. Are the individual's birth parents still living, and, if so, are they still married and where do they live? What are the first names, ages, and locations of siblings? How frequent and what type of contact does the individual have with members of the family of origin, and how satisfying are these relationships? The goal of these questions is not to obtain a detailed family history but, instead, to evaluate (1) overall levels of intimacy or conflict in the family of origin; (2) indicators of emotional or behavioral enmeshment or disengagement; (3) models of emotional expressiveness and conflict resolution; (4) appropriateness and clarity of boundaries; and (5) standards or expectations regarding authority, autonomy, fidelity, and similar themes.

Similar information should be sought regarding previous marriages. For each previous marriage or similar relationship, what were the ages of partners at the time of marriage? How long did the marriage last, and how did it end? Were there children by that marriage and, if so, what are their names, ages, and current living arrangements? How much and what kinds of contact does the individual have with his or her former partner(s) and any children from those relationships, and how satisfying or conflicted are these relationships? Who else does the therapist need to know about because of their impact on the individual or couple's relationship (e.g., current or previous affair partner)?

Each partner should be asked questions that screen for factors that could potentially contribute to crises later in the therapy. These include questions concerning history and current patterns of alcohol and other substance use, history or potential for aggressive behavior toward oneself or others, and current or possible future involvement in legal proceedings. In broaching these domains, partners can be reassured of the therapist's concern about times when couple therapy becomes difficult and may exacerbate distress on an intermediate basis, generating a need to evaluate ahead of time any additional stressors that may compromise efforts to contain that distress.

Finally, each partner should be asked, "What else should I know about you that I've neglected to ask, or you'd like me to know about you because of its importance to you personally?"

Understanding the Structure and Organization of the Marriage

Couples come to an initial interview primed to talk about their relationship difficulties, bare their heartaches, and, more often than not, explain why their partner is primarily at fault. Beginning the interview with an emphasis on getting to know each individual helps counteract this tendency. So, too, does helping partners begin talking about their marriage in a more positive manner—recollecting how they met, courted, decided to marry, and (ideally) enjoyed earlier times in their relationship before deterioration or conflict set in. Formats proposed for accomplishing this (cf. Baucom & Epstein, 1990; Jacobson & Margolin, 1979; Karpel, 1994) include inquiring about the following: How did you meet, and what characteristics of your partner did you find especially attractive? What sustained you during your courtship? What were the circumstances that led to your decision to marry? What are your best memories from early in your marriage? Which parts of those experiences have you been able to sustain or resurrect in recent times?

If the couple has not yet described the current nuclear family, information should be obtained regarding children, their ages and relationships if from a previous marriage, and their general psychosocial functioning. Are there any especially noteworthy facts about the children, such as serious medical or psychological problems (Karpel, 1994)? Who is considered a member of the family, and who is not (e.g., a child from a previous marriage living out-of-state with an ex-spouse)? Also relevant is preliminary information regarding the structure of affect and decision making in the family (L'Abate, 1994). Who does what in the family? Have there been recent role changes? Who is close to whom? Who is in conflict with whom? Who makes the decisions in various areas of their family life (e.g., management of finances, child rearing matters)? Again, a general question can be used to invite important information not elicited by specific questions posed by the therapist. "What do I need to know about your family that I don't know yet in order to understand better the kinds of difficulties the two of you are having?"

Learning about Current Relationship Difficulties

"Tell me why you're here." Couples invariably recognize this directive as indicating the occasion for them to describe their current relationship difficulties and their decision to seek assistance. Because communication difficulties are frequently cited as the cause for seeking therapy, and because this response reveals little about the specific nature of communication deficits or specific domains in which communication difficulties are experienced, specific questions are needed to delineate the precise nature of relationship distress, its evolution, and previous efforts to address these difficulties (L'Abate, 1994).

How does the couple define their primary difficulties? Who has defined the problem? Is one partner more involved in or more distressed by the problem than the other and, if so, why? What does each partner identify as the primary contributing factors to their current struggles? How do partners agree or disagree on their definition and understanding of their difficulties? What experiences and discussions have led them to define their relationship problems in this way? What solutions have they tried in the past, and how did they decide to seek outside assistance at this time? What does each individual believe it would require from him- or herself to promote positive change in the marriage?

Although presenting marital difficulties extend across an infinite range of specific content, Karpel (1994) has identified common themes that can often guide the assessment process. These include the following: (1) repetitive unresolved conflicts, either focusing on one issue or generalized across multiple issues; (2) emotional distance or disaffection that is related to persistent remoteness, excessive demands, relentless criticism, or physical or emotional abuse; (3) stable but devitalized relationships that are characterized by an absence of intimacy, passion, or joy; (4) difficulties with third parties, including in-laws, affair partners, or children; and (5) acute crises including alcohol or substance abuse, major psychopathology, sudden financial stressors, death of a family member, or similar concerns.

L'Abate (1994) noted that the therapist should attend to important relationship dynamics that transcend the specific content of a couple's difficulties. Among these are the following:

- To what degree do intergenerational ties exist? How open is the couple to input from outside the system? To what extent do outside influences function as a resource or a stressor?
- What types of communication-relational patterns exist between partners? To what degree have partners been able to develop a coalition, enabling them to set goals, solve problems, negotiate conflicts, handle crises, and complete individual and family developmental tasks?
- To what extent do redundant, cyclical interactional patterns prevent partners from setting goals, solving problems, negotiating conflict, overcoming crises, and achieving family tasks?
- To what extent have the spouses and all family members been able to negotiate mutually acceptable patterns of separateness (distance) and connectedness (closeness)? To what extent are members emotionally supportive of each other?
- What are the recurrent themes in the marriage and the extended family? What are the personal, conjugal, and family myths that prevent family members from setting goals and solving problems effectively?

Reaching an Informed Decision about Couple Therapy

The assessment interview with a couple—whether conducted in one or multiple sessions—should conclude with a comprehensive and realistic formulation of the couple's difficulties that emphasizes both individual and relationship resources that the couple can mobilize and direct toward strengthening their marriage and reducing relationship distress. It is rare that *no* redeeming features of a relationship can be identified in the initial interview, or that individual or relational characteristics are so irreparably toxic as to preclude encouragement toward an initial trial of 4 to 6 sessions of couple therapy. Exceptions might include instances of sexual or physical abuse by an unremorseful partner or severe substance abuse, both of which mandate intensive individual treatment before couple therapy can be a viable alternative or adjunctive intervention.

Baucom and Epstein (1990) emphasize the importance of constructing an integrative formulation that incorporates both discrete information that is disclosed during the interview and covert impressions that are acquired through observation. They advocate integrating behavioral, cognitive, and affective components at the individual and dyadic levels—taking into account current and historical or developmental considerations. Equally important to an analysis of presenting difficulties is a formulation that incorporates individual and relationship strengths, as well external resources.

Stuart (1980) suggests several formulations that potentially reframe existing struggles in more benevolent terms and promote change. For example: To what extent can the couple be helped to recognize and draw comfort from their similarities and to relabel differences as opportunities for growth or stimulation? Can role shifts associated with modal developmental changes in the family be "normalized" and ways be found to compensate without the level of negative attributions and subjective cost?

Finally, therapists should assess each individual's expectations regarding their own responsibilities and readiness for change, expectations for their partner's change, and anticipated or desired roles of the therapist. Ground rules regarding attendance by one or both partners at each session, along with limits to verbal aggression, confidentiality, and so forth, are likely to vary as a function of treatment modality and individual differences in therapist training, and these must be conveyed clearly to both partners.

The Family Genogram

Virtually every approach to couple therapy acknowledges to some degree the importance of the family of origin in contributing to current relationship patterns. Whether from observational learning of dysfunctional attitudes and behaviors, from attachment theory and relationship schema, or from object relations theory and pathogenic introjects, early experiences from intimate relationships can have enduring effects on individuals' approaches to intimacy, autonomy, affect regulation, and conflict resolution. The family genogram comprises a graphic means of depicting the transgenerational family structures, dynamics, and critical family events that potentially influence family members' interactions with one another (McGoldrick, Gerson, & Shellenberger, 1999). The genogram is constructed from information derived from an extended clinical interview regarding family history—and it both directs the interview content and evolves in response to new information that is gleaned during the course of therapy.

McGoldrick et al. (1999) present a sample genogram for Harry Stack Sullivan (1892–1949), founder of interpersonal psychotherapy and a systematic theory of personality and development emphasizing social interactions as the foundation of a self-system that ultimately governs individuals' interactions with significant others (see Figure 10.2). Sullivan and his parents are depicted in the genogram, along with his paternal and maternal

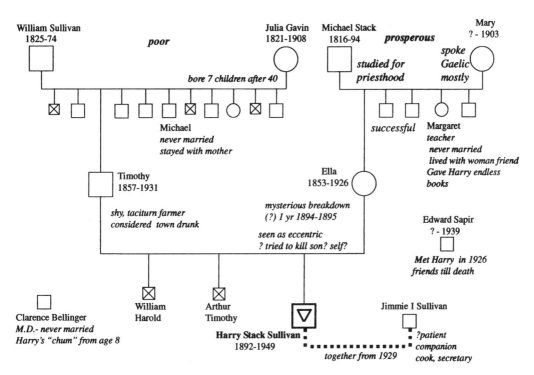

FIGURE 10.2. Genogram for Harry Stack Sullivan. From McGoldrick and Gerson (1985). Copyright 1985 by Monica McGoldrick and Randy Gerson. Reprinted by permission of W. W. Norton & Company, Inc.

grandparents. As his parents' only surviving child, how did Sullivan integrate the contrasting family themes carried forward by his shy alcoholic father—himself the product of a poor family bearing children quite late in life—and his eccentric mother, the oldest daughter of a wealthy family, who appeared emotionally brittle and may have tried to kill both herself and Sullivan when he was 3 years old? To what extent was Sullivan's emotional resilience attributable to his maternal aunt, Margaret, who may have adopted Harry as her own? Answers to such questions are often illuminated by examining individual and relational dynamics in greater detail across the family generations.

The genogram reflects a family systems perspective, positing that relationship patterns in previous generations may provide implicit models for family functioning in the next generation. Structural organization and functional dynamics are viewed both horizontally across the family context and vertically through the generations. As such, the genogram provides a subjective, interpretive tool and helps the therapist delineate contrasts and consistencies within and between the partners' extended families of origin.

Observational Techniques

Heyman (2001) notes that virtually all theories of relationship dysfunction and couple therapies emphasize communication deficits as a common pathway to relationship problems. Consequently, the field has emphasized both formal and informal observational techniques for gaining an understanding of couples' specific communication difficulties and planning appropriate interventions. These range from (1) observing characteristics of couples' emotional expressiveness and problem-solving behaviors during the initial interview and subsequent treatment sessions, to (2) directing the couple to discuss a specific conflict in a clinical setting while the therapist refrains from intervention and takes notes to provide subsequent feedback, or (3) videotaping structured problem-solving tasks in research settings and subjecting partners' interactions to elaborate systems of coding verbal and nonverbal behavior.

Unlike self-report measures, observational assessment provides direct samples of relevant behaviors in a controlled setting that ideally generalize to current or future behavior in the couple's natural environment (Haynes, 2001). Thus, observing a married couple in a therapeutic context while intervening to promote conflict resolution is less relevant for assessing problematic communication patterns than directing the couple to discuss a moderate- or high-conflict issue for 10 minutes without therapist intervention. Observation of a couple's communication, when applied idiographically, can facilitate hypotheses about factors that maintain a couple's communication difficulties that affect both treatment process and outcome. To apply such observations normatively—that is, to evaluate the extent to which a couple's interactions mirror common patterns of either distressed or nondistressed couples—it is necessary that therapists be familiar with communication behaviors that characterize or reliably distinguish clinic from nonclinic populations. Thus, we describe next some of the better-known systems for observing and coding couples' interactions, and then we discuss the common empirical findings that are derived from these and their clinical implications.

Observational Coding Systems

Since the late 1960s, a variety of coding systems have been developed for categorizing and analyzing couples' verbal and nonverbal communication behaviors. A comprehensive review of psychometric findings regarding these systems is provided by Heyman (2001). The earlier systems tended to be more microanalytic, generating a wealth of information about communication patterns of distressed couples but typically requiring inordinate time and coding resources (e.g., teams of highly trained coders requiring as many as 10 hours to code each hour of interaction). More recent coding systems and adaptations of earlier systems have tended to be macroanalytic, emphasizing more global affective or behavioral components of couples' exchanges and promoting a more intuitive nomenclature of communication behaviors that have relevance to couple therapists.

The Marital Interaction Coding System (MICS; Hops, Wills, Patterson, & Weiss, 1972; Weiss, 1992; Heyman, Weiss, & Eddy, 1995), now in its fourth iteration (MICS-IV) is the best known and most widely used of couple observational coding systems. The MICS includes 37 codes of both verbal and nonverbal behavior, such as criticism, disagreement, negative affect, problem description, acceptance of responsibility, agreement, and humor. Numerous studies have supported both the interrater reliability, temporal stability, and discriminant validity of the MICS. Factor analysis of the 37 microanalytic codes resulted in four broad categories: hostility, constructive problem discussion, humor, and responsibility discussion (Heyman, Eddy, Weiss, & Vivian, 1995).

Two macroanalytic adaptations of the MICS have been proposed. Heyman and colleagues described a "rapid" MICS (RMICS) system based on factor-analytic findings for the MICS but integrating additional broad-band codes from other coding systems and empirical developments regarding couples' attributions. The RMICS (Heyman, Vivian, Weiss, Hubbard, & Ayerle, 1993) comprises nine codes: hostility, dysphoric affect, withdrawal, problem discussion, self-disclosure, acceptance, humor, distress-maintaining attributions, and relationship-enhancing attributions. Heyman et al. (1993) provide evidence for both the reliability and discriminant validity of the RMICS and note that it takes approximately 30 minutes to code one 15-minute sample compared to roughly 2 hours for the complete MICS.

A second alternative to the MICS proposed by Weiss and Tolman (1990)—the MICS-Global (MICS-G)—has six global rating categories: conflict, problem solving, validation, invalidation, facilitation, and withdrawal. Each category reflects a composite of microanalytic codes. For example, conflict reflects a composite of complaints, criticism, negative attributions, insults, negative commands, hostility, and sarcasm. Category ratings are made using a 6-point scale ranging from 0 ("none") to 5 ("very high"). The authors present findings supporting the intraobserver reliability, as well as both convergent and discriminant validity data for the MICS-G.

Another microanalytic coding scheme is the Couples Interaction Scoring System (CISS; Gottman, 1979) that categorizes nonverbal behavior of both speaker and listener as negative, neutral, or positive and classifies verbal behavior of the speaker into one of eight categories: agreement, disagreement, communication talk, mindreading, proposing a solution, summarizing other, summarizing self, and problem information or feelings. Although it is less widely used than the MICS, Gottman and colleagues have conducted extensive research with the CISS on the topography of couples' communication patterns and their development over time. As with the MICS, various adaptations of the CISS have been proposed. The best known of these is the Specific Affect Coding System (SPAFF; Gottman & Krokoff, 1989) that classifies speakers' affect as affectively neutral, as one of five negative affects (anger, disgust or contempt, sadness, fear, whining), or as one of five positive affects (affection, humor, interest, anticipation, excitement or joy).

Independent of the coding system employed, specific instructions used to generate couples' observational data will strongly influence both their representativeness and their clinical utility, but not necessarily in the same direction. For example, partners who report infrequent but intense disagreements about their sexual relationship might be directed to "replay" a memorable high-conflict exchange in this domain, even though such exchanges may not characterize their marriage more generally. Moreover, they might be asked to reenact their "best" discussions of their sexual disagreements, as well as their "typical" or "worst" discussions, as a way of distinguishing between their optimal ability versus the modal performance of communication behaviors.

Observational Findings and Clinical Implications

From more than 30 years of observational research, several conclusions can be drawn about distressed couples' communication. Specifically, compared to nondistressed couples from the community, distressed couples are more hostile; start their conversations with greater hostility and maintain more hostility during the course of conversation; are more likely to reciprocate and escalate their partner's hostility; are less likely to edit their behavior during conflict, resulting in longer negative reciprocity loops; emit less positive behavior; and are more likely to show "demand → withdraw" patterns, in which one partner engages in negative interaction (such as demanding, blaming, or accusing) while the other avoids and withdraws from the interaction (Heyman, 2001). By contrast, little is known about the normative communication patterns of nondistressed couples. What little research in this area does show is that nondistressed couples do not naturally paraphrase their partners' statements nor reflect their partners' implied feelings.

Weiss and Heyman (1997) review each of these findings and their clinical implications. Above all, they note the importance of integrating 5- to 10-minute observations of non-structured problem-solving discussions without therapist intervention into the initial assessment process. Heyman (2001) recommends the following questions to guide informal observation: How does the conversation start? Does the level of anger escalate, and what happens when it does? Do the partners enter repetitive negative loops? Are the couple's communication patterns consistent across different domains of conflict? Do their behaviors differ when it is "her" topic versus "his"? Do partners label the other person or their communication process as the "problem"?

Independent of the answers to these questions for any given couple, general implications from observational findings are that clinicians need to reduce the level of overt hostility and hostile withdrawal early in the therapy. Negativity is like a "black hole" that quickly absorbs distressed couples from which they have difficulty escaping. Specific techniques for disrupting negative escalations, getting back on track, or resuming discussions at a later time are essential. Distressed couples need to be taught specific skills in appropriate editing, as well as metacommunication to modify faulty patterns (e.g., "We're getting off track; let's try to refocus on the problem we started with"). Equally important to disrupting negative communication patterns is promoting positive communication behaviors, including emotional expressiveness, validation, and problem-solving skills.

Self-Report Techniques

The use of self-report measures to assess couples' interactions extends as far back as Terman's (1938) seminal research on the psychological and sexual correlates of marital happiness. Terman constructed self-report measures to assess individuals' sociodemographic background, descriptions of their parents and own childhood, psychological factors emphasizing emotionality and general likes and dislikes, views about the ideal marriage, and appraisals of their current marriage and sexual relationship. The rationale underlying self-report strategies in couples assessment is that such techniques (1) are convenient and relatively easy to administer, obtaining a wealth of information across a broad range of issues germane to clinical assessment or research objectives; (2) lend themselves to collection of large normative samples serving as a reference or comparison group facilitating interpretation; (3) allow disclosure about events and subjective experiences respondents may be reluctant to discuss; and (4) provide important data concerning internal phenomena opaque to observational approaches including values and attitudes, expectations and attributions, and satisfaction and commitment.

However, the limitations of traditional self-report measures also bear noting. Specifically, such instruments (1) exhibit susceptibility to both deliberate and unconscious efforts to bias self- and other-presentation in either a favorable or unfavorable manner; (2) are vulnerable to individual differences in stimulus interpretation and errors in recollection of objective events; (3) may inadvertently influence respondents' nontest behavior in unintended ways; and (4) typically provide few fine-grained details concerning moment-to-moment interactions (Grotevant & Carlson, 1989; Jacob & Tennenbaum, 1988; Jacobson & Margolin, 1979; Snyder et al., 1995).

Because of their potential advantages and despite their limitations, self-report techniques of marital and family functioning have proliferated, with published measures numbering well over 1,000 (Touliatos, Perlmutter, & Straus, 1990). However, relatively few of these measures have achieved widespread adoption. Straus (1969) found that 80% of measures had been used only once. Bonjean, Hill, and McLemore (1967) found that only 2% of measures had been used more than five times. Chun, Cobb, and French (1975) found that 63% of measures they reviewed had been used only once, with only 3% being used 10 times or more. Fewer than 40% of marital and family therapists regularly use *any* standardized instruments (Boughner, Hayes, Bubenzer, & West, 1994). Although these surveys are now dated, it seems unlikely that these trends have changed significantly. Contributing to these findings is the inescapable conclusion that the majority of measures in this domain demonstrate little evidence regarding the most rudimentary psychometric features of reliability or validity, let alone clear evidence supporting their clinical utility (Snyder & Rice, 1996).

In the following paragraphs, we describe a small subset of self-report measures that have been selected on the basis of their representativeness across behavioral, cognitive, and affective domains of couples' interactions, potential clinical utility, and at least moderate evidence of reliability and validity across multiple investigations. More comprehensive bibliographies of self-report marital and family measures are available elsewhere (e.g., Corcoran & Fischer, 2000; Davis, Yarber, Bauserman, Schreer, & Davis, 1998; Fredman & Sherman, 1987; Grotevant & Carlson, 1989; Jacob & Tennenbaum, 1988; L'Abate & Bagarozzi, 1993; Touliatos et al., 1990). Other recent texts on couple therapy emphasize the clinical use of self-report measures as an integral component of planning and evaluating couple interventions (cf., Baucom & Epstein, 1990; Epstein & Baucom, in press; Gottman, 1999).

Measures of Behavior

Although distinctions among measures of behavior, cognition, and affect are imperfect, we focus here on measures that purport to assess couples' behavior exchanges, communication, verbal and physical aggression, and sexual intimacy. Among measures of behavior exchange, one of the earliest and most widely used is the Spouse Observation Checklist (SOC; Birchler, Weiss, & Vincent, 1975), a list of 400 discrete behaviors divided on an a priori basis into 12 categories such as affection and physical intimacy, companionship, communication, parenting, finances, and division of household responsibilities. Although specific administration instructions may vary, each individual is asked to complete the checklist over a specific time period (e.g., the previous 24 hours), indicating which behaviors their partner had emitted and whether these were experienced as pleasing or displeasing. As a clinical tool, the SOC generates menus of individual reinforcers and has the potential to delineate relative strengths and weaknesses in the relationship, thus transforming diffuse negative complaints into specific requests for positive change.

Two measures have been developed for evaluating partners' recreational patterns and use of leisure time. The Marital Activities Inventory (MAI; Weiss, Hops, & Patterson, 1973) and the Leisure Activity Interaction Index (LAII; Orthner, 1975) both present individuals with lists of potential recreational activities and ask them to indicate how often they've engaged in these activities over some specified time period and whether alone, with their partner, or with someone other than their partner. Such measures can be useful in educating couples about the relative advantages of parallel versus joint activities as a means of strengthening the relationship at times of varying distress. For example, research has found relationship satisfaction to be positively related to the proportion of time spent together in joint behaviors, negatively related to time spent alone, and only marginally related to time spent together in parallel but noninteractive activity (Orthner, 1975; Smith, Snyder, Trull, & Monsma, 1988).

Other behavioral measures attempt to identify specific areas of desired change, the amount and direction of change desired, the congruence of desired change across partners, and individuals' accuracy in perceiving their partner's wishes. The older of these two, the Areas of Change Questionnaire (ACQ; Weiss & Birchler, 1975), presents each partner with two identical lists of 34 specific behaviors (e.g., helping with housework or spending more time in outside activities) and asks individuals to indicate whether they would like their partner to increase or decrease that behavior, and whether an increase or decrease in his or her own rate of that behavior would be pleasing to the partner. Scoring algorithms for the ACQ have been described for evaluating overall levels of desired change, congruence of partners' desired change in specific behaviors, as well as perceptual accuracy of each individual's understanding of his or her partner's wishes. A recent alternative to the ACQ, Gottman's (1999) Areas of Change Checklist, adopts a simpler approach in listing 36 potential relationship problems and asking respondents to rate the level of desired change for each item on a 5-point scale.

A variety of self-report measures of communication have been developed, several of which are described in an excellent review by Sayers and Sarwer (1998). The Communication Patterns Questionnaire (CPQ; Christensen, 1987) measures the temporal sequence of couples' interactions by soliciting partners' perceptions of their communication patterns before, during, and after conflict. Scores on the CPQ can be used to assess characteristics of the demand → withdraw pattern that is frequently observed among distressed couples. An alternative measure of couples' communication is the Styles of Conflict Inventory (SCI; Metz, 1993), a 126-item inventory that elicits individuals' descriptions of their own behavior in response to a conflict situation, as well as thoughts and perceptions of their partner's behavior. Scores on the SCI permit comparisons of partners' appraisals with each other, as well as comparisons to a standardization sample along dimensions that reflect frequency and intensity of relationship conflicts, and attributions regarding responsibility for relationship conflicts.

Screening for relationship aggression by self-report measures assumes particular importance because of some individuals' reluctance to disclose the nature or extent of such aggression during an initial conjoint interview. By far the most widely used measure of couples' aggression is the Conflict Tactics Scale (CTS). The original CTS (Straus, 1979) included 19 Likert items that assess three modes of conflict resolution: reasoning, verbal aggression, and physical aggression. The revised instrument (CTS2; Straus, Hamby, Boney-McCoy, & Sugarman, 1996) adds scales of sexual coercion and physical injury, as well as additional items to better differentiate between minor and severe levels of verbal and physical aggression.

Gottman (1999) presented an alternative measure, the Waltz–Rushe–Gottman Emotional Abuse Questionnaire (EAQ), a 66-item inventory designed to assess less tangible expressions of psychological abuse including social isolation, degradation, sexual coercion, and destruction of property. A third measure of relationship aggression, the Aggression (AGG) scale of the Marital Satisfaction Inventory—Revised (MSI-R; Snyder, 1997), has 10 items that reflect psychological and physical aggression experienced from one's partner. Similar to the CTS, evidence has been obtained for both the reliability and validity of the AGG scale, and interpretive guidelines are designed to be sensitive to even modest levels of relationship aggression as an indicator for more in-depth evaluation of abuse potential. Advantages of the AGG scale as a screening measure include its relative brevity and its inclusion in a multidimensional measure of couples' relationships (the MSI-R) described later in this chapter.

As with issues of aggression, some people may be reluctant to disclose intimate details of their sexual relationship during an initial interview. Numerous measures of sexual attitudes, behaviors, and conflicts have been developed (Davis et al., 1998). Two more widely used self-report techniques in this domain include the Sexual Interaction Inventory (SII; LoPiccolo & Steger, 1974) and the Derogatis Sexual Functioning Inventory (DSFI; Derogatis & Melisaratos, 1979; Derogatis, Lopez, & Zinzeletta, 1988). The SII is a 102-item measure that asks the individual to rate the frequency of activity and levels of satisfaction, both real and ideal, for both self and partner, across 17 behaviors that range from intercourse to nudity and nonsexual physical intimacy. By comparison, the DSFI includes 254 items comprising 10 scales that reflect such areas as sexual knowledge, range of sexual experiences, and sexual attitudes and drive, as well as psychological symptoms in nonsexual domains. Although concerns have been raised in the literature regarding the veridicality of self-reports, particularly regarding specific sexual practices (cf. McConaghy, 1998), both the SII and DSFI have garnered support for their reliability and discriminant validity, and responses to either measure can be used to introduce sensitive issues during a clinical interview.

Measures of Cognition

In the conceptual model of assessment presented earlier in this chapter, we noted the importance of evaluating couples' assumptions, standards, attentional sets, expectancies, and attributions for relationship events. Several self-report measures have been developed to assist in this process. The Dyadic Attributional Inventory (DAI; Baucom, Sayers, & Duhe, 1989) is a 24-item measure that asks respondents to imagine hypothetical marital events and then, for each event, to generate attributions for their partner's behavior in that situation with regard to source of influence (self, partner, or external factors), stability or instability of causal factors, and their specificity or globality. The DAI assists in identifying and modifying dysfunctional attributional sets that contribute to subjective negativity surrounding specific relationship events.

An alternative measure, the Relationship Attribution Measure (RAM; Fincham & Bradbury, 1992), also presents hypothetical situations but asks respondents to generate responsibility attributions to indicate the extent to which the partner intentionally behaved negatively, was selfishly motivated, and was blameworthy for the event. A third attributional measure, the Marital Attitude Survey (MAS; Pretzer, Epstein, & Fleming, 1992), elicits attributions along six dimensions reflecting causal influence from one's own behavior or personality, the partner's behavior or personality, and attributions regarding the partner's malicious intent or lack of love. The moderating role of these dimensions was demonstrated in a study in which the relation of marital distress to depressive symptomatology was greater for wives who attributed marital difficulties to their own behavior but not to their husbands' behavior (Heim & Snyder, 1991).

Separate from attributional measures have been those that examine unrealistic relationship assumptions or standards. An early measure in this domain, the Relationship Beliefs Inventory (RBI; Eidelson & Epstein, 1992), assesses five dysfunctional ideas about marriage—for example, that disagreements are necessarily destructive or that spouses should know each other's feelings and thoughts without asking. A more recent measure of standards, the Inventory of Specific Relationship Standards (ISRS; Baucom, Epstein, Rankin, & Burnett, 1996), assesses partners' individual boundaries and level of influence, as well as their personal investment in the relationship. Scores on the ISRS can be used to guide clinical interventions—for example, couples reporting fewer individual boundaries, egalitarian decision making, and high relationship investment were more likely to have higher relationship satisfaction.

Measures of Affect

Measures of relationship satisfaction and global affect abound. The two oldest and most widely used are the Locke–Wallace Marital Adjustment Test (MAT; Locke & Wallace, 1959) and the Dyadic Adjustment Scale (DAS; Spanier, 1976). The MAT is a 15-item questionnaire that asks partners to rate their overall happiness in their relationship, as well as their extent of agreement in key areas of marital interaction. Displacing the MAT as the most frequent global measure of relationship satisfaction is the DAS, a 32-item instrument that purports to differentiate among four related subscales that reflect cohesion, satisfaction, consensus, and affectional expression. A third global measure of relationship satisfaction gaining increasing use is the Global Distress (GDS) scale of the MSI-R (Snyder, 1997), a 22-item true–false measure that has been shown to discriminate reliably among varying levels of relationship conflict and distress. In addition to the advantage of its inclusion in a multidimensional measure of couples' interaction, the GDS scale has been recommended as a more sensitive measure of treatment response than alternative global measures (Whisman & Jacobson, 1992).

For abbreviated screening measures of marital distress, several alternatives are available. The Relationship Satisfaction Scale (RSAT; Burns & Sayers, 1992) is a 13-item Likert-type measure that assesses satisfaction in such areas as handling of finances and degree of affection and caring. The Quality of Marriage Index (QMI; Norton, 1983) is a 6-item Likert-type measure that asks respondents to rate their overall level of marital happiness and the accuracy of additional descriptors of overall relationship stability and accord. An even shorter measure, the Kansas Marital Satisfaction Scale (KMSS; Schumm et al., 1986) includes three Likert items that assess satisfaction with marriage as an institution, the marital relationship, and the character of one's spouse. In general, abbreviated scales of global relationship satisfaction are adequate as initial screening measures in primary care or general psychiatric settings, but, due to their brevity, they lack the ability to distinguish reliably among finer gradations of relationship distress among partners who present for couple therapy.

Multidimensional Measures

Well-constructed multidimensional measures of couples' interactions have the potential to discriminate among various sources of relationship strength and conflict. Several such measures have received fairly widespread attention. The PREPARE and ENRICH inventories by Fowers and Olson (1989, 1992) were developed for use with premarital and married couples, respectively; each includes 125 items rated on a 5-point scale to assess relationship accord in such domains as communication, conflict resolution, the sexual relationship, and finances. A computerized interpretive report identifies areas of "strength" and "potential growth" and directs respondents to specific items that reflect potential concerns.

Also widely used in both clinical and research settings is the Marital Satisfaction Inventory—Revised (MSI-R; Snyder, 1997), a 150-item inventory that was designed to identify both the nature and the intensity of relationship distress in distinct areas of interaction. The MSI-R includes 2 validity scales, 1 global scale, and 10 specific scales to assess relationship satisfaction in such areas as affective and problem-solving communication, aggression, leisure time together, finances, the sexual relationship, role orientation, family of origin, and interactions regarding children. More than 20 years of research have supported the reliability and construct validity of the MSI-R scales (cf., Snyder & Aikman, 1999). A computerized interpretive report for the MSI-R draws on actuarial validity data to provide descriptive comparisons across different domains, both within and between partners.

LINKING ASSESSMENT TO TREATMENT

Empirically Supported Couple Therapies

Recent reviews of the marital therapy outcome literature consistently affirm the efficacy of couple therapy (Baucom et al., 1998; Christensen & Heavey, 1999; Shadish et al., 1993; Whisman & Snyder, 1997). Christensen and Heavey (1999) concluded that "in virtually every instance in which a bona fide treatment has been tested against a control group, the treatment has shown reliable change" (p. 167). In their meta-analysis of 27 controlled trials of couple therapy, Shadish et al. (1997) found an average effect size of 0.60; effects were somewhat greater for measures of global marital satisfaction than they were in studies that examined communication and specific problem-solving complaints. Overall, approximately 65% of couples in marital therapy improved, compared to 35% in control conditions.

Few, if any, reliable findings on the differential efficacy of couple treatment approaches exist. Collapsed across studies, there are somewhat stronger effects for behavioral approaches that emphasize positive behavior-exchange strategies and communication skills training. Cognitive-behavioral approaches tend to produce specific gains in domains that have been targeted by that modality (e.g., attributions and assumptions) but without increased gains in overall relationship satisfaction beyond those that are afforded by traditional behavioral techniques. Jacobson and colleagues (Jacobson, Christensen, Prince, Cordova, & Eldridge, 2000) reported somewhat greater efficacy for an approach that combines social-exchange and communication strategies with interventions emphasizing emotional acceptance of enduring differences. Several trials have supported the enhanced efficacy of approaches specifically targeting emotional expressiveness and empathy from an attachment theory perspective (Johnson & Whiffen, 2000), and one trial indicates the enhanced long-term effects of an approach emphasizing insight into developmental origins of relationship patterns and sensitivities (Snyder, Wills, & Grady-Fletcher, 1991).

Despite consistent findings supporting the overall efficacy of couple therapy, it is clear that many couples fail to achieve significant gains from existing approaches. Approximately 35% of couples fail to show significant improvement based on partners' averaged scores on outcome measures. In only 50% of treated couples do *both* partners show significant improvement in marital satisfaction at termination, and in only 40% of treated couples does the level of marital satisfaction at termination approach the average level of marital satisfaction among community (nontherapy) couples. Moreover, follow-up studies show significant deterioration in 30% to 50% of treated couples by two or more years after termination of treatment (Jacobson et al., 1987; Snyder et al., 1991). Cookerly's (1980) 5-year follow-up of couples treated by a variety of marital therapies revealed a separation/divorce rate of 44%.

A Pluralistic, Hierarchical Approach

There is growing evidence that various aspects of both individual and relationship functioning predict treatment outcome (Snyder, Cozzi, & Mangrum, in press; Snyder, Mangrum, & Wills, 1993). Because the functional sources of couples' distress vary so dramatically, the critical mediators or mechanisms of change can also be expected to vary, as should the therapeutic strategies that are intended to facilitate positive change. Based on this conclusion, Snyder (1999, 2000) argued, particularly complex or difficult cases may benefit most from an informed, pluralistic strategy that draws from both conceptual and technical innovations from diverse theoretical models that are relevant to different components of a couple's struggles. Snyder (1999) advocated conceptualizing the therapeutic tasks of couple therapy as comprising six levels of intervention (see Figure 10.3): developing a collaborative alliance, containing disabling relationship crises, strengthening the marital dyad, promoting relevant relationship skills, challenging cognitive components of relationship distress, and examining developmental sources of relationship distress.

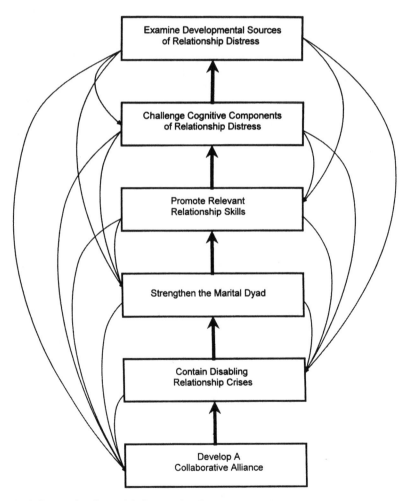

FIGURE 10.3. A hierarchical model for a pluralistic approach to couple therapy. From Snyder (1999). Copyright 1999. Reprinted by permission of Wadsworth, an imprint of the Wadsworth Group, a division of Thomson Learning.

Not all couples require each of the treatment components outlined in this sequential model. Although the sequence of interventions generally advances from crisis containment to promoting relevant skills and examining developmental sources of relationship distress, both external stressors and regressive responses to internal anxiety frequently require a return to interventions that operate at a more fundamental level in the strategic hierarchy. Couples enter treatment at varying levels of functioning and require different initial interventions. Couples also proceed along the continuum of overall functioning during treatment, both requiring and enabling interventions of increasing depth and emotional challenge. Therapeutic movement is rarely linear and an ability to recycle through more fundamental interventions to facilitate the couple's preparedness for conceptually more challenging work is the hallmark of effective treatment.

Linking Assessment to Treatment Planning

Given the diversity in couples' needs, effective treatment is most likely to be rendered when the couple therapist has a solid grounding across diverse theoretical approaches, has acquired a rich repertoire of intervention techniques linked to theory, engages in comprehensive assessment of the marital and family system, and selectively draws on intervention strategies across the theoretical spectrum in a manner consistent with an explicit case formulation. For some couples, brief training in communication skills may result in sustained improvement, whereas for others, major restructuring of family organization and boundaries may be essential to successful intervention. Psychoeducational interventions and behavioral parent training may be critical to some couples, whereas cognitive interventions that challenge irrational fears may be crucial to restoring emotional equilibrium for still others. For some couples, interpretation of developmental origins to conflicts that involve intimacy and emotional vulnerability may comprise a potent intervention, whereas for others, the same approach may elicit heightened defensiveness or cognitive deterioration.

The conceptual models presented here for comprehensive assessment across domains and system levels, and for organizing interventions in an hierarchical and pluralistic approach, provide a means for linking assessment findings to specific interventions. The following case example illustrates such a linkage.

Case Study

Rick and Anne, ages 31 and 28, sought couple therapy following Anne's discovery of Rick's brief affair with a woman he met through his work. Rick held a staff appointment in the university's college of engineering and consulted frequently to firms out of town. The woman he had an affair with over a 3-month period worked as an administrative assistant at one of these firms. Anne worked as a lab technician in the physics department. She had an 8-year-old daughter from a previous marriage that had lasted 2 years. This was Rick's first marriage; he and Anne had been married 5 years.

Rick stated that his affair had ended 6 months previous to the initial session and that Anne had discovered the affair in reviewing credit card statements for tax purposes. He acknowledged that the affair was a horrible mistake, and he had retained no involvement with the other woman after ending the affair from feelings of guilt. However, he also acknowledged considerable frustration in the marriage over the prior several years. In particular, he described Anne as demanding and persistently suspicious, and he found her emotional lability increasingly distressing to him. Rick also expressed frustration with Anne's mismanagement of their finances and with the persistent disagreement between them over how to discipline Anne's daughter, Becky.

Anne countered that Becky had an attention-deficit disorder and that Rick was unrealistic in his expectations and was unreasonably harsh. She acknowledged overspending but attributed this in part to coping with frequent feelings of loneliness and finding special activities for herself and Becky during Rick's trips out of town. After discovering Rick's affair, Anne attempted suicide with an overdose of barbiturates, was hospitalized for 2 weeks, and had continued individual treatment in an outpatient aftercare program.

Both partners expressed affection for each other, and they described their sexual relationship as particularly good. They described difficulties in resolving differences and acknowledged that at times their anger escalated to grabbing and pushing by both partners, and occasionally Anne hit Rick with her fist. Between the initial interview and subsequent session, both partners completed the Marital Satisfaction Inventory—Revised (MSI-R); their profiles are shown in Figure 10.4.

Several features of the couple's profiles are noteworthy. Despite being considerably distressed by Rick's affair, Anne's overall level of distress both on the Global Distress (GDS) scale and on scales reflecting specific domains of interaction was lower than is typical for persons entering couple therapy. Her score on the Conventionalization (CNV) scale, although typical of wives from the general community, was atypical of wives entering therapy and suggested a potential reluctance to confront specific relationship difficulties. Anne's profile had only two scores in the highest (most distressed) range—one indicating her substantial distress regarding the lack of leisure time that she and Rick shared (Time Together, TTO), and the other reflecting a fairly extensive history of distress in her family of origin (Family History of Distress, FAM).

By contrast, Rick's MSI-R profile reflected considerable distress in several areas, including his overall unhappiness in the marriage (GDS) and his dissatisfaction with his and Anne's inability to resolve conflicts and their escalation into physical aggression (Problem Solving Communication, PSC; and Aggression, AGG). Rick also expressed considerable concerns regarding his stepdaughter's psychosocial functioning (Dissatisfaction with Children, DSC) and unhappiness with his and Anne's inability to parent collaboratively (Conflict over Child Rearing, CCR).

In discussing these results, the couple came to understand how their different approaches to "caring for the relationship" resulted in polarized and antagonistic perspectives. The more Rick expressed his concerns about their marriage, the more Anne attempted to minimize difficulties—and the more she minimized, the more he escalated in asserting his unhappiness. Over the course of therapy as Anne came to experience greater trust in the therapeutic process and confront marital concerns more directly, Rick softened his descriptions of relationship problems and began to acknowledge strengths each partner brought to the marriage.

Consistent with the three-stage model for working with affair couples articulated by Gordon et al. (2000), initial sessions focused on helping the couple acknowledge and contain the negative impact of Rick's affair. Emotional stabilization occurred more rapidly than usual, in part because the affair had been short-lived and was ended 6 months earlier by Rick on his own, and in part because of Rick's and Anne's strong emotional attachments to each other.

Subsequent interventions emphasized developing a comprehensive formulation for how Rick's affair came about. Rick acknowledged that his unhappiness with the emotional volatility in their marriage was a major influence in his susceptibility to an affair and was the primary factor behind his considering divorce despite his strong feelings for Anne. To her credit, Anne worked very hard in her individual therapy to assume greater responsibility for regulating her own emotions when she felt anxious in the marriage or hurt by Rick. As suggested by her score on the FAM scale, much of Anne's emotional volatility around

MSI-R Profile Form

Douglas K. Snyder, Ph.D.

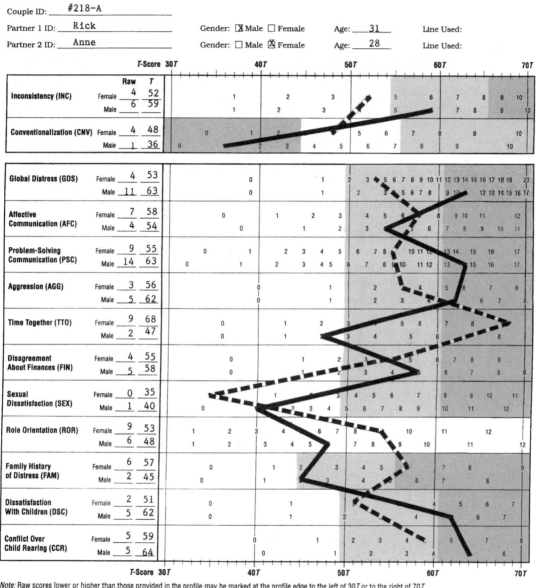

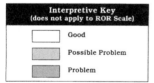

FIGURE 10.4. Couple profiles on the Marital Satisfaction Inventory—Revised (MSI-R) at initial assessment. MSI-R form from Snyder (1997). Copyright 1997 by Western Psychological Services. Reprinted by permission.

the couple's disagreements resulted from a panic rooted in early family experiences of inse-curity and intense conflicts in which parents regularly threatened divorce or emotional withdrawal when displeased with each other or with one of the children. Rick's view of Anne's emotionality softened as he came to appreciate more fully its development sources. Over the months as Anne demonstrated both her commitment and greater ability in regulat-ing her affect, Rick began to trust their conflict discussions more and showed greater re-silience on his own to remain engaged with Anne during these times, even when their dis-cussions became emotionally more intense and uncomfortable. He also worked to take responsibility for his decision to have the affair and to acknowledge its hurtfulness to Anne and its unfairness as his response to his own unhappiness.

The couple's disparity on the TTO scale prompted more detailed exploration of the dy-namics governing their demand $\rightarrow$ withdrawal patterns of interaction. Rick's frequent ab-sences from home and his retreat from Anne when he *was* home exacerbated her fears of being emotionally unimportant to him. The more she sought emotional and behavioral inti-macy, the more he withdrew. Early interventions in the therapy emphasized depolarization in this domain; this helped Anne tolerate some separation and develop social supports of her own outside the marriage, while it encouraged Rick to assume greater responsibility for engaging Anne and planning leisure activities for the two of them.

As the couple's relationship improved, they began to work somewhat more collabora-tively in their parenting of Becky. Because of her own chaotic family history and memories of having felt abandoned emotionally by her parents, Anne tended to be somewhat overly protective of Becky and to undermine Rick's efforts at discipline. As Anne worked to reduce her exaggerated protectiveness, Rick began to examine the rigidity and emotional coldness that characterized his own family. He also began to explore the expectations he had for himself from a somewhat traditional role orientation (ROR scale) and how these attitudes drove him to have unrealistic expectations for Becky's behavior as well. Both partners bene-fited from psychoeducational interventions that emphasized normal child development and more effective parenting techniques.

Over a period of 6 months, the couple came to a better understanding of factors in their marriage, stressors outside their marriage, and aspects of their own individual dynam-ics that contributed to Rick's affair and both partners' marital unhappiness. They made considerable progress in addressing these concerns, and they reached the point where both partners felt ready to "move on" emotionally and experienced confidence in their ability to confront future relationship challenges more effectively.

ASSESSING COUPLES IN MANAGED CARE AND PRIMARY CARE SETTINGS

Screening for Relationship Distress

Not all couples who experience significant relationship distress present themselves as re-questing couple therapy. For example, in primary care settings they may initially present with other emotional or behavioral complaints, including depression, anxiety, and sub-stance abuse. They may first be seen by family practitioners or internists for such somatic complaints as fatigue, chronic headaches, or sleep disturbance. Emergency room personnel may confront persons with severe relationship distress that culminates in physical violence and injuries.

How should medical personnel screen for relationship distress as a contributing or ex-acerbating factor in patients' presenting complaints? In consulting with physicians in a large general hospital and outpatient clinic and helping them screen for relationship distress in order to make appropriate referrals to individual or group couple therapy, we recommend asking patients the following questions:

- On a scale from 1 to 10 (1, very unhappy, to 10, very happy), how happy are you in your relationship?
- Do you and your partner have difficulty communicating?
- Do your arguments ever lead to pushing, slapping, or hitting?
- Do relationship problems contribute to you or your partner feeling depressed, anxious, or lonely? having more difficulty in dealing with your children? feeling less able to deal with such stresses as work, financial difficulties, or health problems? drinking alcohol or using other drugs more than you should?

If the patient rates the relationship from 8 to 10, he or she is unlikely to need couple therapy; however, there still might be benefit from a relationship enhancement program that is designed to make the relationship stronger or more resilient to future stressors. If the patient rates the relationship from 5 to 7, reports significant communication difficulties, or frequently feels depressed, anxious, or lonely in the relationship, the patient and his or her partner may benefit from a relationship enhancement program that teaches more positive ways to interact, understand, and communicate with each other. Finally, if the patient rates the relationship from 1 to 4, if arguments sometimes lead to physical aggression, or if relationship problems affect other areas of the couple's lives, the patient and his or her partner could likely benefit from more focused work with a couples therapist.

A growing number of primary care settings are implementing initial screening surveys that incorporate emotional and behavioral concerns, as well as physical symptoms or complaints, to guide initial assessment, referral, and treatment decisions. We advocate adopting one of the brief relationship satisfaction measures described earlier (e.g., the three-item Kansas Marital Satisfaction Scale, KMSS) as an initial screening device and, for individuals indicating moderate to high levels of global relationship distress, recommending consultation with a mental health professional and following up with a multidimensional self-report measure (e.g., the Marital Satisfaction Inventory—Revised, MSI-R) to differentiate among levels and sources of distress. Independent of the recommendation for further mental health consultation, all medical and allied personnel should be trained to inquire with relationally distressed patients about verbal and physical aggression.

Differential Assessment

As noted earlier in this chapter, previous research has documented the linkage of marital dissatisfaction with the onset, course, and treatment of adult psychiatric disorders (Halford & Bouma, 1997). Because of this, it is important to screen for relationship distress with individuals who present with Axis I or Axis II disorders, as well as to screen for emotional and behavioral concerns among individuals who present primarily with relationship distress. For the former, a standardized brief measure such as the three-item KMSS may be sufficient, or a verbal inquiry that adopts the format we have outlined for physicians described here may suffice. Screening for emotional or behavioral concerns among individuals who present for couple therapy is a more hazardous enterprise. People often enter couple therapy poised to ascribe relationship problems to their partner's personality flaws or presumed psychopathology; consequently, administering measures of personality or psychopathology often heightens defensiveness or promotes toxic attributions. Among standardized measures of emotional and behavioral difficulties, the Symptom Checklist-90—Revised (SCL-90; Derogatis, Meyer, & Gallant, 1977; Derogatis & Savitz, 1999) is perhaps one of the least threatening due to the face validity of its items (e.g., "trouble remembering things" or "feeling hopeless about the future"), each of which is rated on a 5-point scale.

It's important to note that the presence of individual disorders doesn't argue against couple therapy as either a primary or an adjunctive treatment. Couple-based interventions have been shown to be effective for a variety of adult individual disorders, including depression, agoraphobia, obsessive–compulsive disorders, sexual dysfunctions, and alcohol and other substance abuse (Baucom et al., 1998; Christensen & Heavey, 1999).

A couple's own distress both influences, and is influenced by, emotional or behavioral difficulties in their children. In deliberating whether to pursue couple therapy instead of (or in addition to) parent-training or family therapy, a brief screening measure of potential concerns about one or more children can be invaluable. A review of assessment strategies for evaluating emotional and behavioral difficulties in children and adolescents lies outside the scope of this chapter; however, many *couple* measures include one or more items that target concerns about child rearing or children's emotional well-being. For example, the Dissatisfaction with Children (DSC) scale of the MSI-R has been found to relate to a broad range of internalizing and externalizing difficulties indicated on a widely used measure of child and adolescent psychosocial functioning (Snyder, Klein, Gdowski, Faulstich, & LaCombe, 1988).

ADDITIONAL CONSIDERATIONS

Choosing among Assessment Strategies

How should the practitioner choose among the diverse strategies that are available for assessing couples? Criteria noted elsewhere (Jacobson & Margolin, 1979; L'Abate, 1994; Newman, Ciarlo, & Carpenter, 1999; Snyder et al., 1995; Stuart, 1980) for guiding assessment decisions include the following:

• Assessment should be multidimensional and broad-based—extending across multiple domains and addressing individual, dyadic, and family system concerns.

• At the same time, assessment should be parsimonious. This objective can be facilitated by choosing evaluation strategies and modalities that complement each other and by following a sequential approach that uses increasingly narrow-band measures to target problem areas that have been identified by other assessment techniques. We agree with L'Abate and Bagarrozi (1993) that the clinical interview remains the cornerstone of couple assessment. A broadly conceived, semistructured interview allows the practitioner to survey a wide range of potential issues while retaining the flexibility to explore specific concerns of the couple in a more detailed manner. Concurrent with the interview, the clinician should note specific aspects of the couple's communication patterns using guidelines proposed by Heyman (2001) described earlier. The clinical interview and informal observation of couples' communication should be followed by a self-report strategy that adopts a multidimensional measure (e.g., MSI-R; Snyder, 1997) or set of measures (e.g., Gottman, 1999) that differentiate among levels and sources of relationship distress. Areas of individual or relational distress revealed by these approaches can then be assessed further by using structured observations or narrow-band self-report techniques with clear evidence of reliability, validity, and clinical utility.

• Assessment should be linked to theory and an explicit intervention model. Given the diversity of couples' presenting complaints and the multiple factors that contribute to these difficulties, we advocate the pluralistic, hierarchical model presented earlier for organizing interventions in a manner that sequentially addresses the collaborative alliance, initial crises, strengthening of the relationship through systemic and behavioral techniques, teaching specific relationship skills, challenging cognitive components of distress, and exploring developmental sources of dysfunctional relationship patterns.

• Assessment should be therapeutic. This objective is best pursued by including the couple from the outset in the formulation of issues to be addressed and in a discussion of initial assessment findings (Finn & Tonsager, 1977) and by interweaving assessment and interventions throughout the treatment process.

Documenting Therapeutic Change

Among the reasons to engage in empirically grounded couple assessment, L'Abate and Bagarozzi (1993) note the following objectives: to establish a baseline from which to assess therapeutic progress or lack thereof, to identify issues or interaction patterns not otherwise discernable to the therapist, to plan appropriate treatment, and to document the changes that accompany clinical interventions. Clinical practice in a managed care environment demands objective evidence of treatment outcomes. Reliable and valid measures of relationship satisfaction and targeted domains reflecting couples' presenting concerns are essential to documenting therapeutic change.

Couple assessment is qualitatively distinct from assessment of individuals, in that presenting complaints emphasize *relationship* rather than individual components. Unlike individual therapists, couple therapists have a unique opportunity to observe directly the interpersonal exchanges of both individuals and to contrast these patterns of interaction with partners' subjective appraisals of their relationship difficulties. Couple therapists and researchers face a vast array of measurement techniques that are intended to assess relevant behaviors, cognitions, affect, and patterns of interaction relevant to couples' concerns. A constructive assessment strategy is one guided by well-formulated conceptual models of assessment and treatment, use of assessment techniques with demonstrated psychometric adequacy and clinical utility, and an explicit case formulation that links assessment findings to clinical intervention.

REFERENCES

American Psychiatric Association. (1994). *Diagnostic and statistical manual of mental disorders* (4th ed.). Washington, DC: Author.
Baucom, D. H., & Epstein, N. (1990). *Cognitive-behavioral marital therapy.* New York: Brunner/Mazel.
Baucom, D. H., Epstein, N., Rankin, L. A., & Burnett, C. K. (1996). Assessing relationship standards: The Inventory of Specific Relationship Standards. *Journal of Family Psychology, 10,* 72–88.
Baucom, D. H., Epstein, N., Sayers, S., & Sher, T. G. (1989). The role of cognitions in marital relationships: Definitional, methodological, and conceptual issues. *Journal of Consulting and Clinical Psychology, 57,* 31–38.
Baucom, D. H., Sayers, S. L., & Duhe, A. (1989). Attributional style and attributional patterns among married couples. *Journal of Personality and Social Psychology, 56,* 596–607.
Baucom, D. H., Shoham, V., Mueser, K. T., Daiuto, A. D., & Stickle, T. R. (1998). Empirically supported couple and family interventions for marital distress and adult mental health problems. *Journal of Consulting and Clinical Psychology, 66,* 53–88.
Birchler, G. R., Weiss, R. L., & Vincent, J. P. (1975). Multimethod analysis of social reinforcement exchange between maritally distressed and nondistressed spouse and stranger dyads. *Journal of Personality and Social Psychology, 31,* 349–360.

Bonjean, C. M., Hill, R. J., & McLemore, S. D. (1967). *Sociological measurement: An inventory of scales and indices.* San Francisco: Chandler.

Boughner, S. R., Hayes, S. F., Bubenzer, D. L., & West, J. D. (1994). Use of standardized assessment instruments by marital and family therapists: A survey. *Journal of Marital and Family Therapy, 20,* 69–75.

Burman, B., & Margolin, G. (1992). Analysis of the association between marital relationships and health problems: An interactional perspective. *Psychological Bulletin, 112,* 39–63.

Burns, D. D., & Sayers, S. L. (1992). *Development and validation of a brief relationship satisfaction scale.* Unpublished manuscript.

Christensen, A. (1987). Detection of conflict patterns in couples. In K. Hahlweg & M. J. Goldstein (Eds.), *Understanding major mental disorder: The contribution of family interaction research* (pp. 250–265). New York: Family Process Press.

Christensen, A., & Heavey, C. L. (1999). Interventions for couples. *Annual Review of Psychology, 50,* 165–190.

Chun, K., Cobb, S., & French, J. R. P. (1975). *Measures for psychological assessment: A guide to 3,000 original sources and their applications.* Ann Arbor: University of Michigan, Survey Research Center of the Institute for Social Research.

Cookerly, J. R. (1980). Does marital therapy do any lasting good? *Journal of Marital and Family Therapy, 6,* 393–397.

Corcoran, K., & Fischer, J. (2000). *Measures for clinical practice: A sourcebook.* Vol. 1. *Couples, families, and children.* New York: Free Press.

Davis, C. M., Yarber, W. L., Bauserman, R., Schreer, G., & Davis, S. L. (1998). *Handbook of sexuality-related measures.* Thousand Oaks, CA: Sage.

Derogatis, L. R., Lopez, M. C., & Zinzeletta, E. M. (1988). Clinical applications of the DSFI in the assessment of sexual dysfunctions. In R. A. Brown & J. R. Field (Eds.), *Treatment of sexual problems in individual and couples therapy* (pp. 167–186). Costa Mesa, CA: PMA.

Derogatis, L. R., & Melisaratos, N. (1979). The DSFI: A multidimensional measure of sexual functioning. *Journal of Sex and Marital Therapy, 5,* 244–281.

Derogatis, L. R., Meyer, J. K., & Gallant, B. W. (1977). Distinctions between male and female invested partners in sexual disorders. *American Journal of Psychiatry, 134,* 385–390.

Derogatis, L. R., & Savitz, K. L. (1999). The SCL–90–R, Brief Symptom Inventory, and matching clinical rating scales. In M. E. Maruish (Ed.), *The use of psychological testing for treatment planning and outcomes assessment* (2nd ed., pp. 679–724). Mahway, NJ: Erlbaum.

Eidelson, R. J., & Epstein, N. (1982). Cognitive and relationship maladjustment: Development of a measure of dysfunctional relationship beliefs. *Journal of Consulting and Clinical Psychology, 50,* 715–720.

Epstein, N., & Baucom, D. H. (in press). *Treating couples in context: Innovations in cognitive-behavioral therapy.* Washington, DC: American Psychological Association.

Fincham, F. D., & Bradbury, T. N. (1992). Assessing attributions in marriage: The Relationship Attribution Measure. *Journal of Personality and Social Psychology, 62,* 457–468.

Finn, S. E., & Tonsager, M. E. (1997). Information-gathering and therapeutic models of assessment: Complementary paradigms. *Psychological Assessment, 9,* 374–385.

Fowers, B., & Olson, D. (1989). ENRICH marital inventory: A discriminant validity study. *Journal of Marital and Family Therapy, 15,* 65–79.

Fowers, B., & Olson, D. (1992). Four types of premarital couples: An empirical typology based on PREPARE. *Journal of Family Psychology, 6,* 10–12.

Fraenkel, P. (1997). Systems approaches to couple therapy. In W. K. Halford & H. J. Markman (Eds.), *Clinical handbook of marriage and couples interventions* (pp. 379–413). New York: Wiley.

Fredman, N., & Sherman, R. (1987). *Handbook of measurements for marriage and family therapy.* New York: Brunner/Mazel.

Friedman, H. S., Tucker, J. S., Schwartz, J. E., & Tomilson, K. C. (1995). Psychosocial and behavioral predictors of longevity: The aging and death of the "Termites." *American Psychologist, 50,* 69–78.

Gaskill, S. P., Williams, K., Stern, M. P., & Hazuda, H. P. (June, 2000). *Marital distress predicts the incidence of Type 2 diabetes in Mexican Americans and non-Hispanic whites.* Paper presented at the meeting of the American Diabetes Association, San Antonio, Texas.

Geiss, S. K., & O'Leary, D. (1981). Therapist ratings of frequency and severity of marital problems: Implications for research. *Journal of Marital and Family Therapy, 7,* 515–520.

Gordon, K. C., Baucom, D. H., & Snyder, D. K. (2000). The use of forgiveness in marital therapy. In M. E. McCullough, K. I. Pargament, & C. E. Thoresen (Eds.), *Forgiveness: Theory, research, and practice* (pp. 203–227). New York: Guilford Press.

Gottman, J. M. (1979). *Marital interaction: Experimental investigations.* New York: Academic Press.

Gottman, J. M. (1993). The roles of conflict engagement, escalation, and avoidance in marital interaction: A longitudinal view of five types of couples. *Journal of Consulting and Clinical Psychology, 61,* 6–15.

Gottman, J. M. (1999). *The marriage clinic: A scientifically based marital therapy.* New York: Norton.

Gottman, J. M., & Krokoff, L. J. (1989). Marital interaction and satisfaction: A longitudinal view. *Journal of Consulting and Clinical Psychology, 57,* 47–52.

Grotevant, H. D., & Carlson, C. I. (1989). *Family assessment: A guide to methods and measures.* New York: Guilford Press.

Halford, W. K., & Bouma, R. (1997). Individual psychopathology and marital distress. In W. K. Halford & H. J. Markman (Eds.), *Clinical handbook of marriage and couples interventions* (pp. 291–321). New York: Wiley.

Haynes, S. N. (2001). Clinical applications of analogue behavioral observation: Dimensions of psychometric evaluation. *Psychological Assessment, 13,* 73–85.

Heffer, R. W., & Snyder, D. K. (1998). Comprehensive assessment of family functioning. In L. L'Abate (Ed.), *Handbook of family psychopathology: The relational roots of dysfunctional behavior* (pp. 207–233). New York: Guilford Press.

Heim, S. C., & Snyder, D. K. (1991). Predicting depression from marital distress and attributional processes. *Journal of Marital and Family Therapy, 17,* 67–72.

Heyman, R. E. (2001). Observation of couple conflicts: Clinical assessment applications, stubborn truths, and shaky foundations. *Psychological Assessment, 13,* 5–35.

Heyman, R. E., Eddy, J. M., Weiss, R. L., & Vivian, D. (1995). Factor analysis of the Marital Interaction Coding System. *Journal of Family Psychology, 9,* 209–215.

Heyman, R. E., Vivian, D., Weiss, R. L., Hubbard, K., & Ayerle, C. H. (1993, November). *Coding marital interaction at three levels of abstraction.* Paper presented at the meeting of the Association for Advancement of Behavior Therapy, Atlanta, Georgia.

Heyman, R. E., Weiss, R. L., & Eddy, J. M. (1995). Marital Interaction Coding System: Revision and empirical evaluation. *Behaviour Research and Therapy, 33,* 737–746.

Hops, H., Wills, T. A., Patterson, G. R., & Weiss, R. L. (1972). *Marital interaction coding system.* Eugene: University of Oregon and Oregon Research Institute.

Jacob, T., & Tennenbaum, D. L. (1988). *Family assessment: Rationale, methods, and future directions.* New York: Plenum.

Jacobson, N. S., & Christensen, A. (1996). *Integrative couple therapy: Promoting acceptance and change.* New York: Norton.

Jacobson, N. S., Christensen, A., Prince, S. E., Cordova, J., & Eldridge, K. (2000). Integrative behavioral couple therapy: An acceptance-based, promising new treatment for couple discord. *Journal of Consulting and Clinical Psychology, 68,* 351–355.

Jacobson, N. S., & Margolin, G. (1979). *Marital therapy: Strategies based on social learning and behavior exchange principles.* New York: Brunner/Mazel.

Jacobson, N. S., Schmaling, K. B., & Holtzworth-Munroe, A. (1987). Component analysis of behavioral marital therapy: 2-year follow-up and prediction of relapse. *Journal of Marital and Family Therapy, 13,* 187–195.

Johnson, S. M., & Whiffen, V. E. (2000). Made to measure: Adapting emotionally focused couple therapy to partners' attachment styles. *Clinical Psychology: Science and Practice, 6,* 366–381.

Karpel, M. A. (1994). *Evaluating couples: A handbook for practitioners.* New York: Norton.

Kiecolt-Glaser, J. K., Malarkey, W. B., Cacioppo, J., & Glaser, R. (1994). Stressful personal relationships: Immune and endocrine function. In R. Glaser & J. K. Kiecolt-Glaser (Eds.), *Human stress and immunity* (pp. 321–339). San Diego: Academic Press.

L'Abate, L. (1994). *Family evaluation: A psychological approach*. Thousand Oaks, CA: Sage.

L'Abate, L., & Bagarozzi, D. A. (1993). *Sourcebook of marriage and family evaluation*. New York: Brunner/Mazel.

Laumann, E. O., Gagnon, J. H., Michael, R. T., & Michaels, S. (1994). *The social organization of sexuality*. Chicago: University of Chicago Press.

Lederer, W., & Jackson, D. D. (1968). *The mirages of marriage*. New York: Norton.

Locke, H. J., & Wallace, K. M. (1959). Short marital adjustment and prediction tests: Their reliability and validity. *Marriage and Family Living, 21*, 251–255.

LoPiccolo, J., & Steger, J. C. (1974). The Sexual Interaction Inventory: A new instrument for assessment of sexual dysfunction. *Archives of Sexual Behavior, 3*, 585–595.

Martin, T. C., & Bumpass, L. (1989). Recent trends in marital disruption. *Demography, 26*, 37–51.

McConaghy, N. (1998). Assessment of sexual dysfunction and deviation. In A. S. Bellack & M. Hersen (eds.), *Behavioral assessment: A practical handbook* (4th. ed., pp. 315–341). Boston: Allyn & Bacon.

McGoldrick, M., & Gerson, R. (1985). *Genograms in family assessment*. New York: Norton.

McGoldrick, M., Gerson, R., & Shellenberger, S. (1999). *Genograms: Assessment and intervention*. (2nd ed.). New York: Norton.

Metz, M. E. (1993). *Manual for the Styles of Conflict Inventory*. Palo Alto: Consulting Psychologists Press.

Newman, F. L., Ciarlo, J. A., & Carpenter, D. (1999). Guidelines for selecting psychological instruments for treatment planning and outcome assessment. In M. E. Maruish (Ed.), *The use of psychological testing for treatment planning and outcomes assessment* (2nd. ed., pp. 153–170). Mahway, NJ: Erlbaum.

Norton, R. (1983). Measuring marital quality: A critical look at the dependent variable. *Journal of Marriage and the Family, 45*, 141–151.

Orthner, D. K. (1975). Leisure activity patterns and marital satisfaction over the marital career. *Journal of Marriage and the Family, 37*, 91–102.

Pretzer, J. L., Epstein, N., & Fleming, B. (1992). The Marital Attitude Survey: A measure of dysfunctional attitudes and expectancies. *Journal of Cognitive Psychotherapy, 5*, 131–148.

Sayers, S. L., Baucom, D. H., Sher, T. G., Weiss, R. L., & Heyman, R. E. (1991). Constructive engagement, behavioral marital therapy, and changes in marital satisfaction. *Behavioral Assessment, 13*, 25–49.

Sayers, S. L., & Sarwer, D. B. (1998). Assessment of marital dysfunction. In A. S. Bellack & M. Hersen (eds.), *Behavioral assessment: A practical handbook* (4th. ed., pp. 293–314). Boston: Allyn & Bacon.

Schumm, W. R., Paff-Bergen, L. A., Hatch, R. C., Obiorah, F. C., Copeland, J. M., Meens, L. D., & Bugaighis, M. A. (1986). Concurrent and discriminant validity of the Kansas Marital Satisfaction Scale. *Journal of Marriage and the Family, 48*, 381–387.

Shadish, W. R., Montgomery, L. M., Wilson, P., Wilson, M. R., Bright, I., & Okwumabua, T. (1993). Effects of family and marital psychotherapies: A meta-analysis. *Journal of Consulting and Clinical Psychology, 61*, 992–1002.

Smith, G. T., Snyder, D. K., Trull, T. J., & Monsma, B. (1988). Predicting relationship satisfaction from couples' use of leisure time. *American Journal of Family Therapy, 16*, 3–13.

Snyder, D. K. (1997). *Manual for the Marital Satisfaction Inventory—Revised*. Los Angeles: Western Psychological Services.

Snyder, D. K. (1999). Pragmatic couple therapy: An informed pluralistic approach. In D. M. Lawson & F. F. Prevatt (Eds.), *Casebook in family therapy* (pp. 81–110). Pacific Grove, CA: Brooks/Cole.

Snyder, D. K. (2000). Affective reconstruction in the context of a pluralistic approach to couple therapy. *Clinical Psychology: Science and Practice, 6*, 348–365.

Snyder, D. K., & Aikman, G. G. (1999). The Marital Satisfaction Inventory—Revised. In M. E. Maruish (Ed.), *Use of psychological testing for treatment planning and outcomes assessment* (2nd ed., pp. 1173–1210) Mahwah, NJ: Erlbaum.

Snyder, D. K., Cavell, T. A., Heffer, R. W., & Mangrum, L. F. (1995). Marital and family assessment: A multifaceted, multilevel approach. In R. H. Mikesell, D. D. Lusterman, & S. H. McDaniel (Eds.), *Integrating family therapy: Handbook of family psychology and systems theory* (pp. 163–182). Washington, DC: American Psychological Association.

Snyder, D. K., Cozzi, J. J., Grich, J., & Luebbert, M. C. (2001). The tapestry of couple therapy: Interweaving theory, assessment, and intervention. In S. H. McDaniel, D. D. Lusterman, & C. L. Philpot (Eds.), *Casebook for integrating family therapy* (pp. 33–42). Washington, DC: American Psychological Association.

Snyder, D. K., Cozzi, J. J., & Mangrum, L. F. (in press). Conceptual issues in assessing couples and families. In H. A. Liddle, D. Santisteban, J. H. Bray, & R. F. Levant (Eds.), *Family psychology: Science based interventions*. Washington, DC: American Psychological Association.

Snyder, D. K., Klein, M. A., Gdowski, C. L., Faulstich, C., & LaCombe, J. (1988). Generalized dysfunction in clinic and nonclinic families: A comparative analysis. *Journal of Abnormal Child Psychology, 16,* 97–109.

Snyder, D. K., Mangrum, L. F., & Wills, R. M. (1993). Predicting couples' response to marital therapy: A comparison of short- and long-term predictors. *Journal of Consulting and Clinical Psychology, 61,* 61–69.

Snyder, D. K., & Rice, J. L. (1996). Methodological issues and strategies in scale development. In D. H. Sprenkle & S. M. Moon (Eds.), *Research methods in family therapy* (pp. 216–237). New York: Guilford Press.

Snyder, D. K., Wills, R. M., & Grady-Fletcher, A. (1991). Long-term effectiveness of behavioral versus insight-oriented marital therapy: A four-year follow-up study. *Journal of Consulting and Clinical Psychology, 59,* 138–141.

Spanier, G. B. (1976). Measuring dyadic adjustment: New scales for assessing the quality of marriage and similar dyads. *Journal of Marriage and the Family, 38,* 15–28.

Straus, M. A. (1969). *Family measurement techniques.* Minneapolis: University of Minnesota Press.

Straus, M. A. (1979). Measuring intrafamily conflict and violence: The Conflict Tactics (CT) Scales. *Journal of Marriage and the Family, 41,* 75–88.

Straus, M. A., Hamby, S. L., Boney-McCoy, S., & Sugarman, D. B. (1996). The revised Conflict Tactics Scales (CTS2): Development and preliminary psychometric data. *Journal of Family Issues, 17,* 283–316.

Stuart, R. B. (1980). *Helping couples change: A social learning approach to marital therapy.* New York: Guilford Press.

Swindle, R., Heller, K., Pescosolido, B., & Kikuzawa, S. (2000). Responses to nervous breakdowns in America over a 40-year period: Mental health policy implications. *American Psychologist, 55,* 740–749.

Terman, L. M. (1938). *Psychological factors in marital happiness.* New York: McGraw-Hill.

Touliatos, J., Perlmutter, B. F., & Straus, M. A. (Eds.). (1990). *Handbook of family measurement techniques.* Newbury Park, CA: Sage.

Veroff, J., Kulka, R. A., & Douvan, E. (1981). *Mental health in America: Patterns of help seeking from 1957 to 1976.* New York: Basic Books.

Wallerstein, J. S., Lewis, J., & Blakeslee, S. (2000). *The unexpected legacy of divorce: A 25 year landmark study.* New York: Hyperion.

Weiss, R. L. (1992). *The Marital Interaction Coding System—Version IV.* Eugene: Oregon Marital Studies Program.

Weiss, R. L., & Birchler, G. R. (1975). *Areas of change questionnaire.* Unpublished manuscript, University of Oregon.

Weiss, R. L., & Heyman, R. E. (1997). A clinical-research overview of couples interactions. In W. K. Halford & H. J. Markman (Eds.), *Clinical handbook of marriage and couples interventions* (pp. 13–41). New York: Wiley.

Weiss, R. L., Hops, H., & Patterson, G. R. (1973). A framework for conceptualizing marital conflict, a technology for altering it, some data for evaluating it. In F. W. Clark & L. A. Hamerlynck (Eds.), *Critical issues in research and practice: Proceedings of the Fourth Banff International Conference on Behavior Modification* (pp. 309–342). Champaign, IL: Research Press.

Weiss, R. L., & Tolman, A. O. (1990). The Marital Interaction Coding System—Global (MICS-G): A global companion to the MICS. *Behavioral Assessment, 12,* 271–294.

Whisman, M. A. (1999). Marital dissatisfaction and psychiatric disorders: Results from the National Comorbidity Survey. *Journal of Abnormal Psychology, 108,* 701–706.

Whisman, M. A., & Jacobson, N. S. (1992). Change in marital adjustment following marital therapy: A comparison between two outcome measures. *Psychological Assessment, 4,* 219–223.

Whisman, M. A., & Snyder, D. K. (1997). Evaluating and improving the efficacy of conjoint couple therapy. In W. K. Halford & H. J. Markman (Eds.), *Clinical handbook of marriage and couples interventions* (pp. 679–693). New York: Wiley.

11

Schizophrenia

Sarah I. Pratt
Kim T. Mueser

Schizophrenia is a complex psychiatric disorder that has an influence, either directly or indirectly, on practically every area of functioning, ranging from psychological well-being to social adaptation to health and self-sufficiency. The assessment of the disorder, therefore, is necessarily broad-based, as is treatment planning. In order to understand the wide scope of assessment and treatment planning for schizophrenia, it is crucial to review the core psychopathology that defines the illness, along with the common associated features, including comorbid disorders, which complicate the clinical picture.

We begin this chapter with an overview of schizophrenia, emphasizing the clinical signs and symptoms of the syndrome and the characteristic impairments. We also discuss common associated problems present with schizophrenia, which for some patients dominate many of their treatment needs. We then discuss the epidemiology and course of the disorder. We next provide an overall conceptualization of the principles of assessment for schizophrenia, followed by a review of specific assessment procedures, including the use of standardized instruments. Then, we address the process of treatment planning, which naturally flows from the assessment process, and briefly review the evidence in support of specific interventions. We conclude with a brief consideration of remaining questions and future directions for the assessment and treatment planning for persons with schizophrenia.

OVERVIEW OF SCHIZOPHRENIA

The diagnostic criteria for schizophrenia have changed only slightly over the past two decades according to the two major classification systems, the *Diagnostic and Statistical Manual of Mental Disorders* (DSM; American Psychiatric Association, 1994) and the *International Classification of Diseases* (ICD; World Health Organization, 1992) series. Essentially, both the DSM and ICD series specify that the diagnosis of schizophrenia is based on the presence of specific symptoms, the absence of other symptoms, and psychosocial impairments that persist over a significant period of time. Symptoms and impairments must be present in the absence of medical or other organic conditions (e.g., substance abuse) that could lead to similar problems.

Symptoms of Schizophrenia

There is widespread agreement that the core symptoms of schizophrenia can be divided into three broad types: positive symptoms, negative symptoms, and cognitive impairment (Liddle, 1987). Positive symptoms refer to sensory experiences, thoughts, and behaviors that are present in patients but are ordinarily absent in individuals without a psychiatric illness. The most common types of positive symptoms in schizophrenia include hallucinations (hearing, seeing, feeling, tasting, or smelling sensations in the absence of environmental stimuli), delusions (false or patently absurd beliefs that are not shared by others in the person's environment), and bizarre behavior (strange or apparently purposeless behavior). For many patients, positive symptoms fluctuate in their intensity over time and are episodic in nature, at times requiring temporary hospitalization if they pose a significant threat to the safety of the patient or others. A substantial minority of patients (30% to 40%) experience chronic positive symptoms that are the cause of significant distress (Curson, Patel, Liddle, & Barnes, 1988).

Negative symptoms are defined by the absence or diminution of behaviors and emotions that are ordinarily present in persons without psychiatric disorders. Common examples of negative symptoms include blunted affect (diminished expressiveness of facial expression or voice tone), anhedonia (loss of pleasure), apathy (loss of initiative or ability to follow through on plans), social withdrawal, and alogia (diminished amount or content of speech). All of these negative symptoms are relatively common in schizophrenia, and they tend to be stable over time (Mueser, Bellack, Douglas, & Wade, 1991). Furthermore, negative symptoms have a pervasive impact on the ability of patients to function socially and to sustain independent living (Pogue-Geile, 1989).

Cognitive symptoms refer to impairments in the ability to attend to, process, and retrieve information. Deficits in cognitive functioning in schizophrenia run the gamut from the early stages of information processing (including attention and concentration) to encoding and storage (including speed of information processing and memory) to the more complex, higher cognitive skills or executive functions (including abstraction, planning, and problem solving). While there is evidence that cognitive impairment is common across the range of tests of neuropsychological functions, patients with schizophrenia perform especially poorly on measures that involve social stimuli (i.e., social cognition), which may contribute to their problems in social functioning (Penn, Corrigan, & Racenstein, 1998). Like negative symptoms, cognitive impairment tends to be stable over time.

While positive symptoms, negative symptoms, and cognitive impairment are most characteristic of schizophrenia, factor-analytic studies of symptomatology have also consistently identified affective symptoms (Mueser, Curran, & McHugo, 1997). Common mood problems experienced by patients include depression, anxiety, and anger or hostility. The problem of depression is especially vexing as suicide attempts are common in schizophrenia, and approximately 10% of patients die from suicide (Roy, 1986). Anxiety in schizophrenia has only recently received attention, but evidence suggests that it is both common and debilitating.

Characteristic Impairments

In addition to requiring the presence of specific symptoms, modern diagnostic systems also require evidence of sustained functional impairment (e.g., over 6 months for DSM-IV) for the diagnosis of schizophrenia. Common difficulties in psychosocial functioning include problems fulfilling the roles of a worker, student, or homemaker; poor social relationships and inadequately developed leisure and recreational activities; and inability to care for one-self (e.g., impaired grooming, hygiene, ability to cook, clean, do laundry, attend to health care needs).

Although a large majority of individuals with schizophrenia indicate that competitive employment is a primary goal, a small minority (less than 15%) are actually working at any given time (Cook & Razzano, 2000; Drake, McHugo, et al., 1999; Drake, McHugo, Becker, Anthony, & Clark, 1996). Compared with nonclinical populations, individuals with schizophrenia may be greater than four times as likely to be unemployed (Cook & Razzano, 2000). Consequently, many people with schizophrenia require supplemental income to meet their basic living needs, such as disabilities entitlements and financial support from families. The economic dependence of many patients on their relatives, combined with difficulties in independent living, leads to many patients living at home or maintaining high levels of contact and requiring extensive assistance from relatives to live separately. The social impairments pervasive in schizophrenia create significant dependence on others, which, combined with the unpredictable nature of positive symptoms, cognitive impairments, and mood problems, often leads to high levels of family burden for relatives (Hatfield & Lefley, 1987, 1993). This burden can lead to high levels of interpersonal stress and distress, which may need to be addressed in treatment (Leff & Vaughn, 1985).

Problems in functioning contribute to difficulties in several other areas. The poor financial standing of many patients may cause them to reside in impoverished living conditions—for example, in neighborhoods rife with substance abuse and crime—and to maintain poor dietary practices. Furthermore, poor motivation and other negative symptoms, together with poor insight, often negatively impact the ability to identify health problems and to obtain needed care in a timely fashion, which then results in premature physical deterioration and mortality. Thus, treatment for schizophrenia often requires substantial attention to the most common consequences of impaired functioning, such as unstable or unsafe housing, inadequate food and clothing (especially for homeless persons), and neglected health problems.

Common Comorbid Disorders

Two comorbid disorders are frequently present in schizophrenia: substance use disorders (i.e., alcohol or drug abuse or dependence) and posttraumatic stress disorder (PTSD). Each of these disorders may impact on, or interact with, schizophrenia, and therefore their assessment is important for treatment planning.

Extensive research over the past two decades has documented that the prevalence of substance use disorders is substantially higher in schizophrenia than it is in the general population (Cuffel, 1996; Regier et al., 1990). Estimates across numerous studies indicate that the lifetime prevalence of substance use disorders in patients with schizophrenia is about 50%, and that between 25% and 45% of patients have a current or recent (past 6 months) substance use disorder. Substance abuse in schizophrenia is associated with a wide range of negative consequences, including relapse and rehospitalizations, financial and legal problems, housing instability and homelessness, violence and victimization, higher service utilization costs, and family burden (Drake & Brunette, 1998). Furthermore, substance abuse in schizophrenia increases the chances of developing infectious diseases, including HIV, hepatitis B, and especially hepatitis C (Rosenberg et al., 2001). Many theories have been advanced to account for the high prevalence of substance abuse in patients with schizophrenia, including the hypothesis that patients "self-medicate" their symptoms with alcohol and drugs (Khantzian, 1997). While no single theory can explain all comorbidity, it appears that at least some excess rate is due to the fact that patients with schizophrenia are more sensitive to the effects of psychoactive substances, and therefore they develop substance use disorders as a result of abusing relatively moderate amounts of alcohol and drugs (Mueser, Drake, & Wallach, 1998).

There is growing recognition that, compared to persons in the general population, patients with schizophrenia are more prone to experiencing traumatic events, such as physical and sexual assault and witnessing violence (Goodman, Rosenberg, Mueser, & Drake, 1997). Furthermore, many patients are multiply traumatized throughout the course of their lives (Mueser, Goodman et al., 1998). Some individuals with schizophrenia may be especially vulnerable to victimization, such as homeless women (Goodman et al., 1997). In the general population, a common psychiatric consequence of exposure to traumatic events is the development of PTSD. Studies of PTSD in patients with schizophrenia and other severe psychiatric disorders indicate that, consistent with their high exposure to trauma, these people are also at increased risk for PTSD. The lifetime prevalence of PTSD in the general population is about 10%; in contrast, estimates of the current prevalence of PTSD in patients with severe mental illness range from 29% to 43% (Cascardi, Mueser, DeGirolomo, & Murrin, 1996; Craine, Henson, Colliver, & MacLean, 1988; Mueser, Goodman et al., 1998; Switzer et al., 1999). The clinical implications of PTSD are not well understood at this point. However, based on research showing that stress can worsen the course of schizophrenia (see the following section), it is hypothesized that the experience of chronic stress related to PTSD makes the course of schizophrenia worse (Mueser & Rosenberg, 2001). Successful treatment of PTSD in schizophrenia, therefore, may improve the outcome of the disorder.

Theoretical Framework Guiding Assessment and Treatment

The stress–vulnerability model provides a useful theoretical framework for assessment and intervention in schizophrenia (Liberman et al., 1986; Zubin & Spring, 1977). This model assumes that symptom severity and other characteristic impairments of schizophrenia have genetic and related biological bases (psychobiological vulnerability) that was determined early in life by a combination of genes and early environmental factors, such as the intrauterine hormonal environment and birth complications. The vulnerability, and hence symptom severity and functional impairment, can be decreased by medications and increased by stress and substance abuse. Stress, including discrete events such as traumas and exposure to ongoing conditions such as hostile, overly demanding, or unstructured environments, can impinge on vulnerability, thus precipitating relapses and contributing to impairments in other domains (e.g., social functioning). Finally, coping resources, such as coping skills (e.g., social skills) and the ability to obtain social support, can minimize the effects of stress on relapse and the need for acute care.

From the perspective of the stress–vulnerability model, the outcome of schizophrenia can be improved through interventions that target vulnerability, stress, and coping. Pharmacological interventions (antipsychotics) are effective at reducing biological vulnerability. However, adherence to medication is a common problem in patients with schizophrenia, and improving adherence is an important focus of intervention (Corrigan, Wallace, Schade, & Green, 1994). While medication can decrease vulnerability, substance abuse tends to make it worse, thus underscoring the importance of treating substance abuse (i.e., "dual diagnosis" patients) when it is present. Interventions for schizophrenia frequently focus on minimizing stress and maximizing the supportiveness of environments in which patients live.

Environments that are either overstimulating, such as a harsh and critical social environment, or that lack meaningful structure are most stressful. Broadly speaking, interventions may minimize stress in the environment through improved understanding of schizophrenia and better communication skills (as in family therapy) or engaging the patient in meaningful, but not overdemanding activities (such as work or school). Other sources of stress (e.g., exposure to traumatic events, impoverished living conditions) may also be the focus of intervention. Finally, patients can be taught skills to enhance their ability to deal with internal sources of stress (e.g., coping skills for anxiety, depression, persistent hallucinations), external sources of stress (e.g., social skills for managing interpersonal conflict), or to achieve personal goals (e.g., social skills, problem-solving skills).

EPIDEMIOLOGY

The lifetime prevalence of schizophrenia (including the closely related disorders of schizoaffective disorder and schizophreniform disorder) is approximately 1% (Keith, Regier, & Rae, 1991). In general, the prevalence of schizophrenia is remarkably stable across a wide range of different populations and does not discriminate on the basis of gender, race, or religion (Jablensky, 1999). However, schizophrenia is more common in urban areas of industrialized countries (Peen & Dekker, 1997; Takei, Sham, O'Callaghan, Glover, & Murray, 1995; Torrey, Bowler, & Clark, 1997).

As schizophrenia frequently has an onset during early adulthood, persons with the illness are less likely to marry or remain married, particularly males (Eaton, 1975; Munk-Jørgensen, 1987), and are less likely to complete higher levels of education (Kessler, Foster, Saunders, & Stang, 1995). An association between poverty and schizophrenia has long been present, with people belonging to lower socioeconomic classes more likely to develop the disorder (Hollingshead & Redlich, 1958; Salokangas, 1978). Historically, two theories have been advanced to account for this association. The social drift hypothesis postulates that the debilitating effects of schizophrenia on capacity to work result in a lowering of socioeconomic means, and hence poverty (Aro, Aro, & Keskimäki, 1995). The environmental stress hypothesis proposes that the high levels of stress associated with poverty precipitate schizophrenia in some individuals who would not otherwise develop the illness (Bruce, Takeuchi, & Leaf, 1991). Both of these explanations may be partly true, and longitudinal research on changes in socioeconomic class status and schizophrenia provide conflicting results. For example, Fox (1990) reanalyzed data from several longitudinal studies and found that after controlling for initial levels of socioeconomic class, downward drift was not evident. However, Dohrenwend et al. (1992) did find evidence for social drift, even after controlling for socioeconomic class.

ASSESSMENT

Given the heterogeneous nature of schizophrenia, there is no single "gold standard" treatment for the disorder and its characteristic impairments. Innovations in pharmacological and psychosocial interventions for schizophrenia have enabled mental health professionals to speak of "recovery" as an overarching goal for individuals with schizophrenia—recovery being increased positive functioning and support, decreased stress, rehabilitation of deficient functioning, and prevention of deterioration in quality of life by assuming full utilization of available resources (Anthony, 1993; Carling, 1995; Deegan, 1988). To achieve this, however, individuals with schizophrenia often require a broad range of services and therapies. Selection of the particular ingredients necessary to optimize the success of individual treatment programs depends on a thorough assessment of the nature of the illness, personal strengths and weaknesses, and environmental circumstances. Such an assessment is important to assist mental health professionals in tailoring treatment plans to meet the specific needs of individual clients.

Because the presentation of symptoms and associated problems varies considerably among individuals with schizophrenia, mental health care providers should undertake a careful assessment of the specific deficits and target areas of concern even after the diagnosis has been made. A comprehensive assessment intended for use in treatment planning should commence with evaluation of basic illness characteristics, followed by frequently associated features and then common comorbid diagnoses. Techniques for assessing these areas include semistructured clinical interviews with patients and close informants, behavioral tests, self-report questionnaires, standardized rating scales, cognitive measures, and medical procedures. The instruments and methods that will be presented here are empirically validated and have been used both in the laboratory and in treatment settings.

Core Clinical Symptoms

Traditionally, mental health professionals have overemphasized symptoms and symptom reduction in assessing and treating individuals with schizophrenia (Smith et al., 1999). We have identified several associated features and common comorbid psychiatric problems that should also be included as part of a comprehensive assessment before designing an individualized treatment plan. Nevertheless, examination of the nature and severity of the core symptoms of schizophrenia remains important.

Symptoms not only provide a basis for determining the type and dosage of medications needed but also may affect several important domains of functioning, such as work performance, success of interpersonal relationships, ability to participate in treatment of social skills deficits, and even basic life skills. This is particularly true of negative symptoms (e.g., Breier, Schreiber, Dyer, & Pickar, 1991; Eckman et al., 1992; Glynn, 1998; Herz, 1996; Mueser & Bellack, 1998). For example, individuals who suffer from substantial levels of apathy and anhedonia may not be able to motivate themselves to seek employment on their own, engage in psychosocial treatment, or even attend to their own personal care. Recent research has found that positive symptoms are less predictive of the various facets of adaptive functioning that tend to be impaired in individuals with schizophrenia (e.g., M. Green, 1996; Jonsson & Nyman, 1991; Mueser & Bellack, 1998; Penn, Mueser, Spaulding, Hope, & Reed, 1995; Smith et al., 1999; Tollefson, 1996). However, they certainly warrant an initial evaluation and periodic reassessment, given the evidence that they tend to be predictive of clinical outcome measures, such as relapse and rehospitalization (M. Green, 1996).

Positive and Negative Symptoms

Mental health professionals may use a variety of methods to assess positive and negative symptoms, including personal observation, interviews with collaterals, and standardized scales that are designed to measure either type of symptom or both. The most widely used instruments include the Brief Psychiatric Rating Scale (BPRS; Lukoff, Nuechterlein, & Ventura, 1986; Overall & Gorham, 1962), the Scale for the Assessment of Negative Symptoms (SANS; Andreasen, 1982), the Scale for the Assessment of Positive Symptoms (SAPS; Andreasen, 1984), and the Positive and Negative Syndrome Scale (PANSS; Kay, Fiszbein, & Opler, 1987), all of which are designed to be administered as semistructured clinical interviews. The BPRS was developed as a general measure of severe psychopathology in psychiatric disorders and includes items relevant to positive, negative, disorganization, and mood symptoms. The SANS was developed to measure the negative symptoms of schizophrenia, and factor analyses indicate three correlated clusters of symptoms: apathy–anhedonia, blunted or flattened affect, and alogia–inattention (Sayers, Curran, & Mueser, 1996). The SAPS was developed to assess the positive symptoms of schizophrenia, including hallucinations, delusions, bizarre behavior, and thought disorder. The PANSS incorporates all the items of the BPRS and includes additional items that tap negative symptoms and cognitive impairment.

All of the aforementioned scales include items that rely solely on observation by the interviewer, and all permit the interviewer to obtain relevant information from open charts, other mental health professionals, family, or significant others. This is important because individuals with schizophrenia are sometimes reluctant to admit to positive symptoms, especially if they anticipate medication changes or hospitalization as consequences. Before administering these scales, it is helpful to establish a trusting rapport in order to encourage honesty and openness.

Cognitive Impairment

Effective cognitive functioning is required to successfully navigate the social environment and perform even simple tasks of everyday living. Increasingly, it seems clear that cognitive impairments may help explain poor psychosocial functioning in individuals diagnosed with schizophrenia (Green, Kern, Braff, & Mintz, 2000; Penn et al., 1998). For example, cognitive deficits may limit the rate of skill acquisition in treatments that are designed to improve social competence (Mueser et al., 1991). McEvoy et al. (1996) found that better cognitive functioning was related to good common sense, which was defined as the ability to assess and respond successfully to a variety of situations in everyday life. Brekke, Raine, Ansel, Lencz, & Bird (1997) found that cognitive deficits were related to job functioning, independent living skills, and social skills. Deficits in executive functioning, attention, memory, learning, concentration, and visual perception, in particular, have been documented most frequently in the research literature (Bellack, Sayers, Mueser, & Bennett, 1994; Brekke et al., 1997; Green et al., 2000; Mueser et al., 1991; Penn et al., 1998; Saykin et al., 1991; Strauss, 1993; Tollefson, 1996).

There are no well-established relationships between specific cognitive impairments and particular deficits in adaptive functioning (Bellack et al., 1994; Brekke et al., 1997; M. Green, 1996; Penn et al., 1995; Smith et al., 1999; Tollefson, 1996). However, given Tollefson's (1996) assertion that the "cognitive status of the schizophrenic patient may represent the best window for understanding an individual's capabilities and challenges with respect to successful reintegration into society" (p. 34), assessment of cognitive functioning and potential impairments should be performed to inform the treatment planning process. Identification of a deficit in verbal learning and memory, for example, may have implications for the manner in which new information to be learned is presented in a rehabilitative intervention. Individuals who are made aware of a cognitive deficit may modify their approach to tasks (Penn et al., 1998). There is even evidence to suggest that certain antipsychotic medications may have differential effects on the various domains of cognitive functioning that have been identified as commonly impaired in individuals with schizophrenia (e.g., Keefe, Bollini, & Silva, 1999). Therefore, a cognitive assessment may provide useful information about choice of medication.

Cognitive assessment should include evaluation of those domains most frequently impaired in schizophrenia: executive functioning, verbal memory and learning, and sustained attention. The two types of memory that are most commonly impaired in individuals with schizophrenia are working memory and verbal memory. Working memory is the cognitive capacity that allows for the immediate storage and access of information that is needed to perform various activities, including those required for adequate social and role functioning (Docherty et al., 1996). Penn et al. (1995) suggested that deficits in working memory may help explain the difficulty individuals with schizophrenia experience in keeping track of a conversational topic. More generally, a deficit in working memory hampers an individual's automatic processing of information in the social environment (Penn et al., 1998). The best standardized measures of working memory are the Digit Span subtest (particularly digits backward) of the Wechsler Adult Intelligence Scale–III (WAIS-III; Wechsler, 1997a) and the Letter–Number Sequencing subtest of the WAIS-III. Other neurocognitive tests that assess working memory, among other abilities, include the Trail Making Test (Reitan, n.d.) and the Wisconsin Card Sorting Test (WCST; Berg, 1948).

Verbal memory involves recall and retrieval of information that has been conveyed through language. Deficits in verbal memory are often manifested as rapid forgetting of newly learned information (Saykin et al., 1991; Tollefson, 1996). Poor performance on tests of verbal memory have been significantly correlated with social skill impairments, poor independent functioning in the community, and poor social problem-solving abilities (Bellack et al., 1994; Brekke et al., 1997; M. Green, 1996; Mueser et al., 1991; Penn et al., 1995; Tollefson, 1996). Verbal memory is a strong predictor of learning in skills training (Mueser et al., 1991), and improvements in verbal memory are associated with better social and occupational functioning (Brekke et al., 1997). The California Verbal Learning Test (CVLT; Delis, Kramer, Kaplan, & Ober, 1987) is a widely used test of verbal learning and memory in which immediate recall, recognition, learning, and time-delayed recall may be assessed. Several studies (Bowen et al., 1994; Corrigan et al., 1994; M. Green, 1996) using the CVLT have found that performance on this measure is related to deficits in problem-solving abilities and social skills in individuals with schizophrenia. Another widely used test of verbal memory is the Logical Memory subtest of the Wechsler Memory Scales–III (Wechsler, 1997b).

With respect to sustained attention, individuals with schizophrenia have difficulty paying attention to relevant information while ignoring irrelevant stimuli (Tollefson, 1996). Sustained attention, or vigilance, has been found to be related to social problem solving, processing of social information, behavior on inpatient wards, the ability to manage one's own medication, and the ability to function independently (Brekke et al., 1997; M. Green, 1996; Penn et al., 1995; Strauss, 1993; Tollefson, 1996). Vigilance may also be necessary for learning in skills training programs for schizophrenia (M. Green, 1996). Some researchers (e.g., Selten, Van Den Bosch, & Sijben, 1998) speculate that a fundamental deficit in ability to sustain attention may underlie other types of cognitive dysfunctions. These findings are intuitively appealing given that, in order to perform a variety of tasks, individuals need to be able to pay attention to relevant and ignore irrelevant information. Continuous Performance Tests are the most widely used measures of sustained attention in clinical research (Lezak, 1995). They measure an individual's ability to sustain focused attention over time using a rapidly paced visual discrimination task (Nuechterlein et al., 1990). Detection of brief stimuli viewed as part of a Continuous Performance Test is clearly impaired in individuals with schizophrenia (Nuechterlein, 1991).

Adequate social and role functioning requires not only basic-level neurocognitive functions like memory and attention but also higher-level processing, such as organization, planning, reasoning, information processing, decision making, and mental flexibility. These are all considered executive functions, which are handled primarily in the frontal lobe of the cerebral cortex, an area that also is related to negative symptoms, behavioral deficits, and poor social functioning (Breier et al., 1991; Tollefson, 1996). Studies generally have found that people with schizophrenia suffer significant deficits in this area, and this has been related to poor social adjustment, including for example, occupational functioning (Brekke et al., 1997; Penn et al., 1995; Strauss, 1993; Suslow & Arolt, 1997; Tollefson, 1996). The Wisconsin Card Sorting Test (WCST; Berg, 1948; Heaton, 1981), is a measure of mental flexibility and concept formation that has been used for decades as a standard measure of executive functioning in individuals with schizophrenia (Brewer, Edwards, Anderson, Robinson, & Pantelis, 1996; M. Green, 1996; Green et al., 2000; McEvoy et al., 1996; Penn et al., 1995; Smith et al., 1999; Suslow & Arolt, 1997; Tollefson, 1996). Another common test of executive functioning that particularly assesses planning ability is the Tower of London (Shallice, 1982) test. Two similar, but increasingly more complex tests are the Tower of Hanoi (Glosser & Goodglass, 1990) and the Tower of Toronto (Saint-Cyr & Taylor, 1992).

Associated Features

The nature of schizophrenia is such that the illness often pervades many aspects of an affected individual's life. Therefore, while it is essential to assess core clinical symptoms, it is also crucial to evaluate common associated features of the illness and important life domains that may be contributing to impaired functioning. These include medication noncompliance, age-appropriate social and role functioning, occupational performance, issues related to sexuality, and environmental factors such as housing stability and family environment.

Medication Noncompliance

The discovery of antipsychotic medications in the 1950s forever altered the treatment of schizophrenia by enabling institutionalized individuals to function outside the hospital. Decades of research have demonstrated the benefits of antipsychotic agents, particularly with regard to treating the positive symptoms of the disorder. Many individuals with schizophrenia also receive treatment with a number of other medications, including anti-Parkinsonian medications to treat the extrapyramidal side effects of antipsychotics, antidepressants, mood stabilizers, and benzodiazepines.

Studies have demonstrated that up to 55% of individuals with schizophrenia have significant difficulty following treatment recommendations, including taking medications as prescribed (Fenton, Blyler, & Heinssen, 1997; Weiden et al., 1991). Poor treatment adherence is associated with elevated symptom levels and functional impairments, as well as higher rates of relapse and rehospitalization. Although medications primarily target reduction of positive symptoms and improvement in mood (Herz, 1996), indirect benefits from reduction of these symptoms may be observed in adaptive functioning that is targeted by other forms of treatment, such as social skills training, individual or family therapy, and work. Therefore, a comprehensive assessment of individuals with schizophrenia should include review of medications, consultation with a psychiatrist, and evaluation of compliance with prescribed medication regimens.

Noncompliance with medication is often problematic among individuals with schizophrenia. Estimates of rates of noncompliance range widely, from 11% to 80%. Average noncompliance increases from about 50% at 1 year after discharge from a psychiatric hospitalization to 75% by the second year after discharge (Corrigan, Liberman, & Engel, 1990; Kemp, Hayward, Applewaite, Everitt, & David, 1996; Weiden et al., 1994). This contrasts with noncompliance rates of 18% to 40% for psychosocial aspects of treatment (Corrigan et al., 1990).

Determining the level of compliance with medications is more difficult than measuring cooperation with the nonpharmacological aspects of treatment. Urine and blood samples may be analyzed for presence and level of medications, but the results of these methods often are imprecise. For example, the detection in biological specimens of medications with a long half-life may overestimate compliance and may be ambiguous in the case of partial compliance (Kemp et al., 1996). In addition to routine blood or urine tests, there are other quantitative approaches available to evaluate compliance with medications; the simplest of these involves counting the number of pills in medication bottles and comparing this with the number that should have been taken according to the prescribed regimen (Boczkowski, Zeichner, & DeSanto, 1985; Kemp et al., 1996). Family members or residential counselors who supervise medication administration may also be questioned about any missed doses. Finally, research studies of noncompliance have used medication bottles with special caps that record the date and time of each bottle opening as a means of counting doses taken by subjects (e.g., Cramer & Rosenheck, 1999).

If noncompliance is a significant problem, a more thorough assessment of adherence to medication regimens should include evaluation of barriers to compliance, including (1) unpleasant side effects, (2) complexity of medication regimens, (3) cognitive impairment, (4) poor insight or awareness of illness and the need for treatment, (5) poor alliance with mental health care providers, (6) insufficient supervision during administration, (7) family beliefs about illness and/or medications, (8) mental status or current symptoms—for example, paranoia about medications, and (9) perceived benefit of medications (Boczkowski et al., 1985; Corrigan et al., 1990; Cramer & Rosenheck, 1999; Kemp et al., 1996; Weiden et al., 1994). Standardized scales designed to evaluate compliance and attitudes toward medications may help identify targets for intervention. One measure is the Rating of Medication Influences Scale (ROMI; Weiden et al., 1994). Other instruments include the Drug Attitudes Inventory (Hogan, Awad, & Eastwood, 1983), a self-report measure of willingness to take medications, and the Van Putten and May Neuroleptic Dysphoria Scale (Van Putten & May, 1978), which is designed for use with acutely psychotic individuals.

Social and Role Functioning

Impairment in age-appropriate social and role functioning—including performance of a broad range of behaviors from the basic skills of daily living to the more complex tasks required to achieve goals like maintaining steady employment—is common in schizophrenia. Aside from its inherent importance, information about social functioning and adjustment is important because of its diagnostic and prognostic value. Researchers have found that individuals with schizophrenia who have poor social and role functioning are more vulnerable to relapses and generally experience poorer outcomes (Penn et al., 1995).

Social behavior and functioning in individuals with schizophrenia has been operationalized and measured in a number of ways, including the ability to accurately perceive social cues, solve problems, evaluate behavioral alternatives in social situations, comprehend common social interactions, decode facial and vocal expressions of affect, engage in conversations, maintain interpersonal relationships, and attend to personal needs (e.g., grooming, hygiene, and self-care of medical conditions) (Bellack et al., 1994; McEvoy et al., 1996; Mueser et al., 1996). Skills such as illness self-management, use of leisure time, and occupational functioning have also been included in the broad category of social and role functioning (Becker & Drake, 1994; Drake, Becker, Clark, & Mueser, 1999; Eckman et al., 1992; Marder et al., 1996). Assessment of adaptive social and role functioning merits substantial attention, although the number and range of behaviors that contribute to overall social and role functioning make it a difficult construct to quantify (Glynn, 1998).

Some researchers have argued that dysfunction in social behavior and functioning may be linked to deficits in specific social skills, behavioral practices, and cognitive operations that are necessary for effective, successful social interaction (Bellack et al., 1994). Social skills are defined as concrete behaviors or cognitive-perceptual abilities, including nonverbal and verbal skills, awareness of appropriate situation-specific behaviors, problem-solving skills, and accurate perception of the social cues that are needed to affect others and the environment (Mueser & Bellack, 1998; Mueser & Sayers, 1992). Proficient performance of social skills promotes positive social functioning by enabling individuals to negotiate and advocate for themselves, to maintain interpersonal relationships that can serve as sources of support, and to confront situations that require information processing and decision making.

Given that social and role functioning encompass so many specific behavioral capacities, an assessment of this domain should be organized around a limited number of important questions (Bellack, Mueser, Gingerich, & Agresta, 1997; Mueser & Sayers, 1992). First, it is helpful to identify the content areas in which social and role dysfunctions occur. Important areas to assess, which are frequently impaired, include both basic and more complex conversational skills, interpersonal relationships, social problem solving, use of leisure time, grooming and hygiene, care of personal possessions, money management, and conflict resolution.

Second, it is important to investigate the underlying cause for social and role dysfunctions, which is likely to differ among affected individuals. Some studies suggest that impairments in basic aspects of cognitive functioning may limit an individual's ability to perform the more complex behaviors that are required for adaptive social functioning. Other studies of impaired social and role functioning implicate deficiencies in basic social skills as the root of the problem. Alternatively, poor social functioning may result from an underlying social anxiety, which is common among individuals with schizophrenia, as opposed to actual skill deficits (Bellack et al., 1997; Glynn, 1998). Or, adequate performance of skills that are not reinforced due to environmental factors may prevent success in the social arena. Finally, poor social functioning may be caused by deleterious effects of symptoms, particularly psychosis, on interpersonal skills, the impact of medication side effects such as sedation or restlessness, or demographic factors (e.g., females, on average, tend to have better social skills than males; Mueser, Blanchard, & Bellack, 1995).

Third, it is useful to consider whether deficient functioning is more likely to occur in particular settings or situations (Bellack et al., 1997; Mueser & Sayers, 1992). For example, social or interpersonal functioning may differ at home and at work, in familiar and unfamiliar places, or in a clinic and in the home.

Fourth, it is important to obtain a detailed, behaviorally based description of social and role functioning in order to accurately characterize the nature of the dysfunctions. Obtaining this information will assist in identifying targets for treatment and selecting interventions that will optimize social and role functioning. For example, an individual with social skill dysfunction who suffers from social anxiety may need not only skills training but also supplemental anxiety-reduction strategies.

There are a number of methods for assessing social and role functioning. Inclusion of the greatest variety of perspectives and methods of data gathering will yield the richest data on functional status (Scott & Lehman, 1998). It is advisable to begin by gathering information about general functioning and to proceed with evaluation of successively more specific behaviors (Bellack et al., 1997). Information on general functioning is best acquired through interviews with both patients and significant others who have firsthand knowledge about performance of social skills and behaviors (Bellack et al., 1997; Mueser & Bellack, 1998).

Several standardized instruments may be helpful in structuring such interviews. The Social Behavior Schedule (SBS; Wykes & Sturt, 1986), which is administered to a significant other, assesses domains of interpersonal functioning such as ability to hold conversations, comfort and appropriateness of behavior in social situations, degree of social contact, and interpersonal strife. The Katz Adjustment Scale (Katz & Lyerly, 1963) includes self-reports, as well as ratings by close informants, and assesses social behavior, use of leisure time, and participation in socially expected activities. The patient and family versions of the Social Adjustment Scale–II (Schooler, Hogarty, & Weissman, 1979) are clinician-administered interviews. Both measures elicit information about instrumental role functioning, performance of household chores, finances, relationships with immediate and extended family members, social leisure, friendships and dating, and overall personal well-being. The family version additionally includes questions about family burden, stigma, and attitudes toward the relative with schizophrenia. The Life Skills Profile (Rosen, Hadzi-Pavlovic, & Parker, 1989) contains items that evaluate self-care, social contact, appropriateness of communications, social responsibility, and social turbulence and is completed by a close informant. The Social Functioning Scale (Birchwood, Smith, Cochrane, Wetton, & Copestake, 1990) is completed on the basis of information provided by a close informant and the client and assesses seven areas of functioning: social withdrawal, interpersonal functioning, pro-social activities, recreation, level of independence, level of dependence, and employment. The Social-Adaptive Functioning Evaluation (SAFE; Harvey et al., 1997) was designed as a rating scale for geriatric psychiatric patients, but it may be used with lower-functioning individuals with schizophrenia to assess instrumental and self-care, impulse control, and basic social behaviors such as conversational skills, social engagement, and participation in treatment. Assessment of basic daily living skills may also be accomplished using the self-report and informant versions of the Independent Living Skills Survey (Wallace, Liberman, Tauber, & Wallace, 2000), which includes questions about domains of functioning such as self-care, care of personal possessions, money management, and use of public transportation.

Choice of instrument should be based on a number of factors including which particular aspects of functioning are of interest, the extent to which the resulting data will be used in treatment planning, and practical issues such as cost, time, and available staff (Scott & Lehman, 1998). Awareness of neurocognitive impairments and lack of awareness of illness may also influence the decision about whether to rely on self-administered questionnaires or to conduct interviews with knowledgeable informants (Scott & Lehman, 1998).

Another useful technique to evaluate social skills is performance in role plays (Benton & Schroeder, 1990; Eckman et al., 1992; Mueser & Bellack, 1998; Mueser & Sayers, 1992). To ensure that poor performance is not the result of lack of understanding or anxiety, mental health professionals using this method to assess individuals with schizophrenia should do the following before commencing a role play. First, the evaluator should identify a relevant situation that is similar to one that patients may encounter in their daily lives and that includes the opportunity to demonstrate skills that have been identified as potentially deficient (Bellack et al., 1997; Mueser & Sayers, 1992). If specific skill deficits have not been identified, less-scripted role plays may be conducted; these should be designed to evaluate impairments that are frequently observed in individuals with schizophrenia such as body posture; eye contact; amount, content, and appropriateness of verbalizations; pacing of conversation; voice volume; and expression of affect. Second, a description of the scenario that is to be enacted should be provided; this should include the roles that will be played by the confederate(s) and the patient, the length of time for the role play, the patient's goal in the interaction, and who will start the dialogue. Because individuals with schizophrenia are often particularly sensitive to criticism, the role play should be conducted in a relaxed atmosphere and appropriate performance of skills, or effort, should be rewarded with positive verbal praise. Individuals who express anxiety about performing a role play should be reminded of the value of participating in terms of identifying areas of need and practicing social interactions. Behaviors of interest during the role play may be assessed in a number of ways, including frequency counts, Likert-style ratings, or simple ratings of the presence or absence of skills (Bellack et al., 1997; Mueser & Sayers, 1992). Evaluation may be performed during the role play, or more in-depth analyses of skills may be conducted if patients consent to audio or videotaping (Bellack et al, 1997; Mueser & Bellack, 1998).

Role plays may assist with differentiation of skill deficits from performance deficits in individuals who display appropriate behaviors and skills in the context of the role play but not in natural settings. At initial assessment role plays also have the benefit of serving as a baseline with which future performance of skills may be compared if they are repeated periodically throughout the course of treatment. Finally, role plays are standardized measures that have the advantage of controlling extraneous situational factors that may affect the performance of social skills. Research supports the validity of role-play tests in patients with schizophrenia, and therefore they are strongly recommended as a means of identifying deficits in social skills (Bellack et al., 1997; Mueser & Sayers, 1992).

The Role Play Task (RPT), which is part of the Social Problem Solving Battery (SPSB) designed by Sayers, Bellack, Wade, Bennett, and Fong (1995), is a tool that consists of six 3-minute standardized role plays enacted with a confederate. The RPT evaluates the ability to generate solutions to social problems. Specifically, it assesses the ability to initiate and maintain conversations; stand up for personal rights; and use persuasion, negotiation, and compromise in an interpersonal context. For example, one role play requires clients to act out a situation in which the confederate plays the role of a family member with whom they are having a conversation to try to decide on a movie to select in a video store. These role plays are videotaped for detailed evaluation of skill performance by a trained clinician. The Response Generation Task (RGT) is also part of the SPSB and represents an effective method for evaluating problem-solving ability. Patients begin by viewing several short video segments in which two individuals are having a disagreement. After each segment, the clinician stops the tape and asks the patient a series of questions about the goals of the individual who was visible on the screen, how the goal could be achieved, and what could go wrong if the strategy identified was implemented.

Finally, social skills may be evaluated through direct observation of individuals in their natural settings (Mueser & Bellack, 1998; Mueser & Sayers, 1992). The main advantages of this approach over role play are in terms of the ecological validity of the assessment and the opportunity to observe a wider range of behaviors for a longer period of time. Naturalistic observation also provides information about the environmental response to behavior, which cannot be obtained in a standardized role play, and may identify individuals who do not suffer skill deficits but lack success in social functioning because of unrewarding or unreinforcing environments. The disadvantages over role play include the time-consuming nature of such an evaluation, the inability to control extraneous factors that may affect skill performance, the reality that some situations are impossible to observe, and the fact that individuals often behave differently when they know they are being observed.

Occupational Functioning

As stated, there is a high rate of unemployment in patients with schizophrenia, and research indicates that competitive employment may improve overall adaptive functioning. Employment helps increase daily activity, social contact, self-esteem, involvement in other community activities, community tenure, and quality of life and helps decrease the use of mental health services and reliance on mental health professionals (Drake et al., 1996; Torrey,

Becker, & Drake, 1995). Therefore, desire for work should be included in a comprehensive assessment that is designed to assist the treatment planning process.

Although capacity for work used to be the primary vocational assessment goal for persons with schizophrenia, research indicating that supported employment programs are helpful in improving vocational outcomes in a wide variety of patients (Drake, Becker et al., 1999) has shifted the emphasis of assessment to understanding work history, interest in work, and preferences for type of work desired. Rather than attempting to determine whether patients are capable of work, assessment explores the types of work and patient interests most likely to result in a successful work experience. Other correlates of work may also be assessed, but more for the purposes of informing the job search and need for supports than for determining appropriateness of involvement in supported employment.

The assessment should include key predictors of work performance: symptoms, social skill deficits, and cognitive functioning (Cook & Razzano, 2000). High levels of negative symptoms, as well as florid psychotic symptoms, tend to be associated with poorer outcomes in the workplace (Cook & Razzano, 2000; Glynn, 1998), but not necessarily in supported employment programs (e.g., Mueser, Becker et al., 1997). The specific social skill deficits that may negatively affect work performance include communication skills, accurate perception of coworkers' behaviors, problem-solving ability, and sociability. With respect to deficits in social skills, it may be useful to perform observations and ratings of job behaviors and attitudes in actual or simulated work environments. All of the cognitive deficits most commonly observed in schizophrenia have been found to affect outcome in studies of occupational functioning (Cook & Razzano, 2000), so cognitive functioning may need to be assessed. It is also important to assess variables such as motivation to work and ability to manage money. This information will inform the rehabilitation team about the nature of supports a patient will need in order to make work a successful and satisfying experience.

Housing Stability

In the past, large numbers of individuals diagnosed with schizophrenia were housed for long periods of time in mental hospitals or asylums. Many such buildings were erected in rural areas with working farms on the premises, and the institutions provided for the work, leisure, and social life of the residents (Wykes, 1998). In 1955, the number of patients with schizophrenia housed in public psychiatric hospitals in the United States was 559,000 (Torrey, 1995). Today, only about 100,000 individuals with schizophrenia are living on inpatient wards (Torrey, 1995), yet the U.S. population has increased from approximately 166 million in 1955 to 258 million in 1993. Estimates indicate that 30% to 60% of individuals with severe mental illness reside at home (Mueser, Bond, & Drake, 2001). The remainder of nonhospitalized severely mentally ill people live alone or with one or more roommates in independent or supported housing, in group homes or community residences, or in nursing homes or long-term care facilities.

Housing stability and time spent in the hospital are correlated, with greater stability in housing associated with less time in the hospital (Bond, Drake, Mueser, & Latimer, 2001). This may be due to the difficulty maintaining a room in a community residence or a private apartment during a prolonged hospital stay. Hospitalized individuals who rely on social service benefits as their sole source of income are at risk for losing not only their housing but also their belongings because they are often unable to afford to move and pay storage fees for their possessions. For example, if individuals remain in the hospital for longer than 3 months, their Supplemental Security Income (SSI) is automatically terminated (Social Security Administration, 2001). Furthermore, the ability to maintain a stable residence removes the stress associated with searching for housing and adjusting to novel environments, which may exacerbate symptoms and lead to relapse.

Family Environment

Consideration of the family environment is particularly important for individuals with schizophrenia who live at home, but even for those who do not, contact with family members may affect adaptive functioning (Herz, 1996). Assessment of family environment may be accomplished by interviewing individual family members, holding family meetings, observing family interactions in the home, or administering standardized measures that can provide information about the role of the family in either promoting or jeopardizing the well-being of the member with schizophrenia. Important aspects of family functioning to consider include the potential stress, emotional distress, and burden experienced by the family in response to the patient's behaviors, needs, and symptoms, as well as other stressors that may be present. It is also useful to evaluate family knowledge, attributions, expectations, and beliefs about the illness (Clare & Birchwood, 1998). Before deciding whether to include family work as part of the overall treatment plan, it is important to consider the level of interest of the family and patient, the extent and quality of the family contact, and the ability of the family as a whole to identify outcomes that could serve as goals of family therapy (Dixon, Adams, & Lucksted, 2000).

The Relatives Assessment Interview (Barrowclough & Tarrier, 1992) is a structured clinical interview that elicits information regarding the patient's psychiatric history and social functioning, the relatives' responses to the patient, the perceived impact of the illness, attempts at coping, and areas of difficulty and tension in the family. The Family Questionnaire (Barrowclough & Tarrier, 1992) is a checklist of behaviors to be completed by relatives; it provides an overview of perceived problems that is particularly useful as an outcome measure or as a repeated measure of change. Family members' knowledge about schizophrenia may be assessed using the Information Questionnaire—Relative Version (McGill, Falloon, Boyd, & Wood-Siverio, 1983), the Knowledge about Schizophrenia Interview (Barrowclough & Tarrier, 1992), or the Knowledge Questionnaire (Birchwood & Smith, 1987). Negative attitudes toward patients, which may adversely affect patient functioning, may be assessed with the Patient Rejection Scale (Kreisman et al., 1988).

Sexuality and Family Planning

Because increasing numbers of individuals with schizophrenia reside in the community rather than in hospitals, the rates of HIV infection and unwanted pregnancies in this population have likewise risen (Coverdale & Grunebaum, 1998). Before deinstitutionalization, sexuality and family planning were not routinely included in the psychiatric treatment of individuals with schizophrenia. Studies demonstrating that many people with schizophrenia have misconceptions, misinformation, and delusional beliefs about sex and pregnancy, together with the problems of sexually transmitted diseases and the effect of psychotropic medications on the fetus, make it ethically necessary for mental health professionals today to evaluate the sexual histories and practices of all patients. This may serve to identify patients who are at risk for contracting a sexually transmitted disease, to detect unknown early pregnancies so that potentially harmful medication may be stopped and obstetrical evaluations can be performed, and to provide factual information regarding sexual matters that would not otherwise be offered. After adequate therapeutic rapport has been established, an assessment should include questions about current sexual practices, including number and gender of partners; contraceptive use and general knowledge about contraceptive methods; desire for children; and values regarding contraception, pregnancy, and parenting. Female clients should also be asked about the nature of their menstrual cycles, the date of their most recent gynecological exam, and the number of pregnancies they have had and the results thereof (Coverdale & Grunebaum, 1998).

Comorbid Psychiatric Conditions

High rates of concurrent depression, anxiety, substance abuse, and trauma in individuals with schizophrenia require assessment of potential comorbid psychiatric disorders before formulating an individualized treatment plan (Glynn, 1998). Given the differences in the nature and methods used to assess these commonly comorbid conditions, each is discussed separately.

Mood and Anxiety Disorders

Individuals with schizophrenia disproportionately suffer from a lack of positive feelings (anhedonia) and high levels of negative affect, in particular depression, anxiety, and hostility (Blanchard & Panzarella, 1998; Glynn, 1998). With respect to positive affect, studies have demonstrated that social activity is associated with greater well-being. Because social withdrawal and social anxiety are common features of schizophrenia, it is not surprising that positive affect would therefore be deficient. However, as with negative affect, it is unclear whether deficiencies in positive affect leave individuals less likely to seek social activity or whether social withdrawal reduces the experience of positive affect (Blanchard & Panzarella, 1998). Regardless of the directionality of the effect, mood and level of anxiety are important domains to assess in formulating a treatment plan, particularly with the evidence that negative affect is associated with a poorer clinical course in individuals with schizophrenia (Blanchard & Panzarella, 1998).

A number of instruments may be used to assess mood and anxiety, and many of them are mentioned in other chapters of this book. Two well-known instruments with attributes of ease of administration, scoring, and interpretation are the Beck Depression Inventory, second edition (BDI-II; Beck, Steer, & Brown, 1996) and the Beck Anxiety Inventory (BAI; Beck & Steer, 1990). The BDI-II and BAI also have the advantage of being empirically validated and may be repeated frequently to monitor depression and anxiety throughout the course of treatment.

Substance Abuse

Evidence from large-scale studies of substance use demonstrates that the rate of lifetime substance use disorders in individuals with schizophrenia is substantially higher than in the general population (Cuffel, 1996; Regier et al., 1990). Consistent with the general population, substance use disorders in individuals with schizophrenia tend to be chronic, relapsing problems. However, unlike individuals in the general population, people with schizophrenia have greater sensitivity to the psychoactive effects of substances; a lower capacity to engage in controlled use of alcohol and drugs; a greater vulnerability to risk factors such as poverty, poor education, unemployment, and living situations that increase opportunities and pressures to use substances; and increased likelihood to suffer adverse consequences of substance use, such as hospitalization, infectious diseases, homelessness, involvement in the criminal justice system, and suicide (Drake & Brunette, 1998; Drake & Mueser, 2000;

Mueser, Drake, & Noordsy, 1998). Despite the obvious importance of identifying and treating substance use disorders in individuals with schizophrenia, these disorders are often undetected by mental health professionals either because of denial or minimization of use, the tendency to focus on symptom reduction in acutely ill individuals, medical tests that provide data only on recent use, or the reality that screening often is not conducted (Drake & Mueser, 2000; Rosenberg et al., 1998).

Because of the high prevalence of substance abuse in schizophrenia, a comprehensive assessment should explore psychoactive substance use, both past and present. Because many screening instruments for identifying substance abuse in the general population are not sensitive in persons with schizophrenia, alternative instruments have been developed for use with severely mentally ill populations. One such instrument, the Dartmouth Assessment of Lifestyle Instrument (DALI; Rosenberg et al., 1998), is an interviewer-administered scale that may be completed in approximately 6 minutes and was designed as a brief screen for detecting substance use disorder in individuals with severe mental illness, including schizophrenia. Items on the DALI address patterns of substance use, loss of control, consequences of use, dependence in terms of physiological syndromes, and subjective distress.

Even if substance use is denied, some measure of suspicion should be maintained, particularly for young, single males with lower than average levels of education, given that these individuals have the highest rates of comorbidity (Mueser et al., 2000). If substance use is suspected, random urine drug screens and interviews with close informants may be conducted to confirm current substance use. Individuals who acknowledge a history of substance use should be monitored closely because of the chronic, relapsing nature of substance use disorders. More specialized assessment in clients with confirmed substance abuse can be undertaken with the Clinicians' Rating Scales for Alcohol Use Disorder (AUS) and Drug Use Disorder (DUS) (Mueser, Drake, et al., 1995). The AUS and DUS are 5-point rating scales and pertain to the degree of substance use over the preceding 6 months; it is completed by a clinician (or team) based on all available information. Further assessment may include evaluation of patterns of use; motivations for use; awareness of the negative consequences of using; insight regarding the seriousness of the problem; the interaction of substance use with other functional domains such as housing, interpersonal relationships, illness management, and work; and willingness to engage in treatment.

Posttraumatic Stress Disorder

With the recent data that indicate high rates of trauma exposure of individuals with severe mental illness (Goodman et al., 1997), it is important to assess trauma and PTSD in all patients, and a number of standardized instruments are designed to assess trauma exposure and PTSD. The Trauma History Questionnaire (B. Green, 1996) may be used to evaluate exposure to traumatic events in both childhood and adulthood and to identify which events continue to cause the most current distress. The PTSD Checklist (PCL; Blanchard, Jones-Alexander, Buckley, & Forneris, 1996) is a self-report measure that requires respondents to rate the degree to which they experience each of the 17 PTSD symptoms identified in DSM-IV in relation to a prespecified traumatic event. If the results of these screening measures suggest the possibility that an individual may meet diagnostic criteria for PTSD, the Clinician-Administered PTSD Scale (CAPS; Blake et al., 1990) may be used to make a definitive diagnosis. The CAPS is a semistructured interview based on DSM-IV criteria for the disorder and is considered the gold standard for assessing PTSD. Both the PCL and the CAPS have been found to be reliable in patients with severe mental illness and thus demonstrate convergent validity (Mueser, Salyers et al., 2001).

TREATMENT PLANNING AND OUTCOME EVALUATION

Given the substantial variability in presentation of symptoms, associated features, and co-morbid diagnoses in schizophrenia, planning treatment for individuals with this illness must be guided by information obtained from a comprehensive assessment that identifies specific disabilities to serve as targets for change. Because schizophrenia often has a chronic course, evaluation of outcome may be better conceived as regular, periodic monitoring and re-assessment of target problems to determine the effectiveness of treatments that were de-signed to address them. The success of treatment interventions should be assessed no later than the end of the first year of implementation and at least annually thereafter. For the most part, the same assessment strategies employed at the initial evaluation may be repeat-ed when functioning is reassessed. Some of the domains described here may require more close monitoring, depending on the nature of the problems and the interventions used to treat them. For example, medication noncompliance and substance abuse may need more frequent monitoring than do cognitive impairments and housing stability. Most of the treat-ments described next relate directly to impairments that may be identified in an assessment of the various domains already discussed; however, some interventions address more than one problem or target of change.

Medication Compliance Therapy

The success of antipsychotic medications in reducing the positive symptoms of schizophre-nia make them an essential component of treatment. Medication noncompliance should be considered in the presence of an increase in previously controlled positive symptoms or un-remitting, severe symptoms. Several strategies for treating medication noncompliance are available. Boczkowski et al. (1985) describe an example of the psychoeducational approach to noncompliance. This method involves engaging individuals in discussions about their di-agnoses, the positive effects of taking medications, and the negative consequences of not taking medication. Individual medication regimens are carefully reviewed, and understand-ing thereof is verified. Individuals are also provided with written materials that contain im-portant information about their medications.

Behavioral tailoring interventions (e.g., Boczkowski et al., 1985; Cramer & Rosen-heck, 1999) focus on helping patients develop specific cues that incorporate aspects of their daily routine or environment to facilitate medication compliance. For example, patients may be encouraged to pair medication intake with a particular part of their daily routine, to identify a highly visible location for medication bottles, or to design a calendar with re-minders that are to be removed after the administration of each dose. Finally, Kemp et al. (1996) describe an approach to improving compliance based on the principles of motiva-tional interviewing (Miller & Rollnick, 1991). Their approach, coined "compliance thera-py," involves a 4- to 6-session intervention using psychoeducation and cognitive-behavioral techniques to provide information about the benefits and side effects of medications; to highlight discrepancies between patients' actions and beliefs, providing positive reinforce-ment for adaptive behaviors; to emphasize the value of staying well; and to encourage self-efficacy with respect to taking medication.

Medication noncompliance can often persist long enough to produce substantial in-creases in the positive or negative symptoms of schizophrenia that render individuals inca-pable of caring for themselves. Inpatient hospitalization is necessary when individuals pose a threat to themselves or others due to symptom exacerbations, which are frequently caused by medication noncompliance. For the most part, inpatient stays are designed to stabilize symptoms (Herz, 1996), often by restarting or adjusting medication regimens, to facilitate rapid reentry into the community.

Assertive Community Treatment

People with schizophrenia who require assistance with several aspects of daily functioning (such as work, housing, transportation, and money management) may need aid from a variety of social service agencies, including the Social Security Administration, the Federal Department of Housing and Urban Development, the state welfare board, and a number of mental health professionals, including psychiatrists, psychologists, social workers, rehabilitation therapists, and occupational therapists. Coordination of the various services and service providers that are often essential for adaptive functioning in the community can be complex, confusing, and time-consuming. Recognition of the difficulty inherent in simultaneously accessing services from a variety of sources led to the development of a new service, case management, and a new mental health professional, the case manager.

A variety of models of case management have developed over the past three decades, including the brokered model, the clinical case management model, and the assertive community treatment (ACT) model. In the brokered model, case managers essentially function as independent consultants, providing assessment of needs, referrals to services, and ongoing coordination and monitoring of treatment—all independent of clinical care settings (Mueser, Bond, Drake, & Resnick, 1998). In the clinical model, case managers provide clinical services such as psychoeducation and psychotherapy in addition to linking clients with other mental health professionals and necessary services (Mueser, Bond et al., 1998). The most well studied model of case management is ACT, which was designed to be even more comprehensive than the brokered or clinical models in terms of meeting the diverse and multiple needs of patients with severe psychiatric impairments (Mueser, Bond, & Drake, 2001; Mueser, Bond, et al., 1998). ACT is provided by a team of mental health professionals, including psychiatrists, nurses, and case managers, who work at the same facility. Because most mental health services are delivered directly by the ACT team members and not brokered to other providers, both coordination and continuity of care are greatly facilitated. Case loads are shared across clinicians so that one individual is not solely responsible for coordinating the care of a particular group of clients, and ACT teams generally have lower client to case manager ratios (e.g., 10:1 rather than 30:1), allowing for more time to be spent assisting each individual. ACT teams typically offer 24-hour coverage and provide most services in the community.

ACT addresses several of the problem domains that may be identified in a comprehensive assessment of adaptive functioning, and it often serves as a critical foundation for other treatment approaches that are intended to target those impairments. For example, case managers are in an excellent position to monitor problems such as noncompliance with prescribed medications and substance use. Assistance with practical needs of daily living such as housing, transportation, and shopping undoubtedly helps individuals maintain stable living arrangements and reduce stress, which is related to reduced time spent in hospitals and perhaps greater subjective quality of life (Mueser, Bond et al., 1998). Case managers also reduce stress by helping patients navigate the complexities of social service agencies. Finally, assuming a positive working relationship, case managers may be able to convince reluctant patients to participate in useful treatment such as skills training, family work, or cognitive-behavioral therapy, and they may be instrumental in encouraging competitive employment.

Perhaps because ACT has focused on meeting the basic needs of individuals, research on this model has not found substantial effects on social or vocational functioning. This may suggest the need to include more specialized professionals on ACT teams such as employment experts (Bond et al., 2001). Some have expressed concern that ACT will engender dependency in individuals with schizophrenia who rely heavily on services provided by the teams. This concern may be addressed through incorporation of formal skills training and requirements that independent living skills be practiced in natural settings. Or, a program of tiered case management services may be offered to encourage progressively more independence (Mueser & Bond, 2000). ACT treatment manuals and fidelity scales have been developed to facilitate adaptation of the model to individual mental health care settings (Allness & Knoedler, 1998; Stein & Santos, 1998).

Cognitive-Behavioral Therapy

Prior to the introduction of neuroleptic medications, the symptoms of schizophrenia were treated with traditional forms of psychodynamic psychotherapy. The demonstrated effectiveness of medications in reducing the positive symptoms of schizophrenia led to a transition to biological treatments and the emergence of the stress–vulnerability model of the illness. This shifted the focus of psychotherapy from psychodynamic models to supportive models that are designed to encourage the use of medications and help patients avoid or reduce the negative effects of stress by developing more effective coping strategies (Davidson, Lambert, & McGlashan, 1998).

One obvious source of stress for individuals with schizophrenia is the emotional distress that is associated with the experience of positive symptoms, along with the concomitant disturbances in mood that are usually manifested as depression, anxiety, or both. Negative symptoms produce some subjective distress (Mueser, Valentiner, & Agresta, 1997), but positive symptoms are generally accepted to be even more distressing. Cognitive-behavioral techniques may be used to treat comorbid depression and anxiety in individuals with schizophrenia in much the same way as with people who have primary mood or anxiety disorders. The goal of cognitive-behavioral therapy for psychosis is reduction of distress and interference with functioning that is caused by delusions and hallucinations (Garety, Fowler, & Kuipers, 2000).

Aaron Beck, who was influential in developing the cognitive theory of psychopathology, began using structured, cognitive-behavioral approaches to identify and reduce the core symptoms and behaviors that are associated with psychosis as early as the 1950s (Garety et al., 2000). The basic assumptions that serve as the foundations for cognitive-behavioral theory are twofold: (1) individuals develop and maintain cognitive sets, or schemata, that are used to make sense of their experience; and (2) the therapist's role is to challenge dysfunctional or distorted schemata with rational, observable evidence in an effort to change the cognitive sets. Consistent with this theory, delusions and hallucinations may be conceptualized as distorted perceptions and beliefs that are resistant to disconfirmation and that produce misinterpretations of new data in accordance with the set belief system, but which may be altered by reviewing objective evidence and encouraging consideration of alternative perspectives.

Although the basic theory behind cognitive-behavioral interventions is the same, implementation of cognitive-behavioral therapy for psychosis is somewhat different than for depression or anxiety. Most important, in working with psychotic individuals, the initial engagement and rapport-building phase of treatment will likely require more time (Garety et al., 2000). It is particularly important for patients to feel supported and understood before addressing and exploring the evidence that supports psychotic material. An individual therapist is often a very important person in the lives of those who have few social contacts.

People with schizophrenia often seek tolerance, acceptance, respect, validation, compassion, and clarity in communications and expectations from individual therapists (Davidson, Stayner, & Haglund, 1998). While challenges to psychotic beliefs should be avoided until trust has been established, the initial engagement period should include assessment of delusions and hallucinations, along with evaluation of the conviction of beliefs (Davidson, Lambert, & McGlashan, 1998). The engagement phase may also include exploration of the patients' perspectives on their illness, including discussion of factors that produce difficulty or distress, coping strategies that have helped in the past, and expectations for the future. The goals of this exercise are to encourage some acknowledgement of personal dysfunction, to foster the sense that the therapist is collaborating on agenda and goal setting, and to engender feelings of personal control and hope (Garety et al., 2000).

After a trusting alliance has been firmly established, therapists may begin to gently encourage patients to explore the evidence supporting psychotic beliefs, first targeting those that were identified as least firmly held. Consistent with traditional cognitive-behavioral therapy, therapists use Socratic questioning to help patients evaluate evidence, pointing out discrepancies and erroneous reasoning in an effort to dispute misperceptions and encourage reconsideration of beliefs in light of rational evidence. Therapists may need to suggest more alternative explanations for psychotic interpretations and beliefs in light of the greater cognitive rigidity that is sometimes observed in individuals with schizophrenia (Garety et al., 2000). It is important to remember that low self-esteem in schizophrenia may be chronic, particularly, for example, in the case of individuals who have experienced self-deprecatory voices. Negative self-appraisals may be addressed by encouraging a view of the self as an individual who has struggled heroically in the face of considerable adversity (Garety et al., 2000).

Following verbal challenging, therapists may encourage patients to conduct behavioral experiments outside the session that will serve as opportunities for planned reality testing and for attempting the new behavioral alternatives and coping strategies discussed in sessions (Davidson, Lambert, & McGlashan, 1998). These experiments should be reviewed in subsequent sessions. A final phase of cognitive-behavioral therapy involves reviewing the work that has been accomplished and establishing short-, medium-, and long-term goals for the future in light of what was learned in therapy. In their review of outcome studies of cognitive-behavioral therapy for psychosis, Garety et al. (2000) noted that this method has demonstrated substantial benefits in terms of symptom reduction, particularly negative symptoms and depression, which have been maintained as long as 1 year after treatment. Cognitive-behavioral therapy has also been associated with shorter lengths of stay in inpatient facilities.

Social Skills Training

Many individuals with schizophrenia experience significant interruptions or complete deficits in healthy, "normal" social, life-skill, and interpersonal functioning, which represents a domain that is considered independent of symptoms (Bellack et al., 1994; Cyr, Toupin, Lesage, & Valiquette, 1994; Penn et al., 1995; Smith et al., 1995, 1999). Individuals with schizophrenia also experience considerable difficulty behaving appropriately in social situations and often report feeling significant discomfort and unease in the social environment. This may lead to social withdrawal and impairments in age-appropriate social and role functioning. The lack of adequate performance of social skills by many individuals with schizophrenia may represent a significant source of stress and cause for low subjective quality of life and relapse (Bellack et al., 1994; Penn et al., 1995).

Over the past three decades, treatment for schizophrenia has increasingly focused on promoting independence and rehabilitation of social and role functioning through training of basic functional living skills and more complex social skills. Although training of deficient social skills have been delivered in a variety of different ways, most are based on behavioral theories of operant conditioning and social learning theory, which break complex target behaviors into component parts that are taught in incremental steps (Heinssen, Liberman, & Kopelowicz, 2000; Marder et al., 1996). Skills trainers generally take an educational approach and use active teaching methods such as didactic instruction, modeling, behavioral rehearsal, corrective feedback, role play, contingent social reinforcement, and homework. In developing a skills training curriculum, it is important to consider a number of practical issues such as group composition, group size, duration of groups, frequency and length of meetings, setting, timing, and incentives for attendance and participation (Bellack et al., 1997). Skills training programs for individuals with schizophrenia should include opportunities to repeatedly discuss and practice the skills. This overlearning of material will improve the likelihood that the skill will be included in the individual's behavioral repertoire after formal skills training has ended. Ongoing assessment of progress and evaluation of whether clients are actually learning skills is essential and may be determined through observation of role plays or conversations with significant others who routinely observe clients' behavior such as family members, therapists, case managers, and community residence staff. If skills are not being demonstrated, trainers may need to allow more time for practice, to break down complex skills into more manageable segments, or to teach more basic skills that serve as a foundation for complex skills (Bellack et al., 1997).

Skills training programs vary in length and intensity. Acquisition of skills usually requires at least 6 months, with at least two sessions each week (Smith, Bellack, & Liberman, 1996); a meta-analysis of the skills training literature found that weeks of training was positively correlated with size of treatment effects (Dilk & Bond, 1996). Skills training is generally administered in a group format because the behaviors being taught are those that will be used in an interpersonal context. The group can serve as a safe setting in which to practice skills and receive feedback without fear of negative consequences. Although some basic skills will be beneficial to all group members, it is important to identify the particular skill deficits and personal goals of each individual before treatment begins. This knowledge may be used to tailor the skills training to the needs of the individual group members, which helps make the learning process more relevant and motivating.

Several skills training modules have been developed by the Clinical Research Center for Schizophrenia and Psychiatric Rehabilitation at UCLA. These modules have been empirically validated and used in several countries around the world (Chambon & Marie-Cardine, 1998; Liberman et al., 1986; Liberman, DeRisi, & Mueser, 1989; Liberman, Wallace, Blackwell, MacKain, & Eckman, 1992; Liberman et al., 1998). Symptom self-management, recreation for leisure, medication self-management, community reentry, job seeking, workplace fundamentals, basic conversation skills, and friendship and dating are among the modules that are available, all of which use the same teaching techniques, including didactic instruction, role play, problem solving, homework, and in vivo behavioral rehearsal. These modules have been demonstrated to be effective in promoting significant learning of social and independent living skills in individuals with schizophrenia (Liberman et al., 1998; Marder et al., 1996) and, given their user-friendly nature, may be administered by a broad array of mental health professionals.

Some evidence exists that cognitive deficits, particularly in verbal learning and memory, may limit the effectiveness of skills training (Kern, Green, & Satz, 1992; Mueser et al., 1991; Silverstein, Schenkel, Valone, & Nuernberger, 1998). This potential problem may be addressed in a variety of ways:

1. The treatment environment may be altered to accommodate cognitive deficits—for example, training should be conducted in a minimally distracting environment to maximize attention to learning.
2. The treatment room should be arranged to facilitate eye contact with the trainer, and visual cueing devices such as posters, labels, schedules and signs may be used to assist individuals with memory impairments.
3. Shaping procedures may also be used to improve attention, which may facilitate learning, such as rewarding good eye contact, appropriate responses to instructions, or comments reflecting accurate tracking of the group topic with tokens (Heinssen et al., 2000).
4. Between-session reviews may be helpful in promoting learning and memory of skills learned in group (Eckman et al., 1992).
5. Social skills training may be accompanied by adjunctive therapy that is designed to address cognitive deficits by targeting more basic skills such as social perception, verbal communication, and cognitive processing. Integrated Psychological Therapy, which is described more fully later in this chapter, represents one such augmentation strategy (Brenner, Hodel, Roder, & Corrigan, 1992; Brenner et al., 1994).

The UCLA modules described here address potential cognitive impairments in individuals with schizophrenia by using a highly structured format, frequent repetition of information, auditory and visual presentation of material, immediate verbal reinforcement for attention and participation, in vivo modeling, and over-learning.

Evaluation of treatment programs designed to teach specific skills have generally found that many individuals with schizophrenia are able to learn the tasks and perform well on posttest measures of competence for the particular behaviors targeted in the therapy (Arns & Linney, 1995; Cook, Pickett, Fitzgibbon, Jonikas, & Cohler, 1996; Cyr et al., 1994; Herz, 1996; Liberman et al., 1986; Marder et al., 1996; Penn & Mueser, 1996; Smith et al., 1996; Wallace, Liberman, MacKain, Blackwell, & Eckman, 1992). However, generalization of the learning beyond the treatment milieu or to other behaviors may be minimal and does not seem to occur spontaneously. In other words, people do not always incorporate the behaviors they learn in therapy, particularly complex behaviors or generic as opposed to narrowly defined skills, into their daily functioning in the real world (Arns & Linney, 1995; Cook et al., 1996; Liberman et al., 1986; Penn & Mueser, 1996; Smith et al., 1996). There is some evidence that performance of skills in natural settings may occur if the skills are trained (or practiced) in the settings in which they are to be used (Dilk & Bond, 1996; Heinssen et al., 2000). Training significant others, such as case managers, in the principles of skills training facilitates the generalization of behaviors taught in session, resulting in better outcomes than those produced by skills training alone (Heinssen et al., 2000).

Research on social skills training clearly indicates that it is an effective and useful modality for improving adaptive social and role functioning (e.g., Penn & Mueser, 1996; Dilk & Bond, 1996). While skills training has not been demonstrated to substantially affect relapse rates, it may help individuals view themselves as more assertive, less socially anxious, better able to cope with symptoms, and more effective in dealing with treatment providers (Benton & Schroeder, 1990; Douglas & Mueser, 1990; Eckman et al., 1992; Liberman et al., 1992, 1998; Marder et al., 1996; Penn & Mueser, 1996). Questions that remain to be answered about social skills training concern issues such as pacing (e.g., Which skills should be taught and when? How intensive should skills training be? How long should training last?) and the importance of factors that may affect success in skills training, such as cognitive limitations, motivation, and stress tolerance (Heinssen et al., 2000; Smith et al., 1996).

Family Interventions

The theoretical rationale for including family therapy derived from research suggesting that individuals living in families with high expressed emotion (EE)—that is, overt attitudes indicating criticism, dissatisfaction, hostility, and overinvolvement—were more vulnerable to relapse and rehospitalization (Budd & Hughes, 1997; Butzlaff & Hooley, 1998; Linszen et al., 1997). Family intervention was therefore designed to teach more adaptive, less stressful communication skills and problem solving through instruction and modeling of appropriate skills by a therapist. Over the past 20 years, several types of family intervention for schizophrenia have been developed. Common components that are offered in varying amounts include education about the illness; practical and emotional support; and skill development in communication, problem solving, and crisis management (Dixon et al., 2000; Mueser & Bond, 2000). Most successful family intervention programs are offered for a relatively long period of time (more than 6 months) by mental health professionals who are involved in their patients' treatment. Research has demonstrated that family interventions may help lower relapse rates (Dixon et al., 2000; Mueser, Sengupta et al., 2001).

Some frequently used models of family therapy (which can be administered as single- or multiple-family group interventions in homes, clinics, or other sites) include the supportive family model and the behavioral family therapy model. Supportive family therapy primarily involves provision of psychoeducation and emotional support (Kuipers, Leff, & Lam, 1992) and may employ strategies adapted from family systems interventions (Anderson, Reiss, & Hogarty, 1986). When supportive family intervention is provided in the context of a multiple-family group, family members, including relatives and patients, derive much support from other families with similar experiences, as well as coping strategies for dealing with common problems (McFarlane et al., 1991).

Like supportive family therapy, behavioral family interventions include psychoeducation about schizophrenia, but they also systematically teach skills aimed at enabling the family to more effectively manage the illness (Barrowclough & Tarrier, 1992; Falloon, Boyd, & McGill, 1984; Mueser & Glynn, 1999). For example, behavioral family therapy (BFT) involves teaching information about schizophrenia, medications used to treat it, and the stress–vulnerability model, as well as training in communication and problem-solving techniques (Falloon et al., 1984; Mueser & Glynn, 1999). Aside from its emphasis on skills training, BFT may be distinguished from other family interventions for schizophrenia in a number of other ways. First, there is greater emphasis on the individual functioning and well-being of all family members, both patients and caregivers alike, rather than an exclusive focus on the patient (Falloon, 1990). Second, BFT focuses to a larger extent on promoting the coping capacity of the patient by including skills training, not only for the patient but also for family members, to address deficient areas of functioning. The format for the skills training is similar to that described here in that therapists use modeling, role plays, positive and corrective feedback, and homework as teaching tools. The training on problem solving is more structured, and the emphasis on the use of this technique for reducing stress in the family environment is greater in BFT than other types of family therapy. Third, clinicians who provide BFT emphasize fostering a collaborative relationship between themselves, the treatment team, and the family in order to more effectively manage the psychiatric illness and achieve personal and shared goals of family members.

Integrated Dual Diagnosis Treatment

Historically, treatment for individuals dually diagnosed with schizophrenia and a substance use disorder was either sequential or parallel (Drake & Mueser, 2000; Mueser, Drake, &

Noordsy, 1998). Sequential treatment was based on the assumption that treatment of one condition was a necessary prerequisite for treatment of another. For example, the belief that substance use precluded prescription of medication to treat schizophrenia or, conversely, that florid psychosis inherently hampered techniques designed to treat substance use, reflect this perspective. Parallel treatment of dual disorders stems from the traditional separation of mental health and substance abuse services and the assumption that different training and methods are needed to treat the two disorders. The failure of either model to effectively treat patients with dual disorders led to the development of integrated models for mental health and substance abuse treatment (Carey, 1996; Drake & Mueser, 2000; Mueser, Drake, & Noordsy, 1998). Research on integrated treatment models has found that these programs have been able to engage dually diagnosed patients in treatment for at least 1 year or more, thus producing greater improvement in substance use outcomes (Drake, Mercer-McFadden, Mueser, McHugo, & Bond, 1998).

Several different programs based on the integrated approach have been developed with the primary goal of including an awareness of the implications of the substance use disorder into all aspects of the mental health treatment program. Despite differences in the specific aspects of these programs, the common philosophies and ingredients shared by many include assertive outreach, comprehensiveness, family involvement, long-term commitment, a stage approach, and pharmacotherapy (Drake & Mueser, 2000; Mueser, Drake, & Noordsy, 1998). Because patients with dual disorders often drop out of treatment, they require outreach to engage them and significant others in treatment, along with close monitoring over time of mental health and substance abuse.

The most effective integrated treatment models are comprehensive in that they target not only the substance use but also the multitude of other behaviors and life circumstances, such as living environment or social networks, that may be maintaining it. Family involvement is based on the important role relatives can play in giving support and in helping patients get on the road to recovery by developing motivation to work on their dual disorders and self-management strategies. For many patients, both disorders are chronic and stable, and therefore their treatment usually requires a long-term approach (Mueser, Drake, & Noordsy, 1998).

Increasingly, mental health professionals appreciate that successful treatment often progresses in stages. Dually diagnosed patients progress through four main stages of treatment: engagement (when the focus is on developing a therapeutic relationship with a clinician), persuasion (when the focus is on helping the client understand the effect of substance abuse on his or her life and become motivated to address it), active treatment (when the focus shifts to reducing substance use or achieving abstinence), and relapse prevention (when treatment focuses on maintaining awareness of the potential for relapse and addressing other areas of functioning, such as work or relationships). When designing treatment plans for dually diagnosed patients, it is particularly important to consider motivation for change. In the case of individuals with little or no expressed desire to address substance use (i.e., in the engagement and persuasion stages), establishment of a therapeutic rapport and work on other goals that may reduce the opportunity or motivation to use substances, such as finding a stable job or seeking safer housing, may be pursued. Individuals with little motivation for change may also be encouraged to consider how their substance use interferes with achievement of important life goals.

Finally, integrated treatment models must take a careful approach with respect to prescription medications. This includes recognizing the signs and symptoms of withdrawal and drug interactions and avoiding using medications with higher potentials for addiction and abuse (e.g., benzodiazepines), while ensuring that severe psychiatric symptoms such as psychosis are adequately treated. Clinicians need to encourage open communication with patients to enable frank discussion of the compromising effects of substances on schizophrenia. Compliance with prescribed medications should also be monitored closely as many individuals who are actively abusing substances fear drug interactions and therefore do not adhere consistently to medication regimens.

Vocational Rehabilitation

Given the potential benefits of work in terms of increasing activity, socialization, financial status, self-esteem, community tenure, and self-reported quality of life, stable employment should be included as a treatment goal if the patient expresses an interest in it. Historically, vocational rehabilitation programs have followed a stepwise model, relying on extensive pre-employment testing, counseling, training, sheltered employment, and work adjustment trials to prepare individuals for competitive jobs, often called the "train–place" approach (Drake, Becker et al., 1999). This model has been based on a fear of rapid change and has emphasized a slow, safe, sheltered transition to work that places minimal expectations on clients at each stage of the process. However, research on train–place models has failed to support their effects on improving vocational outcomes of patients with schizophrenia (Bond, 1992).

The Individual Placement and Support (IPS) model is based on the "place–train" approach to vocational rehabilitation. IPS is characterized by rapid attainment of competitive jobs in the community, the provision of support and training as needed after work has commenced, and attention to patient preferences in terms of type of job sought and the nature of support provided (Becker & Drake, 1994). To ensure integration of vocational rehabilitation and clinical treatment, in the IPS model, the employment specialist performs all the vocational support functions (i.e., assessment, job search, and support) while working as an integral member of the patient's clinical treatment team. Controlled research on the IPS model has shown that it dramatically increases rates of employment, compared to traditional train–place models or day treatment programs with adjunctive vocational rehabilitation (Cook & Razzano, 2000; Drake et al., 1994, 1996; Drake, Becker et al., 1999; Drake, McHugo et al., 1999).

Cognitive Rehabilitation

Treatments aimed at improving cognitive functioning have been developed to address the adverse impact of cognitive impairments on the ability to perform tasks and to enact the behaviors required for adequate social competence. The first such treatments primarily consisted of repeated practice and coaching of skills identified as deficient through formal assessment of cognitive functioning (Spaulding, Reed, Sullivan, Richardson, & Weiler, 1999). Although many people who received this cognitive remediation performed better on tests of particular skills such as reaction time, vigilance, memory, and cognitive flexibility after training, there was little evidence for generalized improvements in social functioning (Hogarty & Flesher, 1999a). Other programs of cognitive rehabilitation, including Integrated Psychological Therapy (IPT; Brenner et al., 1994) and Cognitive Enhancement Therapy (CET; Hogarty & Flesher, 1999b) represent more ecologically meaningful clinical approaches, using behavioral exercises in a group context to reinforce skill acquisition.

IPT is a highly structured treatment, based on a manual, that is designed for administration to groups of five to seven patients in 30- to 60-minute sessions three times per week. The program is divided into five subsections: cognitive differentiation, social perception, verbal communication, social skills, and interpersonal problem solving. The creators of the program advise that patients be grouped according to an overall assessment of cognitive functioning before treatment begins (Brenner et al., 1994). The first three subsections address cognitive impairments and consist of activities, directed by a therapist, that are designed to combine cognitive operations with social interaction. For example, the verbal communication subsection includes activities designed to exercise attentional skills and short-term memory in a group setting. Patients are required to listen carefully to statements by their peers, then attempt verbatim repetitions and paraphrasing of the information. The fourth and fifth subsections target social interactions and are similar to skills training programs that do not necessarily include an explicit cognitive component.

The CET program is based on an understanding of cognitive impairments in schizophrenia as being developmental in origin (Hogarty & Flesher, 1999a). Therefore, the goal is to facilitate attainment of social cognitive milestones, beginning with teaching effortful and active processing of information that is typically acquired no later than early adulthood, then encouraging cognitive flexibility, perspective taking, and the ability to think abstractly and, finally, using unrehearsed exercises to help individuals tolerate ambiguity and uncertainty (Hogarty & Flesher, 1999b). The program is administered each week in two 60- to 90-minute sessions. Before the program, patients are assessed with a battery of neuropsychological tests in order to identify individual cognitive impairments. Next, patients work with their treatment team to develop specific goals. The first year of treatment involves the use of software programs and exercises that target impairments in attention, memory, and problem solving, many of which were originally designed to rehabilitate skills in individuals with traumatic brain injuries. After the initial assessment, patients are placed in pairs to collaborate on these exercises for approximately 3 months, at which point three or four pairs are combined into a group and work on the software exercises for another 3 months. This use of pairing and grouping encourages social interaction, empathic peer assistance, group problem solving, negotiation, perspective taking, and context appraisal.

After the first year of CET, enhancement of social cognition using several group exercises is added to the practice of specific cognitive skills (Hogarty & Flesher, 1999b). Patients attend social cognitive group sessions that include a psychoeducational presentation by the therapist, review of homework based on the previous presentation, and work on a social cognitive task. The latter task usually involves two patients discussing the intellectual and emotional issues involved in a proposed situation, and it requires that each take the other's perspective. The group sessions are "chaired" by the patients, each of whom takes a turn acting as chairperson. This experience enables individuals to practice paying attention (e.g., maintaining vigilance as to whose hands are raised), keeping the discussion targeted, and facilitating appropriate social exchanges among the other group members. CET has primarily been used with less severely impaired individuals whose behavior is not significantly impacted by positive symptoms (Hogarty & Flesher, 1999b).

Sexuality, Family Planning, and Parenting

Because sexuality and family planning are only beginning to gain recognition as important areas to address in individuals with schizophrenia, empirically validated treatment interventions have yet to be developed. Mental health professionals have traditionally viewed sexuality and family planning as involving medical issues that should be handled by health care providers. However, referrals to separate agencies or offices for obstetrical or gynecological care increases the chance that appointments will be missed due to low motivation, fear, or lack of transportation. In fact, data suggest that many women with schizophrenia receive inadequate gynecological care and that adverse outcomes of pregnancy are more common due to poor prenatal care, delusions that may endanger the fetus, or even psychotic denial of pregnancy (Coverdale & Grunebaum, 1998). Many women with schizophrenia ultimately cannot care for their children, and they are placed in foster care or adopted away, leaving substantial feelings of loss and failure in the mothers.

These circumstances necessitate that mental health professionals assume some responsibility for providing information and support regarding sexuality, family planning, and parenting. This can be accomplished by placing posters and brochures on these issues in waiting rooms to indicate receptiveness of staff members to discuss sexual matters and by introducing such matters in regular discussions with patients. Sexually active patients should be educated about contraception and advised of the consequences of not using protection in terms of sexually transmitted diseases and unwanted pregnancies. In-service training may be provided for mental health staff who do not feel competent to provide family planning advice (Coverdale & Grunebaum, 1998). Parenting issues may be addressed through family intervention involving the patient's partner and parenting classes.

Posttraumatic Stress Disorder

Because the substantial rates of trauma exposure and increased risk for PTSD have only recently been identified in individuals with schizophrenia, empirically validated treatment for this comorbid disorder is still in the early stage of development. Researchers who have started to consider appropriate and effective modes of intervention have suggested that psychoeducation regarding what constitutes a traumatic event, common symptoms associated with the disorder, and what steps to take if PTSD is suspected is an initial step in treating individuals with schizophrenia who may meet diagnostic criteria for the disorder (Mueser & Rosenberg, 2001). This type of education should be provided to both patients and mental health care providers.

Traditional methods for treating PTSD may be adapted for persons with schizophrenia. Exposure-based methods (e.g., imaginal exposure) may need to be titrated to avoid unduly stressful effects on clients. Cognitive restructuring may be useful, but it must progress slowly due to the cognitive impairments that are characteristic of schizophrenia. Clinicians treating PTSD in patients with schizophrenia need to be mindful of the multiproblem nature of the illness, limited coping resources, and presence of risk factors such as lower level of education, housing instability, and poor social judgment that may leave individuals more vulnerable to retraumatization (Mueser & Rosenberg, 2001). An alternative to the focus on treating PTSD symptoms in persons with schizophrenia is to take a broader approach to addressing the consequences of trauma in this population, including skills deficits and poor self-esteem (Harris, 1998).

CASE EXAMPLE

The following case example is provided to illustrate the assessment and treatment approaches described in this chapter.

Twenty-four-year old Mr. N, who resides with his mother, younger sister, and two nephews in rural Vermont, recently returned home from his third hospitalization following a suicide attempt. He was diagnosed with schizophrenia at age 19 after suffering a psychotic break during his sophomore year of college. His compliance with medications and psychotherapy were inconsistent for the next 5 years, during which time he spent most days isolated in his bedroom watching television and smoking cigarettes.

Mr. N's aftercare following his most recent hospitalization was largely planned by members of an assertive community treatment (ACT) team, which included a psychiatrist, a case manager, a vocational specialist, a therapist, and a nurse, at the local mental health center. Members of the team performed an intake that included lengthy interviews with Mr. N and his mother, consultation with a vocational specialist to assess job interests and motivation for work, and a meeting with a case manager. After Mr. N's core symptomatology, which included mild thought disorder, apathy, and a low level of paranoia was assessed, his ability to perform basic life skills (such as taking care of health, appearance, and personal belongings), substance use issues, and social skills were evaluated by using standardized clinical instruments and information from the intake interviews. Mr. N described occasional alcohol and marijuana use, but his mother reported that he used both substances frequently, and she suggested that his substance abuse contributed to relapses and rehospitalizations. He was referred for neuropsychological testing following his complaints of forgetfulness, distractibility, and confusion.

After the intake evaluation, Mr. N, with the help of the vocational specialist, applied for and obtained a job sorting and stocking produce at a local supermarket. He began by working 16 hours per week. The ACT team decided that he should spend one day each week at the community mental health center attending skills training groups, including illness self-management and anger management, as well as participating in a "persuasion group" designed to create motivation to address substance abuse as a problem (Mueser & Noordsy, 1996). He was also scheduled for weekly meetings with his case manager, which usually took place in the community, and his therapist. Mr. N also met with his psychiatrist once a month for evaluation of his medication regimen.

Because of his history of noncompliance with medications, Mr. N was expected to bring his medication bottles to his weekly meetings with his case manager in order to conduct a pill count. He also obtained assistance from his case manager with money management and budgeting, and he submitted to random urine drug screens if he appeared to be abusing substances. Mr. N's therapist used cognitive-behavioral techniques to challenge his persistent persecutory delusions. The therapist also used motivational interviewing strategies to help Mr. N identify personal goals to work toward, and to evaluate whether taking medication would be helpful in achieving those those goals (Kemp, Kirov, Everitt, Hayward, & David, 1998). Weekly sessions were also used to reinforce material and skills taught in the illness management and anger management groups. Mr. N's therapist periodically administered the Beck Depression Inventory (second edition) given his chronic, baseline level of depression and history of suicide attempts.

Mr. N's treatment plan was reviewed formally by the ACT team every 3 months. His ability to manage his paranoia at his job slowly improved over time, and he agreed to gradual increases in his work hours up to 24 per week. Given Mr. N's difficulty coping with his young nephews' mischievous behavior, he began, with the help of his case manager, to work on completing an application for a Section 8 certificate so that he could obtain his own apartment. His attendance at groups and weekly appointments remained somewhat inconsistent, prompting clinic staff to either directly provide transportation or to initiate phone call reminders prior to scheduled activities. Periodic evaluation of Mr. N's attitudes toward taking medications using the Rating of Medication Influences scale (Weiden et al., 1994) indicated low initial perception of benefit of taking medications and deference to medical authority as the reason for compliance. Over time, Mr. N's adherence to medication improved as he began to see it as a tool for helping him achieve the goal of completing his undergraduate degree.

SUMMARY

Schizophrenia is a multifaceted, heterogeneous psychiatric illness that affects practically all aspects of the individuals' lives, from the ability to hold a conversation to the ability to hold a job. The diagnostic criteria for schizophrenia include a range of emotional, cognitive, and

TABLE 11.1 Summary List of Assessment Domains, Assessment Strategies, and Treatment Approaches

Important domains for assessment	Assessment tools and strategies	Treatment approaches
Core clinical symptoms		
Positive and negative symptoms	Brief Psychiatric Rating Scale Scale for the Assessment of Positive Symptoms Scale for the Assessment of Negative Symptoms Positive and Negative Syndrome Scale	Cognitive-behavioral therapy
Cognitive impairment	Trail Making Test Digit Span subtest of Wechsler Adult Intelligence Scale–III Letter–Number Sequencing subtest of WAIS–III Wisconsin Card Sorting Test Tower Tests Continuous Performance Tests California Verbal Learning Test Logical Memory Subtest of Wechsler Memory Scales–III	Integrated psychological therapy Cognitive enhancement therapy
Commonly associated features		
Medication noncompliance	Blood and urine tests Pill counts Rating of Medication Influences scale Drug Attitudes Inventory Van Putten and May Neuroleptic Dysphoria Scale	Psychoeductaion Behavioral tailoring Compliance therapy
Social and role functioning	Role play Naturalistic observation of functioning Social Behavior Schedule Katz Adjustment Scale Social Adjustment Scale–II Life Skills Profile Social Functioning Scale Social–Adaptive Functioning Evaluation Independent Living Skills Survey Role Play Task Response Generation Task	Assertive community treatment Social skills training
Family environment	Relatives Assessment Interview Family Questionnaire Information questionnaire—Relative Version Knowledge about Schizophrenia Interview The Knowledge Questionnaire Patient Rejection Scale	Supportive family therapy Behavioral family therapy
Sexuality and family planning	Interview regarding current sexual practices, knowledge about contraception, desire for children	Psychoeducation

TABLE 11.1 *(continued)*

Important domains for assessment	Assessment tools and strategies	Treatment approaches
Comorbid psychiatric conditions		
Mood and anxiety disorders	Beck Depression Inventory Beck Anxiety Inventory	Cognitive-behavioral therapy
Substance abuse	Dartmouth Assessment of Lifestyle Instrument Clinician's rating scales for alcohol use disorder and drug use disorder Random urine drug screens	Integrated dual diagnosis treatment
Posttraumatic stress disorder	Trauma History Questionnaire PTSD Checklist Clinician-Administered PTSD Scale	Psychoeducation Cognitive restructuring
Occupational functioning	Evaluation of work history, interest in work, predictors of work, and ability to manage money	Assertive community treatment

behavioral dysfunctions that fall into two broad categories: positive and negative symptoms. Additionally, establishment of the diagnosis requires "marked" impairment in the social or occupational domains. Many individuals with schizophrenia struggle with a number of commonly associated problems, such as impaired cognitive functioning, unstable housing status, inadequate attention to medical conditions, and increased risk for contraction of infectious diseases, which may occur as a direct or indirect result of the characteristic features of the illness. Comorbid psychiatric disorders including substance use and posttraumatic stress disorder often complicate the clinical picture. Management of the unique presentation of the illness in a given individual therefore involves assessment and treatment not only of core symptoms but also of the entire person. A summary list of the important domains for assessment, suggested assessment tools and strategies, and recommended treatment approaches discussed in this chapter are presented in Table 11.1.

The empirical literature suggests that the best treatment for individuals with schizophrenia involves a combination of pharmacotherapy and a number of the psychosocial interventions described in this chapter. Given the heterogeneous nature of the illness, mental health professionals should strive to design interventions that are tailored to compensate for individual deficits and capitalize on clients' strengths. Appropriate combinations of pharmacologic and psychosocial treatments based on thorough assessment of core symptoms, impairments in social and role functioning, associated problems, and common comorbid disorders can substantially reduce the burden imposed by schizophrenia and enable countless individuals with the illness to enjoy considerable improvements in positive functioning and overall well-being.

REFERENCES

Allness, D. J., & Knoedler, W. H. (1998). *The PACT model of community-based treatment for persons with severe and persistent mental illness: A manual for PACT start-up.* Arlington, VA: National Alliance for the Mentally Ill.

American Psychiatric Association. (1994). *Diagnostic and statistical manual of mental disorders* (4th ed.). Washington, DC: Author.

Anderson, C. M., Reiss, D. J., & Hogarty, G. E. (1986). *Schizophrenia and the family: A practitioner's guide to psychoeducation and management.* New York: Guilford Press.

Andreasen, N. C. (1982). Negative symptoms in schizophrenia: Definition and reliability. *Archives of General Psychiatry, 39,* 784–788.

Andreasen, N. C. (1984). *The scale for the assessment of positive symptoms (SAPS).* Iowa City: University of Iowa.

Anthony, W. A. (1993). Recovery from mental illness: The guiding vision of the mental health service system in the 1990s. *Psychosocial Rehabilitation Journal, 16,* 11–23.

Arns, P. G., & Linney, J. A. (1995). Relating functional skills of severely mentally ill clients to subjective and societal benefits. *Psychiatric Services, 46,* 260–265.

Aro, S., Aro, H., & Keskimäki, I. (1995). Socio-economic mobility among patients with schizophrenia or major affective disorder: A 17-year retrospective follow-up. *British Journal of Psychiatry, 166,* 759–767.

Barrowclough, C., & Tarrier, N. (1992). *Families of schizophrenic patients: Cognitive behavioral intervention.* London: Chapman & Hall.

Beck, A. T., & Steer, R. A. (1990). *Manual for the Beck Anxiety Inventory.* San Antonio, TX: Psychological Corporation.

Beck, A. T., Steer, R. A., & Brown, G. K. (1996). *Beck Depression Inventory Manual* (2nd. ed.). San Antonio, TX: Psychological Corporation.

Becker, D. R., & Drake, R. E. (1994). Individual placement and Support: A community mental health center approach to vocational rehabilitation. *Community Mental Health Journal, 30,* 193–205.

Bellack, A. S., Mueser, K. T., Gingerich, S., & Agresta, J. (1997). *Social skills training for schizophrenia: A step-by-step guide.* New York: Guilford Press.

Bellack, A. S., Sayers, M. D., Mueser, K. T., & Bennett, M. (1994). Evaluation of social problem solving in schizophrenia. *Journal of Abnormal Psychology, 103,* 371–378.

Benton, M., K., & Schroeder, H. E. (1990). Social skills training with schizophrenics: A meta-analytic evaluation. *Journal of Consulting and Clinical Psychology, 58,* 741–747.

Berg, E. A. (1948). A simple objective technique for measuring flexibility in thinking. *Journal of General Psychology, 39,* 15–22.

Birchwood, M., & Smith, J. (1987). *Schizophrenia and the family.* Baltimore: Johns Hopkins University Press.

Birchwood, M., Smith, J., Cochrane, R., Wetton, S., & Copestake, S. (1990). The Social Functioning Scale: The development and validation of a new scale of social adjustment for use in family intervention programmes with schizophrenic patients. *British Journal of Psychiatry, 157,* 853–859.

Blake, D. D., Weathers, F. W., Nagy, L. M., Kaloupek, D. G., Klauminzer, G., Charney, D. S., & Keane, T. M. (1990). A clinician rating scale for assessing current and lifetime PTSD: The CAPS-1. *Behavior Therapist, 13,* 187–188.

Blanchard, E. B., Jones-Alexander, J., Buckley, T. C., & Forneris, C. A. (1996). Psychometric properties of the PTSD Checklist. *Behaviour Research and Therapy, 34,* 669–673.

Blanchard, J. J., & Panzarella, C. (1998). Affect and social functioning inschizophrenia. In K. T. Mueser & N. Tarrier (Eds.), *Handbook of social functioning in schizophrenia* (pp. 181–196). Boston: Allyn & Bacon.

Boczkowski, J. A., Zeichner, A., & DeSanto, N. (1985). Neuroleptic compliance among chronic schizophrenic outpatients: An intervention outcome report. *Journal of Consulting and Clinical Psychology, 53,* 666–671.

Bond, G. R. (1992). Vocational rehabilitation. In R. P. Liberman (Ed.), *Handbook of psychiatric rehabilitation* (pp. 244–275). New York: Macmillan.

Bond, G. R., Drake, R. E., Mueser, K. T., & Latimer, E. (2001). Assertive community treatment for people with severe mental illness: Critical ingredients and impact on clients. *Disease Management and Health Outcomes, 9,* 141–159.

Bowen, L., Wallace, C. J., Glynn, S. M., Nuechterlein, K. H., Lutzker, J. R., & Keuhnel, T. G. (1994). *Journal of Psychiatric Research, 28,* 289–301.

Breier, A., Schreiber, J. L., Dyer, J., & Pickar, D. (1991). National Institute of Mental Health longitudinal study of chronic schizophrenia. *Archives of General Psychiatry, 48,* 239–246.

Brekke, J. S., Raine, A., Ansel, M., Lencz, T., & Bird, L. (1997). Neuropsychological and psychophysiological correlates of psychosocial functioning in schizophrenia. *Schizophrenia Bulletin, 23,* 19–28.

Brenner, H. D., Hodel, B., Roder, V., & Corrigan, P. (1992). Treatment of cognitive dysfunctions and behavioral deficits in schizophrenia. *Schizophrenia Bulletin, 18,* 21–26.

Brenner, H. D., Roder, V., Hodel, B., Kienzle, N., Reed, D., & Liberman, R. P. (1994). *Integrated psychological therapy for schizophrenic patients (IPT).* Seattle, WA: Hogrefe & Huber.

Brewer, W. J., Edwards, J., Anderson, V., Robinson, R., & Pantelis, C. (1996). Neuropsychological, olfactory, and hygeine deficits in men with negative symptom schizophrenia. *Biological Psychiatry, 40,* 1021–1031.

Bruce, M. L., Takeuchi, D. T. & Leaf, P. J. (1991). Poverty and psychiatric status: Longitudinal evidence from the New Haven epidemiologic catchment area study. *Archives of General Psychiatry, 48,* 470–474.

Budd, R. J., & Hughes, I. C. T. (1997). What do relatives of people with schizophrenia find helpful about family intervention? *Schizophrenia Bulletin, 23,* 341–347.

Butzlaff, R. L., & Hooley, J. M. (1998). Expressed emotion and psychiatric relapse. *Archives of General Psychiatry, 55,* 547–552.

Carey, K. B. (1996). Substance use reduction in the context of outpatient psychiatric treatment: A collaborative, motivational, harm reduction approach. *Community Mental Health Journal, 32*(3), 291–306.

Carling, P. J. (1995). *Return to community: Building support systems for people with psychiatric disabilities.* New York: Guilford Press.

Cascardi, M., Mueser, K. T., DeGirolomo, J., & Murrin, M. (1996). Physical aggression against psychiatric inpatients by family members and partners: A descriptive study. *Psychiatric Services, 47,* 531–533.

Chambon, O., & Marie-Cardine, M. (1998). An evaluation of social skills training modules with schizophrenia inpatients in France. *International Review of Psychiatry, 10,* 26–29.

Clare, L., & Birchwood, M. (1998). Social adjustment of patients living at home. In K. T. Mueser & N. Tarrier (Eds.), *Handbook of social functioning in schizophrenia* (pp. 79–98). Boston: Allyn & Bacon.

Cook, J. A., Pickett, S. A., Fitzgibbon, G., Jonikas, J. A., & Cohler, J. J. (1996). Rehabilitation services for persons with schizophrenia. *Psychiatric Annals, 26,* 97–104.

Cook, J. A., & Razzano, L. (2000). Vocational rehabilitation for persons with schizophrenia: Recent research and implications for practice. *Schizophrenia Bulletin, 26,* 87–103.

Corrigan, P. W., Liberman, R. P., & Engel, J. D. (1990). From noncompliance to collaboration in the treatment of schizophrenia. *Hospital and Community Psychiatry, 41,* 1203–1211.

Corrigan, P. W., Wallace, C. J., Schade, M. L., & Green, M. F. (1994). Learning medication self-management skills in schizophrenia: Relationships with cognitive deficits and psychiatric symptoms. *Behavior Therapy, 25,* 5–15.

Coverdale, J. H., & Grunebaum, H. (1998). Sexuality and family planning. In K. T. Mueser & N. Tarrier (Eds.), *Handbook of social functioning in schizophrenia* (pp. 224–237). Boston: Allyn & Bacon.

Craine, L. S., Henson, C. E., Colliver, J. A., & MacLean, D. G. (1988). Prevalence of a history of sexual abuse among female psychiatric patients in a state hospital system. *Hospital and Community Psychiatry, 39,* 300–304.

Cramer, J. A., & Rosenheck, R. (1999). Enhancing medication compliance for people with serious mental illness. *Journal of Nervous and Mental Disease, 187,* 53–55.

Cuffel, B. J. (1996). Comorbid substance use disorder: Prevalence, patterns of use, and course. In R. E. Drake & K. T. Mueser (Eds.), *Dual diagnosis of major mental illness and substance abuse: Vol. 2. Recent research and clinical implications: New directions for mental health services* (pp. 93–105). San Francisco: Jossey-Bass.

Curson, D. A., Patel, M., Liddle, P. F., & Barnes, T. R. E. (1988). Psychiatric morbidity of a long-stay hospital population with chronic schizophrenia and implications for future community care. *British Medical Journal, 297,* 819–822.

Cyr, M., Toupin, J., Lesage, A. D., & Valiquette, C. A. M. (1994). Assessment of independent living skills for psychotic patients. *Journal of Nervous and Mental Disease, 182,* 91–97.

Davidson, L., Lambert, S., & McGlashan, T. H. (1998). Psychotherapeutic and cognitive-behavioral treatments for schizophrenia: Developing a disorder-specific form of psychotherapy for persons with psychosis. In C. Perris & P. D. McGorry (Eds.), *Cognitive psychotherapy of psychotic and personality disorders.* New York: Wiley.

Davidson, L., Stayner, D., & Haglund, K. E. (1998). Phenomenological perspectives on the social functioning of people with schizophrenia. In K. T. Mueser & N. Tarrier (Eds.), *Handbook of social functioning in schizophrenia* (pp. 66–78). Boston: Allyn & Bacon.

Deegan, P. E. (1988). Recovery: The lived experience of rehabilitation. *Psychosocial Rehabilitation Journal, 11,* 11–19.

Delis, D. C., Kramer, J. H., Kaplan, E., & Ober, B. A. (1987). *California Verbal Learning Test: Adult Version.* San Antonio, TX: Psychological Corporation.

Dilk, M. N., & Bond, G. R. (1996). Meta-analytic evaluation of skills training research for individuals with severe mental illness. *Journal of Consulting and Clinical Psychology, 64,* 337–346.

Dixon, L., Adams, C., & Lucksted, A. (2000). Update on family psychoeducation for schizophrenia. *Schizophrenia Bulletin, 26,* 5–20.

Docherty, N. M., Hawkins, K. A., Hoffman, R. E., Quinlan, D. M., Rakfeldt, J., & Sledge, W. H. (1996). Working memory, attention, and communication disturbances in schizophrenia. *Journal of Abnormal Psychology, 105,* 212–219.

Dohrenwend, B. R., Levav, I., Shrout, P. E., Schwartz, S., Naveh, G., Link, B. G., Skodol, A. E., & Stueve, A. (1992). Socioeconomic status and psychiatric disorders: The causation-selection issue. *Science, 255,* 946–952.

Douglas, M. S., & Mueser, K. T. (1990). Teaching conflict resolution skills to the chronically mentally ill. *Behavior Modification, 14,* 519–547.

Drake, R. E., Becker, D. R., Biesanz, J. C., Torrey, W. C., McHugo, G. J., & Wyzik, P. F. (1994). Rehabilitation day treatment vs. supported employment: I. Vocational outcomes. *Community Mental Health Journal, 30,* 519–532.

Drake, R. E., Becker, D. R., Clark, R. E., & Mueser, K. T. (1999). Research on the individual placement and support model of supported employment. *Psychiatric Quarterly, 70,* 289–301.

Drake, R. E., & Brunette, M. F. (1998). Complications of severe mental illness related to alcohol and other drug use disorders. In: M. Galanter (Ed.), *Recent developments in alcoholism: Vol. XIV. Consequences of alcoholism* (pp. 285–299). New York: Plenum.

Drake, R. E., McHugo, G. J., Bebout, R. R., Becker, D. R., Harris, M., Bond, G. R., & Quimby, E. (1999). A randomized clinical trial of supported employment for inner-city patients with severe mental disorders. *Archives of General Psychiatry, 56,* 627–633.

Drake, R. E., McHugo, G. J., Becker, D. R., Anthony, W. A., & Clark, R. E. (1996). The New Hampshire study of supported employment for people with severe mental illness. *Journal of Consulting and Clinical Psychology, 64,* 391–399.

Drake, R. E., Mercer-McFadden, C., Mueser, K. T., McHugo, G. J., & Bond, G. R. (1998). Review of integrated mental health and substance abuse treatment for patients with dual disorders. *Schizophrenia Bulletin, 24,* 589–608.

Drake, R. E., & Mueser, K. T. (2000). Psychosocial approaches to dual diagnosis. *Schizophrenia Bulletin, 26,* 105–118.

Eaton, W. W. (1975). Marital status and schizophrenia. *Acta Psychiatrica Scandinavica, 52,* 320–329.

Eckman, T. A., Wirshing, W. C., Marder, S. R., Liberman, R. P., Johnston-Cronk, K., Zimmerman, K., & Mintz, J. (1992). Technique for training schizophrenic patients in illness self-management: A controlled trial. *American Journal of Psychiatry, 149,* 1549–1555.

Falloon, I. R. H. (1990). Behavioral family therapy with schizophrenic disorders. In M. I. Herz, S. J. Keith, & J. P. Docherty (Eds.), *Handbook of schizophrenia: Vol. 4. Psychosocial treatment of schizophrenia* (pp. 135–151). New York: Elsevier Science.

Falloon, I. R. H., Boyd, J. L., & McGill, C. W. (1984). *Family care of schizophrenia: A problem-solving approach to the treatment of mental illness.* New York: Guilford Press.

Fenton, W. S., Blyler, C. R., & Heinssen, R. K. (1997). Determinants of medication compliance in schizophrenia: Empirical and clinical findings. *Schizophrenia Bulletin, 23*, 637–651.

Fox, J. W. (1990). Social class, mental illness, and social mobility: The social selection-drift hypothesis for serious mental illness. *Journal of Health and Social Behavior, 31*, 344–353.

Garety, P. A., Fowler, D., & Kuipers, E. (2000). Cognitive-behavioral therapy for medication-resistant symptoms. *Schizophrenia Bulletin, 26*, 73–86.

Glosser, G., & Goodglass, H. (1990). Disorders in executive control functions among aphasic and other brain-damaged patients. *Journal of Clinical and Experimental Neuropsychology, 12*, 485–501.

Glynn, S. M. (1998). Psychopathology and social functioning in schizophrenia. In K. T. Mueser & N. Tarrier (Eds.), *Handbook of social functioning in schizophrenia* (pp. 66–78). Boston: Allyn & Bacon.

Goodman, L. A., Rosenberg, S. D., Mueser, K. T., & Drake, R. E. (1997). Physical and sexual assault history in women with serious mental illness: Prevalence, impact, treatment, and future directions. *Schizophrenia Bulletin, 23*, 685–696.

Green, B. L. (1996). Trauma History Questionnaire (Self-report). In B. H. Stamm (Ed.), *Measurement of stress, trauma, and adaptation* (pp. 366–368). Lutherville, MD: Sidran.

Green, M. F. (1996). What are the functional consequences of neurocognitive deficits in schizophrenia? *American Journal of Psychiatry, 153*, 321–330.

Green, M. F., Kern, R. S., Braff, D. L., & Mintz, J. (2000). Neurocognitive deficits and functional outcome in schizophrenia: Are we measuring the "Right Stuff"? *Schizophrenia Bulletin, 26*, 119–136.

Harris, M. (1998). *Trauma Recovery and Empowerment: A Clinician's Guide for Working with Women in Groups*. New York: Free Press.

Harvey, P. D., Davidson, M., Mueser, K. T., Parrella, M., White, L., & Powchik, P. (1997). Social-Adaptive Functioning Evaluation (SAFE): A rating scale for geriatric psychiatric patients. *Schizophrenia Bulletin, 23*, 131–145.

Hatfield, A. B., & Lefley, H. P. (Eds.). (1987). *Families of the mentally ill: Coping and adaptation*. New York: Guilford Press.

Hatfield, A. B., & Lefley, H. P. (1993). *Surviving mental illness: Stress, coping, and adaptation*. New York: Guilford Press.

Heaton, R. K. (1981). *Wisconsin Cart Sorting Test Manual*. Odessa, FL: Psychological Assessment Resources.

Heinssen, R. K., Liberman, R. P., & Kopelowicz, A. (2000). Psychosocial skills training for schizophrenia: Lessons from the laboratory. *Schizophrenia Bulletin, 26*, 21–46.

Herz, M. I. (1996). Psychosocial treatment. *Psychiatric Annals, 26*, 531–535.

Hogan, T. P., Awad, A. G., & Eastwood, R. (1983). A self-report scale predictive of drug compliance in schizophrenics: Reliability and discriminative validity. *Psychological Medicine, 13*, 177–183.

Hogarty, G. E., & Flesher, S. (1999a). Developmental theory for a cognitive enhancement therapy of schizophrenia. *Schizophrenia Bulletin, 25*, 677–692.

Hogarty, G. E., & Flesher, S. (1999b). Practical principles of cognitive enhancement therapy for schizophrenia. *Schizophrenia Bulletin, 25*, 693–708.

Hollingshead, A. B., & Redlich, F. C. (1958). *Social class and mental illness: A community study*. New York: Wiley.

Jablensky, A. (1999). Schizophrenia: Epidemiology. *Current Opinion in Psychiatry, 12*, 19–28.

Jonsson, H., & Nyman, A. K. (1991). Predicting long-term outcome in schizophrenia. *Acta Psychiatrica Scandinavica, 83*, 342–346.

Katz, M. M., & Lyerly, S. B. (1963). Methosa for measuring adjustment and social behavior in the community: 1. Rationale, description, descriminative validity and scale development. *Psychological Reports, 13*, 503–535.

Kay, S. R., Fiszbein, A., & Opler, L. A. (1987). The positive and negative symptom scale (PANSS) for schizophrenia. *Schizophrenia Bulletin, 13*, 261–276.

Keefe, R., S., E., Bollini, A. M., & Silva, S. G. (1999). Do novel antipsychotics improve cognition? A report of a meta-analysis. *Psychiatric Annals, 29*, 623–629.

Keith, S. J., Regier, D. A., & Rae, D. S. (1991). Schizophrenic disorders. In L. N. Robins & D. A. Regier (Eds.), *Psychiatric disorders in America: The Epidemiologic Catchment Area Study* (pp. 33–52). New York: Free Press.

Kemp, R., Hayward, P., Applewaite, G., Everitt, B., & David, A. (1996). Compliance therapy in psychotic patinets: Randomized controlled trial. *British Medical Journal, 312,* 345–349.

Kemp, R., Kirov, G., Everitt, B., Hayward, P., & David, A. (1998). Randomised controlled trial of compliance therapy: 18-month follow-up. *British Journal of Psychiatry, 173,* 271–272.

Kern, R. S., Green, M. F., & Satz, P. (1992). Neuropsychological predictors of skills training for chronic psychiatric patients. *Psychiatry Research, 43,* 223–230.

Kessler, R. C., Foster, C. L., Saunders, W. B., & Stang, P. E. (1995). Social consequences of psychiatric disorders: I. Educational attainment. *American Journal of Psychiatry, 152,* 1026–1032.

Khantzian, E.J. (1997). The self-medication hypothesis of substance use disorders: A reconsideration and recent applications. *Harvard Review of Psychiatry, 4,* 231–244.

Kreisman, D., Blumenthal, R., Borenstein, M., Woerner, M., Kane, J., Rifkin, A., & Reardon, G. (1988). Family attitudes and patient social adjustment in a longitudinal study of outpatient schizophrenics receiving low-dose neuroleptics: The family's view. *Psychiatry, 51,* 3–13.

Kuipers, L., Leff, J., & Lam, D. (1992). *Family work for schizophrenia: A practical guide.* London: Gaskell.

Leff, J., & Vaughn, C. (1985). *Expressed emotion in families: Its significance for mental illness.* New York: Guilford Press.

Lezak, M. D. (1995). *Neuropsychological assessment* (3rd ed.). New York: Oxford University Press.

Liberman, R. P., DeRisi, W. J., & Mueser, K. T. (Eds.). (1989). *Social skills training for psychiatric patients.* New York: Pergamon.

Liberman, R. P., Mueser, K., Wallace, C. J., Jacobs, H. E., Eckman, T., & Massel, H. K. (1986). Training skills in the psychiatrically disabled: Learning coping and competence. *Schizophrenia Bulletin, 12,* 631–647.

Liberman, R. P., Wallace, C. J., Blackwell, G., Kopelowicz, A., Vaccaro, J. V., & Mintz, J. (1998). Skills training versus psychosocial occupational therapy for persons with persistent schizophrenia. *American Journal of Psychiatry, 155,* 1087–1091.

Liberman, R. P., Wallace, C. J., Blackwell, G., MacKain, S., & Eckman, T. A. (1992). Training social and independent living skills: Applications and impact in chronic schizophrenia. In J. Cottraux, P. Legeron, & E. Mollard (Eds.), *Which psychotherapies in year 2000?* (pp. 65–90). Amsterdam: Swets & Zeitlinger.

Liddle, P. F. (1987). Schizophrenic syndromes, cognitive performance and neurological dysfunction. *Psychological Medicine, 17,* 49–57.

Linszen, D. H., Dingemans, P. M., Nugter, M. A., Van der Does, A. J. W., Scholte, W. F., & Lenoir, M. A. (1997). Patient attributes and expressed emotion as risk factors for psychotic relapse. *Schizophrenia Bulletin, 23,* 119–130.

Lukoff, D., Nuechterlein, K. H., & Ventura, J. (1986). Manual for expanded Brief Psychiatric Rating Scale (BPRS). *Schizophrenia Bulletin, 12,* 594–602.

Marder, S. R., Wirshing, W. C., Mintz, J., McKenzie, J., Johnston, K., Eckman, T. A., Lebell, M., Zimmerman, K., & Liberman, R. P. (1996). Two-year outcome of social skills training and group psychotherapy for outpatients with schizophrenia. *American Journal of Psychiatry, 153,* 1585–1592.

McEvoy, J. P., Hartman, M., Gottlieb, D., Godwin, S., Apperson, L. J., & Wilson, W. (1996). Common sense, insight, and neuropsychological test performance in schizophrenia patients. *Schizophrenia Bulletin, 22,* 635–641.

McFarlane, W. R., Deakins, S. M., Gingerich, S. L., Dunne, E., Horan, B., & Newmark, M. (1991). *Multiple-family psychoeducational group treatment manual.* New York: New York State Psychiatric Institute.

McGill, C. W., Falloon, I. R. H., Boyd, J. L., & Wood-Siverio, C. (1983). Family educational intervention in the treatment of schizophrenia. *Hospital and Community Psychiatry, 34,* 934–938.

Miller, W. R., & Rollnick, S. (1991). *Motivational interviewing: Preparing people to change addictive behavior.* New York: Guilford Press.

Mueser, K. T., Becker, D. R., Torrey, W., Xie, H., Bond, G. R., Drake, R. E., & Bradley, J. D. (1997). Work and nonvocational domains of functioning in persons with severe mental illness: A longitudinal analysis. *Journal of Nervous and Mental Disease, 185,* 419–426.

Mueser, K. T., & Bellack, A. S. (1998). Social skills and social functioning. In K. T. Mueser & N. Tarrier (Eds.), *Handbook of social functioning in schizophrenia* (pp. 79–98). Boston: Allyn & Bacon.

Mueser, K. T., Bellack, A. S., Douglas, M. S., & Wade, J. H. (1991). Prediction of social skill acquisition in schizophrenic and major affective disorder patients from memory and symptomatology. *Psychiatry Research, 37,* 281–296.

Mueser, K. T., Blanchard, J. J., & Bellack, A. S. (1995). Memory and social skill in schizophrenia: The role of gender. *Psychiatry Research, 57,* 141–153.

Mueser, K. T., & Bond, G. R. (2000). Psychosocial treatment approaches for schizophrenia. *Current Opinion in Psychiatry, 13,* 27–35.

Mueser, K. T., Bond, G. R., & Drake, R. E. (2001). Community-based treatment of schizophrenia and other severe mental disorders. *Medscape Mental Health (online journal), 6,* (http://www.medscape.com/medscape/psychiatry/journal/2001/v06.n01/mh3418.mues/).

Mueser, K. T., Bond, G. R., Drake, R. E., & Resnick, S. G. (1998). Models of community care for severe mental illness: A review of research on case management. *Schizophrenia Bulletin, 24,* 37–74.

Mueser, K. T., Curran, P. J., & McHugo, G. J. (1997). Factor structure of the Brief Psychiatric Rating Scale in schizophrenia. *Psychological Assessment, 9,* 196–204.

Mueser, K. T., Doonan, R., Penn, D. L., Blanchard, J. J., Bellack, A. S., Nishith, P., & DeLeon, J. (1996). Emotion recognition and social competence in chronic schizophrenia. *Journal of Abnormal Psychology, 105,* 271–275.

Mueser, K. T., Drake, R. E., Clark, R. E., McHugo, G. J., Mercer-McFadden, C., & Ackerson, T. (1995). *Toolkit for evaluating substance abuse in persons with severe mental illness.* Cambridge, MA: Evaluation Center at Human Services Research Institute.

Mueser, K. T., Drake, R. E., & Noordsy, D. L. (1998). Integrated mental health and substance abuse treatment for severe psychiatric disorders. *Practical Psychiatry and Behavioral Health, 4,* 129–139.

Mueser, K. T., Drake, R. E., & Wallach, M. A. (1998). Dual diagnosis: A review of etiological theories. *Addictive Behaviors, 23,* 717–734.

Mueser, K. T., & Glynn, S. M. (1999). *Behavioral family therapy for psychiatric disorders.* Oakland, CA: New Harbinger.

Mueser, K. T., Goodman, L. B., Trumbetta, S. L., Rosenberg, S. D., Osher, F. C., Vidaver, R., Auciello, P., & Foy, D. W. (1998). Trauma and posttraumatic stress disorder in severe mental illness. *Journal of Consulting and Clinical Psychology, 66,* 493–499.

Mueser, K. T., & Noordsy, D. L. (1996). Group treatment for dually diagnosed clients. In R. E. Drake & K. T. Mueser (Eds.), *New directions in mental health services: Vol. 70. Dual diagnosis of major mental illness and substance abuse disorder II: Recent research and clinical implications* (pp. 33–51). San Francisco: Jossey-Bass.

Mueser, K. T., & Rosenberg, S. D. (2001). Treatment of PTSD in persons with severe mental illness. In J. P. Wilson, M. J. Friedman, & J. D. Lindy (Eds.), *Treating psychological trauma and PTSD* (pp. 354–382). New York: Guilford Press.

Mueser, K. T., Salyers, M. P., Rosenberg, S. D., Ford, J. D., Fox, L., & Carty. P. (2001). A psychometric evaluation of trauma and PTSD assessments in persons with severe mental illness. *Psychological Assessment, 13,* 110–117.

Mueser, K. T., & Sayers, M. D. (1992). Social skills assessment. In D. J. Kavanagh (Ed.), *Schizophrenia: An overview and practical handbook* (pp. 182–205). New York: Chapman & Hall.

Mueser, K. T., Sengupta, A., Schooler, N. R., Bellack, A. S., Xie, H., Glick, I. D., & Keith, S. J. (2001). Family treatment and medication dosage reduction in schizophrenia: Effects on patient social functioning, family attitudes, and burden. *Journal of Consulting and Clinical Psychology, 69,* 3–12.

Mueser, K. T., Valentiner, D. P., & Agresta, J. (1997). Coping with negative symptoms of schizophrenia: Patient and family perspectives. *Schizophrenia Bulletin, 23,* 329–339.

Mueser, K. T., Yarnold, P. R., Rosenberg, S. D., Swett, C., Miles, K. M., & Hill, D. (2000). Substance use disorder in hospitalized severly mentally ill psychiatric patients: Prevalence, correlates, and subgroups. *Schizophrenia Bulletin, 26,* 179–192.

Munk-Jørgensen, P. (1987). First-admission rates and marital status of schizophrenics. *Acta Psychiatrica Scandinavica, 76,* 210–216.

Nuechterlein, K. H. (1991). Vigilance in schizophrenia and related disorders. In H. A. Nasrallah (Series Ed.) & S. R. Steinhauer, J. H. Gruzelier, & J. Zubin (Vol. Eds.), *Handbook of schizophrenia: Vol. 5. Neuropsychology, psychophysiology and information processing* (pp. 397–433). Amsterdam: Elsevier.

Nuechterlein, K. H., Dawson, M. E., Ventura, J., Fogelson, D., Gitlin, M., & Mintz, J. (1990). Testing vulnerability models: Stability of potential vulnerability indicators across clinical state. In H. Hafner & W. F. Gattaz (Eds.), *Search for the causes of schizophrenia* (Vol. 2, pp. 177–191). Berlin: Springer-Verlag.

Overall, G., & Gorham, D. (1962). The Brief Psychiatric Rating Scale. *Psychological Reports, 10,* 799–812.

Peen, J., & Dekker, J. (1997). Admission rates for schizophrenia in The Netherlands: An urban/rural comparison. *Acta Psychiatrica Scandinavica, 96,* 301–305.

Penn, D. L., Corrigan, P. W., & Racenstein, J. M. (1998). Cognitive factors and social adjustment in schizophrenia. In K. T. Mueser & N. Tarrier (Eds.), *Handbook of social functioning in schizophrenia* (pp. 213–223). Boston: Allyn & Bacon.

Penn, D. L., & Mueser, K. T. (1996). Research update on the psychosocial treatment of schizophrenia. *American Journal of Psychiatry, 153,* 607–617.

Penn, D. L., Mueser, K. T., Spaulding, W., Hope, D. A., & Reed, D. (1995). Information processing and social competence in chronic schizophrenia. *Schizophrenia Bulletin, 21,* 269–281.

Pogue-Geile, M. F. (1989). The prognostic significance of negative symptoms in schizophrenia. *British Journal of Psychiatry* (Suppl. 7), 123–127.

Regier, D. A., Farmer, M. E., Rae, D. S., Locke, B. Z., Keith, S. J., Judd, L. J., & Goodwin, F. K. (1990). Comorbidity of mental disorders with alcohol and other drug abuse: Results from the Epidemiologic Catchment Area (ECA) study. *Journal of the American Medical Association, 264,* 2511–2518.

Reitan, R. M. (n.d.). *Instructions and procedures for administering the psychological test battery used at the Neuropsychology Laboratory, Indiana University Medical Center, Indianapolis, IN.* Unpublished manuscript.

Rosen, A., Hadzi-Pavlovic, D., & Parker, G. (1989). The Life Skills Profile: A measure assessing function and disability in schizophrenia. *Schizophrenia Bulletin, 15,* 325–337.

Rosenberg, S. D., Drake, R. E., Wolford, G. L., Mueser, K. T., Oxman, T. E., Vidaver, R. M., Carrieri, K., & Luckoor, R. (1998). Dartmouth Assessment of Lifestyle Instrument (DALI): A substance use disorder screen for people with severe mental illness. *American Journal of Psychiatry, 155,* 232–238.

Rosenberg, S. D., Goodman, L. A., Osher, F. C., Swartz, M., Essock, S. M., Butterfield, M. I., Constantine, N. T., Wolford, G. L., & Salyers, M. P. (2001). Prevalence of HIV, Hepatitis B and Hepatitis C in people with severe mental illness. *American Journal of Public Health, 91,* 31–37.

Roy, A. (Ed.) (1986). *Suicide.* Baltimore: Williams & Wilkins.

Saint-Cyr, J. A., & Taylor, A. E. (1992). The mobilization of procedural learning: The "key signature" of the basal ganglia. In L. R. Squire & N. Butters (Eds.), *Neuropsychology of memory* (2nd ed., pp. 188–202). New York: Guilford Press.

Salokangas, R. K. R. (1978). Socioeconomic development and schizophrenia. *Psychiatria Fennica,* 103–112.

Sayers, M. D., Bellack, A. S., Wade, J. H., Bennett, M. E., & Fong, P. (1995). An empirical method for assessing social problem solving in schizophrenia. *Behavior Modification, 19,* 267–289.

Sayers, S. L., Curran, P. J., & Mueser, K. T. (1996). Factor structure and construct validity of the Scale for the Assessment of Negative Symptoms. *Psychological Assessment, 8,* 269–280.

Saykin, A. J., Gur, R. C., Mozley, D., Mozley, L. H., Resnick, S. M., Kester, D. B., & Stafiniak, P.

(1991). Neuropsychological function in schizophrenia: Selective impairment in memory and learning. *Archives of General Psychiatry, 48,* 618–624.

Schooler, N., Hogarty, G., & Weissman, M. (1979). Social Adjustment Scale II (SAS-II). In W. A. Hargreaves, C. C. Atkisson, & J. E. Sorenson (Eds.), *Resource materials for community mental health program evaluations* (pp. 290–303). (DHEW Publication No. (ADM) 79-328.) Rockville, MD: National Institute of Mental Health.

Scott, J. E., & Lehman, A. F. (1998). Social functioning in the community. In K. T. Mueser & N. Tarrier (Eds.), *Handbook of social functioning in schizophrenia* (pp. 1–19). Boston: Allyn & Bacon.

Selten, J-P. C. J., Van Den Bosch, R. J., & Sijben, A. E. S. (1998). The subjective experience of negative symptoms. In X. F. Amador & A. S. David (Eds.), *Insight and psychosis* (pp. 78–90). New York: Oxford University Press.

Shallice, T. (1982). Specific impairments of planning. *Philosophical Transactions of the Royal Society of London, 298,* 199–209.

Silverstein, S. M., Schenkel, L. S., Valone, C., & Nuernberger, S. W. (1998). Cognitive deficits and psychiatric outcomes in schizophrenia. *Psychiatric Quarterly, 69,* 169–191.

Smith, T. E., Bellack, A. S., & Liberman, R. P. (1996). Social skills training for schizophrenia: Review and future directions. *Clinical Psychology Review, 16,* 599–617.

Smith, T. E., Hull, J. W., Goodman, M., Hedayat-Harris, A., Willson, D., Israel, L., & Munich, R. (1999). The relative influences of symptoms, insight, and neurocognition on social adjustment in schizophrenia and schizoaffective disorder. *Journal of Nervous and Mental Disease, 187,* 102–108.

Smith, T. E., Shea, M. T., Schooler, N. R., Levin, H., Deutsch, A., & Grabstein, E. (1995). Studies of schizophrenia: Personality traits in schizophrenia. *Psychiatry, 58,* 99–112.

Social Security Administration. (2001). *Social Security handbook: Your basic guide to the Social Security programs* (14th ed., SSA Publication No. 65-008). Baltimore: Author.

Spaulding, W. D., Reed, D., Sullivan, M., Richardson, C., & Weiler, M. (1999). Effects of cognitive treatment in psychiatric rehabilitation. *Schizophrenia Bulletin, 25,* 657–676.

Stein, L. I., & Santos, A. B. (1998). *Assertive community treatment of persons with severe mental illness.* New York: Norton.

Strauss, M. E. (1993). Relations of symptoms to cognitive deficits in schizophrenia. *Schizophrenia Bulletin, 19,* 215–231.

Suslow, T., & Arolt, V. (1997). Paranoid schizophrenia: Non-specificity of neuropsychological vulnerability markers. *Psychiatry Research, 72,* 103–114.

Switzer, G. E., Dew, M. A., Thompson, K., Goycoolea, J. M., Derricott, T., & Mullins, S. D. (1999). Posttraumatic stress disorder and service utilization among urban mental health center clients. *Journal of Traumatic Stress, 12,* 25–39.

Takei, N., Sham, P. C., O'Callaghan, E., Glover, G., & Murray, R. M. (1995). Schizophrenia: Increased risk associated with winter and city birth—a case-control study in 12 regions within England and Wales. *Journal of Epidemiology and Community Health, 49,* 106–109.

Tollefson, G. D. (1996). Cognitive function in schizophrenic patients. *Journal of Clinical Psychiatry, 57,* 31–39.

Torrey, E. F. (1995). *Surviving schizophrenia: A manual for families, consumers and providers* (3rd ed.). New York: HarperPerennial.

Torrey, E. F., Bowler, A. E., & Clark, K. (1997). Urban birth and residence as risk factors for psychoses: An analysis of 1880 data. *Schizophrenia Research, 25,* 169–176.

Torrey, W. C., Becker, D. R., & Drake, R. E. (1995). Rehabilitative day treatment vs. supported employment: II. Consumer, family and staff reactions to a program change. *Psychosocial Rehabilitation Journal, 18,* 67–75.

Van Putten, T., & May, P. R. A. (1978). Subjective response as a predictor of outcome in pharmacotherapy. *Archives of General Psychiatry, 35,* 477–480.

Wallace, C. J., Liberman, R. P., MacKain, S. J., Blackwell, G., & Eckman, T. A. (1992). Effectiveness and replicability of modules for teaching social and instrumental skills to the severely mentally ill. *American Journal of Psychiatry, 149,* 654–658.

Wallace, C. J., Liberman, R. P., Tauber, R., & Wallace, J. (2000). The Independent Living Skills Survey: A comprehensive measure of the community functioning of severely and persistently mentally ill individuals. *Schizophrenia Bulletin, 26,* 631–658.

Wechsler, D. (1997a). *Wechsler Adult Intelligence Scale—Third edition: Administration and scoring manual.* San Antonio, TX: Psychological Corporation.

Wechsler, D. (1997b). *Wechsler Memory Scale—Third Edition.* San Antonio, TX: Psychological Corporation.

Weiden, P., Dixon, L., Frances, A., Appelbaum, P., Haas, G., & Rapkin, B. (1991). Neuroleptic noncompliance in schizophrenia. In C. A. Tamminga & S. C. Schulz (Eds.), *Advances in neuropsychiatry and psychopharmacology: Schizophrenia research* (pp. 285–296). New York: Raven Press.

Weiden, P., Rapkin, B., Mott, T., Zygmut, D., Horvitz-Lennon, M., & Frances, A. (1994). Rating of Medication Influences (ROMI) Scale in schizophrenia. *Schizophrenia Bulletin, 20,* 297–307.

World Health Organization. (1992). *International classification of diseases* (10th ed.). Washington, DC: Author.

Wykes, T. (1998). Social functioning in residential and institutional settings. In K. T. Mueser & N. Tarrier (Eds.), *Handbook of social functioning in schizophrenia* (pp. 20–38). Boston: Allyn & Bacon.

Wykes, T., & Sturt, E. (1986). The measurement of social behaviour in psychiatric patients: An assessment of the reliability and validity of the S.S. schedule. *British Journal of Psychiatry, 148,* 1–11.

Zubin, J., & Spring, B. (1977). Vulnerability: A new view of schizophrenia. *Journal of Abnormal Psychology, 86,* 103–123.

12

Substance Use Disorders

Jalie A. Tucker
Rudy E. Vuchinich
James G. Murphy

OVERVIEW OF SUBSTANCE USE DISORDERS

Conceptions of and interventions for substance-related problems are evolving as research findings accrue and as political, economic, and social forces shape government drug policy and drug-related laws. The latter contextual forces are powerful, pervasive, and largely punitive, and they can heavily influence interactions with substance abusers in clinical settings. More so than many medical and mental health problems, substance abuse, particularly of illicit drugs, carries risks of loss of employment, child custody, driving or professional licenses; fines and imprisonment; and social stigmatization, in addition to whatever other substance-related personal, interpersonal, financial, and health problems the individual may be experiencing. Depending on the setting and the nature and goals of an intervention, coercive or punitive elements may exist throughout the clinical interaction and may affect assessment data collection. Even when legal involvement is absent, many clients are coerced or pressured into treatment by employers, family members, or friends. Many clients and some clinicians therefore understandably view the assessment and intervention process as more of an adversarial proceeding than as a collaborative partnership.

A key contextual issue for assessment quality is the extent to which adversarial elements can be neutralized and a partnership can be cultivated. This is not always possible, particularly in legal situations, but the potential to do so in other contexts is often greater than conventional views of substance abuse might suggest. Contrary to the commonly held belief that substance abusers generally lie about or deny their substance misuse and related problems, the accuracy of their reports tends to vary reliably with the consequences of reporting use and with other identifiable features of the assessment context (Babor, Stephens, & Marlatt, 1987; Vuchinich, Tucker, & Harllee, 1988). A major point of this chapter is that contextual features during data collection with substance abusers are influential determinants of assessment quality and utility, regardless of the assessment procedures employed and their quality as judged by psychometric standards.

The punitive consequences of substance misuse also have influenced the nature of relevant services and patterns of utilization. As discussed later in this chapter, the population of substance abusers is much larger and more heterogeneous than clinical impressions suggest. Most treatments are intensive and abstinence-oriented, and they do not well serve the needs of substance abusers with mild to moderate problems or those who want to reduce the harm associated with substance use but who do not or cannot abstain (Tucker, Donovan, & Marlatt, 1999). This underserved majority may surface in a wide range of medical, vocational, and community settings, and they understandably may be reluctant to participate in substance-related services that they did not seek. These trends have important implications for screening, assessment, referral, and intervention activities that go beyond conventional diagnostic workups of clients who present for specialized services.

Another theme guiding this chapter, therefore, is that the heterogeneity of substance-related problems requires a set of similarly diverse interventions (Institute of Medicine, 1990; Tucker et al., 1999). Today's managed health care environment offers opportunities to extend the reach and effectiveness of substance-related services by moving the locus of care from inpatient to outpatient settings and by integrating screenings and brief interventions for substance-related problems into primary care and emergency department settings. Implementing an optimal continuum of care will depend heavily on effective assessment that supports rational choices among a range of service options and on continued monitoring of participants' progress to assure that they are receiving the least intensive and costly, but a sufficiently effective, intervention (Sobell & Sobell, 1999).

The chapter is organized as follows. The first section summarizes the epidemiology of substance abuse, basic information about the U.S. service delivery system, and treatment outcomes. The second section is a selective review of the literature on assessment procedures for alcohol and drug problems. The third section discusses practical recommendations for effective assessment, with an emphasis on contextual variables. The final sections address the integration of assessment with treatment planning and the development of a continuum of care.

THE NATURE OF SUBSTANCE-RELATED PROBLEMS, INTERVENTION OPTIONS, AND OUTCOMES

Epidemiology of Substance Abuse and Patterns of Service Utilization and Remission

Data from clinical samples yields an impression of substance use disorders that is different from population-based survey findings. First, compared to the population of substance abusers, clinical samples tend to have more severe and chronic problems, to be older and disproportionately male, and to be more homogenous regarding the nature and developmental course of problems (Marlatt, Tucker, Donovan, & Vuchinich, 1997). Nevertheless, clinical samples show considerable variability in substance use practices, dependence levels, and related problems, and these dimensions often are not highly correlated.

Second, because substance use disorders are among the most prevalent mental disorders, affected persons are common in the general population and in general clinical practice, even if they go unrecognized (e.g., Kessler et al., 1994). The three most prevalent mental disorders in the Epidemiologic Catchment Area (ECA) study (Narrow, Regier, Rae, Manderscheid, & Locke, 1993; Regier et al., 1993) were anxiety (12.6%), affective (9.5%), and substance use (9.5%), with alcohol abuse being the most common of the latter (7.4%). Commonly misused illicit drugs include marijuana, cocaine, narcotics, and polydrug abuse (including alcohol) (Fischman & Johanson, 1996). Moreover, substance use disorders often are comorbid with affective, anxiety, and antisocial personality disorders (Regier et al., 1990) and with physical disorders, including sexually transmitted diseases (STDs) such as HIV/AIDS, accidents and trauma, and with a range of acute and chronic liver, cardiac, gastrointestinal, and neurological problems. Knowledge of these base rates and comorbid conditions is necessary to guide the focus and scope of screening and assessment procedures, especially in nonspecialized health care and other community settings.

Third, substance use shows reliable trends as a function of age and gender (White & Bates, 1995; Williams & DeBakey, 1992) that should inform screening and intervention planning. Substance use and abuse peak during adolescence and early adulthood and then decrease with age. Males at all ages use and abuse alcohol and other drugs more than females. Relations with ethnicity are more complex, and generalizations are difficult due to large variations in use and abuse within different ethnic groups (U.S. Department of Health and Human Services, 1997).

Fourth, positive changes in substance misuse, including full remissions, can occur without interventions (Tucker & King, 1999). Other substance abusers who receive interventions make positive changes well before or after the treatment. Untreated "natural resolutions" are more common than intervention-assisted resolutions for problem drinking and smoking, and, in the case of problem drinking, natural resolutions yield a higher ratio of moderation to abstinent outcomes than do treatment-assisted resolutions (Sobell, Cunningham, & Sobell,1996). For all drugs of abuse, considerable variability exists in the pathways to successful change (e.g., abrupt abstinence, gradual reductions in use, transitioning from a more to a less dangerous drug class). Although persons who resolve on their own tend to have less serious problems than those who enter treatment, they often fulfill clinical diagnostic criteria for substance use disorders.

Finally, many substance abusers have multiple intervention episodes before they make stable changes. Therefore, a full understanding of relations between interventions and positive change requires an expansion of outcome research beyond evaluations of single treatment episodes to include the study of change over multiple episodes and among samples who did not seek treatment. Adopting such a "career" perspective on the change process and the role of interventions in promoting it is a recent development and one that is sensitive to the chronic nature of these problems in many, but not all, substance abusers.

U.S. System of Care for Substance Use Disorders

Fewer than 25% of persons with problems seek substance-focused services (Marlatt et al., 1997). Substance abuse services are distributed across a pluralistic system that spans the professional and voluntary sectors. Care options variously include substance abuse treatment programs, professional counseling, and mutual help groups, as well as informal help from family, friends, and clergy (Narrow et al., 1993). Very few substance abusers receive specialized services from qualified professionals or as part of their routine health care. Mutual help groups have been a mainstay resource for substance abuse since Alcoholics Anonymous (AA) was organized in the mid–1930s, and recently several other groups (e.g., Rational Recovery, Moderation Management, Women for Sobriety, and SMART Recovery) have emerged and offer approaches other than the 12-step recovery program of AA. The more recent development of professional services for substance use disorders coincided with the articulation and widespread acceptance of disease and addiction models of substance misuse within the medical community (Jellinek, 1960; Peele, 1991). Professional services in the United States continue to be dominated by these models and emphasize permanent abstinence as the primary goal of treatment. Abstinence is often required for treatment entry and retention, which deters participation (Marlatt et al., 1997).

In contrast, many other developed countries have expanded the range of treatment options and goals to include harm reduction alternatives (Marlatt, 1998). This approach values any change that reduces the harm or risk of harm of substance use, including but not limited to sustained abstinence. Examples of harm-reduction programs variously include clean needle exchanges, condom distribution, pharmaco-substitutes for drugs of abuse (e.g., methadone maintenance, nicotine replacement products), and interventions aimed at reducing drug use in high risk situations (e.g., drinking and driving). The approach has gained support in several developed countries (e.g., Australia, Canada, the Netherlands), but remains controversial in the United States and is at odds with the zero tolerance approach of the U.S. war on drugs. Nevertheless, scientific evidence continues to accrue to support the effectiveness of harm reduction programs like clean needle exchanges in reducing the rate of spread of HIV/AIDS without increasing drug use and abuse (National Institutes of Health, 1997).

These different approaches to drug treatment and policy vary in the emphasis and value they place on different parameters of substance misuse. In most any program, reductions in drug use and abuse are a major goal, and pertinent assessment data may variously involve use, dependence levels, and problems that result from use. Additional variables are of interest in harm-reduction programs, which also focus on promoting changes in life functioning (e.g., employment and good health status) and high-risk behaviors other than drug misuse (e.g., risky sex, needle sharing, criminal activity). Positive change on the latter dimensions are valued in their own right, as are reductions in drug use or risky drug-taking practices, even if they fall short of abstinence. In contrast, abstinence-oriented programs, primarily value eliminating substance use, and any use typically is viewed as a negative outcome. Thus, understanding a program's theory and value system with respect to different parameters of substance misuse is a fundamental part of the assessment and evaluation process (McEldowney & Heilman, 1999).

Patterns and Determinants of Intervention Outcomes

Thirty years of controlled treatment outcome studies in the substance abuse area have yielded the following generalizations. First, outcomes are not strongly related to technical variations among competently delivered treatments (e.g., McLellan et al., 1994; Project MATCH Research Group, 1997). This general finding has led to the formulation of research-based treatment principles (National Institute on Drug Abuse, 1999) that supersede earlier efforts to identify the single best treatment and instead emphasize the need for a range of interventions and increasing access to them. Second, outcomes are not highly related to treatment intensity and duration, and many clients with mild to moderate problems improve after a one- to two-session brief intervention (Zweben & Fleming, 1999). Third, longer term outcomes are more related to clients' personal resources and life circumstances during the post-treatment interval than to treatment or client characteristics at intake (e.g., Moos, Finney, & Cronkite, 1990). Fourth, considerable variability exists in the temporal patterning of abstinence, substance use, and misuse over time, both within and across individuals, and this variability is due more to changing environmental circumstances and personal resources than to earlier treatment experiences. Fifth, substance abusers seek or are forced into interventions at variable points in the behavior change process. Some are coerced into interventions before they are motivated to change; others make substantial positive changes on their own and then seek services to support and consolidate the changes; and many enter interventions ambivalent about change (Prochaska & DiClemente, 1986).

Collectively, these findings highlight several issues for clinical assessment and outcome evaluations. Foremost is the variable nature of substance-related problems and motivation for change. These are not static attributes of people but are temporally extended and dynamic behavioral processes. Developing effective interventions that "meet the clients where they are" requires assessment information that is sensitive to the dynamic quality of the problem and the changeable nature of motivation for treatment participation and behavior change (Miller & Rollnick, 1991). In a related vein, patterns of substance use and abuse are embedded in individuals' life contexts, and complex contingencies often exist between substance use, misuse, and abstinence and individuals' access to valued activities (e.g., marital satisfaction; stable employment; physical, mental, and spiritual health). Intervention planning requires assessment of these environment–behavior relations, which also are dynamic in nature.

ASSESSMENT PROCEDURES FOR ALCOHOL AND OTHER DRUG PROBLEMS

The dynamic nature of substance abuse and the many contexts in which it may surface have spurred the development of a range of assessment procedures that serve different purposes at different points in the therapeutic interaction. The following review is necessarily selective because of the breadth and volume of relevant work (e.g., see books and reviews by Allen & Columbus, 1995; Babor, Brown, & Del Boca, 1990; Babor et al., 1987; Donovan, 1999; Donovan & Marlatt, 1988; Maisto, Connors, & Allen, 1995; Sobell, Toneatto, & Sobell, 1994; Vuchinich et al., 1988; Wolff et al., 1999), and it focuses on procedures that have good empirical support and clinical utility and that address relevant issues in the different phases of working therapeutically with substance abusers. Selecting, planning, and evaluating interventions requires the use of a range of assessment procedures that are responsive to the heterogeneity of problems. The nature and goals of assessment will vary according to the problem severity, the setting and population characteristics (e.g., primary care, general inpatient, or specialized clinical setting), the available resources (e.g., time, access to medical equipment), and the purpose of the assessment (e.g., screening, diagnosis and treatment planning, forensic evaluation). Assessment is usually a sequential process (Donovan, 1999) that includes detection of a substance use problem (screening), evaluation of problem severity (e.g., diagnosis, substance use patterns, related adverse consequences), and assessment of factors related to treatment planning and outcomes (e.g., readiness to change, alcohol or drug effect expectancies). The review is organized around this sequential process and is followed by a discussion of considerations for special populations. Table 12.1 summarizes the main features of the measures discussed in the following sections.

Screening

Despite growing evidence that substantial numbers of untreated substance abusers flow through nonspecialty medical settings (Goldberg, Mullen, Ries, Psaty, & Ruch, 1991), only 40% of general medical patients and fewer than 25% of trauma patients are screened for alcohol use or problems (Deitz, Rohde, Bertolucci, & Dufour, 1994). Evidence that brief, primary care interventions can result in reduced drinking and related problems (reviewed by Buchsbaum, 1994) makes screening in those settings a key element in providing a continuum of care for substance abusers, and persons with more serious problems require referral for specialized interventions. Identifying patients with substance abuse also is important for medical management and averting future health problems. For example, alcohol abuse is associated with a higher incidence of postdischarge infections

TABLE 12.1. Summary of Assessment Measures for Substance Misuse and Related Problems

Assessment domain	Measure	Type of measure	Target population(s)	Time to complete	Specialized skills required to administer or score	Clinical utility
Collateral information	Comprehensive Drinker Profile Collateral Interview	Interview	Adults	30 min	Yes	Provides record of drinking history that can corroborate client reports; more detailed past year information can be obtained with collateral version of the TLFB
	Form-90 Collateral Interview	Interview	Adults	30 min	Yes	Uses combination of "grid averaging" and calendar based (i.e., TLFB) method of ascertaining drinking (and drug use) patterns
	TimeLine FollowBack (TLFB)	Interview	Adults/adolescents	360 days = 30 min	Yes	Provides retrospective measure of daily drinking or drug use to supplement client report; more sensitive to variability in consumption patterns than other measures
Screening measures—alcohol	Alcohol Use Disorders Identification Test (AUDIT)	Self-report	Adults/college students	2 min	No	Useful for detection of heavy drinking in diverse populations (e.g., women, minorities); contains three consumption questions (AUDIT-C) that can be used independently as a rapid screen for heavy drinking
	Michigan Alcoholism Screening Test (MAST)	Self-report	Adults	10 min	No	Widely used screening tool for lifetime alcohol abuse/dependence; recommended with psychiatric and alcohol treatment patients; less useful for detecting heavy drinking
	CAGE	Self-report	Adults	1 min	No	Useful as an extremely brief measure of lifetime abuse/dependence; less useful for detecting heavy drinking
	MacAndrew Alcoholism Scale—Revised of the MMPI-2 (MAC-R)	Self-report	Adults	10 min (if administered apart from full MMPI	No	Empirically derived "covert content" items identify individuals with characteristics associated with alcoholism (e.g., cognitive impairment, risk taking); less useful with minorities and women

						Useful with minorities and women
	Rapid Alcohol Problems Screen (RAPS)	Self-report	Adults	1 min	No	
	T-ACE	Self-report	Adults	1 min	No	Screening tool for identifying risky drinking in pregnant woman
	TWEAK	Self-report	Adults	1 min	No	Developed to identify risky drinking during pregnancy; can also be used with nonpregnant women and with men
	U-OPEN	Self-report	Older adults	1 min	No	Sensitive to alcohol problems in older adults
	Michigan Alcoholism Screening Test (MAST)	Self-report	Older adults	10 min	No	Sensitive to alcohol problems in older adults
	Young Adult Alcohol Problem Screening Test (YAAPST)	Self-report	Adolescents/college students	10 min	No	Assesses lifetime and past year alcohol-related consequences common to college students; useful for diagnosing alcohol abuse
	Rutgers Alcohol Problem Index (RAPI)	Self-report	Adolescents/college students	10 min	No	Assesses lifetime and past year alcohol-related consequences common to college students; useful for diagnosing alcohol abuse
Screening measures—drugs	Drug Abuse Screening Test (DAST)	Self-report	Adults	10 min	No	Modeled after the MAST; highly correlated with DSM-III-R abuse/dependence diagnosis
	Drug Use Screening Inventory (DUSI)	Self-report	Adults/adolescents	20 min	No	Evaluates the severity of substance abuse and related impairment across nine life domains
Substance use diagnosis	Comprehensive Drinker Profile (CDP)	Interview	Adults	2 hr	Yes	Provides information on alcohol related diagnosis, drinking history, motivation, and self-efficacy; corresponding follow-up and collateral interviews increase research utility
	Structured Clinical Interview for DSM-IV Axis I Disorders (SCID)	Interview	Adults	1–5 hr	Yes	Comprehensive structured interview; adheres closely to DSM-IV decision trees for alcohol, drugs and comorbid psychiatric disorders
	Alcohol Use Disorders and Associated Disabilities Interview Schedule (AUDASIS)	Interview	Adults	1–2 hr	Yes	Most frequently used in clinical research; can be administered by trained lay interviewers; provides diagnostic information on alcohol, drugs, and comorbid psychiatric disorders

(continued)

421

TABLE 12.1. (*continued*)

Assessment domain	Measure	Type of measure	Target population(s)	Time to complete	Specialized skills required to administer or score	Clinical utility
Substance use diagnosis (*cont.*)	Psychiatric Research Interview for Substance and Mental Disorders (PRISM)	Interview	Adults	1–5 hr	Yes	Widely used with alcohol and drug clinical samples
	Adolescent Diagnostic Interview (ADI)	Interview	Adolescents	45 min	Yes	Provides reliable info on substance use diagnosis; also evaluates interpersonal, social, and school functioning
Dependence symptoms—alcohol	Alcohol Dependence Scale (ADS)	Typically self-report, can use interview format	Mainly adults, some use with adolescents	5 min	Some minimal training required for interview format	Used in a variety of settings to assess alcohol dependence symptoms; score of 9 or more is predictive of dependence diagnosis
Negative consequences—alcohol	Drinking Problems Index (DPI)	Self-report	Older adults	3–5 min	No	17 items cover alcohol-related consequences common to older adults (e.g., falls, confusion)
	Drinking Problems Scale (DPS)	Self-report	Adults	5 min	No	Assesses extent of alcohol-related problems in six areas of life–health functioning
	Drinker Inventory of Consequences from Project MATCH (DrInC)	Self-report	Adults/college students	10 min	No	Covers a range of adverse consequences, from relatively mild problems to indicators of dependence
Negative consequences—alcohol and drugs	Addiction Severity Index (ASI)	Interview; also laboratory tests of drug use	Adults	30–45 min	Yes	Assesses current and lifetime impact of alcohol and drug use on seven domains; provides info on client's level of concern about drug use
	Problem-Oriented Screening Instrument for Teenagers (POSIT)	Self-report	Adolescents	20–25 min	No	Assesses impact of substance use on a number of life domains; available in English and Spanish
	Personal Experience Inventory (PEI)	Self-report	Adolescents	10–20 min	No	Multidimensional screening tool designed to compliment the Adolescent Diagnostic Interview (ADI)

Category	Measure	Format	Population	Time		Description
Alcohol consumption measures	TimeLine FollowBack (TLFB)	Interview or self-report	Adults/adolescents	360 days = 30 min	Yes	Provides detailed information on drinking patterns; can also be used to obtain drug use patterns
	Form-90 from Project MATCH	Interview	Adults	Variable, depends on drinking pattern	Yes	Uses combination of "grid averaging" and calender based (i.e., TLFB) method of ascertaining drinking patterns; baseline and follow-up versions provide continuous measure; also gathers psychosocial and drug use information
	Lifetime Drinking History (LDH)	Interview	Adults/adolescents	20 min	Yes	Brief method of summarizing lifetime drinking; reliance on averaged patterns limits sensitivity to variability within phases
Drug consumption measures	Drug History Questionnaire (DHQ)	Self-report	Adults/adolescents	20 min	No	Provides info on types of drugs used, routes of administration, frequency of use, etc
Comorbidity	Structured Clinical Interview for the DSM-IV Axis I Disorders (SCID)	Interview	Adults	1–5 hr	Yes	Comprehensive structured interview; adheres closely to DSM-IV decision trees for alcohol, drugs, and comorbid psychiatric disorders
	Personality Assessment Inventory (PAI)	Self-Report	Adults/college students	45–90 min	No	Objective personality inventory with a number of clinical and validity scales
	Symptom Checklist-90 (SCL-90)	Self-report	Adults/college students	10–15 min	No	Brief and widely used measure of clinically significant psychiatric symptoms with global scale and nine clinical scales
	Beck Depression Inventory (BDI-II)	Self-report	Adults/college students	5 min	No	Provides a reliable and valid measure of cognitive, affective, physiological, and motivational components of depression
Neuropsychological screening	Trail Making Test (TMT)	Individually administered performance task	Adults	5–10 min	Yes	Provides a brief measure of perceptual-motor functioning; useful initial screen for neuropsychological impairment
	Digit Symbol subscale of Wechsler Adult Intelligence Scale—Revised (WAIS-III)	Individually administered performance task	Adults	5–10 min	Yes	Provides a brief measure of perceptual-motor functioning; useful initial screen for neuropsychological impairment

(continued)

TABLE 12.1. (continued)

Assessment domain	Measure	Type of measure	Target population(s)	Time to complete	Specialized skills required to administer or score	Clinical utility
Neuropsychological assessment	Halstead–Reitan Neuropsychological Test Battery	Individually administered test battery	Adults	> 2 hr	Yes	Comprehensive test of neuropsychological impairment
Readiness to change	Readiness To Change Questionnaire (RTCQ)	Self-report	Adults/adolescents	2–3 min	No	Used widely to assess readiness to change in drinkers not seeking treatment
	Stages of Change Readiness and Treatment Eagerness Scale (SOCRATES)	Self-report	Adults/adolescents	5 min	No	Used widely to assess readiness to change and treatment readiness in treatment samples
	University of Rhode Island Change Assessment (URICA)	Self-report	Adults/adolescents	5 min	No	Assesses beliefs and behaviors related to change process for both alcohol and drug users
Alcohol expectancies	Alcohol Effects Questionnaire (AEFQ)	Self-report	Adults/adolescents	5–10 min	No	Brief measure of both positive and negative alcohol expectancies
	Alcohol Expectancy Questionnaire (AEQ)	Self-report	Adults	20–30 min	No	Assess alcohol expectancies in six domains; widely used in both clinical and research settings
	Effects of Drinking Alcohol (EDA)	Self-report	Adults	5–10 min	No	Focuses on measuring negative expectancies associated with drinking
Cocaine expectancies	Cocaine Effects Expectancy Questionnaire (CEEQ)	Self-report	Adults/adolescents	5–10 min	No	Brief measure of both positive and negative cocaine expectancies

Construct	Measure	Method	Population	Time		Description
Marijuana Expectancies	Marijuana Effects Expectancy Questionnaire (MEEQ)	Self-report	Adults/adolescents	5–10 min	No	Brief measure of both positive and negative marijuana expectancies
Situational antecedents to alcohol use	Inventory of Drinking Situations (IDS)	Self-report	Adults/college students	15 min	No	Provides measure of contexts associated with heavy drinking
Situational antecedents to drug use	Inventory of Drug Taking Situations (IDTS)	Self-report	Adults/college students	15 min	No	Provides measure of contexts associated with drug use; can be used with variety of illicit drugs and tobacco
Self-efficacy—alcohol	Situational Confidence Questionnaire (SCQ)	Self-report	Adults	8–10 min	No	Measures individual's confidence in his/her ability to resist drinking, or heavy drinking, in a number of situations
Self-efficacy—drugs	Drug-Taking Confidence Questionnaire (DTCQ)	Self-report	Adults	8–10 min	No	Measures individual's confidence in his/her ability to resist drug use in a number of situations
Craving—alcohol	Desires for Alcohol Questionnaire (DAQ)	Self-report	Adults	15–30 min	No	Provides psychometrically sound measure of alcohol craving; clinical utility not well established
Craving-cocaine	Cocaine Craving Questionnaire (CCQ)	Self-report	Adults	15–30 min	No	Provides psychometrically sound measure of cocaine craving; clinical utility not well established

and other complications (Jurkovich et al., 1993), and trauma patients admitted with a positive blood alcohol concentration (BAC) are two to three times more likely to be readmitted for a second traumatic incident (Rivera, Koepsell, Jurkovich, Gurney, & Soderberg, 1993; Sims et al., 1989).

Useful measures are brief; validly establish the likely presence and type of substance misuse; can be easily administered and interpreted by nonspecialists; and typically employ verbal reports or biological tests, or both. When screenings are conducted by someone other than the treatment provider, obtaining information beyond what is needed for detection and referral for services unnecessarily lengthens the assessment. When potential providers conduct screenings, such information can advance treatment planning or can be used as part of a brief intervention for individuals with mild to moderate problems (Dimeff, Baer, Kivlahan, & Marlatt, 1999; Miller & Rollnick, 1991). By definition, however, screening measures cannot provide information on key consumption parameters such as quantity consumed, duration of episodes, temporal patterning, or topographical features of use, all of which are important for assessment and treatment planning.

Verbal Report Screening Measures for Alcohol Problems

Self-administered and interview-based screening measures for alcohol-related problems generally assess the presence of medical and psychosocial consequences of drinking and dependence symptoms (reviewed by Carey & Teitelbaum, 1996; Connors, 1995). Good screening measures include the Michigan Alcoholism Screening Test (MAST; Selzer, 1971), the CAGE (acronym for Cut down on drinking, Annoyed by criticism of drinking, Guilty about drinking, and Eye-opener; Mayfield, McLeod, & Hall, 1974), and the Alcohol Use Disorders Identification Test (AUDIT; Saunders, Aasland, Babor, DeLaFuente, & Grant, 1993). All take less than 10 minutes, are easily scored with minimal training, and have been used in diverse settings.

The MAST provides lifetime information on alcohol problems, correctly identifies from 50% to 100% of persons with problems, and is not easily influenced by response sets (Crist & Milby, 1990; Teitelbaum & Mullen, 2000). A recent meta-analysis (Teitelbaum & Mullen, 2000) further showed that the MAST effectively identified the presence of alcohol problems among psychiatric patients, which recommends the MAST for screening in psychiatric settings. Two MAST short forms also have been developed: the 10-item Brief MAST (BMAST) and the 13-item Short MAST (SMAST). Since the BMAST is highly correlated with the full MAST (.95–.99), it can be used instead of the MAST when time is limited (Pokorny, Miller, & Kaplan, 1972). The SMAST performs similarly to the CAGE in terms of sensitivity and specificity and is effective for identifying patients with lifetime alcohol abuse or dependence (Maisto et al., 1995).

The four-item CAGE works well in medical care settings where patient contact time is short, and it performs similarly to the MAST in identifying medical patients with current alcohol dependence (Magruder-Habib, Stevens, & Alling, 1993). However, neither scale distinguishes between current and lifetime problems and thus may yield false positives among persons who have stable resolutions. The AUDIT assesses early signs of problem drinking better than the MAST or CAGE and is recommended for screening populations that have higher proportions of persons with less serious problems (e.g., younger adults) (Carey & Teitelbaum, 1996; Cherpitel, 1998). Another benefit of the AUDIT is that it provides scores for both past year and lifetime use (Saunders et al., 1993).

The 49-item MacAndrew Alcoholism Scale—Revised (MAC-R) of the Minnesota Multiphasic Personality Inventory-2 (MMPI-2; Butcher, Dahlstrom, Graham, Tellegen, & Kaemmer, 1989) has been used for screening purposes and found to discriminate alcoholics from other psychiatric patients (Graham, 2000). The MAC-R measures characteristics common to alcoholics (e.g., cognitive impairment, interpersonal competence, risk taking), but provides no information on drinking patterns or problems. It has poor internal consistency, questionable reliability, and limited utility with minorities and women. Thus, the MAC-R should be reserved for use only when the MMPI-2 data are already available or when assessment of psychiatric disorders is indicated.

Choosing among measures will depend on the screening goals (e.g., sensitivity versus specificity), the characteristics of population and setting, and the available resources for scoring and feedback (Conners, 1995). For a population with a relatively low base rate of alcohol problems (e.g., primary care settings), use of a highly sensitive measure that will maximize the number of true positives is appropriate. Individuals identified with a highly sensitive initial screen (e.g., CAGE with a cut-point of 1) then can be further assessed with a more specific measure (e.g., MAST). Population characteristics (e.g., gender, ethnicity, age) also influence test utility. As discussed later under special populations, most screening measures were developed using white males in treatment, and the usefulness of these data for other groups with less severe problems is not well established (Ames, Schmidt, Klee, & Saltz, 1996; Cherpital, 1998).

Verbal Report Screening Measures for Drug Abuse

Few self-report screening measures for illicit drug abuse exist, and their use with clients who did not present for drug treatment may entail ethical and legal concerns because individuals are being asked for reports about illegal activities (Sobell et al., 1994). The 20-item Drug Abuse Screening Test (DAST; Gavin, Ross, & Skinner, 1989) was modeled after the MAST, assesses the consequences of drug use during the past year, and correlates highly with diagnoses according to the revised third edition of *Diagnostic and Statistical Manual of Mental Disorders* (DSM-III-R; American Psychiatric Association, 1987) of drug abuse and dependence (Donovan, 1999; Sobell et al., 1994). The Drug Use Screening Inventory (DUSI; Tarter & Kirisci, 1997) evaluates the severity of substance abuse (both alcohol and illicit drug use) and substance-related impairment in nine life-health areas (e.g., health status, social competence, work adjustment, family system). Both adult and adolescent versions are available and take about 20 minutes to complete. Tarter and Kirisci (1997) reported that the DUSI was reliable and correctly classified 80% of substance abusers and 100% of normal controls.

Biological Tests for Alcohol and Drug Use

Numerous biological tests are useful as screening measures for substance use and for monitoring use during and after treatment (reviewed by Anton, Litten, & Allen, 1995; Wolfe et al., 1999). Their advantages include the ease of obtaining them in medical settings and their utility as a supplement to self-reported information. Their limitations include cost, lack of specificity, and sensitivity to recent substance use only.

Alcohol breathalyzer tests are used in various contexts (e.g., police or hospital settings) to obtain accurate and easily interpretable estimates of current BAC. Positive BAC or urine readings upon hospital admission indicate that further assessment is warranted but are by no means diagnostic of alcohol abuse or dependence. Conversely, a zero BAC estimate does not assure the absence of substance misuse. For example, only 20% of trauma patients with a positive BAC were found to meet criteria for alcohol abuse or dependence (Cherpitel, 1995), but almost half of trauma patients who had negative BACs met DSM-III-R criteria for alcohol dependence (Soderstrom et al., 1992). Thus, biological tests for recent alcohol use are a useful component in the screening process but cannot stand alone as definitive indicators.

Biological tests for chronic alcohol abuse measure tissue damage that results from years of heavy drinking (Anton et al., 1995; Salaspuro, 1994), and they better reflect sustained heavy drinking. Commonly used blood tests for chronic alcohol abuse include the liver enzyme gamma-glutamyl transferase (GGT), red blood cell mean corpuscular volume (MCV), and carbohydrate-deficient transferrin (CDT), a liver-synthesized protein that may be a precursor to liver cell damage. Because these biological measures generally have poor sensitivity in populations with low base rates of alcohol abuse, it is advantageous to use marker combinations in order to improve sensitivity. Several studies have shown that combining markers as part of discriminate function techniques increases sensitivity to around 90% (Salaspuro, 1994). Anton et al. (1995) recommended a sequential process in which preliminary screening with the more sensitive GGT is followed by testing with the more specific CDT.

Urinalysis reliably detects most drugs of abuse, but its utility varies with the half-life of the drug (e.g., 1 to 3 days for cocaine, 1 to 2 weeks for marijuana), the selected cutpoint for a positive result, and the amount and duration of drug use (Wolff et al., 1999). Urinalysis is usually done in a two-stage process: a relatively inexpensive initial screen (e.g., enzyme immunoassay) is followed by a more elaborate confirmatory test (gas chromatography–mass spectrometry). This two-stage process accurately detects $\geq$ 95% of drug-positive urines for most drug classes (Cook, Bernstein, Arrington, Andrews, & Marshall, 1995), but false negatives are a concern because urine samples can be purposively contaminated (e.g., with soap, bleach, or vinegar), diluted with water, or "flushed" from the body using readily available products designed for this purpose (Wolff et al., 1999). Also of concern is the potential for false positives that result from a range of prescribed or over-the-counter (OTC) medications to foods that contain poppy seeds.

Hair analysis confers an advantage of a longer detection window (up to a year, depending on the length of the hair). However, Wolff et al. (1999) noted many disadvantages, including lack of quality control and standardized analysis procedures; variability in sensitivity due to hair length, growth cycles, and possibly color; potential false positives that result from passive exposure to marijuana or crack smoke; and the possible effects of hair products. Thus, hair samples can yield false positives in non-users and cannot reliably distinguish recent and remote use among users.

Summary

Screening information obtained from self-reports, breath analysis, urinalysis, and hair analysis generally provide convergent information (Cook et al., 1995; Donovan, 1999), although discrepancies can arise from differences in the assessment time frame of biological and self-report measures, false positive urine or hair analysis results for reasons other than illicit drug use, and the failure to self-report substance use (Cook et al., 1995). Thus, no single screening measure can function alone as a "gold standard," and each has advantages and limitations.

Diagnosis and Assessment for Intervention Planning and Implementation

Individuals identified in screenings typically are referred for further assessment to facilitate treatment selection and planning (Allen, Columbus, & Fertig, 1995). The assessment usually involves a diagnostic evaluation, including measurement of substance use, dependence levels, associated negative psychosocial consequences, and comorbid psychopathology (Donovan, 1999).

Diagnostic and Clinical Interview Protocols

Similar diagnostic criteria for substance use disorders are specified in DSM-IV (American Psychiatric Association, 1994) and *International Classification of Diseases,* 10th edition (ICD-10) (World Health Organization, 1990) manuals, which are based on the substance dependence syndrome outlined by the World Health Organization in 1981. The syndrome is characterized by loss of control over use, continued use despite adverse consequences, strong cravings to use, tolerance, and withdrawal symptoms (Maisto & McKay, 1995; World Health Organization, 1981). One key difference between DSM-IV and previous editions is that tolerance and withdrawal are no longer required for the diagnosis of dependence, which is based on the presence of any three of the following seven criteria: (1) tolerance; (2) withdrawal; (3) substance often taken in larger amounts or over a larger time than intended; (4) persistent desire or unsuccessful attempts to cut down or control substance abuse; (5) considerable time spent in activities required to obtain the substance, use it, or recover from use; (6) important social, occupational, or recreational activities curtailed or given up because of substance use; and (7) continued use despite persistent or recurrent physical or psychological problems caused or exacerbated by use (American Psychiatric Association, 1994). Another difference between DSM-IV and DSM-III-R is that the substance abuse diagnosis is no longer a residual category and is now defined as a pattern of problem use lasting at least 12 months, based on recurrent adverse consequences related to use and functional impairment without the presence of tolerance, withdrawal, or a pattern of "compulsive" use.

Substance use disorders usually are diagnosed through a structured interview administered by trained professionals (see Maisto and McKay, 1995, for a review of diagnostic interviews). General psychiatric diagnostic interviews that yield substance-specific DSM diagnoses include the Structured Clinical Interview for DSM-IV Axis I Disorders (SCID; First, Spitzer, Gibbon, & Williams, 1996) and the Psychiatric Research Interview for Substance and Mental Disorders (PRISM; Hasin et al., 1996). Other diagnostic interviews focus specifically on substance abuse and assess lifetime and current alcohol and drug dependence constructs such as withdrawal, craving, and tolerance. For example, the Alcohol Use Disorders and Associated Disabilities Interview Schedule (AUDASIS; Grant & Hasin, 1990) provides DSM and ICD diagnoses for illicit drugs, alcohol, and common comorbid psychiatric disorders (e.g., depression, antisocial personality disorder); demographic information and risk factors (e.g., family history, medical conditions); and drug and alcohol consumption information. The AUDASIS can be administered by trained lay interviewers. Another structured interview that provides a multitude of pertinent data for treatment planning is the Comprehensive Drinker Profile (CDP; Miller & Marlatt, 1984), which assesses drinking patterns, history, motivation to change, self-efficacy, and family history. Versions of the CDP are available for follow-up and collateral interviews and for uncooperative respondents.

To facilitate treatment planning and a functional analysis, the assessment should extend beyond the rather narrow conceptualization of dependence that guides many diagnostic interviews and should assess substance use practices, contextual information such as stimulus conditions that precede use, and psychosocial and other consequences of use. Cognitive variables such as expectancies, self-efficacy, and situational coping also can contribute to treatment planning. Obtaining information that extends beyond diagnostic considerations is particularly relevant for persons with less severe problems, who may not have experienced dependence symptoms.

Drinking Practices

Verbal report measures of alcohol and drug use fall into three general categories: retrospective quantity/frequency (Q/F) questionnaires that ask respondents to summarize their use over some time period; retrospective interviews that assess the temporal patterning of use over some time period; and prospective self-monitoring using diaries, handheld computers, or the telephone (see Sobell & Sobell, 1995a, for a review). Q/F measures are mainly useful for screening individuals and characterizing samples and are not discussed further.

Three widely used retrospective interviews that yield information on the temporal patterning of drinking are the TimeLine FollowBack (TLFB; Sobell & Sobell, 1992, 1995b), Form-90 from Project MATCH (Tonigan, Miller, & Brown, 1997), and the Lifetime Drinking History (LDH; Skinner & Sheu, 1982). The TLFB is a daily drinking estimation method in which clients use a calendar to provide retrospective estimates of their daily drinking during the past year or so. The TLFB has good to excellent psychometric properties with several populations (e.g., males/females, clinical/nonclinical) (Sobell & Sobell, 1995b). It usually is administered in an interview but can be self-administered, including by computer (Sobell & Sobell, 1995a).

Form-90 is a "family of structured interviews" (i.e., intake, follow-up, brief telephone interview, collateral interview) developed as outcome measures for Project MATCH (Tonigan et al., 1997). Form-90 is a calendar-based measure similar to the TLFB, but it also uses a "grid averaging" method to allow quick identification of consistent patterns of drinking; then, when needed, it uses the TLFB method to gather detailed daily drinking reports. Form-90 also collects data on psychosocial functioning, health care utilization, and other licit and illicit drug use. Tonigan et al. (1997) found that Form-90 possessed good to excellent reliability for its indices of alcohol use, drug use, and social functioning.

The LDH collects data on drinking patterns over longer intervals than the TLFB or Form-90. It establishes periods of abstinence and stable drinking patterns, or phases, starting from when respondents began drinking on a regular basis to the present. Then, within phases, average frequency and quantity of consumption are assessed during respondents' usual and maximum drinking patterns. Also assessed are the type of beverages consumed and the occurrence of any morning drinking. Although the LDH is a relatively brief method of summarizing lifetime drinking, its sensitivity to changes in drinking patterns is limited by its reliance on averaged patterns over extended timeframes (Sobell & Sobell, 1995a).

When the resources are available, detailed, high-quality information on daily drinking patterns is best obtained through prospective self-monitoring, which can be variously collected using diaries, handheld computers, or the telephone (e.g., Mundt, Searles, Perrine, & Helzer, 1995; Samo, Tucker, & Vuchinich, 1989; Sobell et al., 1994; Tucker, Vuchinich, Harris, Gavornik, & Rudd, 1991). Self-monitoring generally yields more complete and accurate reports, especially for fine-grained dimensions of use (e.g., duration of and quantities consumed during discrete drinking episodes), but for other dimensions (e.g., frequency of drinking days, types of beverages consumed), retrospective methods like the TLFB perform similarly and often are easier to use. Potential limitations of self-monitoring methods variously include the placement of greater demands on participants' time and the need for training patients in the procedures, technical problems, and reactivity. Reactive effects, if they occur, tend to be transitory (Tucker et al., 1991).

Illicit Drug Use

Measures of illicit drug use practices are less common. A basic difference with implications for assessment is that alcoholic beverages come in standard units that are readily observable, whereas illicit drugs often are used in ambiguous or unknown quantities and strengths. Thus, in assessing illicit drug use, emphasis has been placed on measuring frequency of use, route of administration, and related contextual variables (Donovan, 1999; Sobell et al., 1994). Information on route of administration (e.g., intravenous injection, nasal) is especially important, since routes vary in their associated risks (e.g., HIV), speed of onset, and potency of effects (Sobell et al., 1994). The TLFB and self-monitoring procedures have been adapted to collect this kind of information about illicit drug use (Sobell et al., 1994). There also are drug use history profiles, such as the Drug History Questionnaire (DHQ; Sobell, Kwan, & Sobell, 1995), that assess a number of dimensions of use (e.g., age of first use, frequency of use, date of last use) for different drug classes. As mentioned earlier, the AUDASIS also can be used to assess drug use patterns.

Adverse Consequences of Substance Misuse

Considerable variability exists in the extent to which drinking or other drug use results in symptoms of dependence and impairs life-health functioning. Characterizing this variability is critical for making referrals and for treatment planning. The 25-item Alcohol Dependence Scale (ADS; Skinner & Allen, 1982) yields a reliable and valid assessment of dependence symptoms during the past 12 months and is sensitive enough for use with individuals who have mild to moderate alcohol problems (Kivlahan, Sher, & Donovan, 1989; Sobell et al., 1994). The ADS can help determine whether a goal of abstinence or reduced drinking is appropriate (Skinner & Horn, 1984). Higher scorers have been found to report more drinking and related problems, be more likely to accept an abstinence goal, and be less likely to keep therapy appointments compared to lower scorers (Skinner, 1981a, 1981b).

Psychometrically sound (Maisto & McKay, 1995) measures that assess alcohol-related consequences in multiple health and psychosocial domains include the Drinker Inventory of Consequences from Project MATCH (DrInC; Miller, Tonigan, & Longabaugh, 1995), the Addiction Severity Index (ASI; McLellan, Luborsky, Woody, & O'Brien, 1980), and the Drinking Problems Scale (DPS; Cahalan, 1970). The self-administered DrInC, for example, collects information on lifetime and recent alcohol-related consequences in five areas: interpersonal, physical, social, impulsive, and intrapersonal. The ASI is a widely used and reliable structured interview (Hendricks, Kaplan, VanLimbeek, & Geerlings, 1998; Hodgins & El, 1992) that assesses recent and lifetime functioning in seven areas: drug use, alcohol use, psychiatric adjustment, legal problems, social functioning, employment, medical status. It covers objective indicators of drug problems (e.g., laboratory tests), research-based indices of severity for each area, and subjective appraisals of clients' concern with each problem, which can inform treatment selection and potential sources of client motivation for change. An attractive feature of the ASI is its brief follow-up version. Information on problem areas that individuals find particularly troubling can be useful for developing motivational interventions (Miller & Rollnick, 1991) and treatment goals (Sobell et al., 1994). As noted earlier, the DAST and the DUSI also can be used to assess problems from drug abuse in several areas of functioning.

Contexts Surrounding Substance Misuse

Assessment of how substance use and abuse covary with environmental features is critical to formulating a functional analysis to inform behavioral interventions (Marlatt & Gordon, 1985; Sobell et al., 1994). The functional analysis assesses environmental contexts that precede and maintain drug-seeking and use, topographic features of use and associated behaviors, behaviors that regularly precede drug-seeking and use, and the short- and long-term consequences of use. This description guides interventions to disrupt drug-seeking and substance use and to promote incompatible behaviors. The functional analysis usually is based on interview and self-monitored information.

Questionnaires also are available to assess substance use environments and associated emotional and social stimuli, which can identify situations that increase the risk of use and that merit avoidance or the development of alternative coping skills (Marlatt & Gordon, 1985). For example, the Inventory of Drinking Situations (IDS; Annis, Graham, & Davis, 1987) assesses the extent to which heavy drinking during the past year was associated with unpleasant emotions, physical discomfort, pleasant emotions, testing personal control, urges and temptations, conflict with others, social pressure to drink, and pleasant times with others. The corresponding Inventory of Drug Taking Situations (IDTS; Annis, Martin, & Graham, 1992) provides comparable information for a specified illicit drug. Although measures of relapse risk situations can provide useful information for treatment planning, Sobell et al. (1994) have noted that no experimental evidence links the situations identified on these measures with actual relapse events.

Cognitive and Motivational Variables

Motives for and expectancies regarding alcohol and drug use, readiness to change, self-efficacy expectations for behavior change, and urges and cravings are critical elements of cognitive-behavioral treatments that often warrant assessment (see Carroll, 1999, and Donovan, 1995, for reviews). Expectancies about alcohol and drug effects and self-efficacy to abstain or reduce use predict treatment outcomes and high risk situations for substance use (Maisto, Carey, & Bradizza, 1999). These measures therefore can inform efforts aimed at relapse prevention (Donovan, 1995). Measures such as the Alcohol Expectancy Questionnaire (AEQ; Brown, Goldman, Inn, & Anderson, 1980), Alcohol Effects Questionnaire (AEFQ; Rohsenow, 1983), and the Effects of Drinking Alcohol scale (EDA; Leigh, 1987) assess beliefs about various effects of drinking (e.g., tension reduction, sexual enhancement, social and physical pleasure). Similar questionnaires exist for measuring expectancies concerning the effects of cocaine (Cocaine Effects Expectancy Questionnaire—CEEQ; Jaffe & Kilbey, 1994) and marijuana (Marijuana Effects Expectancy Questionnaire—MEEQ; Schafer & Brown, 1991). Because greater positive alcohol expectancies are associated with poorer treatment outcomes (e.g., Brown, 1985), modifying positive expectancies often is an early target of cognitive interventions (Carroll, 1999).

Self-efficacy, which is one's perceived ability to abstain from or reduce substance use, can be assessed with the Situational Confidence Questionnaire (SCQ; Annis et al., 1987) and the Drug Taking Confidence Questionnaire (DTCQ; Annis et al., 1992), which parallel the IDS and IDTS situations and estimate individuals' confidence in being able to resist drinking heavily or using drugs in each situation (Sobell et al., 1994). For alcohol treatment clients with a goal of abstinence, DiClemente, Carbonari, Mongomery, & Hughes (1994) developed the Alcohol Abstinence Self-Efficacy Scale to measure abstinence self-efficacy across the eight relapse categories used on the IDS. These measures can be administered repeatedly during treatment to monitor self-efficacy in situations that pose a risk of relapse (Donovan, 1995). Research generally indicates that self-efficacy is modified by treatment experiences and that posttreatment self-efficacy is positively correlated with outcomes (Maisto et al., 1999).

Several measures of readiness and motivation for change are guided by the Transtheoretical Model of Change (Prochaska & DiClemente, 1986). The Readiness to Change Questionnaire (RTCQ; Rollnick, Heather, Gold, & Hall, 1992) was designed for use with persons who are not yet in substance abuse treatment but are at risk for problems (Donovan, 1999). The Stages of Change Readiness and Treatment Eagerness Scale (SOCRATES; Miller & Tonigan, 1996) assigns drinkers to a stage of change based the Transtheoretical Model and was used in Project MATCH. The University of Rhode Island Change Assessment (URICA; McConnaughy, Prochaska, & Velicer, 1983) does not focus specifically on alcohol problems and thus is suitable for use with drug abusers (Sobell et al., 1994). The

SOCRATES and the URICA have better reliability with treatment samples than does the RTCQ (Donovan, 1995). All these questionnaires are helpful for developing intervention goals that match the client's resources and readiness for change. For example, a problem drinker in the "precontemplation" stage may require motivational enhancement before an intervention (e.g., drink refusal skill training) can be implemented, whereas someone in the "action" stage will be ready to engage.

Finally, addicts often report significant urges to use drugs that disrupt their daily functioning, persist even after extended abstinence, and may be related to the risk of drug use (Tiffany & Carter, 1998). Psychometrically sound scales are available to assess craving for smoking, alcohol, and illicit drugs such as cocaine and heroin (Tiffany, 1997). For example, the 36-item Desires for Alcohol Questionnaire (DAQ; Love, James, & Willner, 1998) assesses four dimensions of craving (intentions to drink, desires to drink, anticipation of positive outcome, and anticipation of relief from negative affect). The Cocaine Craving Questionnaire (CCQ; Tiffany, Singleton, Haertzen, & Henningfield, 1993) is a similar measure of cocaine craving.

Comorbidity

Rates of comorbidity vary widely according to the population studied and are higher in substance abuse treatment samples than in general population samples (Berkson, 1946; Grant & Dawson, 1999). The ECA study found that 37% of alcohol abusers and 53% of drug abusers met criteria for an additional psychiatric disorder (Regier et al., 1990). Common comorbid conditions include major depression (especially among older adults and women) and antisocial personality disorder (especially among men). The National Comorbidity Study (Kessler et al., 1994) found that a current alcohol or drug use diagnosis increased the odds of current major depression by a factor of 2.6 and 3.0, respectively. A lifetime alcohol or drug use diagnosis also was strongly associated with antisocial personality disorder. Substance abusers with another psychiatric diagnosis tend to experience more alcohol-related problems and greater impairment in social and role functioning and physical health than do those without a comorbid diagnosis (Johnson et al., 1995). Structured interviews such as the SCID (First et al., 1996); objective psychopathology measures such as the Personality Assessment Inventory (PAI; Morey, 1996) and the Millon Clinical Multiaxial Inventory (MCMI-II; Millon, 1992); and brief symptom measures such as the Symptom Checklist-90 (SCL-90; Derogatis, 1977) and the Beck Depression Inventory (BDI-II; Beck, Steer, & Brown, 1996) can be used selectively to evaluate comorbid psychopathology.

Family History

Alcohol and drug problems are familial disorders. The genetic component of such familial patterns is stronger in males than females, but environmental factors have considerable influence in both genders (Sher, 1991). Much personal knowledge about drug use and abuse is learned in the home and may affect later substance use. The Family Tree Questionnaire for Assessing Family History of Drinking Problems (Mann, Sobell, Sobell, & Pavin, 1985) is a structured measure of transgenerational patterns of substance abuse in a family. Current and past emotional and physical abuse are related issues that may merit assessment.

Neuropsychological Status

Chronic heavy drinking can produce cognitive deficits that may require rehabilitation beyond routine substance abuse treatment (Sobell et al., 1994; Tarter & Edwards, 1987). For example, Bates (1997) found that over 50% of clients who entered alcohol treatment had neuropsychological deficits. Domains often affected include speech and language, memory, and attention. Functioning may improve with sustained abstinence, but the probability of full recovery declines after age 40 (e.g., Roehrich & Goldman, 1993). Neuropsychological impairment resulting from other drug use is less common but has been associated with polydrug use and chronic cocaine use (Sobell et al., 1994). Tarter and Edwards (1987) recommended a sequential approach to neuropsychological assessment, beginning with brief, highly sensitive instruments such as the Trail Making Test (TMT; Davies, 1968) and the Digit Symbol subscale of the Wechsler Adult Intelligence Scale (WAIS-III; Wechsler, 1997). If these measures suggest impairment, a neuropsychological battery, such as the Halstead–Reitan (Reitan & Davison, 1974) or the Luria–Nebraska Neuropsychological Test Battery (Golden et al., 1982), should be administered.

HIV/AIDS Risk

Individuals who inject drugs are at high risk for HIV/AIDS and hepatitis B and C because of needle sharing and the unsafe sexual practices that are associated with drug-seeking or drug use. Drug abuse services must be sensitive to this increased STD risk and refer clients for discreet and confidential testing when indicated. Programs that serve homeless substance abusers should arrange to screen for tuberculosis (TB), which is prevalent among the homeless.

Summary

Clinicians must be selective in their use of the diverse assessment procedures that are available to assess substance abuse and related problems. Selection should be based on the clinical setting, population served, available resources, and nature and goals of interventions. Because many assessment tools were developed with samples comprised mainly of adult, white males, they should be used cautiously with some of the special populations discussed next.

Special Populations

Adolescents and Young Adults

By 12th grade, a majority of youths have consumed alcohol (61%) and many have tried marijuana (23.9%) or other drugs (e.g., stimulants, 6%; inhalants, 5%) (Johnston, O'Malley, & Bachman, 1995). But alcohol withdrawal is rare among adolescents, and increased tolerance is so common that it has limited specificity as a feature of dependence (Sanjuan & Langenbucher, 1999). Because adolescents are less likely to meet diagnostic criteria for abuse or dependence (6% according to Rohde, Lewinsohn, & Seeley, 1996), many measures developed with adults have limited utility for youths. Alcohol screening measures developed for use with young adults include the Rutgers Alcohol Problem Index (RAPI; White & Labouvie, 1989) and the Young Adult Alcohol Problem Screening Test (YAAPST; Hurlbut & Sher, 1992), which assess alcohol-related problems that are common to college students. Several other adolescent-specific measures provide comprehensive assessments of substance use and age-relevant areas of functioning (e.g., family, school, peers). The Problem Oriented Screening Instrument for Teenagers (POSIT; Rahdert, 1991) assesses substance use and abuse, physical health, mental health, family relationships, peer relations, educational status, vocational status, social skills, leisure and recreation, and delinquency. The Personal Experience Inventory (PEI; Winters & Henly, 1989) measures substance use and psychosocial functioning and is designed to complement the Adolescent Diagnostic Interview (ADI; Winters & Henly, 1993), which yields DSM-III-R substance use diagnoses and ratings of cognitive and global functioning and psychosocial stressors. Expectancy questionnaires also can contribute to treatment planning (Brown, Christiansen, & Goldman, 1987; Schafer & Brown, 1991).

Women

Women with substance use problems are less likely to be detected, and, if identified, they are less likely to be referred for treatment (Bradley, Boyd-Wickizer, Powell, & Burman, 1998), leading to their underrepresentation among clients in treatment (Schober & Annis, 1996). Because of this gender imbalance, special issues among women—such as depression, relationship and child-rearing concerns, spouse abuse, and obstetric and gynecologic care— may not be routinely assessed. Moreover, women often have more barriers to treatment than men do, such as limitations with respect to transportation, child care, finances, or health care coverage, all of which can be especially acute among poor single mothers. The identification of women substance abusers is hindered by the use of measures developed with male treatment samples, which contain items that typically assess overt social, legal, and employment consequences that are less likely to occur in female problem drinkers (Bradley et al., 1998). Bradley et al. (1998) reviewed the utility of alcohol screening measures for women and recommended the AUDIT and the TWEAK (acronym for Tolerance, friends or relatives Worried about your drinking, Eye-opener, Amnesia, and ever attempted to [K]Cut down on drinking; Russell et al., 1991). A medical examination often is indicated due to women's greater risk of adverse medical consequences of substance abuse. Other key assessment areas for women are comorbidity, especially depression; the potential abuse of prescription drugs such as minor tranquilizers and sedatives (Lisansky-Gomberg, 1999); and HIV risk, including during pregnancy.

Substance use During Pregnancy

Drinking among pregnant women increased from 0.8% in 1991 to 3.5% in 1995, and the prevalence of fetal alcohol syndrome increased six-fold from 1970 to 1993 (Chang, Wilkins-Haug, Berman, & Goetz, 1999). Illicit substance use is particularly likely to be underreported due to its severe stigma and to state laws that require physicians to report it to authorities, which may result in prosecution or loss of custody, or both. For example, Skolnick (1990) found that 16% of pregnant women at an urban medical center had drug-positive urinalyses, but only about one-half of them reported drug use. Of the women so identified who accepted treatment (48%), 61% achieved abstinence, whereas only 12% of those who refused treatment abstained; abstinence was associated with increased birth weight and head circumference. These findings underscore the need for assessment and intervention in prenatal settings that emphasize treatment entry and abstinence, rather than legal consequences. Unfortunately, only 34% of obstetric patients are routinely screened for alcohol use (Stratton, Howe, & Battaglia, 1996). Two CAGE derivatives, the TWEAK and the T-ACE (acronym for Tolerance, Annoyed by criticism of drinking, Cut down on drinking, and Eye-opener; Sokol, Martier, & Ager, 1989), are useful for detecting harmful levels of drinking among pregnant women and were normed using African Americans who attended inner-city antenatal clinics.

Ethnic Minorities

Cherpitel (1998) assessed the performance of several screening measures (e.g., breath test, CAGE, MAST, Brief MAST, AUDIT, TWEAK) among blacks, Hispanics, and whites in an emergency room (ER) setting. The tests did not perform equally well across ethnic groups, and all instruments showed greater sensitivity when the criterion was dependence alone, rather than heavy drinking and dependence combined. The Rapid Alcohol Problems Screen (RAPS; Cherpitel, 1995), a five-item scale developed with a primarily black ER population, was the most sensitive measure among blacks (93% for dependence alone, 77% for heavy drinking or dependence). The RAPS also showed the highest sensitivity among women (91% for dependence alone, 67% for heavy drinking or dependence). Across all ethnic groups, both the AUDIT and the RAPS were highly sensitive among males. A positive breath test was not a sensitive indicator of dependence alone or dependence combined with heavy drinking. Another pertinent finding was that multilingual clinical staff in many treatment centers are rare, even when first-generation immigrants are common in the surrounding neighborhoods.

Older Adults

The increasing numbers of older Americans and a 10% prevalence rate of heavy drinkers among the elderly (Helzer, Burnham, & McEvoy, 1991) have made substance abuse services for older adults a priority (Atkinson, 1990). Illicit drug use among the elderly is relatively infrequent, but prescription drugs such as benzodiazepines and narcotic analgesics are widely prescribed and should be carefully monitored for misuse. Elderly problem drinkers are less likely than younger adults to engage in heavy consumption or to experience work-related problems, drunk driving arrests, and marital problems, and they are more likely to experience aging-like symptoms, such as loss of balance, confusion, and depression. Their problems are likely to go undetected in medical settings; e.g., only 21% of elderly ER patients with alcohol problems were correctly identified (Adams, Magruder-Habib, Trued, & Broome, 1992). The MAST is insensitive to alcohol abuse in older adults, but the MAST-G, designed for them, is highly sensitive and specific (Blow, 1991). The CAGE and the U-OPEN (acronym for Unplanned use, Objections from family/friends, Preoccupation with drinking, Emotional distress drinking, and Neglect of responsibilities; DeHart & Hoffman, 1995) also are sensitive screening measures of problem drinking among the elderly (Jones, Lindsey, Yount, Soltys, & Farini-Enayat, 1993; Maisto et al., 1995). Among measures of alcohol-related problems, the Drinking Problems Index (DPI; Finney, Moos, & Brennan, 1991)) is noteworthy for its assessment of problems often encountered by older drinkers (e.g., felt confused after drinking, had a fall or accident as a result of drinking).

Drug Testing in Workplace and School Settings

This special population topic is rapidly affecting more individuals, many of whom are abstainers, and raises serious issues about privacy and testing without probable cause. Drug testing in schools is less common than in the workplace, but school-based programs appear to be growing, especially for students who participate in school-sponsored extracurricular activities. In the workplace, suggestions that employee drug use is associated with increased absenteeism, higher accident rates, increased use of medical benefits, and higher rates of job turnover (Cook et al., 1995) have made drug testing ubiquitous. The growth in drug testing continues despite ethical concerns, evidence that costs associated with employee drug use may be overstated, and the absence of evidence that drug testing is cost-effective (Lewis, 1999; Patterson, 1994; Zwerling, Ryan, & Orav, 1990).

Employee drug testing is more justifiable when drug-impaired performance poses serious safety threats (e.g., airline pilots, medical professionals). Due to concerns about the accuracy of self-reports, biological measures are the most widely used indicator of employee drug use. As discussed earlier, the validity of biological and self-reported information can be expected to vary according to the consequences of admitting substance use, which can be harsh. For example, Patterson (1994) surveyed a nationally representative sample of public and private employers and found that 36% of employees who tested positive for drugs were terminated immediately, and only 28% were provided with free substance abuse treatment. To avoid false positives, it is critical that information be collected on factors that can influence test results, such as prescription and OTC medication use (Wolff et al., 1999).

PRACTICAL RECOMMENDATIONS FOR EFFECTIVE ASSESSMENT: THE IMPORTANCE OF CONTEXT

Despite clinical lore that denial is a keystone feature of addiction, a large body of research indicates that the validity of substance abusers' verbal reports is heavily influenced by features of the assessment context and by measurement characteristics (Babor et al., 1990; Maisto, McKay, & Conners, 1990; Vuchinich et al., 1988). Therefore, researchers and clinicians should focus on identifying and implementing techniques that enhance the accuracy of self-reported information rather than concluding that these reports are inevitably fallacious (Maisto et al., 1990). Conditions that promote accurate reporting include (1) the absence of negative consequences for reporting substance use or problems; (2) providing assurances of confidentiality; (3) collecting data from individuals whose sobriety has been verified objectively (e.g., by breath tests); (4) using measures that inquire about observable events and behaviors and that do not require subjective inferences or much "mental averaging"; and (5) when retrospective measures are used, providing clients with recall aids, such as calenders that specify anchoring events for the time period of assessment (Babor et al., 1990; Donovan, 1999; Maisto et al., 1990) .

The influence of contextual variables on the accuracy of self-reported drinking information was illustrated in a recent study (Handmaker, Miller, & Manicke, 1999) that evaluated the efficacy of a brief motivational intervention for pregnant drinkers. Levels of reported alcohol consumption, as assessed during empathic, nonjudgmental interviews, were more than three times greater than levels reported on self-administered screening questionnaires. Moreover, when asked about drinking by their physician shortly before delivery, 74% of the participants reported no alcohol consumption during their pregnancy. These highly discrepant findings underscore the need to obtain alcohol-related information in a warm, nonjudgmental manner (Miller & Rollnick, 1991), particularly from groups for whom reports of drinking may result in serious repercussions.

Because no "gold standard" or unassailably valid measure of drug use currently exists, it is best to gather several lines of evidence and to evaluate the extent of convergence. Clients' informed consent to collect data from all sources is essential, and their knowledge that their reports will be verified may enhance reporting accuracy (the "bogus pipeline" effect). The most commonly used sources of self-report verification are biological assays, which were described earlier, and collateral reports from someone in frequent contact with the substance abuser. Unlike biochemical measures, which often provide only categorical information on drug use (i.e., positive or negative), collateral reports can provide detailed information on drug-taking patterns and problems over variable time frames (Maisto et al., 1990). Collateral information also is inexpensive and does not require laboratory equipment. Procedures such as the TLFB, the Form-90, and the CDP can be completed by collaterals. Good agreement typically is observed between reports of readily observable variables, such as frequency of drinking and abstinent days and types of alcoholic beverages consumed. Agreement tends to decrease, although not always significantly so, for more fine-grained parameters of drinking such as quantities consumed and durations of discrete drinking episodes. When discrepancies occur, it usually is the collateral, not the substance abuser, who reports lower values, which suggests accurate reporting by both parties since individuals have greater access to their own behavior. Official documents, such as hospital and arrest records, also have been used for verification purposes, but they can be incomplete or inaccurate and thus are not as useful as collateral reports.

Although these measures often confirm and extend self-reported information, the reports of substance users remain the most significant and complete source of assessment information. For example, results from Project Match (Babor, Steinberg, Anchor, & Del Boca, 2000) indicated that clients' self reports were more sensitive indicators of drinking than were both collateral reports and biochemical measures of liver functioning. GGT was a particularly insensitive measure. Discrepancies between the three measures were positively correlated with problem severity, pretreatment drinking, treatment history, and cognitive impairment. Babor and associates concluded that, for clinical trials using self-referred participants, "resources devoted to collecting these alternative sources of outcome data might be better invested in interview procedures designed to increase the validity of self-report information" (p. 55).

Understanding the Social Meaning of Substance Use and Abuse

Another contextual feature important for understanding a client's substance abuse and the contingencies that maintain it are social network responses to their drug-taking behavior and the values the network has about abstinence, drug use, and abuse (Milby, Schumacher, & Tucker, in press). Whether defined by age, socioeconomics, or geography, social subgroups influence members' substance use traditions, rituals, and norms. Gender, age, ethnic, and cultural subgroups can vary in their use of drug classes, patterns of use, and routes of administration, and these connections may change over time as drug availability, price, and broader socioeconomic and political conditions change. For example, regardless of intent, the U.S. War on Drugs involves mandatory minimum sentencing laws for drug offenses that have resulted in the disproportionate imprisonment of African American and Hispanic males (Courtland, 1996/1997). Crack cocaine, which is favored by minority groups, carries harsher legal penalties than powdered cocaine, which is favored by middle-class white users. Practitioners should assess such contextual features and attend to the traditions, values, and risks that vary across subgroups.

Role of Coercion and the Criminal Justice System in Substance Abuse Services

Over 20% of the nearly 2 million U.S. prison inmates are incarcerated for drug-related crimes, which is an 800% increase since the intensification of the drug war that began in 1980 during the Reagan administration (McCaffrey, 2000). In an effort to reduce this segment of the prison population, "drug courts" flourished during the 1990s and have diverted an estimated 100,000 drug offenders into substance abuse treatment rather than incarceration. When combined with the heightened risk of HIV transmission in prisons, these trends reveal a pressing need for the involvement of substance abuse professionals in the criminal justice system. Substance abuse treatment in prisons improves postrelease outcomes (Wexler & Sacks, 2000), as do postrelease aftercare and relapse prevention programs (Brown, 2000). Furthermore, court-mandated treatment does not produce outcomes that are worse than for clients who enter treatment under less extreme pressure (Stitzer & Mc-Caul, 1987).

These trends have several implications for assessment and treatment. First, individuals legally coerced into treatment are likely to be younger and to have a different clinical presentation than other clients (Schmidt & Weisner, 1999). For example, their substance use practices may be less of a problem than the functional consequences of use, especially in the legal arena, and treatment goals will need to be adjusted accordingly. Second, for people who are incarcerated, assessing their postrelease community and family environment and their functional living skills is critical to planning interventions. Third, the contingencies operating on individuals who are coerced into treatment require very careful assessment. If understood and used properly, they can enhance clients' motivation for treatment and behavior change. To the extent possible, using them in a positive incentive system to promote change and to help clients' gain access to valued nondrug activities and reinforcers is preferable to using them in a response cost or punishment scheme. Finally, limitations on confidentiality must be fully understood by the client and provider alike. Even in court- and employer-referred cases, there usually is some reasonable measure of protection of confidentiality, as long as the client is attending sessions sober.

INTEGRATING ASSESSMENT WITH INTERVENTIONS AND OUTCOME EVALUATION

Using the Assessment Process to Promote a Continuum of Care

More members of the population with substance-related problems need to be reached through screening in nonspecialized health care settings. Persons with problems are common, but their utilization of substance-focused services is not. For example, individuals with accidental or traumatic injuries, or who have been involved in episodes of crime, violence, or sexual assault, should be routinely screened for alcohol or drug involvement, as should clients who present with complaints or symptoms that often are comorbid with substance abuse (e.g., depression, anxiety, memory problems, tremor). Substance use by pregnant women also should be assessed routinely early in pregnancy.

Screening will be helpful to identified individuals only if diverse services that meet the heterogeneous needs are available. An ideal continuum of care would range from brief interventions in nonspecialized settings through outpatient specialized services to inpatient and residential treatment facilities. The proper use of assessment procedures for substance use disorders is central to selecting, implementing, and monitoring whatever intervention is appropriate for a given individual. An important organizing concept is the "stepped care" intervention management approach (Abrams, Clark, & King, 1999; Sobell & Sobell, 1999), in which assessment information is used to select the least intensive and costly intervention that is likely to be effective. Progress is monitored and, if the client fails to improve after a reasonable trial, the level of care is intensified or "stepped up." For example, many persons with less severe problems improve after a brief motivational intervention using feedback from assessment results that is delivered in an objective and empathic manner (reviewed by Bien, Miller, & Tonigan, 1993; Zweben & Fleming, 1999). Such interventions are flexible and can be delivered by nonspecialists in primary care, ER, worksite, and other community settings. For clients with more serious problems, such as alcohol-dependent individuals, brief interventions can facilitate referrals to specialized treatment, which often is needed to resolve their more extensive problems. In other cases, substance abusers who are not presently motivated to change may later use the information provided in the brief intervention to facilitate positive change, with or without specialized care.

The stepped-care concept is not new in medicine, but its application to substance-related problems has been delayed because their heterogeneity was not recognized or reflected in intervention options. The field is moving away from the "one size fits all" abstinence-oriented approach to treatment that has dominated services in the United States for several decades. As discussed next, exploiting these developments on behalf of clients depends on detailed assessment information that continues throughout the therapeutic interaction.

Integrating Assessment into Interventions

Initial assessment information will help establish which aspects of a client's substance-related behaviors should be targeted for interventions, their motivation (or lack thereof) for change in each identified area, the resources available to support specific changes, and the urgency for change due to risks associated with failing to change. Both short- and long-term intervention goals will be developed accordingly, and continued assessment will allow the modification of goals over time, depending on changes in behavior or the lack thereof.

Identification of high-risk behaviors requires early attention. Common risky behaviors among substance abusers include drinking and driving; unsafe sex; injection drug use, especially needle sharing; substance use during pregnancy; and polydrug abuse. For example, lowering the risk of HIV infection to self and others by reducing, if not eliminating, injection drug use, needle sharing, and unprotected sex should be an intervention priority, and HIV testing should be encouraged for as long as the client engages in risky behavior. Assessing and intervening to constrain potentially lethal behaviors to self and others take precedence over other intervention goals, including the conventional treatment goal of the immediate elimination of all substance use. This is a major principle of harm-reduction programs and one that is sensitive to the relative risk of continued engagement in different behaviors (Marlatt, 1998).

A second area for early consideration is the formulation of goals regarding substance use, which is a basic problem parameter in most cases and requires ongoing monitoring. Despite the emphasis on immediate and permanent abstinence in 12-step treatment programs and mutual help groups guided by the principles of AA, the research literature on resolution patterns has revealed several pathways to successful change. For example, "warm-turkey" resolutions that involve gradual reductions from problem to nonproblem alcohol use or abstinence are well known (King & Tucker, 2000; Miller & Page, 1991). In the drug abuse literature, there are reports of opiate addicts who gradually transitioned from heroin use to abstinence with an intervening period of a year or more when they used a range of other drugs (e.g., alcohol, marijuana, hypnotics) (Tucker & King, 1999). Marijuana, in particular, appears to function as a "reverse" gateway drug when drug abusers try to stop using more harmful drugs like opiates (Marlatt, 1998). Thus, with respect to goal setting, a greater range of behavioral possibilities should be entertained and evaluated based on clients' past substance use practices, risks associated with continued use (e.g., health and legal risks), environmental support for different goals, and client preferences. In the case of alcohol abuse, moderation drinking is a reasonable initial goal choice for clients with mild to moderate problems who prefer it and, should they fail to drink moderately after a reasonable trial, are likely to be more receptive to a goal of abstinence. Guidelines for safe alcohol use are available (e.g., Sanchez-Craig, Wilkinson, & Davila, 1995) and are important for use in brief interventions. See Rosenberg (1993) for a review of predictors of moderation outcomes.

Other problem parameters that merit ongoing assessment during interventions will vary across clients, depending on the nature of their problems. For example, some clients will have long-standing, complex contingencies between their substance abuse and specific areas of functioning, such as their marriage or job, and the resolution of these problems will be basic to sustaining overall improvement. Others may have more circumscribed, but nonetheless serious, problems such as drinking to intoxication at social events or failing to use condoms reliably when intoxicated. The nature of the intervention goals will determine the nature of continued assessment with individual clients, and these may change as their goals evolve during treatment.

Outcome Evaluation: Moving beyond a Treatment Efficacy Research Agenda

Assessment obviously plays a key part in any outcome evaluation for clinical purposes and in research to evaluate whether interventions produce beneficial changes in behavioral, health status, and cost-related variables. Detailed discussion of evaluation research is beyond our scope (see also Abrams et al., 1999; Seligman, 1995; Tucker, 1999; Yates, 1995), but a noteworthy trend is the expansion of evaluation questions beyond experiments on treatment efficacy to include studies of the utility and ease of implementation of interventions in usual care settings. These health services research initiatives of the 1990s include evaluations of intervention efficacy, effectiveness, cost-effectiveness, and target population impact. Efficacy studies, typically randomized clinical trials, evaluate the effects of interventions under highly controlled and constrained conditions with homogeneous samples so that the "true" effects of the intervention can be detected. Effectiveness studies evaluate intervention effects under usual care conditions with heterogeneous samples and may or may not involve an experimental manipulation. Cost-effectiveness studies evaluate the relative monetary costs and benefits of interventions in order to identify which intervention produces the best cost/benefit ratio. Target population impact studies include some elements of efficacy, effectiveness, and cost-effectiveness studies and evaluate how well an intervention reaches or "covers" a target population, as well as the magnitude and cost of desirable health or behavioral outcomes that result from the intervention on a per person and population basis.

More is currently known in the substance abuse area about intervention efficacy and cost-effectiveness than about effectiveness and maximizing population impact. Like the general psychotherapy literature, "horse-race" comparisons of different treatments have dominated evaluation research in the substance abuse area, and, also like the psychotherapy literature, outcomes are similar across treatments. Thus, continuing to search for differences based on technical variations in interventions is no longer as compelling as investigating how to lower barriers to services and to reach more of the target population with a range of interventions that better match their diverse needs. One exception to this trend is the recent efficacy evaluations of combining various pharmacotherapies with psychosocial treatments of known efficacy.

Research also has shown that substance abuse interventions are relatively cost-effective in reducing drug-related problems and associated costs. For example, cocaine treatment is more cost-effective than are border interdiction, drug source country eradication programs, and police actions (e.g., RAND Corporation, 1995). In addition, the cost-offset benefits of including substance abuse treatment in comprehensive health plans have been documented for years (Holder, Lennox, & Blose, 1992). Relative to interventions for many health and behavioral health problems, treating substance abuse is cheap and generally yields large benefits in averting future health care and other economic costs (Tengs et al., 1995).

Less research is available on intervention effectiveness and health services research questions, including barriers to and incentives for help-seeking; treatment engagement and retention; how compliance relates to outcome; and how clients' life circumstances interact with intervention entry, engagement, and outcomes (Longabaugh, Wirtz, Zweben, & Stout, 1998; Moos et al., 1990). This complex research agenda departs from conventional efficacy studies and requires the use of different methods. Such research is needed to support the development of a range of interventions that collectively provide cost-effective coverage and rational resource allocation across the continuum of care required by the heterogeneous needs of substance abusers.

There is an array of excellent measures that span the relevant dependent variable domains of substance use practices; related problems, including functional impairment and dependence levels; and the cognitive, affective, and motivational states that have been found to be predictive of outcomes. We also know that several treatment approaches work relatively well for this often chronic behavioral health problem, but that only a small segment of population in need uses them. We know less about how to dimensionalize, assess, and change the natural environments within which substance use is embedded and how features of the health care system interact with person-specific attributes and problems and with their surrounding social and economic environment. Investigating these issues is basic to broadening interventions for substance abuse beyond specialized clinical treatments to include primary care applications, as well as a range of lower-threshold, community, and Internet-based interventions that are guided by public health principles.

INTEGRATING SUBSTANCE ABUSE SERVICES INTO ROUTINE HEALTH CARE: ASSESSING THE SYSTEM

Substance abuse is a prevalent but stigmatized behavioral health disorder that needs an expansion of relevant services. Some expansion is occurring at the grassroots level, as evidenced by the harm-reduction movement and the proliferation of mutual help groups. The health care system also is changing as a result of managed care and offers opportunities to expand and re-configure the way that professional services for substance abuse have been offered. Because the practice environment continues to evolve rapidly, successful providers must stay abreast of the broader health economic, policy, and reimbursement procedures that surround their professional efforts, in addition to continuing to focus on their clients' needs. Although these fundamental changes have been distressing to some practitioners, they offer new avenues for service delivery that may prove beneficial, both economically and with respect to expanding access to services.

Until recently, mental health and substance abuse (MH/SA) services have primarily been offered in inpatient units or specialized programs, which are costly, high-threshold, and stigmatizing. This organizational arrangement is a thinly disguised continuation of the "asylum" model of the Victorian era, which segregated persons with these problems in locked institutions (Tucker, 1999). As managed care has come to dominate the health care market, two new trends are discernable in the way MH/SA services are offered: (1) behavioral health carve-outs, which segregate MH/SA services and require approval for services from a primary care or managed care gatekeeper (Anderson, Berland, Mauch, & Maloney, 1996); or (2) integrated behavioral health care, which involves behavioral health providers as part of the primary care health team so MH/SA services are part of routine health care (Strosahl, 1998). Specialized treatment programs remain necessary for persons with more severe problems who cannot be managed effectively in a primary care setting, but such programs are unnecessary for many persons with substance-related problems. Integrated behavioral health care models reflect a growing appreciation for the facts that substance abuse and other behavioral health problems are common, may present in a variety of ways outside of specialized care settings, and may resolve readily with limited interventions. Provision of services for these problems as part of routine health care offers an avenue for increasing access to appropriate services and often yields economic benefits in reducing total health care costs.

Managed care thus offers an unprecedented opportunity to "mainstream" MH/SA services if certain developments are cultivated and others avoided. On the positive side, more insured individuals now have a behavioral health benefit, which should help destigmatize these disorders and make services more accessible. On the negative side, behavioral health benefits usually involve quite restrictive reimbursable services, have higher copayments and deductibles than medical benefits, and are regarded as most dispensable when benefits are cut to reduce costs, even though they account for a small fraction of insurance plan reimbursements (Strum & Wells, 2000). Furthermore, substance abuse services continue to fare poorly even in relation to mental health services; for example, they were omitted in the first federal parity legislation that sought to establish some measure of equivalence between benefits for health and mental health problems.

A related trend is the tendency of managed care plans to reimburse services at fee levels that are acceptable to the lowest competent provider. Doctoral level providers are not needed for competent therapeutic services for many MH/SA problems (e.g., Dawes, 1994), although they clearly are needed for complex cases, to train and supervise subdoctoral service providers on routine cases, to triage clients appropriately, and to implement and manage practice evaluation activities. This economically driven articulation of new service delivery roles has been painful for independent doctoral practitioners, but in the long run it may make better use of their education and entrepreneurial potential and offer new income possibilities.

So what does this have to do with assessment? As discussed in this chapter, in the short run psychologists and other mental professionals have responded to these health care trends by developing sound screening instruments and brief interventions that can be offered in the busy health care environment. The substance abuse field is a model example of this trend and has made considerable progress in being able to offer clinically feasible, effective services in the new practice environment. In the long run, however, doctoral professionals are not needed as direct providers of these services and will function more effectively as coordinators and supervisors of care, as program evaluation experts, and as system managers. Developing partnerships with physicians, other health care workers at both the doctoral and subdoctoral levels, and managed care companies will continue to be challenging, but all are essential to function in the new environment. This does not mean returning to the old subservient role of assessor that psychiatry imposed on psychology during the post–World War II era. It does mean using our assessment skills to understand the complex contingencies that have emerged in today's managed care practice environment and working to assure adequate access to appropriate services for individual clients within that broader system.

ACKNOWLEDGMENT

Manuscript preparation was supported in part by Grant Nos. R01 AA08972 and K02 AA00209 from the National Institute on Alcohol Abuse and Alcoholism.

REFERENCES

Abrams, D. B., Clark, M. M., & King, T. K. (1999). Increasing the impact of nicotine dependence treatment: Conceptual and practical considerations in a stepped-care plus treatment-matching approach. In J. A. Tucker, D. M. Donovan, & G. A. Marlatt (Eds.), *Changing addictive behavior: Bridging clinical and public health strategies* (pp. 307–330). New York: Guilford Press.

Adams, W. L., Magruder-Habib, K., Trued, S., & Broome, H. L. (1992). Alcohol abuse in elderly emergency room patients. *Journal of the American Geriatrics Society, 40*, 1236–1240.

Allen, J. P., & Columbus, M. (Eds.) (1995). *Assessing alcohol problems: A guide for clinicians and researchers* (Treatment Handbook Series No. 4). Bethesda, MD: National Institute on Alcohol Abuse and Alcoholism.

Allen, J. P., Columbus, M., & Fertig, J. B. (1995). Assessment of alcoholism treatment: An overview. In J. P. Allen & M. Columbus (Eds.), *Assessing alcohol problems: A guide for clinicians and researchers* (Treatment Handbook Series No. 4, pp. 1–9). Bethesda, MD: National Institute on Alcohol Abuse and Alcoholism.

American Psychiatric Association. (1987). *Diagnostic and statistical manual of mental disorders* (3rd ed., rev.). Washington DC: Author.

American Psychiatric Association. (1994). *Diagnostic and statistical manual of mental disorders* (4th ed.). Washington DC: Author.

Ames, G., Schmidt, C., Klee, L., & Saltz, R. (1996). Combining methods to identify new measures of women's drinking problems: Part I. The ethnographic stage. *Addiction, 91*, 829–844.

Anderson, D. F., Berland, J. L., Mauch, D., & Maloney, W. R. (1996). Managed behavioral health care services. In P. R. Kongstvedt (Ed.), *The managed health care handbook* (3rd ed.). Gaithersburg, MD: Aspen Publications.

Annis, H. M., Graham, J. M., & Davis, C. S. (1987). *Inventory of Drinking Situations (IDS): Users guide.* Toronto: Addiction Research Foundation of Ontario.

Annis, H. M., Martin, G., & Graham, J. M. (1992). *Inventory of Drug-Taking Situations (IDTS): Users guide.* Toronto: Addiction Research Foundation of Ontario.

Anton, R. F., Litten, R. Z., & Allen, J. P. (1995). Biological assessment of alcohol consumption. In J. P. Allen & M. Columbus (Eds.), *Assessing alcohol problems: A guide for clinicians and researchers* (Treatment Handbook Series No. 4, pp. 31–40). Bethesda, MD: National Institute on Alcohol Abuse and Alcoholism.

Atkinson, R. M. (1990). Aging and alcohol use disorders: Diagnostic issues in the elderly. *International Psychogeriatrics, 2*, 55–72.

Babor, T. F., Brown, J., & Del Boca, F. K. (1990). Validity of self-reports in applied research on addictive behaviors: Fact or fiction? *Addictive Behaviors, 12*, 5–32.

Babor, T. F., Steinberg, K., Anton, R., & Del Boca, F. K. (2000). Talk is cheap: Measuring drinking outcomes in clinical trials. *Journal of Studies on Alcohol, 61*, 55–63.

Babor, T. F., Stephens, R. S., & Marlatt, G. A. (1987). Verbal report methods in clinical research on alcoholism: Response bias and its minimization. *Journal of Studies on Alcohol, 48*, 410–424.

Bates, M. E. (1997). The stability of neuropsychological assessment early in alcoholism treatment. *Journal of Studies on Alcohol, 58*, 617–622.

Beck, A. T., Steer, R. A., & Brown, G. K. (1996). *Beck Depression Inventory, Second Edition Manual.* San Antonio, TX: Psychological Corporation.

Berkson, J. (1946). Limitations of the application of the 4-fold table analysis to hospital data. *Biometrics, 2*, 47–53.

Bien, T. H., Miller, W. R., & Tonigan, J. S. (1993). Brief intervention for alcohol problems: A review. *Addiction, 88*, 315–336.

Blow, F. (1991). *Michigan Alcoholism Screening Test—Geriatric version (MAST-G).* Ann Arbor: University of Michigan Alcohol Research Center.

Bradley, K. A., Boyd-Wickizer, J., Powell, S. H., & Burman, M. L. (1998). Alcohol screening questionnaires in women. *Journal of the American Medical Association, 280*, 166–174.

Brown, B. S. (2000, August). When treatment works but the community fails: The need for aftercare and relapse prevention. *Connection, 4.*

Brown, S. A. (1985). Reinforcement expectancies and alcoholism treatment outcome after a one-year follow-up. *Journal of Studies on Alcohol, 46*, 304–308.

Brown, S. A., Christiansen, B. A., & Goldman, M. S. (1987). The Alcohol Expectancy Questionnaire: An instrument for the assessment of adolescent and adult alcohol expectancies. *Journal of Studies on Alcohol, 48*, 483–491.

Brown, S. A., Goldman, M. S., Inn, A., & Anderson, L. R. (1980). Expectations of reinforcement from alcohol: Their domain and relation to drinking patterns. *Journal of Consulting and Clinical Psychology, 48,* 419–426.

Buchsbaum, D. (1994). Effectiveness of treatment in general medical patients with drinking problems. *Alcohol Health and Research World, 18,* 140–145.

Butcher, J. N., Dahlstrom, W. G., Graham, J. R., Tellegren, A., & Kaemmer, B. (1989). *Manual for administration and scoring: MMPI-2.* Minneapolis: University of Minnesota Press.

Cahalan, D. (1970). *Problem drinkers.* San Francisco: Jossey Bass.

Carey, K. B., & Teitlbaum, L. M. (1996). Goals and methods of alcohol assessment. *Professional Psychology: Research and Practice, 27,* 460–466.

Carrol, K. M. (1999). Behavioral and cognitive behavioral treatments. In B. S. McCrady & E. E. Epstein (Eds.), *Addictions: A comprehensive guidebook* (pp. 187–215). New York: Oxford University Press.

Chang, G., Wilkens-Haug, L., Berman, S., & Goetz, A. (1999). The TWEAK: Application in a prenatal setting. *Journal of Studies on Alcoholism, 60,* 306–309.

Cherpitel, C. J. (1995). Analysis of cut points for screening instruments for alcohol problems in the emergency room. *Journal of Studies on Alcohol, 56,* 695–700.

Cherpitel, C. J. (1998). Differences in performance of screening instruments for problem drinking among blacks, whites, and Hispanics in an emergency room population. *Journal of Studies on Alcohol, 59,* 420–426.

Conners, G. J. (1995). Screening for alcohol problems. In J. P. Allen & M. Columbus (Eds.), *Assessing alcohol problems: A guide for clinicians and researchers* (Treatment Handbook Series No. 4, pp. 17–30). Bethesda, MD: National Institute on Alcohol Abuse and Alcoholism.

Cook, R. F, Bernstein, A. D., Arrington, T. A., Andrews, C. M., & Marshall, G. A. (1995). Methods for assessing drug use prevalence in the workplace: A comparison of self-report, urinalysis, and hair analysis. *International Journal of the Addictions, 30,* 403–426.

Courtland, D. T. (1996/1997). The drug war's hidden toll. *Issues in Science and Technology, 13,* 71–77.

Crist, D. A., & Milby, J. B. (1990). Psychometric and neuropsychological assessment. In W. D. Lerner & M. A. Barr (Eds.), *Hospital based substance abuse treatment* (pp. 18–33). New York: Pergamon.

Davies, A. D. M. (1968). The influence of age on trail making test performance. *Journal of Clinical Psychology, 24,* 96–98.

Dawes, R. M. (1994). *House of cards: Psychology and psychotherapy built on myth.* New York: Free Press.

DeHart, S. S., & Hoffman, N. G. (1995). Screening and diagnosis of "Alcohol abuse and dependence" in older adults. *International Journal of the Addictions, 30,* 1717–1747.

Deitz, D., Rohde, F., Bertolucci, D., & Dufour, M. (1994). Prevalence of screening for alcohol use by physicians during routine physical examinations. *Alcohol Health and Research World, 18,* 162–168.

Derogatis, L. R. (1977). *SCL-90: Administration, scoring and procedures manual for the revised version.* Baltimore: Clinical Psychometrics Research.

DiClemente, C. C., Carbonari, J. P., Mongomery, R. P. G., & Hughes, S. O. (1994). The Alcohol Abstinence Self-Efficacy Scale. *Journal of Studies on Alcohol, 55,* 141–148.

Dimeff, L. A., Baer, J. S., Kivlahan, D. R., & Marlatt, G. A. (1999). *Brief Alcohol Screening and Intervention for College Students (BASICS): A harm reduction approach.* New York: Guilford Press.

Donovan, D. M. (1995). Assessments to aid in the treatment planning process. In J. P. Allen & M. Columbus (Eds.), *Assessing alcohol problems: A guide for clinicians and researchers* (Treatment Handbook Series No. 4, pp. 75–122). Bethesda, MD: National Institute on Alcohol Abuse and Alcoholism.

Donovan, D. M. (1999). Assessment strategies and measures in addictive behaviors. In B. S. McCrady & E. E. Epstein (Eds.), *Addictions: A comprehensive guidebook* (pp. 187–215). New York: Oxford University Press.

Donovan, D. M., & Marlatt, G. A. (Eds.) (1988). *Assessment of addictive behaviors.* New York: Guilford Press.

Finney, J. W., Moos, R. H., & Brennan, P. L. (1991). The Drinking Problems Index: A measure to assess alcohol-related problems among older adults. *Journal of Substance Abuse, 3,* 395–404.

First, M. B., Spitzer, R. L., Gibbon, M., & Williams, J. B. W. (1996). *Structured Clinical Interview for DSM-IV Axis I Disorders—Patient Edition (SCID-I/P, Version 2.0).* New York: Biometrics Research Department, New York State Psychiatric Institute.

Fischman, M., & Johanson, C. (1996). Cocaine. In C. Schuster & M. Kuhar (Eds.), *Pharmacological aspects of drug dependence: Toward an integrated neurobehavior approach* (pp. 159–195). Berlin: Springer Verlag.

Gavin, D. R., Ross, H. E., & Skinner, H. (1989). Diagnostic validity of the Drug Abuse Screening Test in the assessment of DSM-III drug disorders. *British Journal of Addiction, 84,* 301–307.

Goldberg, H. I., Mullen, M., Ries, R. K., Psaty, B. M., & Ruch, B. P. (1991). Alcohol counseling in a general medical clinic. *Medical Care, 29,* 49–56.

Golden, C. J., Ariel, R., McKay, S. E., Wilkening, G. N., Wolf, B. A., & MacInnes, W. D. (1982). The Luria–Nebraska Neuropsychological Battery: Theoretical orientation and comment. *Journal of Consulting and Clinical Psychology, 50,* 291–300.

Graham, J. R. (2000). *MMPI-2: Assessing personality and psychopathology* (pp. 155–160). New York: Oxford University Press.

Grant, B. F., & Dawson, D. A. (1999). Alcohol and drug use, abuse, and dependence: Classification, prevalence, and comorbidity. In B. S. McCrady & E. E. Epstein (Eds.), *Addictions: A comprehensive guidebook* (pp. 9–29). New York: Oxford University Press.

Grant, B. F., & Hasin, D. S. (1990). *The Alcohol Use Disorders and Associated Disabilities Interview Schedule (AUDADIS).* Rockville, MD: National Institute of Alcohol Abuse and Alcoholism.

Handmaker, N. S., Miller, W. R., & Manicke, M. (1999). Findings of a pilot study of motivational interviewing with pregnant drinkers. *Journal of Studies on Alcohol, 60,* 285–287.

Hasin, D. S., Trautman, K. D., Miele, G. M., Samet, S., Smith, M., & Endicott, J. (1996). Psychiatric Research Interview for Substance and Mental Disorders (PRISM): Reliability for substance abusers. *American Journal of Psychiatry, 153,* 1195–1201.

Helzer, J. E., Burnham, A., & McEvoy, L. T. (1991). Alcohol abuse and dependence. In L. N. Robins, & D. A. Regier (Eds.), *Psychiatric disorders in America: The Epidemiologic Catchment Study* (pp. 81–115). New York: Free Press.

Hendricks, V. M., Kaplan, C. D., VanLimbeek, J., & Geerlings, P. (1988). The Addiction Severity Index: Reliability and validity in a Dutch addict population. *Journal of Substance Abuse Treatment, 17,* 606–610.

Hodgins, D. C., & El, G. N. (1992). More data on the Addiction Severity Index: Reliability and validity with the mentally ill substance abuser. *Journal of Nervous and Mental Disease, 180,* 197–201.

Holder, H. D., Lennox, R. D., & Blose, J. O. (1992). The economic benefits of alcoholism treatment: A summary of twenty years of research. *Journal of Employee Assistance Research, 1,* 63–82.

Hurlbut, S. C., & Sher, K. J. (1992). Assessing alcohol problems in college students. *Journal of American College Health, 41,* 49–58.

Institute of Medicine. (1990). *Broadening the base of treatment for alcohol problems.* Washington, DC: National Academy Press.

Jaffe, A. J., & Kilbey, M. M. (1994). The Cocaine Expectancy Questionnaire (CEQ): Construction and predictive utility. *Psychological Assessment, 6,* 18–26.

Jellinek, E. M. (1960). *The disease concept of alcoholism.* New Brunswick, NJ: Hill House Press.

Johnson, J. G., Spitzer, R. L., Williams, J. B. W., Knoenke, K., Linzer, M., Brody, D., DeGruy, F., & Hahn, S. (1995). Psychiatric comorbidity, health status, and functional impairment associated with alcohol abuse and dependence in primary care patients: Findings of the PRIME MD–1000 study. *Journal of Consulting and Clinical Psychology, 63,* 133–140.

Johnston, L. D., O'Malley, P. M., & Bachman, J. G. (1995). *National Survey results on drug use from the monitoring the future study, 1975–1994: Vol. 1. Secondary school students* (NIH Publication No. 95-4026). Washington, DC: U.S. Government Printing Office.

Jones, T. V., Lindsey, B. A., Yount, P., Soltys, R., & Farini-Enayat, B. (1993). Alcoholism screening questionnaires: Are they valid in elderly medical outpatients? *Journal of General Internal Medicine, 8,* 674–678.

Jurkovich, G. J., Rivera, F. P., Gurney, J. G., Fligner, C., Ries, R., Mueller, B. A., & Copass, M. (1993). The effects of acute alcohol intoxication and chronic alcohol abuse on outcome from trauma. *Journal of the American Medical Association, 270,* 51–56.

Kessler, R. C., McGonagle, K. A., Zhao, S. A., Nelson, C. B., Hughes, M., Eshleman, S., Wittchen, H., & Kendler, K. S. (1994). Lifetime and 12-month prevalence of DSM III-R psychiatric disorders in the U.S.: Results from the National Comorbidity Study. *Archives of General Psychiatry, 51,* 8–19.

King, M. P., & Tucker, J. A. (2000). Behavior change patterns and strategies distinguishing moderation drinking and abstinence during the natural resolution of alcohol problems without treatment. *Psychology of Addictive Behaviors, 23,* 537–541.

Kivlahan, D. R., Sher, K. J., & Donovan, D. M. (1989). The Alcohol Dependence Scale: A validation study among inpatient alcoholics. *Journal of Studies on Alcohol, 50,* 170–175.

Leigh, B. C. (1987). Beliefs about the effects of alcohol on self and others. *Journal of Studies on Alcohol, 48,* 467–475.

Lewis, D. C. (1999). Drug testing: The downside of a good technology. *Brown University Digest of Addiction Theory and Application, 18,* 8–11.

Lisansky-Gomberg, E. S. (1999). Women. In B. S. McCrady & E. E. Epstein (Eds.), *Addictions: A comprehensive guidebook* (pp. 9–29). New York: Oxford University Press.

Longabaugh, R., Wirtz, P. W., Zweben, A., & Stout, R. L. (1998). Network support for drinking, Alcoholics Anonymous, and long-term matching effects. *Addiction, 93,* 1313–1333.

Love, A., James, D., & Willner, P. (1998). A comparison of two alcohol craving questionnaires. *Addiction, 93,* 1091–1102.

Magruber-Habib, K., Stevens, H. A., & Alling, W. C. (1993). Relative performance of the MAST, VAST, and CAGE versus DSM-III criteria for alcohol dependence. *Journal of Clinical Epidemiology, 46,* 435–441.

Maisto, S. A., Carey, K. B., & Bradizza, C. M. (1999). Social learning theory. In K. E. Leanard & H. T. Blane (Eds.), *Psychological theories of drinking and alcoholism* (2nd ed., pp. 106–163). New York: Guilford Press.

Maisto, S. A., Conners, G. J., & Allen, J. P. (1995). Contrasting self-report screens for alcohol problems: A review. *Alcoholism Clinical and Experimental Research, 19,* 1510–1516.

Maisto, S. A., & McKay, J. R. (1995). Diagnosis. In J. P. Allen and M. Columbus (Eds.), *Assessing alcohol problems: A guide for clinicians and researchers* (Treatment Handbook Series No. 4, pp. 41–54). Bethesda, MD: National Institute on Alcohol Abuse and Alcoholism.

Maisto, S. A., McKay, J. R., & Conners, G. J. (1990). Self-report issues in substance abuse: State of the art and future directions. *Behavioral Assessment, 12,* 117–134.

Mann, R. E., Sobell, L. C., Sobell, M. B., & Pavin, D. (1985). Family tree questionnaire for assessing family history of drinking problems. In D. J. Lettieri, J. E. Nelson, & M. A. Sayers (Eds.), *Alcoholism treatment assessment research instruments* (NIAAA Treatment Handbook Series No. 2, pp. 162–166). Washington, DC: U.S. Government Printing Office.

Marlatt, G. A. (Ed.) (1998). *Harm reduction: Pragmatic strategies for managing high-risk behaviors.* New York: Guilford Press.

Marlatt, G. A., & Gordon, J. R. (Eds.). (1985). *Relapse prevention: Maintenance strategies in the treatment of addictive behaviors.* New York: Guilford Press.

Marlatt, G. A., Tucker, J. A., Donovan, D. M., & Vuchinich, R. E. (1997). Help-seeking by substance abusers: The role of harm reduction and behavioral-economic approaches to facilitate treatment entry and retention. In L. S. Onken, J. D. Blaine, & J. J. Boren (Eds.), *Beyond the therapeutic alliance: Keeping the drug-dependent individual in treatment* (NIDA Research Monograph No. 165, pp. 44–84). Rockville, MD: U.S. Department of Health and Human Services.

Mayfield, D., McLeod, G., & Hall, P. (1974). The CAGE questionnaire: Validation of a new alcoholism instrument. *American Journal of Psychiatry, 131,* 1121–1123.

McCaffrey, B. R. (2000, August). Drug abuse and the criminal justice system: Saving lives and preventing crime through treatment. *Connection,* 1–2.

McConnaughy, E. A., Prochaska, J. O., & Velicer, W. F. (1983). Stages of change in psychotherapy: Measurement and sample profiles. *Psychotherapy: Theory, Research, and Practice, 20,* 368–375.

McEldowney, R. P., & Heilman, J. G. (1999). Evaluation of substance abuse treatment programs in the era of managed care: The role of cost–benefit analysis. In J. A. Tucker, D. M. Donovan, & G. A. Marlatt (Eds.), *Changing addictive behavior: Bridging clinical and public health strategies* (pp. 344–365). New York: Guilford Press.

McLellan, A. T., Alterman, A. I., Metzger, D. S., Grissom, G. R., Woody, G. E., Luborsky, L., & O'Brien, C. P. (1994). Similarity of outcome predictors across opiate, cocaine, alcohol treatments: Role of treatment services. *Journal of Consulting and Clinical Psychology, 62*, 1141–1158.

McLellan, A. T., Luborsky, L., Woody, G. E., & O'Brien C. P. (1980). An improved diagnostic evaluation instrument for substance abuse patients: The Addiction Severity Index. *Journal of Nervous and Mental Disorders, 168*, 26–33.

Milby, J. B., Schumacher, J. E., & Tucker, J. A. (in press). Substance abuse. In J. Raczynski, L. Bradley, & L. Leviton (Eds.), *Disorders of behavior and health* (Vol. 2). Washington, DC: American Psychological Association.

Miller, W. R., & Marlatt, G. A. (1984). *Manual for the Comprehensive Drinker Profile.* Odessa, FL: Psychological Assessment Resources.

Miller, W. R., & Page, A. C. (1991). Warm turkey: Other routes to abstinence. *Journal of Substance Abuse Treatment, 8*, 227–232.

Miller, W. R., & Rollnick, S. (1991). *Motivational interviewing: Preparing people to change addictive behavior.* New York: Guilford Press.

Miller, W. R., & Tonigan, J. S. (1996). Assessing drinkers' motivation for change: The Stages of Change Readiness and Treatment Eagerness Scale (SOCRATES). *Psychology of Addictive Behaviors, 10*, 81–89.

Miller, W. R., Tonigan, J. S., & Longabaugh, R. (1995). *The Drinker Inventory of Consequences (DrInC): An instrument for assessing adverse consequences of alcohol abuse. Test Manual* (Project MATCH Monograph Series, Vol. 4). Rockville, MD: National Institute on Alcohol Abuse and Alcoholism.

Millon, T. (1992). Millon Clinical Multiaxial Inventory: 1 and 2. *Journal of Counseling and Development, 70*, 421–426.

Moos, R. H., Finney, J. W., & Cronkite, R. (1990). *Alcoholism treatment: Context, process, and outcome.* New York: Oxford University Press.

Morey, L. C. (1996). *An interpretive guide to the Personality Assessment Inventory (PAI).* Sarasota, FL: Psychological Assessment Resources.

Mundt, J. C., Searles, J. S., Perrine, M. W., & Helzer, J. E. (1995). Cycles of alcohol dependence: Frequency-domain analyses of daily drinking logs for matched alcohol-dependent and nondependent subjects. *Journal of Studies on Alcohol, 56*, 491–499.

Narrow, W. E., Regier, D. A., Rae, D. S., Manderscheid, R. W., & Locke, B. A. (1993). Use of services by persons with mental and addictive disorders. *Archives of General Psychiatry, 50*, 95–107.

National Institute on Drug Abuse. (1999). *Principles of drug addiction treatment: A research-base guide* (National Institutes of Health Publication No. 99–4180). Bethesda, MD: Author.

National Institutes of Health (1997). *Interventions to prevent HIV risk behaviors* (NIH Consensus Statement No. 15[2], pp. 1–41). Bethesda, MD: Author.

Patterson, D. (1994). Drug testing technology: A matter of choice. *Behavioral Health Management, 14*, 26–30.

Peele, S. (1991). *Diseasing of America: Addiction treatment out of control.* Boston: Houghton Mifflin.

Pokorny, A. D., Miller, B. A., & Kaplan, H. B. (1972). The brief MAST: A shortened version of the Michigan Alcoholism Screening Test. *American Journal of Psychiatry, 129*, 342–345.

Prochaska, J. O., & DiClemente, C. C. (1986). Toward a comprehensive model of change. In W. R. Miller and N. Heather (Eds.), *Treating addictive behaviors: Processes of change* (pp. 3–27). New York: Plenum.

Project MATCH Research Group (1997). Matching alcoholism treatment to client heterogenity: Project MATCH posttreatment drinking outcomes. *Journal of Studies on Alcohol, 58*, 7–29.

Rahdert, E. R. (1991). *The adolescent assessment/referral system manual.* Washington, DC: Alcohol, Drug Abuse, and Mental Health Administration.

RAND Corporation. (1995). *Projecting future cocaine use and evaluating control strategies* (Research Brief No. 6002). Santa Monica, CA: Rand Drug Policy Research Center.

Regier, D. A, Farmer, M. E., Rae, D. S., Locke, B. Z., Keith, S. J., Judd, L. L., & Goodwin, F. K. (1990). Comorbidity of mental disorders with alcohol and other drug abuse: Results from the epidemiologic catchment area (ECA) study. *Journal of the American Medical Association, 264,* 2511–2519.

Regier, D. A., Narrow, W. E., Rae, D. S., Manderscheid, R. W., Locke, B. Z., & Goodwin, R. K. (1993). The de facto U.S. mental and addictive disorders service system. *Archives of General Psychiatry, 50,* 85–94.

Reiten, R. M., & Davison, L. A. (1974). *Clinical neuropsychology: Current status and applications.* Washington, DC: Winston.

Rivera, F. P., Koepsell, T. D., Jurkovich, G. J., Gurney, J. G., & Soderberg, R. (1993). The effects of alcohol abuse on readmission for trauma. *Journal of the American Medical Association, 270,* 1962–1964.

Roehrich, L., & Goldman, M.S. (1993). Experience-dependent neuropsychological recovery and the treatment of alcoholism. *Journal of Consulting and Clinical Psychology, 61,* 812–821.

Rohde, P., Lewinsohn, P. M., & Seeley, J. R. (1996). Psychiatric comorbidity with problematic alcohol use in high school students. *Journal of the American Academy of Child and Adolescent Psychiatry, 35,* 101–109.

Rohsenow, D. J. (1983). Drinking habits and expectancies about alcohol's effects for self versus others. *Journal of Consulting and Clinical Psychology, 51,* 752–756.

Rollnick, S., Heather, N., Gold, R., & Hall, W. (1992). Development of a brief "Readiness to Change" questionnaire for use in brief, opportunistic interventions among excessive drinkers. *British Journal of Addictions, 87,* 743–754.

Rosenberg, H. (1993). Prediction of controlled drinking by alcoholics and problem drinkers. *Psychological Bulletin, 113,* 129–139.

Russell, M., Martier, S. S., Sokol, R. J., Jacobson, S., Jacobson, J., & Bottoms, S. (1991). Screening for pregnancy risk drinking: TWEAKING the tests. *Alcoholism: Clinical and Experimental Research, 15,* 638.

Salaspuro, M. (1994). Biological state markers of alcohol abuse. *Alcohol Health and Research World, 18,* 131–135.

Samo, J. A., Tucker, J. A., & Vuchinich, R. E. (1989). Agreement between self-monitoring, subject recall, and collateral observation measures of alcohol consumption in older adults. *Behavioral Assessment, 11,* 391–409.

Sanchez-Craig, M., Wilkinson, D. A., & Davila, R. (1995). Empirically based guidelines for moderate drinking: 1-year results from three studies with problem drinkers. *American Journal of Public Health, 85,* 823–828.

Sanjuan, P. M., & Langenbucher, J. W. (1999). Age-limited populations: Youth, adolescents, and older adults. In B. S. McCrady & E. E. Epstein (Eds.), *Addictions: A comprehensive guidebook* (pp. 477–498). New York: Oxford University Press.

Saunders, J. B., Aasland, O. G., Babor, T. F., DeLaFuente, J. R., & Grant, M. (1993). Development of the Alcohol Use Disorders Identification Test (AUDIT): WHO collaborative project on early detection of persons with harmful alcohol consumption. *Addiction, 88,* 296–303.

Schafer, J., & Brown, S. A. (1991). Marijuana and cocaine effect expectancies and drug use patterns. *Journal of Consulting and Clinical Psychology, 59,* 558–565.

Schmidt, L. A., & Weisner, C. M. (1999). Public health perspectives on access and need for substance abuse treatment. In J. A. Tucker, D. M. Donovan, & G. A. Marlatt (Eds.), *Changing addictive behavior: Bridging clinical and public health strategies* (pp. 67–96). New York: Guilford Press.

Schober, R., & Annis, H. M. (1996). Barriers to help-seeking for change in drinking: A gender-focused review of the literature. *Addictive Behaviors, 21,* 81–92.

Seligman, M. E. P. (1995). The effectiveness of psychotherapy: The *Consumer Reports* study. *American Psychologist, 50,* 965–974.

Selzer, M. L. (1971). The Michigan Alcoholism Screening Test: The test for a new diagnostic instrument. *American Journal of Psychiatry, 127,* 1653–1658.

Sher, K. J. (1991). *Children of alcoholics: A critical appraisal of theory and research.* Chicago: University of Chicago Press.

Sims, D. W., Bivins, B. A., Obeid, F. N., Horst, H. M., Sorensen, V. J., & Fath, J. J. (1989). Urban trauma: A chronic recurrent disease. *Journal of Trauma, 29,* 940–947.

Skinner, H. A. (1981a). Comparison of clients assigned to inpatient and outpatient treatment for alcoholism and drug addiction. *British Journal of Psychology, 138,* 312–320.

Skinner, H. A. (1981b). Primary syndromes of alcohol abuse: Their measurement and correlates. *British Journal of Addiction, 76,* 63–76.

Skinner, H. A., & Allen, B. A. (1982). Alcohol dependence syndrome: Measurement and validation. *Journal of Abnormal Psychology, 91,* 199–209.

Skinner, H. A., & Horn, J. L. (1984). *Alcohol Dependence Scale (ADS): Users guide.* Toronto: Addiction Research Foundation of Ontario.

Skinner, H. A., & Sheu, W. J. (1982). Reliability of alcohol use indices: The Lifetime Drinking History and the MAST. *Journal of Studies on Alcohol, 43,* 1157–1170.

Skolnick, A. (1990). Drug screening in prenatal care demands objective medical criteria, support services. *Journal of the American Medical Association, 264,* 309–311.

Sobell, L. C., Cunningham, J. A., & Sobell, M. B. (1996). Recovery from alcohol problems with and without treatment: Prevalence in two population studies. *American Journal of Public Health, 86,* 966–972.

Sobell, L. C., Kwan, E., & Sobell, M. B. (1995). Reliability of a drug history questionnaire (DHQ). *Addictive Behaviors, 20,* 233–241.

Sobell, L. C., & Sobell, M. B. (1992). Timeline follow-back: A technique for assessing self-reported alcohol consumption. In R. Litten & J. Allen (Eds.), *Measuring alcohol consumption: Psychosocial and biological methods* (pp. 41–72). Totowa, NJ: Humana Press.

Sobell, L. C., & Sobell, M. B. (1995a). Alcohol consumption measures. In J. P. Allen and M. Columbus (Eds.), *Assessing alcohol problems: A guide for clinicians and researchers* (Treatment Handbook Series No. 4, pp. 55–73). Bethesda, MD: National Institute on Alcohol Abuse and Alcoholism.

Sobell, L. C., & Sobell, M. B. (1995b). *Alcohol Timeline Followback user's manual.* Toronto: Addiction Research Foundation of Ontario.

Sobell, L. C., Toneatto, T., & Sobell, M. B. (1994). Behavioral assessment and treatment planning for alcohol, tobacco, and other drug problems: Current status with an emphasis on clinical applications. *Behavior Therapy, 25,* 533–580.

Sobell, M. B., & Sobell, L. C. (1999). Stepped care for alcohol problems: An efficient method for planning and delivering clinical services. In J. A. Tucker, D. M. Donovan, & G. A. Marlatt (Eds.), *Changing addictive behavior: Bridging clinical and public health strategies* (pp. 331–343). New York: Guilford Press.

Soderstrom, C. A., Dischinger, P. C., Smith, G. S., McDuff, D. R., Hebel, J. R., & Gorelick, D. A. (1992). Psychoactive substance dependence among trauma center patients. *Journal of the American Medical Association, 267,* 2756–2759.

Sokol, R. J., Martier, S.S., & Ager, J. W. (1989). The T-ACE questions: Practical prenatal detection of risk drinking. *American Journal of Obstetrics and Gynecology, 160,* 863–870.

Stitzer, M. L., & McCaul, M. E. (1987). Criminal justice interventions with drug and alcohol abusers. In E. K. Morris & C. J. Braukmann (Eds.), *Behavioral approaches to crime and delinquency: A handbook of application, research, and concepts* (pp. 331–361). New York: Plenum.

Stratton, K., Howe, C., & Battaglia, F. (Eds.). (1996). *Fetal alcohol syndrome: Diagnosis, epidemiology, prevention, and treatment.* Washington DC: National Academy Press.

Strosahl, K. (1998). Integrating behavioral health and primary care services: The primary mental health care model. In A. Blount (Ed.), *Integrated primary care: The future of medical and mental health collaboration* (pp. 139–166). New York: Norton.

Strum, R., & Wells, K. (2000). Health insurance may be improving—but not for individuals with mental illness. *Health Services Research, 35,* 253–262.

Tarter, R., & Edwards, K. (1987). Brief and comprehensive neuropsychological assessment of alcoholism and drug abuse. In L. Hartlage, M. Ashen, & L. Hornsby (Eds.), *Essentials of neuropsychological assessment* (pp. 138–162). New York: Springer.

Tarter, R., & Kirisci, L. (1997). The Drug Use Screening Inventory for adults: Psychometric structure and discriminative sensitivity. *American Journal of Drug and Alcohol Abuse, 23,* 207–219.

Teitelbaum, L., & Mullen, B. (2000). The validity of the MAST in psychiatric settings: A meta-analytic integration. *Journal of Studies on Alcohol, 61,* 254–261.

Tengs, T. O., Adams, M. E., Pliskin, J. S., Safran, D. G., Siegel, J. E., Weinstein, M. C., & Graham, J. D. (1995). Five-hundred life-saving interventions and their cost-effectiveness. *Risk Analysis, 15,* 369–390.

Tiffany, S. T. (1997). New perspectives on the measurement, manipulation and meaning of drug craving. *Human Psychopharmacology, 12,* 103–113.

Tiffany, S. T., & Carter, B. L. (1998). Is craving the source of compulsive drug use? *Journal of Psychopharmacology, 12,* 23–30.

Tiffany, S. T., Singleton, E., Haertzen, C. A., & Henningfield, J. E. (1993). The development and initial validation of a cocaine craving questionnaire. *Drug and Alcohol Dependence, 34,* 19–28.

Tonigan, J. S., Miller, W. R., & Brown, J. M. (1997). The reliability of Form-90: An instrument for assessing alcohol treatment outcome. *Journal of Studies on Alcohol, 58,* 358–364.

Tucker, J. A. (1999). Changing addictive behavior: Historical and contemporary perspectives. In J. A. Tucker, D. M. Donovan, & G. A. Marlatt (Eds.), *Changing addictive behavior: Bridging clinical and public health perspectives* (pp. 3–44). New York: Guilford Press.

Tucker, J. A., Donovan, D. M., & Marlatt, G. A. (Eds.). (1999). *Changing addictive behavior: Bridging clinical and public health strategies.* New York: Guilford Press.

Tucker, J. A., & King, M. P. (1999). Resolving alcohol and drug problems: Influences on addictive behavior change and help-seeking processes. In J. A. Tucker, D. M. Donovan, & G. A. Marlatt (Eds.), *Changing addictive behavior: Bridging clinical and public health perspectives* (pp. 97–126). New York: Guilford Press.

Tucker, J. A., Vuchinich, R. E., Harris, C. V., Gavornik, M. G., & Rudd, E. J. (1991). Agreement between subject and collateral reports of alcohol consumption in older adults. *Journal of Studies on Alcohol, 52,* 148–155.

U.S. Department of Health and Human Services. (1997). *Ninth Special Report to the U.S. Congress on Alcohol and Health* (NIH Publication No. 97–4017). Bethesda, MD: National Institute on Alcohol Abuse and Alcoholism, National Institutes of Health.

Vuchinich, R. E., Tucker, J. A., & Harllee, L. M. (1988). Behavioral assessment. In D. M. Donovan & G. A. Marlatt (Eds.), *Assessment of addictive behaviors: Behavioral, cognitive, and physiological procedures* (pp. 51–93). New York: Guilford Press.

Wechsler, D. (1997). *Manual for the Wechsler Adult Intelligence Scale—third edition.* San Antonio, TX: The Psychological Corporation.

Wexler, H. K., & Sacks, S. (2000, August). Effectiveness of prison substance abuse treatment: A review and research agenda. *Connection, 3,* 8.

White, H. R., & Bates, M. E. (1995). Cessation from cocaine use. *Addiction, 90,* 947–957.

White, H. R., & Labouvie, E. W. (1989). Towards the assessment of adolescent problem drinking. *Journal of Studies on Alcohol, 50,* 30–37.

Williams, G. D., & Debakey, S. F. (1992). Changes in levels of alcohol consumption: United States, 1983–1988. *British Journal of Addiction, 87,* 643–648.

Winters, K. C., & Henly, G. A. (1989). *Personal Experience Inventory (PEI).* Los Angeles: Western Psychological Services.

Winters, K. C., & Henly, G. A. (1993). *Adolescent Diagnostic Interview (ADI).* Los Angeles: Western Psychological Services.

Wolff, K., Farrell, M., Marsden, J., Monteiro, M. G., Ali, R., Welch, S., & Strang, J. (1999). A review of biological indicators of illicit drug use, practical considerations and clinical usefulness. *Addiction, 94,* 1279–1298.

World Health Organization. (1981). Nomenclature and classification of drugs and alcohol-related problems: A WHO memorandum. *Bulletin of the World Health Organization, 59,* 225–242.

World Health Organization. (1990). *International classification of diseases* (10th ed.). Geneva: Author.

Yates, B. T. (1995). Cost-effectiveness analysis, cost-benefit analysis, and beyond: Evolving models for the scientist–manager–practitioner. *Clinical Psychology: Science and Practice, 2,* 385–398.

Zweben, A., & Fleming, M. F. (1999). Brief interventions for alcohol and drug problems. In J. A. Tucker, D. M. Donovan, & G. A. Marlatt (Eds.), *Changing addictive behavior: Bridging clinical and public health strategies* (pp. 251–282). New York: Guilford Press.

Zwerling, C., Ryan, J., & Orav, E. J. (1990). The efficacy of preemployment drug screening for marijuana and cocaine predicting employment outcome. *Journal of the American Medical Association, 264,* 2639–2644.

13

Personality Disorders

Thomas A. Widiger

OVERVIEW OF PERSONALITY DISORDERS

"Personality traits are enduring patterns of perceiving, relating to, and thinking about the environment and oneself that are exhibited in a wide range of social and personal contexts" (American Psychiatric Association, 1994, p. 630). Every individual, including every person who has been diagnosed with a mental disorder, will have had a characteristic manner of thinking, feeling, behaving, and relating to others prior to and during the course of his or her mental disorder. In addition, "when personality traits are inflexible and maladaptive and cause significant functional impairment or subjective distress . . . they constitute Personality Disorders" (American Psychiatric Association, 1994, p. 630), and many of the persons obtaining treatment within clinical settings will be there primarily because of their personality disorder (Widiger & Sanderson, 1997).

A variety of studies have indicated that the presence of a personality disorder can complicate substantially the treatment of an anxiety, mood, or other mental disorder (Reich & Vasile, 1993; Shea, Widiger, & Klein, 1992). Antisocial patients can be irresponsible, unreliable, or untrustworthy; paranoid patients can be mistrustful, accusatory, and suspicious; dependent patients can be excessively needy; passive–aggressive patients can be argumentative and oppositional; and borderline patients can be intensely manipulative and unstable (Millon et al., 1996; Sanderson & Clarkin, 1994; Stone, 1993). Personality disorders are also among the most difficult to treat, in part because they involve pervasive and entrenched behavior patterns that have been present throughout much of a person's life. People consider many of their personality traits to be integral to their sense of self, and they may even value particular aspects of their personality that a clinician considers to be important targets of treatment (Millon et al., 1996; Stone, 1993).

Nevertheless, contrary to popular perception, personality disorders are not untreatable. Maladaptive personality traits are often the focus of clinical treatment (Beck, Freeman, & Associates, 1990; Benjamin, 1993; Linehan, 1993; Millon et al., 1996; Paris, 1998; Shea, 1993; Soloff, Siever, Cowdry, & Kocsis, 1994; Stone, 1993), and there is compelling empirical support to indicate that meaningful responsivity to treatment does occur (Perry,

Banon, & Ianni, 1999; Sanislow & McGlashan, 1998). Treatment of a personality disorder is unlikely to result in the development of a fully healthy or ideal personality structure (whatever that may entail), but clinically and socially meaningful change to personality structure and functioning can occur.

Perry et al. (1999) conducted a sophisticated and detailed meta-analysis of 15 published personality disorder psychotherapy studies. Among their results was the finding that approximately 50% of patients with a personality disorder tend to recover (i.e., no longer meet diagnostic criteria for the respective disorder) after 1 year and 4 months of focused treatment (approximately 93 sessions), whereas a 50% recovery rate would not occur until approximately 10½ years over the natural course of the disorder (which may have included brief periods of unknown treatments). Perry et al. (1999) concluded that "psychotherapy is an effective treatment for personality disorders and may be associated with up to a seven-fold faster rate of recovery in comparison with the natural history of the [personality] disorder" (p. 1312).

Similar conclusions were reached by Sanislow and McGlashan (1998) in their comprehensive review of pharmacologic and psychosocial treatment studies. They indicated that patients do not reach a level of "normalcy," but there is compelling "evidence that effective treatments exist to alleviate symptoms and reduce symptomatic behavior" (Sanislow & McGlashan, 1998, p. 237). Scheel (2000) provided a thorough and detailed critique of almost every empirical study of the effectiveness of dialectical behavior therapy for borderline personality disorder. She was concerned that the effectiveness of dialectical behavior therapy has often been exaggerated, but she also acknowledged that "summarizing published empirical results across studies, standard outpatient dialectical behavior therapy has been associated with lesser parasuicidal behavior, psychiatric hospitalization, anger, and psychotropic medication usage, and with increased client retention, overall level of functioning, overall social adjustment, and employment performance" (Scheel, 2000, p. 76).

In sum, treatment can have a clinically meaningful effect on personality disorder symptomatology, although the presence of this symptomatology will also complicate the treatment of other mental disorders placed on Axis I of the fourth edition of the *Diagnostic and Statistical Manual of Mental Disorders* (DSM-IV; American Psychiatric Association, 1994). Both of these findings argue for the inclusion of measures of personality disorder symptomatology within treatment outcome studies. Even if treatment is not concerned directly with a personality disorder, focusing instead on a mood, anxiety, or other Axis I mental disorder (American Psychiatric Association, 1994), personality disorder symptomatology can go far in explaining why some patients failed to respond as expected to the Axis I treatment (e.g., Shea et al., 1992). Clinicians and researchers who are concerned primarily with the treatment of an Axis I mental disorder would then be well advised to include a measure of personality disorder symptomatology if they intend to fully account for the variation in their patients' treatment responsivity. In addition, clinicians and researchers who are primarily concerned with the treatment of a personality disorder should not assume that their efforts will be ineffective. They are also advised to include objective measures of personality disorder symptomatology to empirically document the effectiveness of their treatment program.

EMPIRICAL LITERATURE ON ASSESSMENT MEASURES

There are many alternative instruments for the assessment of personality disorders, and currently five semistructured interviews are coordinated explicitly with the diagnostic criteria provided within DSM-IV (American Psychiatric Association, 1994): (1) Diagnostic Interview for Personality Disorders (DIPD; Zanarini, Frankenburg, Chauncey, & Gunderson, 1987); (2) International Personality Disorder Examination (IPDE; Loranger, 1999); (3) Personality Disorder Interview–IV (PDI-IV; Widiger, Mangine, Corbitt, Ellis, & Thomas, 1995); (4) Structured Clinical Interview for DSM-IV Axis II Personality Disorders (SCID-II; First, Gibbon, Spitzer, Williams, & Benjamin, 1997); and (5) Structured Interview for DSM-IV Personality Disorders (SIDP-IV; Pfohl, Blum, & Zimmerman, 1997). There are also additional interviews for the assessment of individual personality disorders, such as (but not limited to) the Revised Diagnostic Interview for Borderlines (DIB-R; Zanarini, Gunderson, Frankenburg, & Chauncey, 1989), the Diagnostic Interview for Narcissism (DIN; Gunderson, Ronningstam, & Bodkin, 1990), and the Hare Psychopathy Checklist—Revised (PCL-R; Hare, 1991), as well as interviews for the assessment of alternative dimensional models of personality disorder symptomatology, such as the Structured Interview for the Five-Factor Model (SIFFM; Trull & Widiger, 1997).

There are six inventories that are commonly used for the assessment of the DSM-IV personality disorders: (1) Minnesota Multiphasic Personality Inventory–2 (MMPI-2; Hathaway et al., 1989) personality disorder scales developed originally by Morey, Waugh, and Blashfield (1985) but revised for the MMPI-2 by Colligan, Morey, and Offord (1994); (2) Millon Clinical Multiaxial Inventory–III (MCMI-III; Millon, Millon, & Davis, 1994); (3) Personality Diagnostic Questionnaire–4 (PDQ-4; Hyler et al., 1988; Hyler, 1994); (4) Personality Assessment Inventory (PAI; Morey, 1991); (5) Wisconsin Personality Disorders Inventory (WISPI; Klein et al., 1993); and (6) Coolidge Axis II Inventory (CATI; Coolidge & Merwin, 1992); and, again, questionnaires to assess various components of personality disorder symptomatology, including (but not limited to) the NEO Personality Inventory—Revised (NEO PI-R; Costa & McCrae, 1992), Schedule for Nonadaptive and Adaptive Personality (SNAP; Clark, 1993), Dimensional Assessment of Personality Pathology (DAPP-BQ; Livesley & Jackson, in press), Structural Analysis of Social Behavior (SASB; Benjamin, 1988), Inventory of Interpersonal Problems (IIP; Horowitz, Rosenberg, Baer, Ureno, & Villasenor, 1988), Personality Assessment Form (PAF; Pilkonis, Heape, Ruddy, & Serrao, 1991), and Shedler–Westen Assessment Procedure (SWAP-200; Westen & Shedler, 1999a).

Diversity of Options

Table 13.1 provides a comparative listing of the most commonly used instruments for the assessment of personality disorder symptomatology, along with a brief indication of their advantages and potential disadvantages. It is evident from this table that there is a diversity of options. In addition, all of the semistructured interviews can be administered, with at most only minor modifications, to either the patient or an informed source. Most of the inventories were constructed primarily to be completed by a patient, but some of them include informant versions (e.g., NEO PI-R Form R; Costa & McCrae, 1992). The PAF and the SWAP-200 are perhaps best described as clinician-report inventories. The PAF is a list of the 12 DSM-III-R (American Psychiatric Association, 1987) personality disorders, along with a brief description of each of them. The SWAP-200 is a set of 200 items, approximately half of which are the 94 DSM-IV personality disorder diagnostic criteria; the other half are additional personality disorder symptomatology, defense mechanisms, and adaptive personality traits. The PAF and the SWAP-200 would be completed by a patient's therapist, using his or her own preferred means for the assessment of each item.

The SWAP-200 is also unique in its use of a Q-sort format (Westen & Shedler, 1999a), which is equivalent to using a Likert-scale and requiring that the respondent provide scores that are consistent with a desired distribution. For example, Westen and Shedler (1999b)

TABLE 13.1. Instruments for the Assessment of Personality Disorders (PD)

Title and citation	Acronym	Format	Length	Coverage	Advantages	Potential disadvantages
Coolidge Axis II Inventory (Coolidge & Merwin, 1992)	CATI	SRI	200	DSM-III-R PD diagnostic criteria	Items coordinated with DSM criteria; includes validity and a few Axis I scales	Limited empirical support; not revised for DSM-IV
Diagnostic Interview for Narcissism (Gunderson et al., 1990)	DIN	SSI	105[a]	Narcissistic PD symptoms	Subscales for components of narcissistic symptomatology; only SSI devoted to narcissism	Substantial amount of time to assess for one PD
Diagnostic Interview for Personality Disorders (Zanarini et al., 1987)	DIPD	SSI	398[a]	DSM-IV PD diagnostic criteria	Empirical support; less expensive than other PD SSIs	Used less frequently than other PD SSIs; manual is limited with respect to scoring guidelines
Dimensional Assessment of Personality Pathology (Livesley & Jackson, in press)	DAPP-BQ	SRI	290	PD symptoms	Precise coverage of components of DSM-IV PDs	Absence of DSM-IV PD scales; absence of validity scales
Hare Psychopathy Checklist—Revised (Hare, 1991)	PCL-R	SSI CRI	Unclear	Psychopathy	Substantial empirical support; covers more aspects of psychopathy than DSM-IV	As much a checklist as an interview; relies heavily on legal record
International Personality Disorder Examination (Loranger, 1999)	IPDE	SSI	537[a]	DSM-IV and ICD-10 criteria	Jointly assesses for ICD-10 PDs; good empirical support	More time-consuming than other PD SSIs; relies on DSM-IV questions to assess for ICD-10 criteria
Inventory of Interpersonal Problems (Horowitz et al., 1988)	IIP	SRI	127	PD symptoms	Comprehensive and circumplex assessment of problems in interpersonal relatedness	Absence of scales for PD symptoms that are not interpersonal; absence of DSM-IV PD scales
Millon Clinical Multiaxial Inventory–III (Millon et al., 1994)	MCMI-III	SRI	175	DSM-IV PDs	Empirical support; includes validity and Axis I scales	Relatively expensive; hand-scoring impractical; problematic for higher functioning samples; gender bias
Minnesota Multiphasic Personality Inventory–2 (Hathaway et al., 1989; Colligan et al., 1994)	MMPI-2	SRI	157[b]	DSM-III PDs	Embedded within MMPI-2	May require administration of all 567 MMPI-2 items; unvalidated cutoff points; possible gender bias

456

Instrument	Method	Number	Domain assessed	Strengths	Limitations
NEO Personality Inventory—Revised (Costa & McCrae, 1992)	SRI	240	Normal and abnormal traits	Substantial empirical support; includes traits that may facilitate treatment	Currently inadequate scales for assessment of DSM-IV PDs; validity scales are experimental
Personality Assessment Form (Pilkonis et al., 1991)	CRI	13[c]	DSM-III-R PDs	Requires no systematic interview	Absence of interview questions to ensure systematic and consistent assessments
Personality Assessment Inventory (Morey, 1991)	SRI	344	DSM-III-R PDs	Subscales for borderline and antisocial PDs; psychometrically strong; Axis I and validity scales	Absence of scales for eight of the PDs; not revised for DSM-IV
Personality Diagnostic Questionnaire–4 (Hyler et al., 1988; Hyler, 1994)	SRI	99	DSM-IV PD diagnostic criteria	Brief and inexpensive; item(s) for each DSM-IV PD criterion; used frequently	Psychometrically weak; inconsistent empirical support
Personality Disorder Interview–IV (Widiger et al., 1995)	SSI	325[a]	DSM-IV PD diagnostic criteria	Empirical support; manual provides detailed rationale and guidelines for each diagnostic criterion	Used less frequently than SIDP-IV, IPDE, or SCID-II
Revised Diagnostic Interview for Borderlines (Zanarini et al., 1989)	SSI	106[a]	Borderline PD symptoms	Subscales for components of borderline symptomatology; good empirical support	Original DIB at times preferred over DIB-R; substantial amount of time to assess for one PD
Shedler–Westen Assessment Procedure (Westen & Shedler, 1999a)	CRI Qsrt	200[c]	Abnormal and normal traits and defenses	Requires no systematic interview; includes psychodynamic items	Susceptible to halo effects; forced distribution of items; Q-sorting can require substantial time
Schedule for Nonadaptive and Adaptive Personality (Clark, 1993)	SRI	375	PD symptoms	Precise coverage of components of DSM-IV PDs; validity scales	Empirical support for DSM-IV PD scales is limited
Structured Clinical Interview for DSM-IV Axis II Personality Disorders (First et al., 1997)	SSI	303[a]	DSM-IV PD diagnostic criteria	Screening questionnaire available; empirical support; coordinated with Axis I interview	Perhaps more superficial in questions than most other SSIs; manual limited in its coverage

(continued)

TABLE 13.1. (continued)

Title and citation	Acronym	Format	Length	Coverage	Advantages	Potential disadvantages
Structured Interview for DSM-IV Personality Disorders (Pfohl et al., 1997)	SIDP-IV	SSI	337[a]	DSM-IV and ICD-10 criteria	Good empirical support; support for training	Manual is limited in its instructions for scoring of DSM-IV and ICD-10
Structured Interview for the Five-Factor Model (Trull & Widiger, 1997)	SIFFM	SSI	240[a]	Normal and abnormal traits	Empirical support; includes traits that may facilitate treatment; only SSI for dimensional model	Absence of DSM-IV PD scales; limited usage
Wisconsin Personality Disorders Inventory (Klein et al., 1993)	WISPI	SRI	214	DSM-III-R PD diagnostic criteria	Coordinated with interpersonal, object relational theory; item(s) for each PD diagnostic criterion	Limited usage; some items involve complex concepts; not revised for DSM-IV

Note. Length, relative estimate of length of instrument (for SRIs, number of items; for SSIs, approximate number of questions administered; for CRIs, number of constructs assessed); SRI, self-report inventory; SSI, semistructured interview; CRI, clinician-report inventory; DSM, *Diagnostic and Statistical Manual of Mental Disorders*, either DSM-III, DSM-III-R, or DSM-IV (American Psychiatric Association, 1980, 1987, 1994); PD, personality disorder; ICD-10, *International Classification of Diseases* (World Health Organization, 1992).

[a]Numbers provided for semistructured interviews are only an approximation of the number of questions provided in interview form; the actual number of questions administered will vary, depending on items or questions skipped during interviews and additional follow-up inquiries that might be administered. Many SSIs also require additional observational ratings (e.g., 32 specified for IPDE, 19 for DIPD-IV, 16 for SIDP-IV, 7 for SCID-II, and 3 for PDI-IV).

[b]MMPI-2 includes 567 items, but Morey et al. (1985) PD scales uses only 157 of them.

[c]Number of constructs assessed by interviewer; actual number of questions provided by an interviewer to assess these constructs will vary substantially.

used an 8-point Likert scale (0, not at all descriptive, irrelevant, or inapplicable; 1, applies just a little bit; up to 7, highly descriptive). In this study the clinicians were required to provide a rating of 7 on eight, and only eight, of the 200 items; 10 items were required to receive a rating of 6, and 100 of the 200 items were required to receive a rating of 0. Requiring that a specific distribution of personality disorder ratings be provided is advantageous in minimizing the occurrence of unexpected results (Westen & Shedler, 1999a), although a forced distribution can also fail to provide the most accurate descriptions. For example, clinicians were required by Westen and Shedler (1999a) to rate 100 (half) of the SWAP-200 items as being irrelevant or inapplicable even if most of the items were in fact considered by the clinicians to be relevant and applicable. The SWAP-200 fixed distribution is equivalent to requiring that persons administering a DSM-IV personality disorder semistructured interview rate half of the diagnostic criteria as being absent, no matter what the respondents say in response to an interviewer's questions.

Potential disadvantages are also noted in Table 13.1 for each of the other instruments. No single instrument can be recommended without any reservations, as any particular instrument will have at least one important limitation or concern. For example, the PCL-R (Hare, 1991) is a well-validated instrument for the assessment of psychopathy; however, as suggested by its title, it is perhaps better described as a checklist than as a semistructured interview. Many of its items are scored primarily (if not solely) on the basis of a person's legal, criminal record rather than on the basis of interview questions (e.g., a history of murders or rapes indicates the presence of a lack of empathy; Hare, 1991). The availability of a detailed criminal history within prison settings has contributed to the PCL-R's excellent interrater reliability and predictive validity, but an application of the PCL-R within most other clinical settings will have to rely more heavily on an interview, the administration and scoring of which will be unclear for some PCL-R items (Lilienfeld, 1994; Rogers, 1995).

Most of the instruments listed in Table 13.1 were based on the DSM-IV personality disorder diagnostic criteria (American Psychiatric Association, 1994). However, the CATI (Coolidge & Merwin, 1992), the PAI (Morey, 1991), and the WISPI (Klein et al., 1993) were constructed in reference to the DSM-III-R criteria sets (American Psychiatric Association, 1987), and the Morey et al. (1985) MMPI-2 scales were constructed in reference to the DSM-III criteria sets (American Psychiatric Association, 1980). These self-report inventories have not since been revised to be compatible with the DSM-IV criteria sets, and it is possible that the revisions that have been made to the diagnostic nomenclature would have a significant effect on their validity as instruments for the assessment of the DSM-IV personality disorders (Clark, Livesley, & Morey, 1997).

Even those instruments that are coordinated with DSM-IV might do so from different theoretical perspectives. For example, many of the MCMI-III personality disorder scales (particularly the obsessive–compulsive, antisocial, narcissistic, and histrionic) are slanted somewhat toward the theoretical model of Millon et al. (1996). The WISPI and the SWAP-200 items emphasize an object relational, psychodynamic perspective (Benjamin, 1993; Klein et al., 1993; Westen, 1997); the DIN and the DIB-R represent perspectives on the narcissistic and borderline personality disorders (respectively) of Gunderson and his colleagues (Gunderson et al., 1990; Zanarini et al., 1989); many PAI items emphasize an interpersonal model (Morey, 1991); and the NEO PI-R and SIFFM items assess personality disorder from the perspective of the five-factor model of personality (Costa & McCrae, 1992; Trull & Widiger, 1997).

The diversity of choices can be problematic (Perry et al., 1999; Shea, 1997). Different assessment instruments are unlikely to provide the same results, and it can at times be unclear if the failure to replicate findings across studies is due to an idiosyncratic administration of a particular instrument, differences in setting or population, or fundamental differences among the instruments with respect to the constructs being assessed. Regier et al. (1998) have therefore proposed that researchers in future studies agree to use just one common interview schedule in order to obtain more uniform results. Pilkonis (1997) and Shea (1997) have similarly recommended that treatment outcome researchers agree to use a common core battery of instruments that would cover the important domains of personality functioning in a manner that is reasonably compatible across different theoretical perspectives. Marziali, Munroe-Blum, and McCleary (1999) have developed a set of scales (the Objective Behavioral Index) that they suggest are particularly well suited for the assessment of treatment outcome for borderline personality disorder.

A confinement of methodologies to a common set of instruments would contribute to the obtainment of more uniform results and would substantially improve the comparison and integration of findings across studies (Perry et al., 1999), but confining future research and assessment to just one instrument would also be at the cost of failing to recognize or appreciate the actual extent to which obtained results reflect unique aspects of a particular instrument. In fact, the absence of consistent findings across different instruments (Perry, 1992; Regier et al., 1998) is a strong argument against confining future research to just one instrument. The diversity of options should perhaps be addressed by further research comparing the concurrent, predictive, and construct validity of the alternative instruments, rather than compelling a premature selection of any one of them.

Convergent Validity

A substantial amount of research has been conducted on the convergent validity among the alternative assessment instruments (Kaye & Shea, 2000; Perry, 1992; Widiger & Sanderson, 1995a; Widiger & Saylor, 1998; Zimmerman, 1994). This research has often found weak agreement with respect to categorical diagnoses of individual personality disorders: "The plain news is summarized by the median value across studies of the median kappa within each study (i.e., the median of the median kappa values); median kappa = .25 (range = .08–.54)"; the author concluded that "on average, the chance-corrected agreement between diagnostic methods is poor" (Perry, 1992, p. 1649).

Perry's (1992) negative conclusions have been cited widely, but his review was based on a very limited number of studies ($N = 9$) and he was unable to consider alternative explanations for the poor agreement rates. Table 13.2 provides a more extensive summary available from 35 studies, some of which included three or more instruments and/or analyzed the findings in alternative ways. The results from the 35 studies are organized in Table 13.2 with respect to analyses of (1) categorical diagnoses; (2) quantitative assessments of the extent of personality disorder symptomatology, with at least one of the two instruments being a semistructured interview; and (3) quantitative assessments, with both instruments being self-report inventories.

Dimensional versus Categorical Ratings

Perry (1992) had concluded that "the overall situation is improved only slightly when dimensional scores for different methods are compared" (p. 1650). However, it is evident from Table 13.2 that substantially weaker results are usually obtained when agreement is assessed with respect to categorical diagnoses (exceptions to which are discussed in the following pages). The median convergent validity for categorical diagnoses across all personality disorders is approximately .25 ($N = 122$ correlations), whereas the median convergent validity for the extent to which a personality disorder is present is approximately .42 ($N = 427$ correlations). In fact, two of the studies considered by Perry (1992) had provided both

TABLE 13.2. Concurrent Validity Coefficients for Various Instruments in Personality Disorder

Instrument	PRN	SZD	SZT	ATS	BDL	HST	NCS	AVD	DPD	CPS	PAG
					Disorder						
Categorical diagnoses (kappa)											
SIDP-R/Conf[35]	.04	—	—	.25	.40	.46	.39	.51	.52	.40	.47
PDE/Conf[35]	—	—	—	—	-.06	.24	.20	.37	.09	.51	.11
SCID-II/PDE[24]	.29	.14	.44	.59	.53	.58	.44	.56	.66	.50	.21
PDQ/Clinician[33]	.40	-.16	.01	.07	.46	.15	.10	.10	.08	.08	-.02
PDQ-R/PDE[7]	.12	-.02	.54	.36	.46	.18	.42	.53	.52	.38	.21
PDQ-R/PDE[8]	.10	.26	.00	—	.42	.22	.10	.37	.14	.37	.33
PDQ-R/SCID[7]	.27	.43	.48	.42	.53	.24	.34	.63	.57	.30	.23
PDQ-R/SCID[8]	.25	.00	-.03	—	.37	.32	.23	.46	.53	.42	.46
PDQ-4/SCID[30]	.16	.09	.09	.28	.19	.12	.28	.15	.24	.09	.09
MMPI-2/SCID[25]	.05	.21	.22	.20	.28	-.05	.19	.42	.37	—	.18
MCMI-II/SCID[25]	.05	.21	.24	.10	.34	.12	.37	.28	.13	-.05	.22
MCMI-II/MMPI[25]	.30	.31	.48	.19	.34	.25	.37	.44	.27	—	.25
Median:	.16	.18	.23	.25	.38	.23	.32	.43	.32	.37	.21
Dimensional ratings that included a semistructured interview											
MCMI/SIDP[1]	.29	.40	.31	.23	.32	.05	.04	.53	.51	-.29	.28
MCMI/SIDP[2]	.22	.39	.37	—	.32	.20	.18	.42	.38	-.05	.14
MCMI/SIDP[3]	.28	.20	.15	.30	.80	.22	.14	.31	.38	.15	.50
MCMI/SIDP[4]	.20	.31	.23	.14	.63	.07	.26	.56	.31	.02	.41
MCMI/SIDP[17]	.03	.47	.39	.23	.33	.26	.34	.60	.21	-.04	.17
MCMI/PDI-I[18]	.08	.02	.33	.28	.51	.01	.21	.53	.64	-.32	.15
MCMI-II/SCID[29]	.39	.31	.17	.47	.51	.32	.34	.55	.40	.08	.38
MCMI-II/PDI-II[18]	.30	.52	.21	.32	.63	.24	.32	.64	.36	.11	.64
MCMI-II/PDI-III[19]	.44	.53	.61	.58	.63	.30	.42	.58	.50	-.04	.44
MCMI-II/PDE[5]	.38	.48	.39	.37	.60	.56	.41	.51	.38	-.05	.41
PDQ/SIDP[1]	.56	.33	.49	.78	.64	.47	.53	.51	.59	.52	.46
PDQ/SIDP[6]	.43	.24	.34	.55	.39	.42	.26	.30	.35	.47	.37
PDQ-R/SIDP[20]	.22	.32	.31	.20	.39	.38	.15	.21	.36	.29	.26
PDQ-R/SIDP-R[9]	.31	.60	.32	.44	.48	.40	.38	.35	.55	.47	.43
PDQ-4/SCID[30]	.36	.19	.20	.37	.40	.29	.42	.36	.39	.28	.30
MMPI/SIDP-R[9]	.33	.47	.35	.53	.66	.31	.10	.47	.40	.24	.47
WISPI/PAF[27]	.23	.21	.40	.41	.27	.36	.49	.28	.37	.26	.40
WISPI/SCID-II[28]	.43	.40	.51	.24	.61	.29	.15	.65	.49	.59	.46
WISPI/PDE[28]	.11	.36	.18	.39	.47	.22	.38	.58	.51	.40	.54
SCID-II/PDE[24]	.68	.58	.72	.87	.76	.77	.80	.78	.81	.77	.74
Median:	.30	.34	.34	.37	.50	.30	.33	.52	.40	.20	.41
Dimensional ratings that were confined to self-report inventories											
MCMI/PDQ[1]	.30	.28	.38	.15	.47	.15	.47	.68	.53	-.47	.59
MCMI/MMPI[10]	.33	.64	.41	.30	.55	.61	.66	.62	.52	-.38	.51
MCMI/MMPI[11]	.44	.35	.51	.14	.28	.66	.55	.65	.68	-.42	.50
MCMI/MMPI[12]	.69	.68	.78	.25	.54	.71	.55	.76	.68	-.31	.48
MCMI/MMPI[13]	.45	.61	.55	.14	.49	.71	.70	.77	.60	-.49	.70
MCMI/MMPI[13]	.19	.22	.57	.13	.49	.44	.49	.69	.59	-.50	.65
MCMI/MMPI[14]	.08	.67	.74	.15	.42	.68	.78	.82	.50	-.30	.57
MCMI/MMPI[21]	.32	.74	.53	.25	.37	.69	.73	.79	.67	-.27	.46
MCMI/MMPI[21]	.26	.71	.44	.20	.52	.64	.61	.67	.67	-.24	.46
MCMI/MMPI[22]	.27	.62	.48	.09	.46	.63	.66	.76	.53	-.13	.50
MCMI-II/MMPI[15]	.50	.73	.86	.57	.68	.74	.65	.87	.56	-.04	.70
MCMI-II/MMPI2[32]	.52	.66	.68	.46	.68	.57	.68	.76	.63	-.10	.62
MCMI-II/CATI[31]	.58	.22	.65	.57	.87	.72	.38	.80	.43	.10	.86

(continued)

TABLE 13.2. *(continued)*

Instrument	Disorder										
	PRN	SZD	SZT	ATS	BDL	HST	NCS	AVD	DPD	CPS	PAG
	Dimensional ratings that were confined to self-report inventories *(cont.)*										
MCMI-II/CATI[34]	.55	−.13	.57	.70	.88	.10	.40	.55	.20	−.11	.77
MMPI/PDQ-R[16]	.42	.26	.46	.51	.75	.32	−.04	.57	.60	.36	.62
MMPI/PDQ-R[23]	.61	.23	—	.63	—	−.04	.24	.73	.58	.47	.57
MMPI/PDQ-R[26]	.38	.31	.50	.50	.53	.09	−.12	.56	.35	.19	.20
WISPI/PDQ[27]	.66	.37	.72	.68	.54	.79	.67	.75	.79	.57	.67
WISPI/MCMI[27]	.38	.48	.43	.32	.14	.10	.57	.79	.68	−.26	.50
Median:	.42	.48	.54	.30	.53	.63	.57	.75	.59	−.24	.57

Note. PRN, paranoid; SZD, schizoid; SZT, schizotypal; ATS, antisocial; BDL, borderline; HST, histrionic; NCS, narcissistic; AVD, avoidant; DPD, dependent; CPS, obsessive–compulsive; PAG, passive–aggressive. Conf, Consensus conference ratings based in part on the respective semistructured interview findings (Pilkonis et al., 1995); Clinician, rating for each personality disorder provided by patient's therapist; acronyms for each instrument are provided in Table 13.1.
[1]Reich et al. (1987); [2]Torgersen and Alnaes (1990); [3]Nazikian et al. (1990); [4]Jackson et al. (1991); [5]Soldz et al. (1993); [6]Zimmerman and Coryell (1990); [7]Hyler et al. (1990); [8]Hyler et al. (1992); [9]Trull and Larsen (1991); [10]Streiner and Miller (1988); [11]Dubro and Wetzler (1989); [12]Morey and LeVine (1988); [13]Zarrelle et al. (1990); [14]McCann (1989);[15]McCann (1991); [16]Trull (1993); [17]Hogg et al., 1990; [18]Widiger and Freiman (1988); [19]Corbitt (1995); [20]Yeung et al. (1993); [21]Schuler, Snibbe, and Buckwalter (1994); [22]Wise (1994); [23]Trull et al. (1993);[24]Skodol et al. (1991); [25]Hills (1995); [26]O'Maille and Fine (1995); [27]Klein et al. (1993); [28]Barber and Morse (1994); [29]Marlowe et al. (1997); [30]Fossati et al. (1998); [31]Coolidge and Merwin (1992); [32]Wise (1996); [33]Hyler et al. (1989); [34]Silberman, Roth, Segal, and Burns (1997); [35]Pilkonis et al. (1995).

categorical and dimensional analyses (i.e., Skodol, Oldham, Rosnick, Kellman, & Hyler, 1991; Zimmerman & Coryell, 1990), and the authors of both studies had concluded that there was significant improvement when the personality disorders were considered dimensionally rather than categorically. Zimmerman and Coryell (1990), for example, indicated that "the dimensional scores of the two measures were significantly correlated; however, concordance for categorical diagnoses was poor" (p. 528); Skodol et al. (1991) concluded that "the correlations between the dimensional scores derived from the two interviews were substantially better" (p. 18).

Heumann and Morey (1990) provided clinicians with information about hypothesized correlates of borderline personality disorder to investigate whether their judgments would be more reliable when they were categorical or quantitative: "The results obtained in this study support the often cited contention that dimensional ratings of personality disorder are more reliable than categorical ones" (Heumann & Morey, 1990, p. 499). The improvement obtained with dimensional scores is not due simply to a statistical artifact. If the distinctions being made by the dimensional analyses (within a group of persons diagnosed with or without the respective personality disorder) were not reliable or valid, then no increase in the convergence of measures would be obtained.

> The greater agreement shown by comparing dimensions of disorder than by comparing strict categorical diagnoses suggests that patients are providing interviewers with reliable information about areas of difficulty in personality functioning . . . However, when information is combined into diagnoses either by complex, multi-item algorithms or by fixed and somewhat arbitrary cutpoints in polythetic criteria sets, the agreement is lost. (Skodol et al., 1991, pp. 22–23).

"The diagnostic approach used [in DSM-IV] represents the categorical perspective that Personality Disorders represent qualitatively distinct clinical syndromes" (American Psychiatric Association, 1994, p. 633), but the empirical support for this perspective does appear to be minimal relative to the alternative perspective that personality disorders are on a continuum with one another, with other mental disorders, and with normal personality functioning (Livesley, 1998; Widiger & Sanderson, 1995b). Personality and personality disorders appear to be the result of a complex interaction of biogenetic dispositions and environmental experiences that result in an array of possible constellations of adaptive and maladaptive personality traits (Clark et al., 1997; Widiger, 1997; Widiger & Sanderson, 1997). Providing a diagnosis that refers to a particular constellation of traits can be useful in highlighting particular features that would be evident within a prototypic case (e.g., Widiger & Lynam, 1998), but a categorical diagnosis will suggest the presence of features that are not in fact present and will fail to identify important features that are present (Widiger, 1993).

Structured versus Unstructured Assessments

Perry's (1992) review of the assessment research has also been interpreted as indicating weak empirical support for the convergent validity of structured assessments. Westen (1997), for example, concluded from Perry's review that "self-report measures have tended to perform particularly poorly" (p. 896). Perry (1992) had indeed stated "that interview methods demonstrated higher levels of concordance with one another than with self-report instruments" (p. 1650). Perry and Westen have argued for instruments modeled more closely on unstructured clinical interviews: "The problems . . . may stem in part from the fact that these instruments bear little resemblance to the way clinicians actually draw inferences about personality" (Westen, 1997, p. 896).

However, it is also evident from Table 13.2 that convergent validity generally improves as the degree of structure increases. Self-report inventories are the most heavily structured assessment instruments, and, in fact, they can be characterized as being equivalent to fully structured interviews that are self-administered (Loranger, 1992; Widiger & Saylor, 1998). The median convergent validity coefficient for quantitative assessments across all personality disorders when semistructured interviews are used is .34 ($N = 220$ correlations), whereas the median convergent validity coefficient when self-report inventories are used is .54 ($N = 207$ correlations). If one confines the comparison to the nine studies considered by Perry (1992), the worst median convergent validity coefficient was obtained in the only study to have used unstructured interviews by practicing clinicians (i.e., Hyler et al., 1989). The agreement (with a self-report measure) for the clinicians' personality disorder diagnoses ranged in this study from a low of −.16 to a high of only .46, with the median kappa being the lowest obtained across all 35 studies (i.e., only .08). In marked contrast, the highest median kappa was obtained in the only study that had assessed the agreement between two different semistructured interviews (Skodol et al., 1991). The kappa values in this study ranged from a low of .14 (higher than the median value obtained with an unstructured clinical interview in Hyler et al., 1989), to a high of .66, with a median kappa of .54. A median kappa of .54 for a categorical diagnosis is not outstanding, but it is comparable to that obtained for Axis I disorders (Loranger, 1992).

In sum, no matter how one does the comparison, convergent validity increases as the amount of structure in the assessment increases. Contrary to the conclusions of Perry (1992) and Westen (1997), it is not the case that findings have been particularly poor when self-report inventories have been used. In fact, the findings have been particularly best when self-report inventories have been used.

There are a few exceptions to the general finding that dimensional and structured assessments obtain better convergent validity than the categorical and unstructured assessments (respectively). For example, it appears from Table 13.2 that better convergent validity is obtained for the assessment of obsessive–compulsive personality disorder symptomatology with categorical diagnoses than with dimensional ratings, and better agreement when semistructured interviews rather than self-report inventories are used. However, this curious anomaly appears to be due primarily to the weak validity provided for that personality disorder by one particular self-report inventory, the MCMI (Millon et al., 1994). The MCMI assessment of obsessive–compulsive symptomatology typically obtains a significant negative correlation with other self-report inventories (Widiger & Sanderson, 1995a). The median convergent validity for self-report inventories other than the various editions of the MCMI is .42 (N = 4). The median convergent validity when one of the editions of the MCMI is correlated with another self-report inventory is −.27 (N = 15); the median convergent validity coefficient of the MCMI with a semistructured interview is −.01 (N = 10). In other words, it might be the case that the correlation of the MCMI obsessive–compulsive scale with semistructured interviews tends to be zero rather than negative because the semistructured interviews are providing less reliable assessments of this disorder than is provided by self-report inventories. Self-report inventories do appear to provide a more convergent assessment of the obsessive–compulsive personality disorder than the semistructured interviews, which, in turn, provide a more valid assessment than the unstructured clinical interviews; however, if the self-report inventory is one of the editions of the MCMI, then the most reliable finding might be to obtain a negative convergent validity coefficient.

The weaker results obtained with unstructured clinical interviews is not surprising, as unstructured clinical interviews are often unreliable (Kirk & Kutchins, 1992; Mellsop, Varghese, Joshua, & Hicks, 1982) and are highly susceptible to primacy effects, halo effects, false expectations, misleading assumptions, and confirmatory biases (Dawes, 1994; Garb, 1998; Widiger & Saylor, 1998), due in large part to a failure to conduct systematic, replicable, or comprehensive assessments. A variety of studies have indicated that clinicians relying on unstructured clinical interviews routinely fail to assess for the presence of the specified diagnostic criteria (Widiger & Saylor, 1998). One of the more compelling demonstrations of this failure was provided by Morey and Ochua (1989). Morey and Ochua provided 291 clinicians with the 166 DSM-III (American Psychiatric Association, 1980) personality disorder diagnostic criteria and asked them to indicate both which DSM-III personality disorder(s) were present in one of their patients and which of the 166 DSM-III personality disorder diagnostic criteria were present. Kappa for the agreement between their diagnoses and the diagnoses that would be given based on the diagnostic criteria they indicated to be present was poor, ranging from .11 (schizoid) to .58 (borderline), with a median kappa of only .25. In other words, their clinical diagnoses agreed poorly with their own assessments of the diagnostic criteria for each of the personality disorders. These findings were subsequently replicated: "It appears that the actual diagnoses of clinicians do not adhere closely to the diagnoses suggested by the [diagnostic] criteria" (Blashfield & Herkov, 1996, p. 226).

Self-report inventories and semistructured interviews go far in ensuring that a systematic and comprehensive assessment has been conducted. Many patients will meet the DSM-IV diagnostic criteria for more than one personality disorder (Bornstein, 1998; Lilienfeld, Waldman, & Israel, 1994; Shea, 1995), yet clinicians will typically provide only one personality disorder diagnosis to each patient (Gunderson, 1992). Clinicians tend to diagnose personality disorders hierarchically. Once a patient is identified as having a particular personality disorder (e.g., borderline), clinicians will often fail to assess whether additional personality traits are present (Herkov & Blashfield, 1995). Adler, Drake, and Teague (1990) provided 46 clinicians with case histories of a patient that met the DSM-III criteria for four personality disorders: histrionic, narcissistic, borderline, and dependent. "Despite the directive to consider each category separately . . . most clinicians assigned just one [personality disorder] diagnosis" (Adler et al., 1990, p. 127); 65% of the clinicians provided only one diagnosis, 28% provided two, and none provided all four.

Comorbidity among mental disorders is a pervasive phenomenon that can have substantial significance and importance to clinical treatment and outcome research (Clark, Watson, & Reynolds, 1995; Lilienfeld et al., 1994; Widiger & Clark, 2000), yet it may be grossly under-recognized in general clinical practice. Zimmerman and Mattia (1999b) compared the Axis I clinical diagnoses provided for 500 patients who were assessed with unstructured clinical interviews with the diagnoses provided by a semistructured interview that systematically assessed for the presence of the diagnostic criteria. More than 90% of the patients receiving the unstructured clinical interview were provided with only one Axis I diagnosis, whereas more than one-third of the patients assessed with the semistructured interview were discovered to have met the diagnostic criteria for at least three different Axis I mental disorders. Zimmerman and Mattia (1999a) also reported that clinicians diagnosed only 0.40% of the patients with borderline personality disorder; whereas 14.40% were diagnosed with this disorder when the semistructured interview was implemented. Zimmerman and Mattia (1999a) then provided the clinicians with the additional information obtained by the more systematic semistructured interview. They found that "providing the results of [the] semistructured interview to clinicians prompts them to diagnose borderline personality disorder much more frequently" (Zimmerman & Mattia, 1999a, p. 1570). The rate of diagnosis increased from 0.4% to 9.2%, which they felt was "inconsistent with the notion that personality disorder diagnoses based on semistructured interviews are not viewed as valid by clinicians" (Zimmerman & Mattia, 1999a, p. 1570). If clinicians are provided with systematic and comprehensive assessments of personality disorder symptomatology, they do recognize the value of this information.

PRACTICAL RECOMMENDATIONS

The primary method for the assessment of personality disorders in general clinical practice is an unstructured interview (Watkins, Campbell, Nieberding, & Hallmark, 1995; Westen, 1997), whereas most researchers rely primarily on semistructured interviews (Rogers, 1995; Zimmerman, 1994). The failure of clinicians to use semistructured interviews might be due in part to a failure of training programs to adequately develop an appreciation of the importance and benefits of conducting systematic and thorough interview assessments. Equally important, however, is the impracticality of administering an entire semistructured interview in routine clinical practice.

Semistructured interviews that cover all of the DSM-IV personality disorder diagnostic criteria will typically require about 2 hours of administration (with the SCID-II requiring the least amount of time and the IPDE requiring the most; Widiger & Saylor, 1998). Two hours to administer a semistructured interview might appear to be excessive, but 2 hours to assess 94 DSM-IV personality disorder diagnostic criteria is still spending only 90 seconds (on average) to assess each diagnostic criterion. One probably should be spending more time than simply 90 seconds to assess for the presence of a borderline identity disturbance, a narcissistic lack of empathy, or a schizotypal social anxiety. The PAF and the SWAP-200 require only 30 to 45 minutes to complete, as no interview questions are provided or required for the scoring of their items. The SWAP-200 will take somewhat longer than the PAF to complete because it includes more items and, more important, items will need to be rescored to conform to the required distribution of scoring. Self-report inventories will require very little time or effort on the part of the clinician to administer, but they can require considerable time and expense to score. For example, computer scoring of the MCMI-III is expensive, and hand-scoring MCMI-III personality disorder scales can take as long as 30 to 45 minutes per patient. There are no computer or hand-scoring templates for the Colligan et al. (1994) MMPI-2 personality disorder scales.

The administration of a semistructured interview can also be perceived and experienced as being simply a lengthy, mindless, and superficial symptom counting (Westen & Shedler, 1999a). Most clinicians prefer to follow leads that arise during the course of an interview, adjusting the content and style to facilitate rapport, responding to the particular needs of an individual patient, and exploring some areas of functioning in substantially more depth than others (Westen, 1997). The administration of a complete personality disorder semistructured interview is probably unrealistic and impractical in routine clinical practice, particularly if the bulk of the time is spent in determining which diagnostic criteria are not present. Rapport can be undermined by a repetitive and seemingly endless survey of 94 diagnostic criteria, many of which are not present.

However, the amount of time required for the administration of a semistructured interview can be reduced substantially by first administering a self-report inventory as a screening instrument to identify which personality disorders should be emphasized during an interview and which disorders could be ignored with minimal risk (Widiger & Sanderson, 1995a). A potential advantage of the SCID-II (First et al., 1997) and the IPDE (Loranger, 1999), relative to the other semistructured interviews, is that they provide easily hand-scored, self-report screening instruments constructed to err in the direction of false positives (Jacobsberg, Perry, & Frances, 1995; Lenzenweger, Loranger, Korfine, & Neff, 1997). The screening questionnaires can be used to eliminate a substantial proportion of the personality disorder interview and to identify the major domains of functioning that should be investigated, some of which were perhaps not originally anticipated. For example, the interviewer might focus on just the two to four personality disorder diagnoses that obtained the highest elevations on the screening instrument, thereby considerably reducing the amount of time that is needed for the administration of a semistructured interview, yet still covering domains of functioning that might have been missed in the process of an unstructured interview.

A variety of other approaches to screening instruments are also being explored (e.g., Dowson, 1992). Some researchers are exploring whether just 11 questions from the SIDP-IV semistructured interview can be used to identify whether any one of the DSM-IV personality disorders is likely to be present (Langbehn et al., 1999). Others have been conducting studies to try to reduce the 127-item IIP (Horowitz , Rosenberg, Baer, Ureno, & Villasenor, 1988) to a much briefer set of items (e.g., 25) that would identify effectively whether any one of the 10 DSM-IV personality disorders is likely to be present (e.g., Kim & Pilkonis, 1999; Pilkonis, Kim, Proietti, & Barkham, 1996; Scarpa et al., 1999). A hypothesis of this project is that personality disorders are primarily disorders of interpersonal relatedness (Benjamin, 1993; Pilkonis, 1997); therefore, an instrument that provides a comprehensive assessment of the different ways in which a person can be interpersonally dysfunctional might serve as an effective, if not optimal, screening device.

Another approach would be to administer as a screening device a self-report inventory that was constructed to provide a comprehensive assessment of the DSM-IV personality disorder symptomatology, such as any of the CATI, MCMI-III, MMPI-2, PDQ-4, or WISPI. No self-report inventory should be used as the sole, authoritative, or final basis for a clinical diagnosis. Although none of them are so valid that they can be relied on to provide a clinical diagnosis, many of them could be used as screening instruments before administering a semistructured interview. For example, the PDQ-4 (Hyler, 1994) is as brief as the screening questionnaires for the SCID-II (First et al., 1997) and the IPDE (Loranger, 1999), and it has been researched much more heavily. There is little advantage in using a weakly validated screening instrument in preference to a more strongly validated inventory that was constructed to provide a comprehensive assessment. In contrast, the PDQ-4 has obtained some of the weakest convergent validity results (see Table 13.2). Fossati et al. (1998) even concluded that "the PDQ-4 did not appear as an adequate instrument to assess DSM-IV personality disorders, even for screening purposes" (p. 178).

The most effective approach would be to use a more strongly validated self-report measure that will effectively screen for all of the DSM-IV personality disorders, erring in the direction of false positives rather than false negatives. A follow-up semistructured interview can then confirm the diagnoses by conducting a systematic assessment of each diagnostic criterion. The administration of a semistructured personality disorder interview will be particularly advantageous in clinical situations in which the credibility or the validity of the assessment might be questioned (e.g., forensic or disability evaluations), because the administration of the interview will ensure and document that the assessment was indeed comprehensive, replicable, and objective.

INTEGRATING ASSESSMENT WITH TREATMENT PLANNING AND OUTCOME MEASUREMENT

A number of issues should be considered when conducting assessments of personality disorders for treatment planning and outcome measurement. Many of these are not unique to the assessment of personality disorders, but some might be of particular importance for personality disorders. Discussed next are issues concerning age of onset, duration of symptomatology, distortions in self-perception, and the pervasive or multifactorial nature of personality structure.

Age of Onset

Personality disorders, by definition, must have an onset that "can be traced back at least to adolescence or early adulthood" (American Psychiatric Association, 1994, p. 633). DSM-IV does not recognize the existence of a personality disorder with an onset occurring within adulthood, unless its etiology can be attributed to the neurophysiological effects of a known medical condition. A DSM-IV personality disorder must be evident at least since young adulthood. In contrast, the World Health Organization's International Classification of Diseases (ICD-10; World Health Organization, 1992) does include diagnoses for personality change secondary to catastrophic experiences (Shea, 1996) or secondary to the experience of a severe mental disorder (Triebwasser & Shea, 1996).

A reason for the DSM-IV restriction is to avoid confusing the assessment of a mood, anxiety, substance dependence, or other Axis I mental disorder with a personality disorder. One of the more well-established and consistently replicated findings is the considerable effect of Axis I psychopathology on the assessment of personality (Widiger & Sanderson, 1995a; Zimmerman, 1994). It is likely that the majority of persons with a personality disorder will seek treatment at a time when they are in crisis or at least experiencing substantially increased levels of distress, anxiety, or depression (Shea, 1997), and persons who are significantly anxious, depressed, angry, or distraught will often fail to provide an accurate description of their usual way of thinking, feeling, behaving, and relating to others. Requiring that the assessment of a personality disorder document its presence since late childhood is one means by which to ensure that the personality disorder was indeed present before the onset of a current Axis I disorder (Triebwasser & Shea, 1996).

Personality disorder assessment instruments, however, vary substantially in how they operationalize the age of onset requirement. For example, the PDI-IV (Widiger et al., 1995) encourages the interviewer to document that each diagnostic criterion has been evident throughout much of the person's adult life, whereas the IPDE (Loranger, 1999) requires only that one of the diagnostic criteria for a respective personality disorder be present since the age of 25; all of the other diagnostic criteria can be evident only within the past few years. Self-report instruments are generally very weak in addressing age of onset. The MMPI-2 makes no reference to age of onset in its instructions to respondents (Hathaway et al., 1989); the PDQ-4 indicates that respondents should describe themselves in reference to how they have been over the past several years (Hyler, 1994); and the MCMI-III instructs respondents to answer the questions in reference to their current problem(s) (Millon et al., 1994). The instructions to MCMI-III test respondents are to describe their "feelings and attitudes" and "to be honest and serious as you can in marking the statements since the results will be used to help your doctor in learning about your problems." There is no instruction to describe one's characteristic manner of thinking, feeling, behaving, or relating to others prior to the onset of a recent mental disorder. In response to such MCMI-III borderline personality disorder items as "I have tried to commit suicide" and "I have given serious thought recently to doing away with myself" (Millon et al., 1994, p. 99), test respondents are unlikely to make any distinction between a suicidality secondary to a recent depressive mood disorder from the self-destructive behavior evident within a borderline personality disorder.

Instruments that lack an age of onset requirement or otherwise emphasize current functioning for their assessment of personality are likely to be susceptible to mood state and other Axis I confusions. The initial elevations on their scales at the beginning of a treatment may say more about an Axis I mental disorder than a personality disorder, and decreases in elevations over the course of treatment can also reflect the effective treatment of the Axis I disorder rather than actual changes to personality functioning (Hirschfeld et al., 1989). For example, Piersma (1989) reported significant decreases on the MCMI-II schizoid, avoidant, dependent, passive-aggressive, self-defeating, schizotypal, borderline, and paranoid personality disorder scales over the course of a brief inpatient treatment. Piersma (1989) concluded that "the MCMI-II is not able to measure long-term personality characteristics ('trait' characteristics) independent of symptomatology ('state' characteristics)" (p. 91).

Comparable results have also been obtained with semistructured interviews. For example, Loranger et al. (1991) compared IPDE assessments obtained at an inpatient admission to those obtained 1 week to 6 months later and reported that "there was a significant reduction in the mean number of criteria met on all of the personality disorders except schizoid and antisocial" (p. 726). They also argued that the reduction was not due to an inflation of scores at the beginning of treatment secondary to depressed or anxious mood because the change in personality disorder scores was not correlated with change in scores on anxiety or depression. However, an alternative perspective is that the study simply lacked sufficiently sensitive or accurate measures to adequately explain why there was a substantial decrease on 10 of the 12 personality disorder scales. It is unlikely that 1 week to 6 months of treatment resulted in the extent of changes to personality that were indicated by the IPDE (the change scores also failed to correlate with length of treatment). It is noteworthy in this respect that four patients were diagnosed with a histrionic personality disorder at admission, whereas eight patients were diagnosed with this disorder at discharge (despite the decrease in mean number of histrionic symptoms across all patients). If the changes in IPDE scores are valid, then treatment apparently created histrionic personality disorders in four of the patients.

Comparable increases after treatment on selected personality disorder scales were also reported by Piersma (1989) with the MCMI-II. Scores decreased with treatment on eight of the personality disorder scales but increased on the MCMI-II histrionic and narcissistic scales. The MCMI-III (Millon et al., 1994) and the MMPI-2 (Colligan et al., 1994) histrionic and narcissistic scales include many items that appear to be assessing adaptive self-confidence, assertiveness, and gregariousness, such as MCMI-III items no. 35 (keyed false), "I often give up doing things because I'm afraid I won't do them well"; no. 57, "I think I am a very sociable and outgoing person"; no. 40 (keyed false), "I guess I'm a fearful and inhibited person"; and no. 84 (keyed false), "I'm too unsure of myself to risk trying something new" (Millon et al., 1994). Such items will not lack validity in identifying maladaptive narcissism (as arrogant persons will endorse these items), but it might also be easy for such items to confuse adaptive confidence with narcissistic arrogance or to confuse a healthy sense of efficacy and self-worth with a grandiose sense of self-importance. Lindsay, Sankis, and Widiger (2000) suggested that "in order for the MCMI-III or MMPI-2 narcissistic scales to show a significant decrease in narcissistic personality disorder symptomatology after treatment of the disorder, the patient would have to endorse after successful treatment items indicating the absence of normal, healthy self-confidence and self-esteem" (p. 228).

Duration of Symptoms

Personality disorders, by definition, involve traits that are "stable and of long duration" (American Psychiatric Association, 1994, p. 633). However, the frequency with which various diagnostic criteria will be evident over any particular period of time can vary substantially (Loranger, 1999; Widiger et al., 1995). For example, borderline feelings of emptiness are likely to be evident more continuously or frequently than are borderline expressions of suicidality. Persons will feel empty much more often than they will commit suicidal acts. There will even be variability within a diagnostic criterion for different expressions of a respective personality trait. For example, one may need more instances of overspending than of unsafe sex to attribute borderline impulsivity to a respondent. And, personality disorder instruments again vary substantially in the time durations that are required. For example, the SCID-II and the IPDE generally require that each diagnostic criterion be evident over a 5-year period, whereas the DIPD generally requires only 2 years.

The duration requirement is of considerable importance to clinicians and researchers who are attempting to assess treatment effectiveness. Borderline self-destructiveness must be evident for at least 5 years to indicate its presence on the SCID-II, but it is unclear how long it should not be present to indicate its absence. Simply because a person does not report being suicidal at the end of treatment does not necessarily suggest that this trait of borderline personality disorder is no longer present. The suicidality of a person with borderline personality disorder will not be evident every day, every week, or even every month (Gunderson, 1987). One month of no suicidal ideation may indicate an improvement in functioning during that period of time, but it may not indicate an actual or sustained change to personality functioning. Personality traits are enduring characteristics of the self, not temporary or transient improvements to functioning secondary to a situational alteration, such as a temporary stabilization of a marriage or mood. If persons must evidence self-destructiveness over a 5-year period to indicate the presence of borderline suicidality, perhaps they should also evidence the absence of self-destructiveness over a 5-year period to indicate the successful treatment of this borderline suicidality.

However, requiring that a maladaptive personality trait be absent for 5 years before one considers it to be absent may substantially complicate the cost of conducting outcome studies for the treatment of personality disorders. Instruments that require substantial durations in time will be much less sensitive to actual changes in personality functioning than are instruments that require shorter durations in time (Costa & McCrae, 1994). Requiring only a brief period of time (e.g., the last few weeks of clinical treatment) can exaggerate the extent and stability of change, but only somewhat longer durations of time might be acceptable for an indication that a personality disorder is in partial or full remission (American Psychiatric Association, 1994). In any case, the time duration for judgments of change to personality functioning should at least consider how frequently the symptom or trait was evident prior to treatment.

Self-Perception Distortions

A personality disorder will often include a gross, or at least pathologic, distortion in a person's manner of "perceiving and interpreting self, other people, and events" (American Psychiatric Association, 1994, p. 63,3). "Antisocial persons will tend to be characteristically dishonest or deceptive in their self-descriptions, dependent persons may self-denigrate, paranoid persons will often be wary and suspicious, borderline persons will tend to idealize and devalue, narcissistic persons will often be arrogant or self-promotional, and histrionic persons will often be overemotional, exaggerated, or melodramatic in their self-descriptions" (Widiger & Saylor, 1998, p. 151). The self-perception of a person with a personality disorder should not be taken at face value (Benjamin, 1993), but instruments again vary in the extent to which they attempt to address this concern (Westen, 1997).

The degree of structure involved in an assessment may correlate with the extent to which an instrument accepts respondents' answers at face value (Bornstein, 1997; Westen, 1997). Self-report inventories and fully structured interviews will tend to have the most number of direct inquiries (e.g., simply asking respondents whether a diagnostic criterion is present); semistructured interviews will include many direct inquiries; unstructured interviews will still be predominated by direct inquiries but may include more open-ended questions and observations; some projective tests may have no direct inquiries (Widiger & Saylor, 1998). However, it is not the case that self-report inventories or semistructured interviews rely solely on direct inquiry. Many self-report inventories include a substantial proportion of subtle, indirect items, as well as validity scales that are used to detect distortion, denial, and exaggeration that may themselves suggest the presence of personality disorder symptomatology. In addition, semistructured interviews include many open-ended questions, indirect inquiries and observations of the respondents' manner of relating to the interviewer. Interviewers administering a semistructured interview do not simply record respondents' answers to queries but are instead using their clinical expertise to rate each diagnostic criterion based in part on direct, indirect, and open-ended questions that have been found by experienced investigators to be effective for assessing whether a particular diagnostic criterion is present.

The administration of an interview or a self-report inventory to someone other than the person who is the focus of the assessment (e.g., a spouse, close friend, or colleague) is another way of addressing distortion and dissimulation in respondents' self-descriptions. Self and informant assessments of personality disorder symptomatology will often fail to agree, and it is not yet certain which perspective should be considered to be more valid than the other (Bernstein et al., 1997; Dowson, 1992; Dreesen, Hildebrand, & Arntz, 1998; Riso, Klein, Anderson, Ouimette, & Lizardi, 1994; Zimmerman, Pfohl, Coryell, Stangl, & Corenthal, 1988). Spouses, close friends, and colleagues will not provide an entirely accurate description of an identified patient, as they will not be familiar with all aspects of the person's functioning and they may have their own axes to grind. Nevertheless, they do provide a useful source of additional information; they may have known a patient's characteristic manner of functioning well before the onset of a recently developed mental disorder;

and they may lack the distortions, denials, and exaggerations that characterize the patient's personality disorder. Interviews with informants might be particularly useful after treatment has ended to offset a tendency of persons to exaggerate treatment responsivity. One of the many intriguing results from the meta-analysis of personality disorder psychotherapy studies by Perry et al. (1999) was their finding of an inverse relationship between treatment duration and the self-reported assessments of outcome that was not found with observer ratings of outcome. They offered a number of alternative explanations for this finding, but they emphasized one compelling possibility that self-reports of improvement after brief interventions are still heavily invested by the initial feelings of distress that are particularly responsive to immediate signs of change. In any case, it is perhaps best to include both self and observer perspectives in treatment outcome assessments, and to consider each as providing a degree of useful information that together may provide a more valid description of the identified patient than either perspective considered alone.

Pervasiveness of the Disorder

Personality disorders are, by definition, pervasive. This is operationalized in DSM-IV as being evident "in two (or more) of the following areas: (1) cognition (i.e., ways of perceiving and interpreting self, other people, and events); (2) affectivity (i.e., the range, intensity, lability, and appropriateness of emotional response); (3) interpersonal functioning; [and] (4) impulse control" (American Psychiatric Association, 1994, p. 633). Personality disorders are syndromes or constellations of maladaptive personality traits, and different forms of treatment may affect different aspects of personality. For example, Sanislow and McGlashan (1998) suggested that pharmacologic interventions primarily affect disturbances in mood, affectivity, and cognitive-perceptual aberrations, aspects of personality functioning that are classified within the five-factor model of personality as being within the broad domain of neuroticism (Costa & McCrae, 1992). Psychodynamic, psychosocial, and cognitive-behavioral interventions, in contrast, also focus their interventions on matters of interpersonal relatedness and occupational functioning that are more readily apparent within the other five-factor model personality domains of extraversion, agreeableness, and conscientiousness (Trull & Widiger, 1997).

A treatment outcome assessment that is confined simply to a determination of whether a personality disorder is present or absent will fail to adequately recognize or appreciate the multifactorial nature of personality functioning. Identifying whether or not a person no longer meets the threshold for a DSM-IV diagnosis of a respective personality disorder is informative with respect to a medical concept of caseness or disorder (Regier et al., 1998), but persons meet and fail to meet DSM-IV diagnostic thresholds for a variety of different reasons (Shea, 1995; Widiger & Sanderson, 1995b). For example, persons who no longer meet the DSM-IV diagnostic criteria for borderline personality disorder could still evidence inappropriate or intense anger, frantic efforts to avoid abandonment, unstable and intense relationships, and affective instability—all traits that will have substantial importance to functioning and to the evaluation of treatment effectiveness (Skodol, 1989). Dialectical behavior therapy has been shown empirically to have a significant and meaningful effect on much of the symptomatology of borderline personality disorder, but Linehan, Tutek, Heard, and Armstrong (1994) emphasize that the treatment does not, in fact, cure persons of this disorder. "Dialectical behavior therapy may have been most effective in increasing distress tolerance and associated control of maladaptive behavior and least successful in actually increasing satisfaction and happiness" (Linehan et al., 1994, p. 1775). Dialectical behavior therapy is effective in anger reduction, social adjustment, and impulsivity, but it may not be as effective in the treatment of feelings of depressiveness or hopelessness (Scheel, 2000).

One approach to addressing the heterogeneity in symptomatology of persons with (and without) respective personality disorders is to analyze and report results for individual diagnostic criteria. Some of the personality disorders have relatively homogeneous diagnostic criteria sets (e.g., paranoid), but most of the criteria sets are quite heterogeneous in both form and content (Shea, 1992). For example, personality disorder diagnostic criteria vary in the extent to which they are behaviorally specific (e.g., borderline recurrent suicidal ideation) or require clinical inference and judgment (e.g., borderline identity disturbance); in the extent to which they might overlap with Axis I disorders (e.g., borderline transient, stress-related paranoid ideation versus histrionic perception of relationships being more intimate than they actually are); and in the aspect of personality functioning that is involved (cognitive, affective, behavioral, or interpersonal). The reliability of individual diagnostic criterion assessments can at times be quite weak, but analyses at the criterion level will at least suggest which aspects of the symptomatology were more or less responsive to treatment.

Instruments that include subscales for different components of various personality disorders, such as the subscales for borderline personality disorder in the PAI (Morey, 1996) and the DIB-R (Zanarini et al., 1989) will provide more reliable and valid assessments than analyses of individual diagnostic criteria. Even more informative would be the administration of inventories and interviews that provide separate scales for different domains of personality functioning, such as the SNAP (Clark, 1993), DAPP-BQ (Livesley & Jackson, in press), NEO PI-R (Costa & McCrae, 1992), SIFFM (Trull & Widiger, 1997), IIP (Horowitz et al., 1988), SASB (Benjamin, 1988), or SWAP-200 (Westen & Shedler, 1999a). These latter instruments can be problematic for the provision of DSM-IV diagnoses, but they may in fact be more useful than DSM-IV instruments by providing more precise information with respect to clinically significant domains of functioning. For example, rather than indicate whether a person no longer meets the DSM-IV criteria for the histrionic, borderline, and antisocial personality disorders, assessment with the SNAP will indicate whether there has been a clinically significant decrease in the more specific components of manipulation, self-harm, exhibitionism, or impulsivity, accompanied perhaps by no meaningful changes in dependency or entitlement.

The scales of the NEO PI-R and the SIFFM are particularly advantageous by including the assessment of adaptive personality traits that may facilitate treatment responsivity (Harkness & Lilienfeld, 1997; Sanderson & Clarkin, 1994), as well as by providing scales for the assessment of maladaptive personality traits that will complicate or undermine treatment responsivity. In addition, the five-factor model is organized with respect to broad and fundamental domains of personality functioning that may correspond to different aspects of treatment responsivity. For example, distress, dysphoria, and negative affectivity are covered within the domain of neuroticism; interpersonal relatedness is within the domains of extraversion and introversion; and work-related (occupational) behaviors are within the domain of conscientiousness. Each of these broad domains is further differentiated into underlying facets (e.g., neuroticism is differentiated in terms of anxiousness, depressiveness, angry hostility, vulnerability, self-consciousness, and impulsivity).

ASSESSMENT IN MANAGED CARE AND PRIMARY CARE SETTINGS

One central concern for the assessment of personality disorders in managed and primary care settings is the limited amount of time that is available for such assessments. The procedure recommended here—to first administer a self-report inventory as a screening instrument, followed by a semistructured interview that is confined to one or more of the personality disorder scales that are elevated on the screening measure—would be of obvious practical benefit in such settings. Clinicians working within managed care settings might be tempted to rely even more heavily on unstructured clinical interviews, given the limited amount of time available to them. However, unstructured clinical interviews are probably even less reliable and valid when less time is available to the clinician, as less time will contribute to an increased reliance on impressionistic assumptions and biased expectations (Garb, 1998).

Self-report inventories will be particularly advantageous in such settings, alerting clinicians to domains of maladaptive (and adaptive) functioning that they might otherwise have missed. Clinicians within managed and primary care settings might also find the more abbreviated versions of the instruments to be the only realistic options available to them. The MMPI-2 and the MCMI-III require a considerable amount of time for a patient to complete, as well as considerable amount of time for the clinician to score if the clinician cannot expend the amount of money (and time) required for computer scoring.

An additional consideration for clinicians working within managed care settings is to assess for various components of DSM-IV personality disorders, rather than or in addition to categorical diagnoses. Brief clinical treatments are unlikely to cure persons of their personality disorder, if by a cure is meant that a person no longer evidences any of the respective personality disorder symptomatology. Brief clinical treatments may not even result in a person no longer meeting the diagnostic threshold for a respective personality disorder (Perry et al., 1999). However, treatment may result in clinically significant reductions in socially meaningful aspects of personality functioning, such as marital stability, suicidality, physical assaultiveness, or criminal arrest. Rather than confine oneself simply to an assessment of the presence versus absence of a personality disorder, clinicians may find better justification for their practice by assessing the components of maladaptive personality functioning that are contributing to substantial social and public health care costs and that are being effectively addressed or at least diminished significantly through their clinical treatment (Linehan, 1993; Pilkonis, 1997; Shea, 1997).

Clinical treatments of mental disorders are often focused on the immediate concerns or complaints of the individual patient that are diagnosed in DSM-IV on Axis I (American Psychiatric Association, 1994). Personality disorders were placed on a separate axis in DSM-III to encourage clinicians to take a broader perspective (Frances, 1980). A personality disorder may not always be the immediate focus of concern for the patient, but personality disorder symptomatology may have as much, if not more, social, occupational, and public health care costs (Linehan, 1993). Treatment of personality disorders might then be a highly cost-effective approach for managed care, and the inclusion of personality disorder assessments within clinical practice that assess for improvement in functioning that contributes to substantial social and public health care costs may go far in documenting the importance of this treatment.

REFERENCES

Adler, D. A., Drake, R. E., & Teague, G. B. (1990). Clinicians' practices in personality assessment: Does gender influence the use of DSM-III Axis II? *Comprehensive Psychiatry, 31,* 125–133.

American Psychiatric Association. (1980). *Diagnostic and statistical manual of mental disorders* (3rd ed.). Washington, DC: Author.

American Psychiatric Association. (1987). *Diagnostic and statistical manual of mental disorders* (3rd ed., rev.). Washington, DC: Author.

American Psychiatric Association. (1994). *Diagnostic and statistical manual of mental disorders* (4th ed.). Washington, DC: Author.

Barber, J. P., & Morse, J. Q. (1994). Validation of the Wisconsin Personality Disorders Inventory with the SCID-II and PDE. *Journal of Personality Disorders, 8*, 307–319.

Beck, A. T., Freeman, A., & Associates (1990). *Cognitive therapy of personality disorders*. New York: Guilford Press.

Benjamin, L. S. (1988). *Intrex user's manual*. Madison, WI: Intrex Institute.

Benjamin, L. S. (1993). *Interpersonal diagnosis and treatment of personality disorders*. New York: Guilford Press.

Bernstein, D. P., Kasapis, C., Bergman, A., Weld, E., Mitropoulou, V., Horvath, T., Klar, H., Silverman, J., & Siever, L. J. (1997). Assessing Axis II disorders by informant interview. *Journal of Personality Disorders, 11*, 158–167.

Blashfield, R. K., & Herkov, M. J. (1996). Investigating clinician adherence to diagnosis by criteria: A replication of Morey and Ochoa (1989). *Journal of Personality Disorders, 10*, 219–228.

Bornstein, R. F. (1997). Dependent personality disorder in the DSM-IV and beyond. *Clinical Psychology: Science and Practice, 4*, 175–187.

Bornstein, R. F. (1998). Reconceptualizing personality disorder diagnosis in the DSM-V: The discriminant validity challenge. *Clinical Psychology: Science and Practice, 5*, 333–343.

Clark, L. A. (1993). *Manual for the Schedule for Nonadaptive and Adaptive Personality*. Minneapolis: University of Minnesota Press.

Clark, L. A., Livesley, W. J., & Morey, L. (1997). Personality disorder assessment: The challenge of construct validity. *Journal of Personality Disorders, 11*, 205–231.

Clark, L. A., Watson, D., & Reynolds, S. (1995). Diagnosis and classification of psychopathology: Challenges to the current system and future directions. *Annual Review of Psychology, 46*, 121–153.

Colligan, R. C., Morey, L. C., & Offord, K. P. (1994). MMPI/MMPI-2 personality disorder scales: Contemporary norms for adults and adolescents. *Journal of Clinical Psychology, 50*, 168–200.

Coolidge, F. L., & Merwin, M. M. (1992). Reliability and validity of the Coolidge Axis II Inventory: A new inventory for the assessment of personality disorders. *Journal of Personality Assessment, 59*, 223–238.

Corbitt, E. (1995). *Sex bias and the personality disorders*. Unpublished doctoral dissertation, University of Kentucky, Lexington.

Costa, P. T., & McCrae, R. R. (1992). *Revised NEO Personality Inventory (NEO PI-R) and NEO Five-Factor Inventory (NEO-FFI) professional manual*. Odessa, FL: Psychological Assessment Resources.

Costa, P. T., & McCrae, R. R. (1994). Set like plaster? Evidence for the stability of adult personality. In T. F. Heatherton & J. W. Weinberger (Eds.), *Can personality change?* (pp. 21–40). Washington, DC: American Psychological Association.

Dawes, R. M, (1994). *House of cards: Psychology and psychotherapy built on myth*. New York: Free Press.

Dowson, J. H. (1992). Assessment of DSM-III-R personality disorders by self-report questionnaire: The role of informants and a screening test for co-morbid personality disorders (SCTCPD). *British Journal of Psychiatry, 161*, 344–352.

Dreesen, L., Hildebrand, M., & Arntz, A. (1998). Patient–informant concordance on the Structured Clinical Interview for DSM-III-R Personality Disorders (SCID-II). *Journal of Personality Disorders, 12*, 149–161.

Dubro, A. F., & Wetzler, S. (1989). An external validity study of the MMPI personality disorder scales. *Journal of Clinical Psychology, 45*, 570–575.

First, M., Gibbon, M., Spitzer, R. L., Williams, J. B. W., & Benjamin, L. S. (1997). *User's Guide for the Structured Clinical Interview for DSM-IV Axis II Personality Disorders*. Washington, DC: American Psychiatric Press.

Fossati, A., Maffei, C., Bagnato, M., Donati, D., Donini, M., Fiorilli, M., Novella, L., & Ansoldi, M. (1998). Brief communication: Criterion validity of the Personality Diagnostic Questionnaire–4+ (PDQ-4+) in a mixed psychiatric sample. *Journal of Personality Disorders, 12*, 172–178.

Frances, A. J. (1980). The DSM-III personality disorders section: A commentary. *American Journal of Psychiatry, 137*, 1050–1054.

Garb, H. N. (1998). *Studying the clinician: Judgment research and psychological assessment.* Washington, DC: American Psychological Association.

Gunderson, J. G. (1987). Interfaces between psychoanalytic and empirical studies of borderline personality. In J. Grotstein, M. Solomon, & J. Lang (Eds.), *The borderline patient* (Vol. 1, pp. 37–59). Hillsdale, NJ: Analytic Press.

Gunderson, J. G. (1992). Diagnostic controversies. In A. Tasman & M. B. Riba (Eds.), *Review of psychiatry* (Vol. 11, pp. 9–24). Washington, DC: American Psychiatric Press.

Gunderson, J. G., Ronningstam, E., & Bodkin, A. (1990). The diagnostic interview for narcissistic patients. *American Journal of Psychiatry, 47,* 676–680.

Hare, R. D. (1991). *The Hare Psychopathy Checklist—Revised manual.* North Tonawanda, NY: Multi-Health Systems.

Harkness, A. R., & Lilienfeld, S. O. (1997). Individual differences science for treatment planning: Personality traits. *Psychological Assessment, 9,* 349–360.

Hathaway, S. R., McKinley, J. C., Butcher, J. N., Dahlstrom, W. G., Graham, J. R., & Tellegen, A. (1989). *Minnesota Multiphasic Personality Inventory test booklet.* Minneapolis: Regents of the University of Minnesota.

Herkov, M. J., & Blashfield, R. K. (1995). Clinicians' diagnoses of personality disorder: evidence of a hierarchical structure. *Journal of Personality Assessment, 65,* 313–321.

Heumann, K. A., & Morey, L. C. (1990). Reliability of categorical and dimensional judgments of personality disorder. *American Journal of Psychiatry, 147,* 498–500.

Hills, H. A. (1995). Diagnosing personality disorders: An examination of the MMPI-2 and MCMI-II. *Journal of Personality Assessment, 65,* 21–34.

Hirschfeld, R., Klerman, G., Lavori, P., Keller, M., Griffith, P., & Coryell, W. (1989). Premorbid personality assessments of first onset of major depression. *Archives of General Psychiatry, 46,* 345–350.

Hogg, B., Jackson, H. J., Rudd, R. P., & Edwards, J. (1990). Diagnosing personality disorders in recent-onset schizophrenia. *Journal of Nervous and Mental Disease, 178,* 194–199.

Horowitz, L. M., Rosenberg, S. E., Baer, B. A., Ureno, G., & Villasenor, V. S. (1988). Inventory of interpersonal problems: Psychometric properties and clinical applications. *Journal of Consulting and Clinical Psychology, 56,* 885–892.

Hyler, S. E. (1994). *Personality Diagnostic Questionnaire–4 (PDQ-4).* Unpublished test. New York: New York State Psychiatric Institute.

Hyler, S. E., Rieder, R. O., Williams, J. B. W., Spitzer, R. L., Hendler, J., & Lyons, M. (1988). The Personality Diagnostic Questionnaire: Development and preliminary results. *Journal of Personality Disorders, 2,* 229–237.

Hyler, S. E., Rieder, R. O., Williams, J. B. W., Spitzer, R. L., Lyons, M., & Hendler, J. (1989). A comparison of clinical and self-report diagnoses of DSM-III personality disorders in 552 patients. *Comprehensive Psychiatry, 30,* 170–178.

Hyler, S. E., Skodol, A. E., Kellman, H. D., Oldham, J. M., & Rosnick, L. (1990). Validity of the Personality Diagnostic Questionnaire—Revised: Comparison with two structured interviews. *American Journal of Psychiatry, 147,* 1043–1048.

Hyler, S. E., Skodol, A. E., Oldham, J. M., Kellman, H. D., & Doidge, N. (1992). Validity of the Personality Diagnostic Questionnaire—Revised: A replication in an outpatient sample. *Comprehensive Psychiatry, 33,* 73–77.

Jackson, H. J., Gazis, J., Rudd, R. P., & Edwards, J. (1991). Concordance between two personality disorder instruments with psychiatric inpatients. *Comprehensive Psychiatry, 32,* 252–260.

Jacobsberg, L., Perry, S., & Frances, A. (1995). Diagnostic agreement between the SCID-II screening questionnaire and the Personality Disorder Examination. *Journal of Personality Assessment, 65,* 428–433.

Kaye, A. L., & Shea, M. T. (2000). Personality disorders, personality traits, and defense mechanisms. In H. A. Pincus, A. J. Rush, M. B. First, & L. E. McQueen (Eds.), *Handbook of psychiatric measures* (pp. 713–750). Washington, DC: American Psychiatric Association.

Kim, Y., & Pilkonis, P. A. (1999). Selecting the most informative items in the IIP scales for personality disorders: An application of item response theory. *Journal of Personality Disorders, 13,* 157–174.

Kirk, S. A., & Kutchins, H. (1992). *The selling of DSM: The rhetoric of science in psychiatry*. New York: Aldine de Gruyter.

Klein, M. H., Benjamin, L. S., Rosenfeld, R., Treece, C., Husted, J., & Greist, J. H. (1993). The Wisconsin Personality Disorders Inventory: I. Development, reliability, and validity. *Journal of Personality Disorders, 7*, 285–303.

Langbehn, D. R., Pfohl, B. M., Reynolds, S., Clark, L. A., Battaglia, M., Bellodi, L., Cadoret, R., Grove, W., Pilkonis, P., & Links, P. (1999). The Iowa Personality Disorder Screen: Development and preliminary validation of a brief screening interview. *Journal of Personality Disorders, 13, 75–89.*

Lenzenweger, M. F., Loranger, A. W., Korfine, L., & Neff, C. (1997). Detecting personality disorders in a nonclinical population: Application of a 2-stage procedure for case identification. *Archives of General Psychiatry, 54,* 345–351.

Lilienfeld, S. O. (1994). Conceptual problems in the assessment of psychopathy. *Clinical Psychology Review, 14,* 17–38.

Lilienfeld, S. O., Waldman, I. D., & Israel, A. C. (1994). A critical examination of the use of the term "comorbidity" in psychopathology research. *Clinical Psychology: Science and Practice, 1,* 71–83.

Lindsay, K. A., Sankis, L. M., & Widiger, T. A. (2000). Gender bias in self-report personality disorder inventories. *Journal of Personality Disorders, 14,* 218–232.

Linehan, M. M. (1993). *Cognitive-behavioral treatment of borderline personality disorder*. New York: Guilford Press.

Linehan, M. M., Tutek, D. A., Heard, H. L., & Armstrong, H. E. (1994). Interpersonal outcome of cognitive behavioral treatment for chronically suicidal borderline patients. *American Journal of Psychiatry, 151,* 1771–1776.

Livesley, W. J. (1998). Suggestions for a framework for an empirically based classification of personality disorder. *Canadian Journal of Psychiatry, 43,* 137–147.

Livesley, W. J., & Jackson, D. (in press). *Manual for the Dimensional Assessment of Personality Pathology—Basic Questionnaire*. Port Huron, MI: Sigma Press.

Loranger, A. W. (1992). Are current self-report and interview methods adequate for epidemiological studies of personality disorders? *Journal of Personality Disorders, 6,* 313–325.

Loranger, A. W. (1999). *International Personality Disorder Examination (IPDE)*. Odessa, FL: Psychological Assessment Resources.

Loranger, A. W., Lenzenweger, M. F., Gartner, A. F., Susman, V. L., Herzig, J., Zammit, G. K., Gartner, J. D., Abrams, R. C., & Young, R. C. (1991). Trait–state artifacts and the diagnosis of personality disorders. *Archives of General Psychiatry, 48,* 720–729.

Marlow, D. B., Husband, S. D., Bonieskie, L. M., Kirby, K. C., & Platt, J. J. (1997). Structured interview versus self-report test vantages for the assessment of personality pathology in cocaine dependence. *Journal of Personality Disorders, 11,* 177–190.

Marziali, E., Munroe-Blum, H., & McClearly, L. (1999). The Objective Behavioral Index: A measure for assessing treatment response of patients with severe personality disorders. *Journal of Nervous and Mental Disease, 187,* 290–295.

McCann, J. T. (1989). MMPI personality disorder scales and the MCMI: Concurreng validity. *Journal of Clinical Psychology, 45,* 365–369.

McCann, J. T. (1991). Convergnent and discriminant validity of the MCMI-II personality disorder scales. *Psychological Assessment: A Journal of Consulting and Clinical Psychology, 3,* 9–18.

Mellsop, G., Varghese, F. T. N., Joshua, S., & Hicks, A. (1982). The reliability of Axis II of DSM-III. *American Journal of Psychiatry, 139,* 1360–1361.

Millon, T., Davis, R. D., Millon, C. M., Wenger, A. W., Van Zuilen, M. H., Fuchs, M., & Millon, R. B. (1996). *Disorders of personality: DSM-IV and beyond*. New York: Wiley.

Millon, T., Millon, C., & Davis, R. (1994). *MCMI-III manual*. Minneapolis, MN: National Computer Systems.

Morey, L. C. (1991). *The Personality Assessment Inventory professional manual*. Odessa, FL: Psychological Assessment Resources.

Morey, L. C. (1996). *An interpretive guide to the Personality Assessment Inventory (PAI)*. Odessa, FL: Psychological Assessment Resources.

Morey, L. C., & LeVine, D. J. (1988). A multitrait–multimethod examination of Minnesota Multiphasic Personality Inventory (MMPI) and Millon Clinical Multiaxial Inventory (MCMI). *Journal of Psychopathology and Behavioral Assessment, 10,* 333–344.

Morey, L. C., & Ochoa, E. S. (1989). An investigation of adherence to diagnostic criteria: Clinical diagnosis of the DSM-III personality disorders. *Journal of Personality Disorders, 3,* 180–192.

Morey, L. C., Waugh, M. H., & Blashfield, R. K. (1985). MMPI scales for DSM-III personality disorders: Their derivation and correlates. *Journal of Personality Assessment, 49,* 245–251.

Nazikian, H., Rudd, R. P., Edwards, J., & Jackson, H. J. (1990). Personality disorder assessments for psychiatric inpatients. *Australian and New Zealand Journal of Psychiatry, 24,* 37–46.

O'Maille, P. S., & Fine, M. A. (1995). Personality disorder scales for the MMPI-2: An assessment of psychometric properties in a correctional population. *Journal of Personality Disorders, 9,* 235–246.

Paris, J. (1998). Psychotherapy for the personality disorders: Working with traits. *Bulletin of the Menninger Clinic, 62,* 287–297.

Perry, J. C. (1992). Problems and considerations in the valid assessment of personality disorders. *American Journal of Psychiatry, 149,* 1645–1653.

Perry, J. C., Banon, E., & Ianni, F. (1999). Effectiveness of psychotherapy for personality disorders. *American Journal of Psychiatry, 156,* 1312–1321.

Pfohl, B., Blum, N., & Zimmerman, M. (1997). *Structured Interview for DSM-IV Personality.* Washington, DC: American Psychiatric Press.

Piersma, H. L. (1989). The MCMI-II as a treatment outcome measure for psychiatric inpatients. *Journal of Clinical Psychology, 45,* 87–93.

Pilkonis, P. A. (1997). Measurement issues relevant to personality disorders. In H. H. Strupp, M. J. Lambert, & L. M. Horowitz (Eds.), *Measuring patient change in mood, anxiety, and personality disorders: Toward a core battery* (pp. 371–388). Washington, DC: American Psychological Association.

Pilkonis, P. A., Heape, C. L., Proietti, J. M., Clark, S. W., McDavid, J. D., & Pitts, T. E. (1995). The reliability and validity of two structured diagnostic interviews for personality disorders. *Archives of General Psychiatry, 52,* 1025–1033.

Pilkonis, P. A., Heape, C. L., Ruddy, J., & Serrao, P. (1991). Validity in the diagnosis of personality disorders: The use of the LEAD standard. *Psychological Assessment, 3,* 46–54.

Pilkonis, P. A., Kim, Y., Proietti, J. M., & Barkham, M. (1996). Scales for personality disorders developed from the Inventory of Interpersonal Problems. *Journal of Personality Disorders, 10,* 355–369.

Regier, D. A., Kaelber, C. T., Rae, D. S., Farmer, M. E., Knauper, B., Kessler, R. C., & Norquist, G. S. (1998). Limitations of diagnostic criteria and assessment instruments for mental disorders: Implications for research and policy. *Archives of General Psychiatry, 55,* 109–115.

Reich, J., Noyes, R., & Troughton, E. (1987). Lack of agreement between instruments assessing DSM III personality disorders. In C. Green (Ed.), *Conference on the Millon clinical inventories* (pp. 223–234). Minnetonka, MN: National Computer Systems.

Reich, J., & Vasile, R. G. (1993). Effect of personality disorders on the treatment outcome of Axis I conditions: An update. *Journal of Nervous and Mental Disease, 181,* 475–484.

Riso, L. P., Klein, D. N., Anderson, R. L., Ouimette, P. C., & Lizardi, H. (1994). Concordance between patients and informants on the Personality Disorder Examination. *American Journal of Psychiatry, 151,* 568–573.

Rogers, R. (1995). *Diagnostic and structured interviewing: A handbook for psychologists.* Odessa, FL: Psychological Assessment Resources.

Sanderson, C., & Clarkin, J. F. (1994). Use of the NEO-PI personality dimensions in differential treatment planning. In P. T. Costa & T. A. Widiger (Eds.), *Personality disorders and the five-factor model of personality* (pp. 219–235). Washington, DC: American Psychological Association.

Sanislow, C. A., & McGlashan, T. H. (1998). Treatment outcome of personality disorders. *Canadian Journal of Psychiatry, 43,* 237–250.

Scarpa, A., Luscher, K., Smalley, K. J., Pilkonis, P. A., Kim, Y., & Williams, W. C. (1999). Screening for personality disorders in a nonclinical population. *Journal of Personality Disorders, 13,* 345–360.

Scheel, K. R. (2000). The empirical basis of dialectical behavior therapy: Summary, critique, and implications. *Clinical Psychology: Science and Practice, 7*, 68–86.

Schuler, C. E., Snibbe, J. R., & Buckwalter, J. G. (1994). Validity of the MMPI personality disorder scales (MMPI-PI). *Journal of Clinical Psychology, 50*, 220–227.

Shea, M. T. (1992). Some characteristics of the Axis II criteria sets and their implications for the assessment of personality disorders. *Journal of Personality Disorders, 6*, 377–381.

Shea, M. T. (1993). Psychosocial treatment of personality disorders. *Journal of Personality Disorders, 7*(Suppl.), 167–180.

Shea, M. T. (1995). Interrelationships among categories of personality disorders. In W. J. Livelsey (Ed.), *The DSM-IV personality disorders* (pp. 397–406). New York: Guilford Press.

Shea, M. T. (1996). Enduring personality change after catastrophic experience. In T. A. Widiger, A. J. Frances, H. A. Pincus, R. Ross, M. B. First, & W. W. Davis (Eds.), *DSM-IV sourcebook* (Vol. 2, pp. 849–860). Washington, DC: American Psychiatric Association.

Shea, M. T. (1997). Core battery conference: Assessment of change in personality disorders. In H. H. Strupp, L. M. Horowitz, & M. J. Lambert (Eds.), *Measuring patient changes in mood, anxiety, and personality disorders: Toward a core battery* (pp. 389–400). Washington, DC: American Psychological Association.

Shea, M. T., Widiger, T. A., & Klein, M. H. (1992). Comorbidity of personality disorders and depression: Implications for treatment. *Journal of Consulting and Clinical Psychology, 60*, 857–868.

Silberman, C. S., Roth, L., Segal, D. L., & Burns, W. J. (1997). Relationship between the Million Clinical Multiaxial Inventory-II and Coolidge Axis II Inventory in chronically mentally ill older adults: A pilot study. *Journal of Clinical Psychology, 53*, 559–566.

Skodol, A. E. (1989). *Problems in differential diagnosis: From DSM-III to DSM-III-R in clinical practice.* Washington, DC: American Psychiatric Press.

Skodol, A. E., Oldham, J. M., Rosnick, L., Kellman, H. D., & Hyler, S. E. (1991). Diagnosis of DSM-III-R personality disorders: A comparison of two structured interviews. *International Journal of Methods in Psychiatric Research, 1*, 13–26.

Soldz, S., Budman, S., Demby, A., & Merry, J. (1993). Diagnostic agreement between the Personality Disorder Examination and the MCMI-II. *Journal of Personality Assessment, 60*, 486–499.

Soloff, P. H., Siever, L., Cowdry, R., & Kocsis, J. H. (1994). Evaluation of pharmacologic treatment in personality disorders. In R. F. Prien & D. S. Robinson (Eds.), *Clinical evaluation of psychotropic drugs: Principles and guidelines* (pp. 651–673). New York: Raven.

Stone, M. H. (1993). *Abnormalities of personality: Within and beyond the realm of treatment.* New York: Norton.

Streiner, D. L., & Miller, H. R. (1988). Validity of the MMPI scales for DSM-III personality disorders: What are they measuring? *Journal of Personality Disorders, 2*, 238–242.

Torgersen, S., & Alnaes, R. (1990). The relationship between the MCMI personality scales and DSM-III, Axis II. *Journal of Personality Assessment, 55*, 698–707.

Triebwasser, J., & Shea, M. T. (1996). Personality change resulting from another mental disorder. In T. A. Widiger, A. J. Frances, H. A. Pincus, R. Ross, M. B. First, & W. W. Davis (Eds.), *DSM-IV sourcebook* (Vol. 2, pp. 861–868). Washington, DC: American Psychiatric Association.

Trull, T. J. (1993). Temporal stability and validity of two personality disorder inventories. *Psychological Assessment, 5*, 11–18.

Trull, T. J., Goodwin, A. H., Schopp, L. H., Hillenbrand, T. L., & Schuster, T. (1993). Psychometric properties of a cognitive measure of personality disorders. *Journal of Personality Assessment, 61*, 536–546.

Trull, T. J., & Larsen, S. L. (1991, August). *External validity of two personality disorder inventories.* Paper presented at the 99th Annual Meeting of the American Psychological Association, San Francisco, CA.

Trull, T. J., & Widiger, T. A. (1997). *Structured Interview for the Five-Factor Model of Personality.* Odessa, FL: Psychological Assessment Resources.

Watkins, C. E., Campbell, V. L., Nieberding, R., & Hallmark, R. (1995). Contemporary practice of psychological assessment by clinical psychologists. *Professional Psychology: Research and Practice, 26*, 54–60.

Westen, D. (1997). Divergences between clinical and research methods for assessing personality disorders: Implications for research and the evolution of Axis II. *American Journal of Psychiatry, 154,* 895–903.

Westen, D., & Shedler, J. (1999a). Revising and assessing Axis II: Part I. Developing a clinically and empirically valid assessment method. *American Journal of Psychiatry, 156,* 258–272.

Westen, D., & Shedler, J. (1999b). Revising and assessing Axis II: Part II. Toward an empirically based and clinically useful classification of personality disorders. *American Journal of Psychiatry, 156,* 273–285.

Widiger, T. A. (1993). The DSM-III-R categorical personality disorder diagnoses: A critique and an alternative. *Psychological Inquiry, 4,* 75–90.

Widiger, T. A. (1997). Mental disorders as discrete clinical conditions: Dimensional versus categorical classification. In S. M. Turner & M. Hersen (Eds.), *Adult psychopathology and diagnosis* (3rd ed., pp. 3–23). New York: Wiley.

Widiger, T. A., & Clark, L. A. (2000). Toward DSM-V and the classification of psychopathology. *Psychological Bulletin, 126,* 946–963.

Widiger, T. A., & Freiman, K. (1988). *Personality Interview Questions–II: Reliability, validity, and methodological issues.* Paper presented at the National Institute of Mental Health Workshop on Assessment of Personality Disorders, Bethesda, Maryland.

Widiger, T. A., & Lynam, D. R. (1998). Psychopathy and the five-factor model of personality. In T. Millon, E. Simonsen, M. Birket-Smith, & R. D. Davis (Eds.), *Psychopathy: Antisocial, criminal, and violent behavior* (pp. 171–187). New York: Guilford Press.

Widiger, T. A., Mangine, S., Corbitt, E. M., Ellis, C. G., & Thomas, G. V. (1995). *Personality Disorder Interview—IV: A semistructured interview for the assessment of personality disorders. Professional manual.* Odessa, FL: Psychological Assessment Resources.

Widiger, T. A., & Sanderson, C. J. (1995a). Assessing personality disorders. In J. N. Butcher (Ed.), *Clinical personality assessment: Practical approaches* (pp. 380–394). New York: Oxford University Press.

Widiger, T. A., & Sanderson, C. J. (1995b). Toward a dimensional model of personality disorders. In W. J. Livesley (Ed.), *The DSM-IV personality disorders* (pp. 433–458). New York: Guilford Press.

Widiger, T. A., & Sanderson, C. J. (1997). Personality disorders. In A. Tasman, J. Kay, & J. A. Lieberman (Eds.), *Psychiatry* (Vol., 2, pp. 1291–1317). Philadelphia: W. B. Saunders.

Widiger, T. A., & Saylor, K. I. (1998). Personality assessment. In A. S. Bellack & M. Hersen (Eds.), *Comprehensive clinical psychology* (pp. 145–167). New York: Pergamon.

Wise, E. A. (1994). Managed care and the psychometric validity of the MMPI and MCMI personality disorder scales. *Psychotherapy in Private Practice, 13,* 81–97.

Wise, E. A. (1996). Comparative validity of MMPI-2 and MCMI-II personality disorder classifications. *Journal of Personality Assessment, 66,* 569–582.

World Health Organization. (1992). *The ICD-10 classification of mental and behavioural disorders: Clinical descriptions and diagnostic guidelines.* Geneva, Switzerland: Author.

Yeung, A. S., Lyons, M. J., Waternaux, C. M., Faraone, S. V., & Tsuang, M. T. (1993). Empirical determination of thresholds for case identification: Validation of the Personality Diagnostic Questionnaire—Revised. *Comprehensive Psychiatry, 34,* 384–391.

Zanarini, M. C., Frankenburg, F. R., Chauncey, D. L., & Gunderson, J. G. (1987). The Diagnostic Interview for Personality Disorders: Interrater and test–retest reliability. *Comprehensive Psychiatry, 28,* 467–480.

Zanarini, M. C., Gunderson, J. G., Frankenburg, F. R., & Chauncey, D. L. (1989). The Revised Diagnostic Interview for Borderlines: Discriminating BPD from other Axis II disorders. *Journal of Personality Disorders, 3,* 10–18.

Zarrelle, K. L., Schuerger, J. M., & Ritz, G. H. (1990). Estimation of MCMI DSM-III Axis II constructs from MMPI scales and subscales. *Journal of Personality Assessment, 55,* 195–201.

Zimmerman, M. (1994). Diagnosing personality disorders: A review of issues and research methods. *Archives of General Psychiatry, 51,* 225–245.

Zimmerman, M., & Coryell, W. H. (1990). Diagnosing personality disorders in the community: A comparison of self-report and interview measures. *Archives of General Psychiatry, 47,* 527–531.

Zimmerman, M., & Mattia, J. I. (1999a). Differences between clinical and research practices in diagnosing borderline personality disorder. *American Journal of Psychiatry, 156,* 1570–1574.

Zimmerman, M., & Mattia, J. I. (1999b). Psychiatric diagnosis in clinical practice: Is comorbidity being missed? *Comprehensive Psychiatry, 40,* 182–191.

Zimmerman, M., Pfohl, B., Coryell, W., Stangl, D., & Corenthal, C. (1988). Diagnosing personality disorders in depressed patients. A comparison of patient and informant interviews. *Archives of General Psychiatry, 45,* 733–737.

14

Sexual Dysfunction

Markus Wiegel
John P. Wincze
David H. Barlow

OVERVIEW OF SEXUAL DYSFUNCTION

With the success of sildenafil citrate (Viagra) in the treatment of male erectile disorder, and the recent publication of the results from the National Health and Social Life Survey (Laumann, Paik, & Rosen, 1999), sexual dysfunctions have received renewed public and clinical attention. The finding that 43% of women and 31% of men suffered from some type of sexual difficulty in particular received public notice (Laumann et al., 1999, p. 541). In addition, primary care physicians and general practitioners are prescribing Viagra for erectile problems more frequently, and this has resulted in fewer erectile dysfunction cases presenting to urologists and sexual therapy clinics. However, the greater involvement of primary care physicians, who are not specifically trained in the assessment of sexual dysfunction, increases the likelihood that patients receive inappropriate treatment—for example, prescribing Viagra to treat erectile dysfunction in cases due to marital problems. The high prevalence of sexual dysfunction, and the increased number of non–sex therapists and non–urologists as treatment providers, underscores the need for accurate assessment and effective treatment planning.

Most cases of sexual dysfunctions involve multiple contributing and maintaining factors. Sexual dysfunction can result from many possible factors including medical diseases, medication side effects, relationship difficulties, emotional and psychological factors, comorbid Axis I psychiatric disorders, normative age-related changes, lifestyle factors, and, more often than not, a combination of some or all of these. Without an understanding of the contributing causes, the diagnostic categories in the *Diagnostic and Statistical Manual of Mental Disorders,* fourth edition (DSM-IV; American Psychiatric Association, 1994) provide little guidance regarding the most efficacious treatment options for a particular case. To delineate the most relevant contributing causes, the clinician requires a working knowledge of assessment techniques from a variety of areas and disciplines.

The incorporation of assessment results into the treatment plan is particularly important because various contributing and maintaining factors frequently require different treatment interventions. For example, when an assessment determines that arteriosclerosis contributes to erectile difficulties, treatment with either sildenafil citrate (Viagra) or vasoactive injections may be indicated. If the assessment also reveals the presence of chronic low sexual desire in the partner or considerable amounts of marital and relationship distress, simply providing the patient with a functional erection will not resolve the couple's sexual difficulties.

The chapter begins with an overview of diagnostic criteria and the prevalence of sexual dysfunction. Strategies pertinent to the general assessment of sexual dysfunction, including assessment measures, are presented, followed by specific considerations for each dysfunction. Next, case conceptualization, treatment planning, and outcome evaluation are presented, and the chapter closes with a case example that illustrates application of the material presented here.

Diagnostic Criteria

Sexual dysfunction can broadly be defined as "the persistent impairment of the normal patterns of sexual interest or response." DSM-IV organizes sexual dysfunctions according to the sexual response cycle phases: desire, arousal, and orgasm (Masters & Johnson, 1966; Kaplan, 1979). DSM-IV also includes an additional sexual pain disorder category. The specific "A" criteria for each of the 11 sexual dysfunctions are listed in Table 14.1. Uniformly for all sexual dysfunctions, the "B" criterion specifies that the disorder must cause marked distress or interpersonal difficulty. The "C" criterion specifies that the dysfunction should not be better accounted for by another Axis I disorder (except another sexual dysfunction), not result from a general medical condition, or not be due to the effects of a substance. DSM-IV includes specifiers for duration (lifelong vs. acquired), context (generalized vs. specific), and etiology (due to psychological factors vs. due to combined factors). More so than for other mental disorders, the criteria for sexual difficulties are broad and fairly vague, and they often require a large degree of subjective interpretation of contexts by the clinician. The classification of sexual difficulties presents unique challenges because it is highly sensitive to cultural and temporal changes in societal beliefs and attitudes about the "normalcy" and "naturalness" of different sexual behaviors. As attitudes change, so does the nosology (Leiblum, 1999).

Prevalence

In the past decade, several large-scale epidemiological studies of sexual behavior and sexual dysfunction have been published. These studies are reviewed by Simons and Carey (2001) and update the information on prevalence originally reviewed by Spector and Carey (1990) (see Table 14.2). Simons and Carey point out that more than one-third of the 52 studies they reviewed did not provide any operational definition of the dysfunction being investigated, and only 8 studies used DSM criteria. This is an important issue as the prevalence of sexual difficulties (i.e., the symptoms of sexual dysfunction) may occur with a much higher frequency than the sexual dysfunctions as defined by DSM-IV, which require the presence of interference and distress (criterion B). Differences in the operational definition used across studies potentially explain some of the variability in the prevalence rates reported.

Simons and Carey (2001) reported prevalence estimates for female hypoactive sexual desire disorder that ranged from 5% (Ventegodt, 1998) to 46% (Chiechi, Granieri, Lobascio,

TABLE 14.1. Diagnostic Criteria for DSM-IV Sexual Dysfunctions ("A" Criteria)

Disorder	DSM-IV "A" criteria
Hypoactive sexual desire disorder (302.71)	Persistently or recurrently deficient (or absent) sexual fantasies and desire for sexual activity. The judgment of deficiency or absence is made by the clinician, taking into account factors that affect sexual functioning, such as age and the context of the person's life.
Sexual aversion disorder (302.79)	Persistent or recurrent extreme aversion to, and avoidance of, all (or almost all) genital sexual contact with a sexual partner.
Female sexual arousal disorder (302.72)	Persistent or recurrent inability to attain, or to maintain until completion of the sexual activity, an adequate lubrication–swelling response of sexual excitement.
Male erectile disorder (302.72)	Persistent or recurrent inability to attain, or to maintain until completion of the sexual activity, an adequate erection.
Female orgasmic disorder (302.73)	Persistent or recurrent delay in, or absence of, orgasm following a normal sexual excitement phase. Women exhibit wide variability in the type or intensity of stimulation that triggers orgasm. The diagnosis of female orgasmic disorder should be based on the clinician's judgment that the woman's orgasmic capacity is less than would be reasonable for her age, sexual experience, and the adequacy of sexual stimulation she receives.
Male orgasmic disorder (302.74)	Persistent or recurrent delay in, or absence of, orgasm following a normal sexual excitement phase during sexual activity that the clinician, taking into account the person's age, judges to be adequate in focus, intensity, and duration.
Premature ejaculation (302.75)	Persistent or recurrent ejaculation with minimal sexual stimulation before, on, or shortly after penetration and before the person wishes it. The clinician must take into account factors that affect duration of the excitement phase, such as age, novelty of the sexual partner or situation, and recent frequency of sexual activity.
Dyspareunia (not due to a general medical condition) (302.76)	Recurrent or persistent genital pain associated with sexual intercourse in either a male or female.
Vaginismus (306.51)	Recurrent or persistent involuntary spasm of the musculature of the outer third of the vagina that interferes with sexual intercourse.
Sexual dysfunction due to a general medical condition[a,b]	A. Clinically significant sexual dysfunction that results in the marked distress or interpersonal difficulty predominates in the clinical picture. B. There is evidence from the history, physical examination, or laboratory findings that the sexual dysfunction is fully explained by the direct physiological effects of a general medical condition.
Substance-induced sexual dysfunction[a,c]	A. Clinically significant sexual dysfunction that results in marked distress or interpersonal difficulty predominates in the clinical picture. B. There is evidence from the history, physical examination, or laboratory findings that the sexual dysfunction is fully explained by substance use as manifested by either (1) or (2): (1) the symptoms in Criterion A developed during, or within a month of, substance intoxication (2) medication use is etiologically related to the disturbance

[a]Both "A" and "B" criteria are listed.

[b]Indicate the general medical condition and type of dysfunction (female hypoactive sexual desire disorder, 625.8; male hypoactive sexual desire disorder, 608.89; male erectile disorder, 607.84; female dyspareunia, 625.0; male dyspareunia, 608.89; other female sexual dysfunction, 625.8; other male sexual dysfunction, 608.89).

[c]Indicate specific substance (alcohol, 291.8; amphetamines, 292.89; cocaine, 292.89; opioid, 292.89; sedative, hypnotic, or anxiolytic, 292.89; other, 292.89) and specifier (with impaired desire, with impaired arousal, with impaired orgasm, or with sexual pain).

TABLE 14.2. Community Prevalence Rates for Sexual Dysfunctions

Disorder	Men 1990	Men 2001	Women 1990	Women 2001
Hypoactive sexual desire disorder	16%	0–3%	34%	14–33%
Sexual aversion disorder	?	?	?	?
Female sexual arousal disorder/male erectile disorder	4–9%	0–5%	11–14%	6–8%
Orgasmic disorder[a]	4–10%	0–3%	5–10%	7–10%
Premature ejaculation	36–38%	4–5%	—	—
Dyspareunia	?	0.2–8%	8–23%	3–18%
Vaginismus	—	—	?	0.5%

Note. Studies reviewed by Spector and Carey (1990) and Simons and Carey (2001).
[a]The prevalence of female orgasmic disorder varies widely depending on the situation. For example, Hite (1977) reported that 4% of women are nonorgasmic during masturbation (global), whereas up to 70% of women do not reach orgasm during intercourse.

Ferreri, & Loizzi, 1997). Laumann et al. (1999) reported a 1-year prevalence rate of 33%, based on symptom endorsement only. In contrast, Lindal and Stefansson (1993) reported the lifetime prevalence of female hypoactive desire disorder to be 16%, based on DSM-III criteria. The highest prevalence rates were found in samples of postmenopausal women (Simons & Carey, 2001). For female sexual arousal disorder, studies reviewed by Simons and Carey reported prevalence rates from 6% (Lindal & Stefansson, 1993) to 19% (Laumann et al., 1999). The prevalence estimates for female orgasmic disorder ranged from 4% to 7%, whereas Laumann et al. (1999) reported that 24% of women were unable to achieve orgasms. Reports for the prevalence of dyspareunia ranged from 3% to 18%. Simons and Carey (2001) note that the wide range of estimates was primarily influenced by methodological differences. For example, Lindal and Stefansson (1993) reported the lifetime prevalence (3%) and adhered to DSM criteria. In contrast, studies that found higher rates (e.g., 18% reported by Moody & Mayberry, 1993) tended to report point prevalence rates and used non-DSM operational definitions for dyspareunia. Consistently, the lower rates were found in north European samples, while the higher rates were noted in samples from the United States (Simons & Carey, 2001). The available community prevalence estimates for vaginismus ranged from 0.5% to 1% (Fugl-Meyer & Sjogren Fugl-Meyer, 1999; Ventegodt, 1998).

The community prevalence rates for male sexual dysfunction evidenced similar variability. Prevalence rates for male hypoactive sexual desire disorder ranged from 0% to 7% (Simons & Carey, 2001). However, Laumann et al. (1999) reported the 1-year prevalence rate for male complaints of low sexual desire to be 16%. The prevalence rates for male erectile disorder reported by Simons and Carey (2001) ranged from 0% to 10%. Erectile problems become dramatically more frequent with increasing age. The Massachusetts Male Aging Study (Feldman, Goldstein, Hatzichristou, Krane, & McKinlay, 1994) found that that half (52%) of men who were 40 to 70 years old experienced erectile dysfunction, and approximately three times as many older men than younger men experienced moderate to severe erectile problems. The reported prevalence rates of premature ejaculation ranged from 4% to 5% (Simons & Carey, 2001). In contrast, Laumann et al. (1999) found that 29% of men self-reported ejaculating too quickly. Male orgasmic disorder was reported to occur in 0% to 3% of community samples, with a higher prevalence found in samples of gay men (lifetime prevalence of 39%). Simons and Carey (2001) reported that sexual pain is relatively rare in community samples of men (lifetime prevalence of 0.2%). However, Rosser, Metz, Bockting, and Buroker (1997) found a higher current prevalence of pain during insertive (3%) and receptive (16%) anal sex in gay men.

The reported prevalence of a sexual dysfunction may vary, depending on the sample and the diagnostic criteria employed in a particular study. Not everyone who endorses symptoms of sexual dysfunction actually meets DSM-IV criteria for a sexual dysfunction. For example, Fugl-Meyer and Sjogren Fugl-Meyer (1999) found that only 45% of women with orgasmic problems perceived this as problematic. The results of this study underscore the importance of assessing the amount of distress and interference clients experience in regard to their sexual dysfunction before assigning a formal diagnosis. The assessment and diagnosis of sexual dysfunction requires careful consideration of many diverse aspects of the clients' sexual functioning, interference and distress being only a part of these. The following section describes the areas commonly covered in the assessment of sexual dysfunctions and includes a review of commonly used assessment measures.

ISSUES ADDRESSED IN THE ASSESSMENT OF SEXUAL DYSFUNCTION

An assessment of sexual dysfunction should enable the clinician/researcher to (1) determine the current level of sexual functioning, (2) describe the presenting problem and any comorbid problems, (3) formulate working hypotheses of the most relevant etiological and maintaining factors, (4) establish treatment goals and a treatment plan, and (5) be able to provide clear, constructive feedback to the client (Wincze & Carey, 2001). A further function of the assessment is to establish a baseline for comparison with posttreatment evaluations. Therefore, it is important for the assessment to yield both qualitative information that provides rich clinical details and quantitative data using reliable and valid instruments.

Sexual dysfunctions can result from a plethora of potential contributing causes, and sexual functioning in general is influenced by the individual's life context; as a result, it is necessary to cover a diverse number of topics during the course of the assessment. A comprehensive assessment of sexual dysfunction covers the following topic areas: (1) demographics, (2) overview of the problem, (3) current level of sexual functioning and history of the presenting problem (including relevant etiological factors), (4) psychosexual history, (5) history of sexual abuse, (6) medical history, (7) medications, (8) psychological and emotional functioning, (9) current environmental stressors, (10) general relationship with the primary partner, (11) and an interview with the partner. Depending on the case, different areas may require greater emphasis, whereas others may be less relevant. Clinical judgment is required in deciding how much time will be spent assessing each of the different areas. Each of these areas is described in more detail in Wincze and Carey (2001).

ASSESSMENT INSTRUMENTS

Clinical Interviewing

One of the cornerstones of psychological assessment is the clinical interview. It serves as a means of gathering information (self-report and behavioral observations) and provides a means for initially establishing rapport with the client. The interviewer should be able to listen, be non-judgmental, and be comfortable discussing the sexual material (especially when talking about behaviors outside the cultural norms) (Wincze & Carey, 2001). At the beginning of the interview it is important to make the client feel at ease. Prior to beginning the assessment interview, this can be facilitated by introducing oneself, providing information about one's training and experience, previewing the structure of the assessment, and giving explicit permission for clients to be embarrassed or uncomfortable while talking about their sexuality.

A number of instruments are available to clinicians and researchers to aid in the process of assessment. These instruments include semistructured interviews, a variety of questionnaires, and medical assessment techniques. Examples from each of these types of assessment tools will be described in the following section.

Semistructured Clinical Interviews

Derogatis Interview for Sexual Functioning (DISF)

Recently Derogatis (1997, 1998) developed the DISF, a semistructured interview that is designed to assess an individual's current level of sexual functioning. The interview is organized into five domains: sexual cognition and fantasy, sexual arousal, sexual behavior and experiences, orgasm, and sexual drive and relationship. The DISF contains 26 items that are rated by the interviewer on a 4-point scale. Separate male and female versions exist, and separate norms have been developed for males and females. Norms for additional populations (for example, geriatric populations and gay men) are under development. The DISF can be interpreted at the level of the discrete item, the functional domain, and the total score. On the level of the functional domain, scores are transformed to standardized area t-scores, allowing for easy comparison between functional domains intraindividually and across individuals or groups. The DISF has been shown to be both internally stable and reliable. Since the interview has only recently been published, further validation is necessary. However, initial data demonstrated that men and women with and without sexual dysfunctions can be distinguished based on the DISF and that it is sensitive to treatment-related improvements in sexual functioning. The DISF can aid in diagnosis, although it does not assess for DSM-IV criteria specifically.

Self-Report Measures and Questionnaires

The time most clinicians have for completing an assessment is very limited. Since it is often necessary to cover a wide variety of areas from multiple disciplines, it is helpful and often necessary to complement the assessment interview with questionnaires for the client to complete at home.

Questionnaires vary in the scope of their content. Questionnaires may focus on the general level of sexual functioning, cover all of the sexual dysfunctions, restrict themselves to specific sexual dysfunctions, or assess important related areas. A clinician or researcher must make choices about how much time and energy the client will spend completing each type of questionnaire. Having a standard assessment battery that can be augmented with questionnaires that specifically relate to the client's presenting problem can save time in preparing for an assessment. The following section describes some of the most common pen-and-paper measures used for the assessment of sexual dysfunctions. The section organizes the measures by type, starting with global sexual functioning and dysfunction measures, moving on to dysfunction-specific measures, and ending with questionnaires that assess important related areas.

Global Assessment Measures for Sexual Functioning and Dysfunction

Derogatis Sexual Functioning Inventory (DSFI)

One of the best-validated scales for the assessment of sexual functioning is the DSFI (Derogatis & Melisaratos, 1979; Derogatis, Meyer, & Dupkin, 1976). The DSFI is a widely used, omnibus scale of "current sexual functioning." It contains 245 items that measure 10 domains that are considered important for effective sexual functioning: information, experience, drive, attitudes, psychological symptoms, affect, gender-role definition, fantasy, body image, and sexual satisfaction. The different DSFI subscales reflect the multidimensionality of sexuality, and allow the clinician or researcher to plot a profile of the client's strengths and weaknesses in sexual functioning. One of the advantages of the DSFI is that norms and psychometric information are available for each of the subscales, thus allowing them to be used separately or together. The scale was validated with (and different norms exist for) both men and women with and without sexual dysfunctions. However, the DSFI does not assess sexual dysfunctions directly.

Most of the DSFI subscales have high internal consistency and good reliability. Two of the subtests, the Brief Symptom Inventory (BSI; Derogatis & Savitz, 1999; see also Chapter 2, this volume) and the Derogatis Affects Balance Scale (Derogatis & Rutigliano, 1996) have been validated as separate scales for measuring either psychological distress or mood and affect, respectively.

Two separate overall scores can be obtained for the DSFI. The Sexual Functioning Index (SFI) is calculated by summing all of the subtest scores, after they have been converted to *t*-scores (mean = 50, *SD* = 10). The SFI represents the individual's quality of sexual functioning in actuarial terms (Derogatis, 1998). The second overall score, the Global Sexual Satisfaction Index (GSSI) assesses the client's subjective judgment of the quality of sexual functioning. The respondent is asked to indicate, using a single item, the quality of her or his sexual functioning from "could not be worse" to "could not be better."

The DSFI has been used in numerous outcome studies that have confirmed its validity and sensitivity to disease-related declines in sexual functioning. In addition, it has been shown to discriminate between individuals with and without sexual problems. Although the scale takes about an hour to complete, it provides a wealth of information in a succinct manner (e.g., the profile of sexual functioning). It is one of the best-validated scales and one of the few for which norms exist. Thus, the scale allows one to interpret the client's scores relative to known groups. The DSFI assesses current levels of sexual functioning, taking into account the multidimensional nature of sexual behavior and response.

Golombok–Rust Inventory of Sexual Satisfaction (GRISS)

The GRISS (Rust & Golombok, 1986) is intended for heterosexual couples or individuals. It provides both an overall score of the quality of sexual functioning and subscale scores for different areas of sexual functioning. The GRISS is a 28-item scale with separate forms for males and females. The items are presented in a 5-point Likert-type scale that range from "never" to "always." The questionnaire takes about 4 to 10 minutes to complete.

The GRISS was empirically constructed and rigorously validated. Each subscale was constructed to contain four items, and the subscale scores can be plotted in the form of a profile. The following subscales are included in the GRISS: erectile dysfunction, orgasmic disorders, vaginismus, premature ejaculation, male avoidance, female avoidance, male satisfaction, female satisfaction, male nonsensuality, female nonsensuality, sexual infrequency, and noncommunication. Factor analysis and cross sample validation revealed two reliable, stable factors (an overall male score and an overall female score). The GRISS has been shown to be extremely internally consistent (Rust & Golombok, 1986). The test–retest reliability was calculated by using data that were obtained from 41 clinical couples pre- and posttreatment (marital or sex therapy) and are therefore likely underestimations of the stability of the scores. Rust and Golombok (1986) reported a test–retest value of .76 and .65 for the male and female scales, respectively. Both the male and female scales of the GRISS were found to discriminate between clinical and control samples.

Furthermore, the specific GRISS sexual dysfunction subscales were able to discriminate between groups diagnosed by sex therapists with specific sexual difficulties and a control group (Rust & Golombok, 1986). The GRISS has also been shown to be sensitive to improvements during treatment.

The GRISS is a psychometrically sound instrument that has been used widely in both clinical and research work. Its main utility may be as an outcome measure for couples and individuals undergoing sex or marital therapy (Rust & Golombok, 1998).

Sexual Dysfunction Scale (SDS)

The SDS (McCabe, 1994, 1998) is a 348-item self-report measure that assesses various sexual dysfunctions and their associated factors. The scale is divided into different sections that correspond to types of sexual problems: nature of the problem (30 items), premature ejaculation (33 items), erectile dysfunction (33 items), retarded ejaculation (31 items), orgasmic dysfunction (48 items), female unresponsiveness (51 items), vaginismus (31 items), and lack of sexual interest (91 items). All respondents complete the section on the nature of their sexual difficulties and the relevant section(s) that correspond to their sexual dysfunction(s). As a result, the questionnaire can take between 10 to 50 minutes to complete, depending on the number of problems experienced. Each dysfunction-specific section contains items that query the frequency, duration, and severity of the problem, as well as items that relate to medical, relationship, lifestyle, and attitudinal factors. Additional items assess an individual's response to experiencing a sexual dysfunction and the effect the dysfunction has on the relationship (for those currently in a relationship).

The SDS has been carefully developed over the last decade. It was pilot tested and cross-validated on groups that experienced different sexual dysfunctions and on a control group. The measure has been shown to have adequate reliability and validity (McCabe, 1998).

Female Sexual Function Index (FSFI)

The FSFI (Rosen et al., 2000) was developed as a brief, multidimensional self-report instrument for assessing the key dimensions of sexual function in women. The FSFI contains 19 items that assess sexual functioning during the past 4 weeks in the areas of sexual desire, arousal, lubrication, orgasm, satisfaction, and pain. The measure was validated on a sample of women with female sexual arousal disorder (FSAD) and a sample of women without sexual difficulties. Factor analytic studies revealed the FSFI to have a five-factor structure (desire/arousal, lubrication, orgasm, satisfaction, and pain). Based on clinical considerations, the desire and arousal factor was separated into two subscales. The six subscales of the FSFI were shown to have excellent internal reliability (Cronbach's alpha) and good test–retest reliability. All six domains were able to discriminate between the FSAD group and the control group, with the largest mean differences occuring on the lubrication and arousal domains. The Locke–Wallace Marital Adjustment Test (Locke & Wallace, 1959) was used to establish divergent validity. The FSFI is psychometrically sound and easy to administer, and has demonstrated ability to discriminate between clinical and nonclinical populations, thus making it ideal for use as a treatment outcome measure.

Diagnosis-Specific Assessment Measures

International Index of Erectile Functioning (IIEF)

The IIEF (Rosen, Riley et al., 1997) is a brief (15 items), psychometrically sound measure of erectile functioning. The measure has been shown to be sensitive to treatment changes, and it has been translated into 10 different languages. The IIEF is multidimensional and assesses sexual functioning in five domains: erectile functioning, orgasmic functioning, sexual desire, intercourse satisfaction, and overall satisfaction.

The IIEF has excellent psychometric properties, and its factor structure has been confirmed. All domains of the IIEF, except the sexual desire domain, showed excellent ability to discriminate between men with and without erectile problems, thereby establishing discriminant validity. Based on outcome studies that examined treatment of erectile disorder by sildenafil citrate, the sensitivity and specificity to treatment changes were determined. The results indicated that all five domains were sensitive to treatment-related improvements. The specificity was evaluated by a comparison of self-rated treatment nonresponders. None of the pre- to posttreatment comparisons approached statistical significance, which demonstrates good specificity of the IIEF.

More recently, a 5-item, abridged version of the IIEF was developed and provisionally validated (IIEF–5). The items were chosen from the original 15 on their ability to identify presence and severity of erectile problems. The IIEF–5 was shown to have favorable psychometric properties. Using a cutoff score of 21 (range of 5 to 25) the IIEF–5 was shown to have a sensitivity of .98 and a specificity of .88 for classifying individuals with erectile problems.

The IIEF has many advantages. It takes less than 15 minutes to complete, is easily comprehensible, and easily scored. There are separate items for achieving and maintaining erections, and it assesses the ability to achieve erections in nonintercourse sexual activity. There is one item that asks about the respondent's confidence in being able to achieve and maintain an erection, a psychological dimension that has been shown to be related to treatment outcome (Rosen, Leiblum, & Spector, 1994). The IIEF is very specific in that it assesses only current sexual functioning. Assessment of other components associated with sexual functioning and of the relationship by the IIEF is limited. The narrow focus of the measure and its excellent psychometric properties make it an outstanding measure of treatment outcome. One limitation of the IIEF is that it has only been validated on a heterosexual population. The standard instructions define sexual intercourse as "penile–vaginal penetration," making it less applicable to gay or bisexual men.

Sexual Desire Inventory (SDI)

The SDI (Spector, Carey, & Steinberg, 1996, 1998) is a 14-item, self-report inventory that was designed to measure sexual desire in individuals or couples. The inventory defines sexual desire as "interest in or wish for sexual activity" (Spector et al., 1996, p. 178). The SDI contains two scales: interest in partner-related sexual behavior (Dyadic Desire) and interest in self-directed sexual behavior, such as masturbation (Solitary Sexual Desire). The inventory measures sexual desire primarily as a cognitive variable by assessing the frequency and strength of thoughts directed toward approaching or being receptive to sexual stimuli (Spector et al., 1998). By including the two scales, the SDI recognizes the multidimensional aspect of sexual desire. The inventory uses the past month as its reference period and consists of multiple-choice (frequency items) and Likert-type items (strength of desire items). The SDI takes about 5 minutes to complete. Scores are obtained by summing the items for each subscale. For couples, the female partner dyadic score can be subtracted from the male partner dyadic score to derive a measure of discrepancy. The language of the SDI is non-heterosexist, and although it has not been validated in gay, lesbian, or bisexual samples, this measure could in theory be used with these populations.

The SDI has a high internal consistency (Spector et al., 1996). Based on a sample of 380 students, the convergent validity was established by correlating the solitary desire scores with the frequency of solitary sexual behavior ($r = .8$, $p < .0001$) and the dyadic desire scale with the frequency of partner related behavior ($r = .34$, $p < .0001$). Spector et al. (1998) point out that neither scale correlate exactly with behavior, which emphasizes the inaccuracy of using just sexual behavior frequency as a measure of desire. Neither SDI subscale was found to correlate with social desirability, which demonstrates discriminant validity (Spector et al., 1998). Factor analysis supported the presence of the two factors: dyadic desire and solitary desire. The last item (item 14) did not load on either factor (and was not hypothesized to) and asks about distress during abstinence.

Overall, the SDI is a highly reliable, valid measure of sexual desire that is easy to use and score. Unlike scales such as the drive subscale of the Derogatis Sexual Function Inventory, it does not rely primarily on frequency of sexual behavior as a measure of desire; instead, it measures primarily cognitive aspects of sexual desire. Unfortunately, to date no data on norms or base rates have been published.

Sexual Attitudes and Beliefs

Negative attitudes toward sexuality have been theorized to contribute to sexual dysfunction (e.g., Lazarus, 1989; Watters, Askwith, Cohen, & Lamont, 1985) and are associated empirically with the presence of sexual dysfunction in both men and women (McCabe & Cobain, 1998). Furthermore, specific attitudes may directly affect treatment planning. For example, a client who has very negative attitudes or misconceptions about masturbation will be more resistant to behavioral exercises that include nondemand self-touching and masturbatory exercises, which are a common component of sex therapy.

Scales and inventories developed to assess sexual attitudes are plentiful. Unfortunately, norms, base rates, or cutoff scores are lacking for many of these instruments. Without available norms, interpretation of the scores is difficult (and often meaningless) and relegated to an idiographic review of individual item responses. This issue is particularly problematic for assessing sexual attitudes because these are mediated by age, gender, and cultural/societal context.

Sexual Opinion Survey (SOS)

One of the most commonly used and best-validated sexual attitude/belief scales is the SOS (Fisher, 1998; Fisher, Byrne, White, & Kelley, 1988). The SOS is not an attitude scale per se but is theorized to assess the personality dimension of erotophobia–erotophilia, which is described as a learned disposition to respond to sexual stimuli with affect and evaluations that range from negative (erotophobia) to positive (erotophilia). The dimension of erotophobia–erotophilia is theorized to be related to avoidance and approach of sexual situations and stimuli (Fisher, 1998; Fisher et al., 1988; Gilbert & Gamache, 1984). The SOS is a 21-item scale that asks respondents to rate different descriptions of sexual stimuli on a 6-point Likert-type scale that ranges from strongly agree to strongly disagree. The items are presented in the form of opinion statements (e.g., "Pornography is obviously filthy, and people should not try to describe it as anything else") or as more personal statements (e.g., "If people thought I was interested in oral sex, I would be embarrassed"). The scale takes about 10 minutes to complete.

The SOS was found to have good internal consistency (Cronbach's alpha) and 2-month test–retest reliability (r) (Fisher et al. 1988). Two different factor structures have been reported for the SOS. Using a sample of parents, Gilbert and Gamache (1984) found three factors: open sexual display, sexual variety, and homoeroticism. The factor analysis by Rise, Traeen, and Kraft (1993), using a sample of Norwegian adolescents, found evidence for four factors: erotophilia (positive reaction to sexuality), erotophobia (negative reaction), unconventional sex, and homosexual orientation. The construct validity of the SOS is based on more than a decade of empirical and theoretical work. For women, the erotophobia–erotophilia dimension has been associated with frequency of sexual activity, frequency of orgasm, sexual desire, sexual assertiveness, sexual excitability, and sexual satisfaction (Hurlbert, Apt, & Rabehl, 1993). For men, the dimension has been associated with the maximum number of sexual partners per month and lifetime number of sexual partners (Bogaert & Fisher, 1995). Erotophobia–erotophilia has also been linked with individual difference measures of sexual preoccupation, sensation seeking, sexual permissiveness, openness to diverse sexual practices, sexual guilt, homophobia, and authoritarianism (see Fisher, 1998, for a review). Furthermore, individuals who score in the erotophobic range report more negative attitudes toward sexuality, produce briefer or less-explicit sexual fantasies, and have less experience with erotica (Fisher, 1998).

One of the largest advantages to the SOS is that norms have been established for different genders, age groups, religions, and countries (Brazil, Canada, Hong Kong, India, Israel, Japan, and United States). The SOS can be administered to both partners in a couple to ascertain how similar their affective reactions and evaluations of sexual stimuli are. Husband–wife discrepancies on the SOS have been associated with lower sexual satisfaction (Smith, Becker, Byrne, & Przybyla, 1993). Norms for lesbian or gay populations have not been reported in the literature, but since the SOS contains several items that relate to homosexuality, sexual orientation clearly will affect the score.

Sexual Satisfaction

Index of Sexual Satisfaction (ISS)

The ISS (Hudson, 1998; Hudson, Harrison, & Crosscup, 1981) is a brief measure of the general degree of sexual satisfaction within the relationship. It contains 25 Likert-type items on a 7-point scale, with ratings that range from "none of the time" to "all of the time," designed to measure the degree of sexual dissatisfaction. ISS scores range from 0 to 100, where higher scores indicate greater dissatisfaction and scores greater than 30 indicate the presence of clinical levels of sexual discord in the relationship (Hudson, 1998). The ISS takes 7 minutes to complete and can be scored providing at least 80% of the items have been completed.

The ISS has been found to have a high internal consistency. The known groups validity coefficient (troubled and untroubled groups) was found to be .76, as determined by the point biserial correlation between criterion groups (Hudson, 1998). Data regarding the test–retest reliability are unavailable. The scale's brevity makes it suitable for evaluating treatment outcome.

Other Relevant Questionnaires

Early Sexual Experiences Checklist (ESEC)

The ESEC (Miller, Johnson, & Johnson, 1991) provides an efficient, accessible means for detecting unwanted sexual experience that occurred before age 16. The format and language of the ESEC do not require respondents to label themselves as "sexually abused," and the scale avoids pejorative terms or evaluations. Respondents are simply asked to check, from a list of nine items, any specific, unwanted overt sexual experiences that occurred. Respondents may check more than one behavior, write in additional experiences, or check none of the above. A second section includes nine additional items that pertain to the most distressing event. These items ask the respondent to indicate her or his age, the age and relationship of the other party, frequency and duration of the experience, and the degree of distress experienced at the time of the event and currently. The last question represents a checklist regarding the type of coercion involved. The ESEC can be completed in less than 5 minutes.

Miller and Johnson (1998) note that the Early Sexual Experiences Checklist obtains results comparable to more time-consuming and costly face-to-face interviews. In addition, Miller and Johnson (1997, as cited in Miller & Johnson, 1998) found that of those respondents who reported bothersome childhood sexual events, 56% did not explicitly label themselves as sexually abused, indicating that the ESEC is able to detect events, regardless of whether the respondent labels the experiences as sexual abuse. The advantage of the ESEC is its brevity and its avoidance of evaluative labels. As a result, it may provide the client with an opportunity to report childhood sexual abuse without the potential discomfort of doing so in a face-to-face interview.

Sexual Arousability Inventory (SAI) and Sexual Arousability Inventory—Expanded (SAI-E)

The original SAI (Chambless & Lifshitz, 1984; Hoon, Hoon, & Wincze, 1976) is a 28-item, self-report inventory that measures the perceived arousability of a variety of sexual experiences including foreplay, oral–genital sexual activity, erotic materials, and intercourse. The SAI-E is the same instrument, except that each of the 28 items is rated a second time in terms of how much anxiety each activity elicits. Respondents are asked to rate each of the items on a 7-point Likert-type scale (from –1, adversely affects arousal, to 5, always causes arousal, extremely arousing) for arousal and (from –1, relaxing, calming, to 5, always causes anxiety, extremely anxiety producing) for anxiety. Respondents base their ratings on their past experience or how arousing or anxiety producing the activity would be if they were to experience it. The original SAI was designed for and validated with heterosexual and lesbian women, whereas the SAI-E can be completed by both men and women, regardless of sexual orientation or preference. The measure takes about 10 to 15 minutes to complete. A 14-item short version has been developed and takes less than 5 minutes to complete. A Spanish version of the SAI-E has also been initially validated (Aluja & Torrubia, 1994; Aluja, Torrubia, & Gallart, 1990).

The arousability component of the SAI-E (i.e., SAI) has been extensively validated, especially for heterosexual and lesbian women. Reliability and validity data for men are currently not available for either the arousability or anxiety components of the SAI-E. For women, the arousability component has been shown to be very internally consistent and reliable. The construct validity of the arousability component has been established based on correlations with awareness of physiological response, satisfaction with responsiveness, and frequency of and experience with sexual activity (Aluja & Torrubia, 1994; Hoon et al., 1976). Factor-analytic studies found five stable and interpretable factors for heterosexual women and six for lesbian women. In addition, the arousability component of the SAI-E has been shown to discriminate between women with and without sexual dysfunctions. The anxiety component of the SAI-E has received initial validation (Chambless & Lifshitz, 1984).

Normative scores on the SAI-E have been published for heterosexual women, lesbian women, and heterosexual men for arousability and anxiety (heterosexual women only) (Hoon & Chambless, 1998). More comprehensive norms for men and women with sexual dysfunctions would increase the clinical utility of the SAI-E even further.

The SAI and SAI-E are psychometrically valid, clinically useful measures that can assist in identifying specific sexual activities that may be problematic. The arousability scale of the SAI-E, although not empirically validated for this purpose, may also be useful in evaluating increases in "pleasure-focused" approach to sexual activity during treatment.

Other Resources

Two volumes are immensely useful for evaluating and deciding which questionnaires a clinician or researcher may want to use. *Sexuality-Related Measures: A Compendium* (Davis, Yarber, & Davis, 1988) and the more recent *Handbook of Sexuality-Related Measures* (Davis, Yarber, Bauserman, Schreer, & Davis, 1998) provide reviews for a large number of measures. In addition, review articles may provide information about older measures (Conte, 1986; Schiavi, Derogatis, Kuriansky, O'Connor, & Sharpe, 1979; Talmadge & Talmadge, 1990).

Medical, Urological, or Gynecological Examination

Sexual dysfunctions secondary to medical conditions are common. Because sexual response depends on the central and peripheral nervous system, hormones, and the circulatory system, any medical condition that involves these systems has the potential to disrupt sexual functioning. Sexual dysfunction in both men and women has been associated with intracranial diseases, such as epilepsy, encephalopathy, stroke, and Parkinson's disease (Lechtenberg & Ohl, 1994). Strokes, head trauma, and brain surgery, depending on the location of the insults in the brain, may result in either hyposexuality or hypersexuality.

Diabetes mellitus and other peripheral neuropathy (such as Shy–Drager Syndrome) also represent common contributing causes of sexual dysfunction. Over 50% of men with diabetes mellitus eventually develop erectile problems that are associated primarily with nerve damage in the corpora cavernosa but also are related to endocrine and vascular deficiencies (Lechtenberg & Ohl, 1994). Dyspareunia, reduced vaginal lubrication, and orgasmic dysfunction are associated with diabetes mellitus in women, and even mild neuropathic changes can significantly raise stimulatory threshold levels (see Hulter, 1999, for review). Clearly, physical conditions that affect the genital blood supply, such as arteriosclerosis, have a negative effect on sexual arousal. Major risk factors for generalized arteriosclerosis include cigarette smoking, diabetes, and hypertension.

Many medications have side effects that interfere with sexual functioning. A thorough review of hypertensive medications that interfere with sexual functioning can be found in Rosen, Kostis, Jekelis, and Taska (1994). Feliciano and Alfonso (1997) provide an excellent review of the sexual side effects of psychotropic medications. For a general review of the sexual side effects of medications, see Crenshaw and Goldberg (1996) and Finger, Lund, and Slagle (1997).

The medical exam contains some standard tests and procedures and, as the case requires, follow-up tests to confirm the results. Most medical exams include an examination of the external genitalia and laboratory testing of hormone levels, renal function, urinalysis, and glucose tolerance. For men, especially older adults, a prostate exam and for women a pap smear is included in the examination. Since neurological disorders often result in sexual dysfunctions, a screen for neurological pathology and possible referral to a neurologist may also be indicated. For example, 94% of women with hypothalmo-pituitary disorders, 83% of women with multiple sclerosis, and 40% of women with insulin-dependent diabetes mellitus were found to suffer from a sexual dysfunction (decreased desire, insufficient lubrication, or orgasmic difficulties) (Hulter, 1999).

Depending on the nature of the sexual difficulty and the case presentation, additional tests may be necessary. For men with erectile problems, several procedures have been developed to determine the quality of their penile functioning (see the following section on Male Erectile Disorder).

CONSIDERATIONS FOR THE ASSESSMENT
OF SPECIFIC SEXUAL DYSFUNCTIONS

Hypoactive Sexual Desire Disorder

Hypoactive sexual desire disorder (HSDD), one of the most common sexual difficulties, is characterized by the recurrent and persistent absence or deficiency of sexual desire or interest in sexual activity. The accurate assessment of HSDD is complicated by the lack of agreement on a definition of sexual desire itself. Most authors agree that sexual desire is a subjective state and a multifaceted construct that is the endpoint of a series of complex interactions between biological, psychological (cognitive and affective), interpersonal, and sociocultural factors (Beck, 1995; Leiblum & Rosen, 1989; Wincze & Carey, 2001). Unlike with sexual arousal, there are virtually no data available on psychophysiological markers of sexual desire. Also, most experts agree that frequency of sexual behavior is not an accurate indicator of sexual desire (e.g., Beck, 1995, Spector et al., 1996; Wincze & Carey, 2001) because an individual may engage in sexual behavior as a result of partner pressure or due to other motives (e.g., intimacy) (Beck, Bozman, & Qualtrough, 1991; Laan & Everaerd, 1995). Frequently, sexual desire has been assessed using a single-item Likert-type scale. However, this assumes that sexual desire is a unitary construct. Currently, the most common manner of assessing levels of sexual desire use a combination of the frequency of sexual thoughts and fantasies, sexual urges, solitarily sexual behavior, and initiating or being receptive toward sexual activity. No one single behavior or self-report item seems to capture sexual desire accurately.

The diagnosis of HSDD is further complicated because levels of sexual desire vary widely among individuals, between genders, across cultures, and across ages (Leiblum & Segraves, 1995). As is often the case, clients present for treatment due to increasing pressure or ultimatums from their partners. DSM-IV contains no diagnostic category for hyperactive sexual desire disorder; as a result, in couples who present with discrepancies in ideal sexual frequency, the partner with the lower level of sexual desire is often pathologized. Conceptualizing sexual desire problems as a desire *discrepancy* shifts blame away from the individual with lower desire levels and sets the stage for the couple to work together. This may include resolving the discrepancy through compromise, working on other couples' issues that may affect sexual desire (i.e. amount of intimacy, power issues), or accepting their differences in desire and modifying how they interact sexually (as opposed to changing the frequency).

Many different factors can affect one's levels of sexual desire, including age, social and educational factors, and cultural variables (Beck, 1995), and HSDD has consistently been associated with heightened levels of marital or dyadic distress (Beck, 1995). Thus, particular attention to relationship issues is warranted when assessing sexual desire. Repeated pressure from a partner to engage in sexual activity is itself detrimental to sexual desire and satisfaction (Davies, Katz, & Jackson, 1999). Therefore, even when the initial reason for a decline in desire is independent of relational factors, there is a high likelihood that relationship issues play a role in maintaining the difficulty. Decreases in sexual desire may also be due to negative affect, such as anger (Beck & Bozman, 1995), poor body image (Werlinger, King, Clark, Pera, & Wincze, 1997; Wiederman, 2000), and a history of sexual trauma (Becker, Skinner, Abel, Axelrod, & Cichon, 1984; Becker, Skinner, Abel, & Cichon, 1986).

Low levels of sexual interest may also result from chronic illness and emotional difficulties (especially depression and anxiety).

Hormone levels in both men and women also affect sexual desire. Regan (1999) reviewed the literature on endocrine factors and their relationship with sexual desire. For both men and women, sexual desire is to some extent androgen-dependent. The majority of testosterone (96% to 98%) is bound to proteins, primarily to sex-hormone-binding globulin (SHBG) and to albumin, and is therefore not available to exert its affects on target cells. The remaining portion, called "free," "unbound," or "bioavailable" testosterone, is most useful for assessing androgenic influences on sexual response, including desire. However, testosterone does not influence sexual desire in a linear relationship. Bancroft (1988), Campbell and Udry (1994), and Sherwin (1988) have proposed that sexual desire is noticeably affected only when the level of the hormone has dropped below some unspecified critical threshold. At or above this threshold, increasing the level of androgens will have no further influence on desire. Regan (1999) concludes that while a certain level of androgens may be necessary for sexual desire, presence of adequate levels of hormones is not alone sufficient to produce sexual desire.

Low sexual desire is frequently comorbid with other sexual dysfunctions. K. B. Segraves and R. T. Segraves (1991) found that 40% of their female sample with a primary hypoactive sexual desire disorder ($N = 588$) also received a diagnosis of an arousal or orgasmic disorder. At other times, reduced sexual desire results from the frustration and negative affect that are produced by another sexual dysfunction. Therefore, establishing the time course of each sexual dysfunction in clients with multiple sexual problem areas is diagnostically important. For example, a woman who feels pain during sexual activity may lose her sexual desire as a result of repeated unpleasant sexual experiences. However, a woman who engages in sexual activity despite a lack of desire (e.g., due to partner pressure) may experience pain during coitus as a result of reduced lubrication.

Sexual Aversion Disorder

Sexual aversion disorder, which involves fear or disgust and active avoidance of sexual contact, first appeared in the *Diagnostic and Statistical Manual of Mental Disorders,* third edition, revised (DSM-III-R; American Psychiatric Association, 1987). Data on the prevalence and nature of sexual aversion disorder are scarce. Sexual aversion disorder can be conceptualized as being similar to a specific phobia of sexual stimuli and may result from fear of contracting sexually transmitted disease, reminders of past sexual trauma, or feelings of personal inadequacy (Katz, Gipson, & Turner, 1992). Schover and LoPiccolo (1982) conceptualized sexual aversion disorder as occupying the severe end of a continuum that has hypoactive sexual desire disorder at is mild end. Kaplan and Klein (1987) emphasized panic-like states as a possible symptom manifestation. The aversion can be generalized, with the individual responding with fear and avoidance of any situation or behavior that may lead to sexual activity. Alternatively, the aversion may be more specific, being limited to sexual situations involving a partner, the genitalia, or certain aspects such as genital secretions. Thus, some individuals with sexual aversion disorder may experience sexual desire, engage in sexual fantasies, and enjoy autoerotic behavior, yet they may experience intense fear and disgust when confronted by a sexual situation involving a partner. In an early paper on sexual aversion syndrome, Crenshaw (1985) emphasized the importance of distinguishing between lifelong and acquired sexual aversions. She stated that lifelong sexual aversion disorder is more often associated with negative attitudes toward sex, early negative sexual messages, religious orthodoxy, and childhood sexual trauma. Acquired sexual aversion disorder is more frequently associated with the experience of comorbid sexual dysfunction, in particular the sexual pain disorders. A diagnosis of sexual aversion disorder is not made if the avoidance occurs solely in the context of another Axis I disorder, such as post-traumatic stress disorder or depression. Many men may avoid sexual activity as a result of erectile problems or premature ejaculation. Unless the person experiences fear or disgust when confronted with a sexual situation, this would not qualify for an additional diagnosis of sexual aversion disorder. More commonly, individuals develop a sexual aversion as a consequence of repeated painful sexual activity, which at times can be manifested as fear and avoidance of anything that may potentially lead to sexual behavior.

Erectile Dysfunction

Of all the sexual dysfunctions, male erectile disorder has been the most widely researched. Possibly as a result of the greater amount of knowledge, erectile dysfunction exemplifies, par excellence, the reciprocal influence of cognitive, affective, interpersonal, sociological, and biological factors on sexual functioning.

Research has shown that men with and without sexual dysfunction differ in several important ways, including their response to anxiety and performance pressure, affective response to sexual stimuli, and the accuracy of reporting levels of sexual arousal (Cranston-Cuebas & Barlow, 1990). These findings are important to consider during the evaluation of erectile problems. For example, men with erectile dysfunction tend to underestimate their level of erectile response (Sakheim, Barlow, Abrahamson, & Beck, 1987). As a result, it is important to ask clients directly whether they are able to achieve partial erections and to ask the client's partner to estimate the degree of erections that is typically obtained. Men with erectile disorder also tend to focus on performance aspects rather than on erotic cues during sexual activity and approach sex with negative expectations; both of these cognitive biases have been shown to reduce erectile response (Bach, Brown, & Barlow, 1999; Cranston-Cuebas & Barlow, 1990). Asking clients about the type of thoughts or "what they say to themselves" during sexual activity allows the clinician to determine the degree to which concerns about performance and about pleasing the partner, along with failure statements (negative expectancies), interfere with arousal levels.

Determining whether the client has difficulty in getting erections, or in maintaining them, or both, is also important. If the client reports that he is not able to maintain the erection, it is important to determine at what point the erection declines. Surprisingly, many men interpret their loss of an erection after ejaculation, especially if their ejaculatory latency is short, as erectile problems. The differential diagnosis between erectile problems and premature ejaculation is important for other reasons as well. A number of men suffer from both premature ejaculation and erectile problems. In these cases, often the premature ejaculation is lifelong, and the erectile problems develop as a result of attempts by the client to delay ejaculation through distraction (e.g., thinking of baseball scores). The shift away from erotic cues, the increased levels of negative affect, and a focus on performance (delay of ejaculation) often overshoots the client's goal of reducing arousal to delay ejaculation to the point where it is difficult to maintain the erection. When this pattern is repeated over time, the increased anxiety over maintaining erections and the accompanying sympathetic activation may lead to ejaculating more quickly. In these cases, the two sexual problems reinforce and maintain one another.

Assessing whether erectile problems are situational (partner activity only) or global (all situations, including morning erections) gives the clinician a very rough estimate about the likelihood that significant physiological factors are contributing to the erectile problems. In some studies, the complete absence of morning or nighttime erections has been shown to be the single best indicator of significant organic factors that contribute to the problem (Segraves, Segraves, & Schoenberg, 1987).

A number of medical examinations and assessment techniques have been developed for determining the extent and type of organic pathology that may contribute to erectile problems; these are reviewed next.

Nocturnal penile tumescence (NPT) evaluation and penile plethysmography are procedures utilized as screens to determine the presence of organic factors. During the rapid eye movement (REM) sleep phase, men usually experience four or five sleep-related erections that last about 30 minutes each. These erections can be measured in the context of a sleep laboratory or by using an ambulatory monitor, such as the Rigiscan (Bradley, Timm, Gallagher, & Johnson, 1985). Typically, the patient is asked to spend several consecutive nights in a sleep laboratory and the frequency, duration, and rigidity of erections, as well as electroencephalography (EEG) measures, are recorded. NPT assessment in the context of a sleep laboratory is considered the gold standard, but it is also extremely expensive. Gordon and Carey (1995) evaluated the efficacy of assessing sleep-related erections during a morning nap after slight sleep deprivation. The sleep deprivation increased the likelihood that REM sleep would occur during the nap. This outpatient procedure showed potential for offering a cost-effective alternative to overnight evaluations. A further alternative is using a portable monitor during several consecutive nights at home. The Rigiscan, the first commercially available ambulatory NPT monitor, consists of a small computer and two flexible rings that are attached by cords to the tip and base of the penis. Frequency, duration, circumference change, and radial rigidity of sleep-related erections are recorded. The Rigiscan has been criticized on the basis that it assesses radial rigidity, rather than axial rigidity, and that it lacks the additional measurements taken in the sleep laboratory.

In theory, if men are able to obtain erections during sleep, but not during partner stimulation, this is taken as evidence that their erectile function is primarily due to psychological and interpersonal factors. However, sleep-related erections have been shown to be affected by age, sleep apnea, depression, and low hormone levels. In addition, Ghezzi, Malvestiti, Baldini, Zaffaroni, & Zibetti (1995) found normal NPT recordings in 10 out of 14 men with multiple sclerosis. While shortcomings exist in NPT evaluations, it is nonetheless an important source of information in an overall comprehensive evaluation.

The assessment of the penile blood vessels and blood flow uses one or more of the following procedures: penile brachial blood pressure index, duplex ultrasonography (Doppler blood flow analysis), arteriography, cavernosometry, or cavernosography.

The penile–brachial index represents the penile systolic blood pressure divided by the brachial systolic blood pressure. Using a pediatric blood pressure cuff applied to the base of the flaccid penis, the penile blood pressure of each of the dorsal arteries is measured by using a continuous-wave Doppler probe; the reading is compared to brachial systolic pressure reading. The ratio should be around 1 for each of the dorsal arteries, and a ratio of below .7 (i.e., the penile pressure is lower than the brachial pressure) has been used to indicate arteriogenic erectile dysfunction. However, this test has been shown to be unreliable and should not be used as the sole measure.

One of the most versatile vascular diagnostic tests is color duplex ultrasonography (Doppler wave-form analysis). Duplex ultrasonography combined with a vasoactive intravenous injection (15 to 30 milligrams of papaverine or 10 micrograms of alprostadil) provides a quantifiable functional measure of penile arterial blood flow and a high-resolution image of the penile vascular anatomy. The ultrasound probe is able to image the individual cavernous arteries selectively and perform a Doppler blood flow analysis simultaneously. The procedure is performed before and after the injection. The procedure has also been used to assess venous leakage; however, this use is less well established than the assessment of arterial pathology and needs further validation.

In patients where arterial or venous pathology is suspected and vascular surgery is planned, either penile arteriography or cavernosography is used to verify the diagnosis and to identify the site of the vascular blockage or lesion. Both arteriography and cavernosography involve imaging subsequent to infusion of a radio-contrast solution into the pudendal artery and the corpora cavernosa, respectively. These procedures are considered by many the gold standard for assessing vascular penile pathology.

The technological sophistication of many of the medical assessment techniques is undoubtedly impressive, but as Bancroft (1992) points out, "as a diagnostic approach, [their] use has, with few exceptions, been seriously and significantly flawed. These tests are based on the assumption that the erectile machinery and its associated vasculature can be tested and evaluated in isolation from the man and his psychological nature" (p. ix). The temptation to consider the etiological problem solved once *any* organic pathology has been identified is strong (Tiefer & Melman, 1989). This tendency has been reinforced by numerous research studies that attempt to classify patients into nonoverlapping groups of organic and psychogenic erectile dysfunction. Remembering that the physical factors represent one of multiple determinants is crucial in the assessment and treatment of erectile problems (and sexual dysfunction in general).

Female Sexual Arousal Disorder

Female sexual arousal disorder (FSAD) is one of the least studied sexual disorders. A number of reasons may account for lack of clinical research. First, the comorbidity between desire, arousal, and orgasmic disorders makes it difficult, in many cases, to assign arousal difficulties as the primary diagnosis. Lack of sexual desire tends to increase distress in the woman's partner, while orgasm difficulties tend to be distressing to the female client. Thus, when women present with multiple sexual difficulties, the more distressing aspects of their presentation are likely to be given a primary diagnosis. Furthermore, lack of physiological arousal (vaginal lubrication and swelling) is easily self-treated by using commercially available lubricants, and this is another reason that arousal problems may not lead to high levels of distress. Careful assessment of both physiological markers and subjective experiences of sexual arousal is necessary.

The lack of research and low prevalence may be the result of the particular diagnostic criteria used. R. T. Segraves and K. B. Segraves (1991) found that only 8% of 532 women were diagnosed as having FSAD and only 2% received a diagnosis of FSAD without also receiving a secondary diagnosis of low sexual desire or orgasm difficulties. In contrast, when the prevalence of female sexual difficulties is studied in nonclinical samples, the most common sexual complaints are of anxiety and inhibition during sexual activity (38.1%), lack of sexual pleasure (16.3%), and lack of lubrication (13.6%) (Rosen, Taylor, Leiblum, & Bachmann, 1993). The manner in which researchers and clinicians interpret and assimilate these complaints into the current DSM-IV nosology affects their reported prevalence. Nevertheless, inquiries regarding such complaints should be made.

Reductions in estrogen production may result in decreased lubrication in menopausal and postmenopausal women. After menopause, it may also take women longer to become sufficiently lubricated, which may result in pain during intercourse. Additionally, a woman may misinterpret menopausal changes to mean that she is no longer feminine or is less attracted to her partner (Hillman, 2000). Therefore, it is important to differentiate between normal age-related changes that occur as a result of menopause and those that result from FSAD. In addition to reductions and delays in lubrication, other menopause-related changes include reductions in nipple erections, increased skin sensitivity, and loss of vaginal elasticity. In some women the increased skin sensitivity may make breast and clitoral stimulation irritating rather than arousing (Galindo & Kaiser, 1995). However, unlike physical reductions in lubrication, women do not lose their ability to experience subjective sexual arousal or have multiple orgasms. Negative attitudes toward menopause and lack of knowledge about changes (not declines) in sexual functioning may adversely affect an elderly woman's enjoyment of sexuality. During an assessment, it is vital to assess a client's understanding of the normal age-related changes, as well as her expectations for sexual functioning.

Premature Ejaculation

Premature ejaculation (PE) is one of the most common sexual difficulties experienced by men. The reported prevalence rates vary from 1% to 75%. Based on a representative U.S. sample, Laumann et al. (1999) reported that about 30% of men experienced difficulties with early ejaculation. Few questionnaires or inventories exist specifically for the evaluation of premature ejaculation, and there are none that have been adequately validated. The wide range in reported prevalence rates and lack of validated assessment instruments is in part due to the lack of agreement on an operational definition of premature ejaculation.

Some theorists have used the length of time from intromission to ejaculation (ejaculatory latency) as the criteria. For example, Kinsey, Pomeroy, and Martin (1948) found that 75% of the men in the sample ejaculated in less than 2 minutes. Spiess, Geer, and O'Donohue (1984) and Strassberg, Mahoney, Schaugaard, and Hale (1990) also defined ejaculation under 2 minutes as constituting premature ejaculation. However, other theorists have argued for different times. Cooper and Magnus (1984) and Waldinger, Hengeveld, Zwinderman, and Olivier (1998) have defined premature ejaculation as ejaculation that occurs in less than 1 minute. The later study found that 90% of the 140 men with lifelong premature ejaculation who comprised their sample ejaculated in less than 1 minute. Several studies examined the average time to ejaculation in men without any sexual difficulties and found that the average latency fell between 4 to 10 minutes (Gebhard, 1966; Hunt, 1974). Kameya, Deguchi, and Yokota (1997) conducted a well-controlled study in which a trained masseuse manually stimulated blindfolded participants to orgasm on four occasions, each a week apart. The results indicated a mean ejaculatory latency of 156.5 ± 80.7 seconds (about 2.6 minutes). The shorter latencies found in this study were partly due to the age of the sample (29 healthy volunteers ages 18 to 25). As can be seen, using a criterion time to define premature ejaculation is problematic because ejaculatory latency naturally increases as a function of age (Masters & Johnson, 1970, p. 318).

Several alternative criteria have been suggested. Masters and Johnson (1970) defined premature ejaculation as a man's inability to inhibit ejaculation long enough for his partner to reach orgasm 50% of the time. However, by some estimates 70% of women do not reach orgasm during coitus (Hite, 1976), making this definition problematic. Alternatively, the number of intravaginal thrusts has also been suggested as a way of operationalizing premature ejaculation (Colpi, Fanciullacci, Beretta, Negri, & Zanolla, 1986). Kaplan (1989) emphasized the notion of "voluntary control" over ejaculation. This notion is reflected in the DSM-IV criterion A, "[ejaculating] before the person wishes it." However, since ejaculation is the result of a critical level of afferent input that reaches the spinal cord and causes a reflex mediated response (Newman, Reiss, & Northrup, 1982), voluntary control over ejaculation may not be entirely realistic. The notion of "lack of ejaculatory control" has been emphasized in the clinical sex therapy literature. McCarthy (1989) and Zilbergeld (1992, 1999) note that early masturbatory and sexual experiences under rushed, high-anxiety conditions may lead an individual to develop a conditioned quick ejaculatory response. They propose that men with premature ejaculation lack awareness of their arousal level and fail to make adjustments in their speed and intensity of thrusting in order to prolong their ejaculatory latency (see also Kaplan, 1974).

The differences in criteria highlight the different areas that are important to consider in the assessment of premature ejaculation (see Metz, Pryor, Nesvacil, Abuzzahab, & Koznar, 1997 for a review). No single measure (for example, ejaculatory latency or partner satisfaction) is adequate for assessing premature ejaculation. Extreme cases, where the man consistently ejaculates before intromission or as a result of visual stimulation alone, are easily diagnosed. But in the majority of cases, the man's ejaculatory latency is between 1 and 4 minutes, which makes it necessary to consider additional factors. Age, novelty of the situation, time since the last ejaculation, type of behavior (e.g., masturbation, oral or manual stimulation, or intercourse), and medications all influence ejaculation. In addition, it is important to assess the patient's and partner's expectations, because some men with premature ejaculation hold unrealistic expectations (Wincze & Carey, 2001). Last, the amount of distress experienced by the individual and his partner must be taken into account. McCarthy (1989) describes a common pattern of sexual activity during which the couple engages in highly arousing multiple-stimulation activities so that the woman (or partner) is orgasmic, and this is followed by quick, intense intercourse and ejaculation after only a minute of short, rapid stroking (p. 144). He points out that if both partners are satisfied with this pattern, labeling this as premature ejaculation could create an iatrogenic dysfunction. Therefore, it is vital to develop an understanding of the ejaculatory pattern in the couple's sexual relationship, including carefully assessing each partner's pattern of arousal and orgasm, their sexual style, expectations regarding ejaculation and sexual satisfaction, the pattern of intercourse thrusting, the man's sense of awareness and voluntary control over ejaculation, and the time between the beginning of stimulation and ejaculation (McCarthy, 1989, pp. 144–145).

Male Orgasmic Disorder

Male orgasmic disorder, formally inhibited male orgasmic disorder, tends to be fairly rare in community samples (7–9%, Laumann et al., 1999). Many men with male orgasmic disorder do not present for help because they are able to perform sexually, and they often provide enough stimulation for their partner to reach multiple orgasms. Men with inhibited orgasmic disorder have been termed the "workhorse" of sexual relationships. Frequently, the problem starts to interfere and comes to the attention of clinicians when a couple tries to conceive.

Diagnostically it is important to determine whether the problem occurs only with partner sexual activity or whether it is more generalized and present during masturbation. Generalized orgasm and ejaculation problems are frequently the result of prostate surgery or medication side effects. For example, transurethral resection of the prostate (TURP) or equivalent procedures (e.g., radiofrequency transurethral needle ablation of the prostate [TUNA] or transurethral electrovaporization of the prostate [TUVP]) have been associated with ejaculatory problems, mainly retrograde ejaculation, in over 80% of patients (Hammadeh, Madaan, Singh, & Philp, 1998; Perera & Hill, 1998). Montejo-Gonzalez and colleagues (1997) evaluated the incidence of sexual dysfunction resulting from different selective serotonin reuptake inhibitors (SSRIs) and found that over half of the men experienced either delays or absence of ejaculation as a side effect; this effect was particularly pronounced with paroxetine. In these instances, a diagnosis of sexual dysfunction due to a general medical condition or a substance-induced sexual dysfunction would be assigned, not male orgasmic disorder. A diagnosis of male orgasmic disorder is also not assigned if the sexual difficulty includes a pattern of ejaculation without pleasurable orgasm or orgasm without ejaculation, in which case a diagnosis of sexual dysfunction not otherwise specified would be more appropriate.

Apfelbaum (1989) described men who experience ejaculatory difficulties primarily during partner-related sexual activity as frequently preferring autoerotic stimulation to partner stimulation. Apfelbaum (1989) points out that simply having an erection does not mean that the man experiences sexual desire or subjective sexual excitement, and this notion has received empirical support (Delizonna, Wincze, Litz, Brown, & Barlow, 2001). He suggests that male orgasmic disorder should be conceptualized similarly to coital female orgasmic disorder. The discordance between reports of physical and subjective sexual arousal in women is a well-established phenomenon (Laan & Everaerd, 1995). Conceptualizing male orgasmic disorder in this manner, rather than as the man withholding pleasure from his partner, is consistent with models of sexual dysfunction (Barlow, 1986). In male orgasmic disorder, performance-related cognitions shift the attentional focus away from erotic cues, which result in reductions of subjective arousal rather than of physiological arousal, as in male erectile disorder. Thus, contributing factors toward coital male orgasmic disorder would include arousal-interfering situations, performance-related cognitions, and negative affective states (e.g., lack of intimacy).

Female Orgasmic Disorder

Articles like "Sex, What Every Woman Should Know" and "20 Earth-Quaking Moves That Will Make Him Plead for Mercy and Beg for More" appear on the covers of popular magazines such as *Vogue* and *Cosmopolitan*. The message is clear: "In order to have good sex, a woman must be able to perform in bed." Part of that performance for women is having an orgasm (or multiple orgasms) easily and every time. Heiman and Grafton-Becker (1989) point out that female sexual satisfaction has only recently (in the 20th century) become a concern, and the fact that female orgasm problems are recognized and treated is, in part, a cultural accident. There is little doubt that the cultural attitudinal shift away from controlling female sexuality to expectations of satisfaction and orgasm is beneficial to women (and less sexist); however, with it the sexual performance pressures experienced by women have also increased. In contrast to the "sexual fantasy descriptions" found in movies, romance novels, and magazines, the reality is that many women do not experience orgasms from penile–vaginal intercourse. Hite (1976) reported that only 30% to 50% of women experienced orgasm during face-to-face, penile–vaginal intercourse. Summarizing several studies, Haavio-Mannila and Kontula (1997) reported that women experience orgasm only 40% to 80% of the time, regardless of stimulation method. Data originally collected by Kinsey showed that only 14% of women were able to experience multiple orgasms on some occasions (Kinsey, Pomeroy, Martin, & Gebhard, 1953). Therefore, the absence of orgasms during intercourse does not represent a female sexual dysfunction (Andersen & Cyranowski, 1995; Wincze & Carey, 2001).

According to DSM-IV, female orgasmic disorder is defined as the "delay in, or absence of, orgasm following a normal excitement phase. . . ." This criterion is particularly problematic since many women who have difficulties with orgasm report lower levels of sexual arousal. Andersen (1981) found that among women with lifelong female orgasmic disorder, 70% scored below the 50th percentile on the Sexual Arousability Inventory (according to the normative data published by Hoon et al., 1976) and 47% scored below the 25th percentile. The overlap between desire, arousal, and orgasm difficulties in women complicates differential diagnoses.

A wide variety of psychological variables have been hypothesized to contribute to female orgasm dysfunction, including sexual ignorance, sexual skill of the partner, negative attitudes toward sexual activity and masturbation, sex guilt, lack of assertiveness, relationship distress, greater endorsement of sexual myths, negative sexual experiences, religiosity, and global personality structure. Morokoff (1978) reviewed a variety of these and found that no single factor seemed strongly related to orgasmic response and dysfunction in women. However, some differences between women with and without female orgasmic disorder have been found. Women with orgasm difficulties tend to score higher on measures of sex guilt (Derflinger, 1998; Kelly, Strassberg, & Kircher, 1990; Morokoff, 1985), tend to be less sexually assertive (Delehanty, 1982; Newcomb, 1984), and endorse more negative attitudes toward sexual activity and masturbation or endorse more sexual myths (Kelly et al., 1990). Based on statistical analyses, Derogatis, Fagan, Schmidt, Wise, & Gildem (1986) identified two subgroups of anorgasmic women. One subgroup included women who endorsed feelings of inferiority, negative body image, and more psychological symptoms; the other subgroup endorsed more liberal sexual attitudes, higher level of desire, and more extensive sexual fantasies. The authors speculated that orgasm difficulties in the second subgroup were related to interpersonal problems or physiological factors. In a similar study, Derogatis, Schmidt, Fagan, and Wise (1989) identified four subgroups of anorgasmic women: low desire, histrionic/marital conflict, psychiatric disorder, and constitutional. The constitutional subgroup was similar to the second subtype in the 1986 study. Newcomb (1984) examined several attitudinal and behavioral factors in the context of a path analysis. He found that although parental attitudes contributed to orgasm functioning, this relationship was moderated by social and dating assertiveness and actual sexual behavior. Furthermore, women with orgasmic disorder and nondysfunctional women who reach orgasm inconsistently were found to be less aware of the physiological signs of arousal and orgasm (Andersen & Cyranowski, 1995; Hoon & Hoon, 1978). Heiman and Grafton-Becker (1989) discuss that women who have difficulties in reaching orgasm may fear loss of control during orgasm.

In the past, the length of foreplay and orgasm was thought to be significantly related to female orgasmic disorder. However, research has consistently failed to support this notion (Fisher, 1973; Gebhard, 1966; Huey, Kline-Graber, & Graber, 1981; Kinsey et al., 1953). Kelly et al. (1990) reported no differences between women who were anorgasmic in partner sexual situations and those without difficulties on their approval, use, and comfort with sexual activities that involved direct clitoral stimulation (e.g., cunnilingus or manual stimulation). However, women who could not reach orgasm with their partners reported significantly less comfort in communicating about sexual activity, but only about those activities that involved direct clitoral stimulation (i.e., there were no group differences in comfort communicating about intercourse).

Although many studies that examine correlates of orgasm problems do not distinguish between lifelong and acquired or between global and situational, some differences between these subtypes have been found. Women with acquired and situational female orgasmic disorder tend to be more distressed about and less satisfied with their overall relationship (McGovern, Stewart, & LoPiccolo, 1975). Acquired orgasmic dysfunction may also be the result of medication side effects, especially from antidepressants. The distinction between lifelong and acquired difficulties is particularly important for treatment planning. Women with lifelong and global orgasmic dysfunction respond well to treatment with masturbation training (Heiman & Meston, 1997), whereas women with acquired orgasm difficulties tend to do better in treatments that address couples issues (such as communication training).

Dyspareunia

Dyspareunia, more so than most female sexual dysfunctions, requires a multidisciplinary assessment. Dyspareunia may be the result of a variety of factors, both physical or medical and psychosocial. Common physical contributing factors include vulvar vestibulitis, atrophy of the vaginal canal, cervical cancer, local infections (e.g., *Neisseria gonorrhoeae, Candida albicans,* or *Trichomonas vaginalis*), hymenal tags, endometriosis, pelvic tumors, prolapsed uterus, or an allergic or irritative reaction to self-administered feminine-hygiene products. Pelvic inflammatory disease (PID) has also been associated with dyspareunia; however, PID is more likely to provoke unremitting pain rather than pain limited to intercourse (Lechtenberg & Ohl, 1994). Commonly suggested psychosocial factors include negative attitudes toward sexuality, anxiety, depression, relationship maladjustment, and a history of child sexual abuse or sexual trauma (Lazarus, 1989). Clear empirical evidence for these psychosocial factors is still largely lacking.

A thorough medical or gynecological examination is essential during the assessment of dyspareunia in order to rule medical causes in or out. Routinely, the gynecological exam should include visual examination of the vulvar region; palpitation of the vulvar, vaginal, and pelvic regions; and a cotton swab test. The cotton swab test involves applying pressure on a number of sites that surround the vaginal opening in an attempt to localize vaginal entry level pain. In addition to a pap smear, smears for the following cultures should be obtained: general cervical culture, gonorrhea, chlamydia, and ureaplasma or mycoplasma. When the visual exam indicates the possibility of vaginal atrophy, estrogen levels should also be assessed. In cases where there exists the possibility that the pain is related to abnormal pelvic structures, ultrasound can be used to visually inspect the ovaries, uterus, and bladder. As with other sexual dysfunctions, the presence of physical (or psychological) factors does not exclude the presence of the other type of factor. In a study of 112 women who presented with dyspareunia, Meana, Binik, Khalife, and Cohen (1997b) identified four subgroups: vulvar vestibulitis (46%), vulvar/vaginal atrophy (13%), no relevant physical findings (24%), and a mixed subgroup (17%) (a residual category). The most common subtype was the vulvar vestibulitis group, who have a condition that is characterized by sharp burning pain located in and limited to the vulvar vestibule (vaginal opening) that is elicited via pressure applied to this area. A common physical finding in this group is the presence of vulva erythema (redness) of various degrees. Vulvar vestibulitis affects mostly younger women and has no clear etiological determinants, although it has been associated with frequent yeast infections and other urogenital inflammatory conditions (Bergeron et al., 1997). Women in the vulvar/vaginal atrophy group were found to have visually detectible impoverished skin elasticity, turgor, and labial fullness, as well as visible thinning of the vaginal mucosa, all of which are commonly associated with estrogen deficiency.

The DSM-IV criteria and specifiers for dyspareunia provide little information relevant to treatment planning, which, to some extent, is determined by the etiological and contributing factors. Meana et al. (1997b) propose to make use of the rich chronic pain literature to provide better assessment and classification. They point out that dyspareunia is the only pain disorder that is described by the behavior that elicits the pain, rather than the pain itself, which is the defining feature. Chronic pain is traditionally described using four taxa: region, system (in this case urogenital), pattern of occurrence (in this case recurrent), and onset of pain (Meana et al., 1997b). Meana and Binik (1994) developed a classification system that combines the DSM-IV specifiers and that of pain assessment, resulting in the following specifiers: lifelong/acquired, generalized/situational, location of the pain (vaginal vestibule, vaginal canal, and pelvic region), onset of the pain during an episode of intercourse (sexual activity), average duration of pain, and interference of pain with intercourse (sexual activity). Meana et al. (1997b) found that location of pain and onset during an episode of sexual activity best discriminated between the subtypes of dyspareunia (vestibulitis, vaginal atrophy, and no physical findings; the mixed subgroup was excluded from the analysis). Some 92% of the vulvar vestibulitis group and the vaginal atrophy group reported that the pain began at entry (moment of vaginal penetration or contact). The majority of the women in the vulvar vestibulitis subgroup reported that the pain was limited to the vaginal opening (48%) or occurred in the vestibule and within the vaginal canal (32%). In contrast, 86% of the vaginal atrophy subgroup reported that the pain occurred only in the vaginal canal. In contrast, the group of women with dyspareunia but no physical findings reported mixture of pain onset and locations. Meana, Binik, Khalife, and Cohen (1997a) compared 105 women with dyspareunia to matched controls. The results showed that the clinical sample held more negative attitudes toward sexuality and had lower levels of relationship adjustment. More interestingly, when the data were examined by dyspareunia subtype (vulvar vestibulitis and no physical findings), the group without physical findings evidenced more psychological symptoms and worse relationship adjustment, but not significantly lower sexual functioning impairment than the control group. In contrast, the vulvar vestibulitis subgroup demonstrated higher impairment only in sexual functioning than the control group.

Vaginismus

The term "vaginismus" was first coined by Sims in 1861, and descriptions of vaginismus can be found in the literature as early as 1547. However, surprisingly little empirical work has focused on this sexual dysfunction (Reissing, Binik, & Khalife, 1999). The DSM-IV names the "recurrent or persistent involuntary spasm of the musculature of the outer third of the vagina" as the defining characteristic. According to DSM-IV, these spasms are readily observable and in some cases sufficiently severe to cause pain, although pain is not necessary in order to meet the diagnostic criteria. Most often the vaginal spasms are confirmed by a gynecologist during a pelvic floor exam. At times, the diagnosis is made based on the client's inability to tolerate the exam, which could be due to a number of factors, including pain resulting from dyspareunia. Surprisingly, to date only one study has directly assessed vaginal muscle activity; van der Velde and Everaerd (1999) found no differences between 67 women with vaginismus and 43 control participants on their ability to voluntarily control pelvic floor muscles measured via surface electromyography. In a small study, van der Velde, Laan, and Everaerd (in press) presented neutral, erotic, threatening, and sexually threatening film clips to 22 women with vaginismus, while monitoring pelvic floor musculature via vaginal surface electromyography. The results indicated that women who experienced past negative sexual experiences evidenced an increase in involuntary pelvic floor musculature during the sexually threatening film clip. On reviewing this study, Reissing, Flory, and Binik (2000) point out that these results unfortunately did not include a comparison to women with dyspareunia or to control participants.

CASE CONCEPTUALIZATION, TREATMENT PLANNING, THERAPY, AND MEASURING OUTCOME

Once all the necessary assessment information has been collected, one challenge in completing a thorough assessment of sexual dysfunction is integrating information relating to different aspects of sexual functioning from a variety of sources. Tiefer and Melman (1989) point out that sexual arousal is, truly, at least a "Sensorymotorneurohormonalvascularpsychosociocultural interpersonal event!" (p. 210). A case conceptualization should relate the aspects of the client's complaint to one another and explain why the individual developed the sexual dysfunction and how it is maintained (Wincze & Carey, 2001). The treatment plan should build on the case conceptualization by including interventions that address the contributing and maintaining factors that were identified through the assessment.

Case Conceptualization

One of the functions of an assessment is to allow the clinician to form an initial hypothesis and begin to gather information in support of this hypothesis. During the assessment, several potential contributing factors typically emerge. Information gathered from follow-up questions, medical tests, and questionnaires is used to further support the role of these factors (or alternatively rule them out) and to determine their relative severity.

One of the first steps is determining which difficulty causes the most interference and distress. Once the principal diagnosis has been established, all of the potential contributing factors, including other comorbid disorders, are considered. There are several possible ways of organizing the information regarding etiology (contributing factors) for the purpose of constructing the case formulation. One possibility is to view the different components of sexual functioning (physiological, emotional, interpersonal, and psychological) as representing relative strengths and weaknesses that influence each other and affect, either positively or negatively, on the quality of sexual functioning and the sexual relationship. The metaphor of a scale can illustrate how different negative and positive factors tip the scale toward dysfunctional or successful sexual functioning (see Wincze & Barlow, 1996). The different facets of sexual functioning are considered separately and in relation to one another. The advantages of this model are that it considers the multidetermined nature of sexual dysfunctions and incorporates the strengths that the client and the partner bring to the sexual relationship. A sexual problem can result from the aggregation of several mild negative factors (e.g., age-related changes, smoking, negative attitudes toward sex), which considered separately might not be sufficient to cause the problem. Additionally, the fewer positive factors that are present, the greater the likelihood that negative factors will suffice to tip the scale toward problematic sexual functioning (i.e., the presence of positive factors counters the effects of negative factors). Thus, the onset of the sexual dysfunction may result from the loss of a previously present positive factor rather than the occurrence of new negative factors. This model is also a very useful tool for giving feedback to clients and helping them understand the complexities of their sexual dysfunction. Often, clients hold a bias toward conceptualizing their sexual problems as caused by medical conditions or organic pathology. This bias may result from their hope for a quick medical solution (possibly a magic pill) or because an organic etiology is seen as less stigmatizing. Helping clients view their sexuality and sexual difficulties as determined by a composition of factors, including but not limited to medical and physical factors, facilitates their understanding that a medical intervention will most likely not be a fix-all but addresses only one of the contributing factors. Thus, such a case conceptualization provides a rationale for an integrated treatment approach.

A different format for organizing the information is to view the different contributing factors as representing predisposing influences, precipitating events, and maintaining factors (Wincze & Carey, 2001). For example, early negative sexual messages, a history of smoking, rigid narrow views toward sexuality, and poor dyadic communication increase an individual's vulnerability for developing a sexual dysfunction. Common precipitating causes include stress at work, increased marital discord, the birth of a child, depression, local infections, or simply the occasional performance failure. Most men experience occasions during which they are not able to achieve or maintain an erection or occasions when they ejaculate more quickly. In the same manner, women will have experiences when they are unable to reach orgasm or times when they have difficulties becoming aroused. The client's and the partner's reaction to these normal fluctuations may determine whether or not they develop a sexual problem. Worrisome thoughts about sexual performance, poor sexual communication, depression, anger, and resentment may all function as factors that maintain the sexual problems, even when the precipitating cause is no longer present. Some factors may function as both risk factors and maintaining factors. For example, marital discord and poor communication may predispose a couple to have less-satisfying sexual interactions and subsequently leave them with few coping skills to resolve the difficulties. A performance- or goal-driven approach to sexual behavior, or what Masters and Johnson (1970) identified as "performance anxiety," is another example of a factor that may influence both the development and maintenance of a sexual dysfunction. Viewing sexual activity in terms of performance, rather then in terms of pleasure, can result in the individual overvaluing the importance of obtaining lubrication or reaching orgasm (having an erection or delaying orgasm). Once the person experiences a "performance failure," the focus on performance is intensified, thus creating a vicious circle.

The above manner of organizing the assessment information has the advantage that it considers the functional role of different etiological factors. Furthermore, it accounts for the possibility that the primary contributing factors may change over time and that the effects of sexual dysfunctions (e.g., depression, increased performance worry, increased relationship discord) also function to maintain the sexual problems further.

The two above-described methods for organizing the assessment information and case conceptualization can be used in combination to provide a comprehensive picture that includes both strengths and weaknesses, as well as different types of factors (predisposing, precipitating, and maintaining factors). These strategies for organizing the assessment information have the additional advantage that they accommodate a wide variety of theoretical orientations.

Grounding case formulations and treatment recommendations in an empirically supported theoretical model is also very useful for organizing the data collected during the assessment. For example, during the 1980s our laboratory developed a model to describe how the cognitive, emotional, and behavioral factors interact to maintain sexual dysfunctions (Barlow, 1986; Cranston-Cuebas & Barlow, 1990). Over the last decade and a half, this model has received empirical validation. According to the model, cognitive factors such as performance worries, negative expectancies, and perceived lack of control shift the individual's attentional focus away from the erotic cues in the sexual environment. With increased autonomic arousal (either from increased sexual arousal or due to anxiety), the attentional focus narrows, increasing the salience of the nonerotic, performance-related cognitions and further blocking out the erotic cues, thus leading to decreased sexual arousal and dysfunctional performance (i.e., loss of erection or not reaching orgasm). Negative affect related to dysfunctional performance becomes paired with the sexual situation, which further reduces sexual arousal in future sexual interactions. This pattern then functions as a negative feedback loop that eventually leads to the avoidance of sexual situations (see Figure 14.1).

Treatment Goals and Treatment Planning

Frequently, clients' treatment goals include improving their sexual performance, such as being able to delay ejaculation for hours. Adopting performance enhancement as the official goal of treatment may have the unintended effect of reinforcing and strengthening clients' focus on sexual performance rather than on sexual pleasure, thus increasing their performance worries and sexual difficulties. Treatment goals should be constructed in terms of increasing the client's ability to enjoy and derive pleasure from sexual activity or in terms of

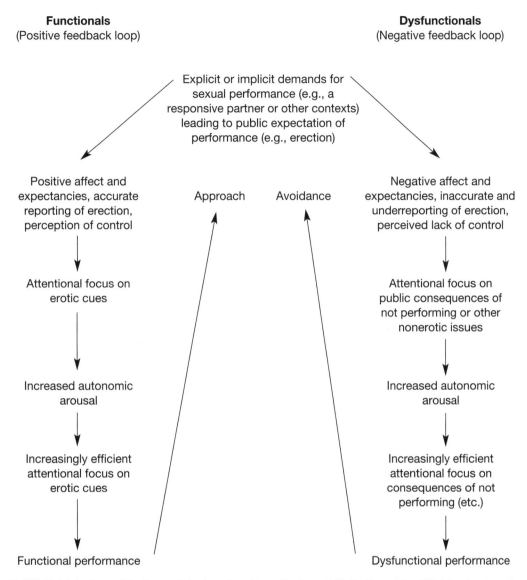

Functionals
(Positive feedback loop)

Dysfunctionals
(Negative feedback loop)

Explicit or implicit demands for sexual performance (e.g., a responsive partner or other contexts) leading to public expectation of performance (e.g., erection)

Positive affect and expectancies, accurate reporting of erection, perception of control

Approach   Avoidance

Negative affect and expectancies, inaccurate and underreporting of erection, perceived lack of control

Attentional focus on erotic cues

Attentional focus on public consequences of not performing or other nonerotic issues

Increased autonomic arousal

Increased autonomic arousal

Increasingly efficient attentional focus on erotic cues

Increasingly efficient attentional focus on consequences of not performing (etc.)

Functional performance

Dysfunctional performance

FIGURE 14.1. A model of sexual dysfunction. From Barlow (1986). Copyright 1986 by the American Psychological Association. Reprinted by permission.

improving the quality of the sexual relationship. For example, rather than setting the attainment of rigid erections (or orgasms) as the goal of treatment, a more appropriate goal would include developing a "pleasure-focused approach" to sexual activity or increasing the client's sexual satisfaction.

The treatment plan functions as a blueprint for the structure and content of treatment. It also serves as a contract between the clinician and the patient by including specific agreed-upon treatment goals and proposing a means of achieving these goals.

The treatment plan follows logically from the case conceptualization by including treatment interventions that are aimed at addressing the contributing and maintaining factors that were identified by the assessment. Determining which specific intervention will be effective for addressing a particular contributing factor is based on the empirical literature and the client's preferences. When possible, treatment interventions with established efficacy are preferred over unvalidated approaches (for reviews of treatment efficacy, see Heiman & Meston, 1997; Segraves & Althof, 1998). Unfortunately, the lack of well-controlled outcome studies for sex therapy does not always permit this.

Treatments for Sexual Dysfunction

Historically, the psychosocial treatment of sexual dysfunctions can be divided into five different epochs: psychoanalytic, early behavioral, Masters and Johnson, neo-Masters and Johnson, and psychobiological (Segraves & Althof, 1998). In 1970, with the publication of Master and Johnson's *Human Sexual Inadequacy,* a new era of sex therapy began. Sex therapy theory and practice embraced the technology of behavior therapy and its directive, symptom-focused treatment exercises. In the beginning, many theorists were skeptical and considered this approach overly simplistic; however, few could argue with the success of Master and Johnson's outcome research (despite methodological criticisms). Twenty years later, Leiblum and Rosen (1989) noted the growing breadth of eclecticism in the field and that few writers would advocate sole reliance on technique-based approaches to the treatment of specific sexual dysfunctions.

Since the 1980s, sexual dysfunction treatment approaches, in particular for erectile problems, have become increasingly more medicalized (Rosen, 1996; Tiefer, 1994). A person who suffers from male erectile disorder can choose among a variety of medical treatments, for example: oral medications (sildenafil citrate), vasoactive intracorporeal injections (papaverine, prostaglandin E1), urethral suppositories (MUSE), vacuum constriction devices, vascular surgery, and penile implants. The success of Viagra has spurred research efforts to develop similar medical treatment options for women. There is no doubt that countless men (and women) have benefited from the medical advances. The publicity of treatment options by the national media about a topic that many clients and some physicians are reluctant to discuss is also a benefit. However, the exclusive genital focus by medical treatments neglects the important emotional and interpersonal aspects of sexual functioning.

Much like in the 1970s, when years of insight-oriented therapy were replaced by couples behavioral homework exercises as the predominant sex therapy paradigm, medical interventions provide a quicker and easier alternative for symptom resolution. With further medical advances, the trend by physicians to prescribe medical treatments for predominantly psychogenic sexual dysfunction will mushroom. What remains are the psychological, emotional, and interpersonal issues that accompany all sexual difficulties, regardless of etiology. Sex therapists have long understood that our biggest sex organs are the brain and the heart, not the clitoris and the penis. The challenge to clinical researchers and practitioners at the beginning of the twenty-first century is the integration of medical advances into the larger theoretical framework of sex therapy.

The essence and overall goal of sex therapy is creating or restoring mutual sexual comfort, satisfaction, and pleasure, as well as reducing distress. More specific treatment components are employed in the service of helping clients develop a "pleasure-focused" approach to sexuality that will replace their "performance-" or "goal"-focused approach. Sensate focus, cognitive restructuring, stimulus control and scheduling, communication training, and education all help clients develop a pleasure-focused approach and represent the cornerstones of sex therapy (for a review of sex therapy interventions, see Leiblum & Rosen, 2000; or Wincze & Carey, 2001). The development of a pleasure-focused approach to sexual activity provides the theoretical framework for incorporating disorder-specific treatment components. As stated earlier, a client's specific treatment plan depends heavily on the contributing and maintaining factors that were identified in the assessment. Contemporary sex therapy integrates components from cognitive therapy, behavioral therapy, systems therapy, marital therapy, interpersonal therapy, and medical treatments. Interventions for particular contributing factors and sexual dysfunctions have been developed. For example, systematic desensitization and exposure exercises employing dilators with increasingly larger circumferences are used to reduce anxiety in the treatment of vaginismus and dyspareunia. Medical interventions, such as hormone therapy, oral medications (Viagra for erectile problems, antidepressants for premature ejaculation), or surgery (for dyspareunia or penile vascular insufficiency) typically address specific symptoms or contributing causes. Medical interventions, rather than being the sole treatment, can be integrated into the treatment plan much like any other treatment component.

Helping clients understand and accept the broader goal of developing a pleasure-focused approach to sexual activity, not just the restoration of functioning (although this may be a pleasant side effect), is the first step in any sex therapy program. Taking the time to explain and outline the rationale for this approach is critical for increasing client compliance and avoiding frustration.

Evaluating Treatment Outcome

The evaluation of treatment outcome starts during treatment planning by operationalizing treatment goals using *specific, measurable* criteria. Newman, Ciarlo, and Carpenter (1999) point out that unlike in treatment efficacy research studies, where treatment dosage levels are fixed (set number of sessions), in clinical practice the clinician works with the client or couple to achieve an agreed-upon level of functioning or reduction in symptoms. The authors emphasize the need for effectiveness studies that can answer the question "What type and how much treatment will achieve a given outcome criteria for X% of clients?" The evaluation of treatment outcomes relies on pre- to posttreatment assessment measure scores and subjective ratings by the client, partner, and clinician. Thus, at pretreatment those questionnaires that will be used at posttreatment need to be known.

An evaluation of treatment outcomes should aim to answer the following questions:

1. To what degree was the presenting problem alleviated?
2. Did treatment work?
3. Were the client and the partner satisfied with the treatment?
4. What was the overall impact of the treatment?

The first and second question may seem redundant, but they are quite separate. Client improvement and resolution of the sexual problem (question 1) is measured by comparing the pre- and posttreatment scores on either a global measure of sexual dysfunction (e.g., the GRISS) or when available, a diagnosis specific measure (e.g., SDI or IIEF). The second question pertains to whether the treatment interventions achieved their designed purpose. The overarching goal of sex therapy is reduction of distress and the restoration or establishment of a mutually satisfying sexual relationship. Therefore, a measure of client and partner sexual satisfaction represents an important component of the outcomes evaluation. In addition, measures evaluating each treatment component (sensate focus, education, communication training, etc.) are needed. For example, if the treatment plan included education and cognitive restructuring to reduce negative sexual attitudes, the degree of change in attitudes must be assessed before one can determine whether treatment worked. The specific questionnaires required to accomplish this end will largely depend on the theorized etiologic contributing factors and the treatment plan. This type of outcomes evaluation is especially important in the field of sex therapy. Due to the lack of large, well-controlled, randomized trials for sex therapy, little is known about which treatment components represent the active ingredients associated with improvement. For example, at one time it was believed that Kegel exercises lead to improvements in orgasmic functioning in the treatment of female orgasmic disorder. However, when Roughan and Kunst (1981) evaluated the effect of Kegel exercises separate from the total treatment package, no increase in orgasm frequency or correlations between change in the strength of the pubococcygeus muscle and frequency of orgasm were found. Thus, treatment outcome evaluations are not only important for working with managed care companies but also contribute to treatment effectiveness research that is critical for advances in the field of sex therapy.

The third and fourth questions pertain to client satisfaction with the treatment and improvements in quality of life. Recently, specific treatment satisfaction and quality of life measures have been developed for clinical trials in the treatment of erectile disorder. Although these questionnaires were developed for evaluating medical treatments, they are also applicable to sex therapy outcome evaluations. The EDITS (Erectile Dysfunction Inventory of Treatment Satisfaction; Althof et al., 1999) assesses the client's and his partner's satisfaction with the erectile dysfunction treatment. The 11-item client version contains items concerning overall satisfaction, treatment side effects, ease of use, and the naturalness and quality of erections. The 5-item partner version contains items relating to partner overall satisfaction and partner satisfaction with the quality of the erection. Both client and partner versions have been shown to have favorable psychometric properties and, more important, a high test–retest reliability.

Quality of life assessments are important because the presence of sexual dysfunctions can negatively affect a person's self esteem, can result in depression, and can increase relationship discord. Rosen (1998) reviewed the quality of life instruments designed specifically for the treatment of erectile disorder. Rosen emphasized the importance of continued development of sexual dysfunction specific quality of life measures since most general quality of life measures were designed for medically ill patients and focus on physical functioning. Wagner, Patrick, McKenna, and Proese (1996) developed a 19-item scale, QOL-MED (Quality of Life—Male Erectile Disorder). The scale contains items pertaining to masculinity issues, emotional response to experiencing erectile problems, and overall life satisfaction. The initial psychometric evaluations of the QOL-MED seem promising.

Assessment Feedback

One of the roles of the case conceptualization is to aid in providing the client coherent feedback about her or his difficulties and the available treatment options. Before giving the client feedback, it is important to set the stage by explaining that the information about contributing causes (case conceptualization) represents hypotheses formed by the assessor and that one of the purposes of providing feedback is to determine whether the case conceptualization is consistent with the client's experiences. Encouraging the client to comment on the assessment results provides the clinician with an opportunity to fine-tune the case conceptualization. Presenting the assessment results can be divided into three parts: reviewing the facts of the presenting problem, outlining the relevant contributing and maintaining factors, and discussing the available treatment options.

At times, the difficulty that is most interfering and in need of treatment may not be the sexual problem for which the client originally sought help. For example, in cases where there is a significant alcohol or substance use disorder, it is usually futile to attempt to work on the sexual problem until the dependence problem has been addressed. In these cases, being able to provide a clear and understandable rationale for why particular problems need to be addressed before working on the sexual problem directly is crucial to facilitating the client's acceptance of treatment recommendations that may be unexpected and often unwelcome.

A great deal of information, and misinformation, regarding medical interventions for sexual problems can be found on television talk shows, in magazine articles, and on the Internet. Many clients are influenced by these sources and will have questions about "the newest treatments." It is important to provide accurate information about medical interventions and how these fit into the particular client's treatment plan.

The assessment of sexual dysfunction, case conceptualization, treatment planning, and client feedback requires the clinician to consider many different aspects of sexual functioning (including physical, emotional, cognitive, and interpersonal aspects of sexuality) and to have a working knowledge of both psychosocial interventions and medical treatments. The following case example illustrates the practical application of the information and strategies presented in this chapter.

CASE EXAMPLE

Background

Demographic Information and Overview

Mr. V is a 53-year-old, college educated, never-married, Caucasian male who presented with lifelong erectile disorder.

Presenting Problem and Current Level of Sexual Functioning

Mr. V reported difficulty achieving an erection 50% of the time and further difficulties maintaining the erection during the remaining time. He stated that he is able to accomplish vaginal penetration only on 10% of occasions that he attempts intercourse. He estimated that during sexual activity he achieves about 60% of a full erection. Mr. V denied any additional sexual problems, except occasional difficulties with inhibited ejaculation. He reported being able to achieve almost a full erection during masturbation, although on occasion maintaining his erection and reaching orgasm were difficult. He reported rare occasions of early morning erections.

History of the Difficulties

Mr. V's erectile problems began at age 33 with his first attempt at intercourse. He described a situation where his "buddies" arranged for a prostitute, and after they had sex with her, it was Mr. V's turn. He remembered being worried about performing as well as his friends and being unsure of exactly what to do. When he was not able to achieve an erection, the prostitute became frustrated and irritated with him, resulting in his feeling embarrassed and inadequate. Since that occasion, Mr. V has had difficulties achieving and maintaining erections in most partner sexual activities.

Psychosexual History

Mr. V described his parents as conservative and strict. Mr. V was raised Catholic, and he recalled that his mother was a devout Catholic. He described his father as a withdrawn and unaffectionate man. He reported that sex was never talked about in the home and that he received most of his sexual information from his male peers. He reported being shy as a child and having no dating experience in high school and college. Due to feeling sexually inadequate, Mr. V began avoiding sexual activity, in particular intercourse. After college, Mr. V was involved in a series of relationships, each of which lasted around 4 months, at which time his partners usually terminated the relationship. In his late 30s, Mr. V met the woman with whom he had his most significant relationship. They dated for 2 years and were engaged to be married for almost 2 years. He stated that his partner called off the engagement due to his lack of interest in sex.

History of Sexual Abuse

Mr. V denied having any unwanted or abusive sexual experiences.

Medical History

Mr. V's medical history revealed that he had undergone transurethral resection of the prostate (TURP) surgery for benign prostatic hyperplasia (BPH) 9 months before this assessment. In addition, Mr. V was taking medication to control his high blood pressure (medium dose of an angiotensin-converting enzyme [ACE] inhibitor).

Psychological/Emotional Functioning

At the time of the assessment, Mr. V described being anxious in a variety of social situations, including parties, public speaking, dating, and assertiveness situations. Mr. V reported quitting or losing several jobs due to his social anxiety. Mr. V was working a minimum-wage job, stocking shelves at a supermarket, much below his educational potential. Based on these observations, Mr. V met the criteria for social phobia, generalized. No other Axis I or Axis II disorders were observed.

Current Relationship

Mr. V reported being in a romantic relationship with a woman 11 years younger for the past 14 months. He described a good relationship, which was confirmed by his score on the Dyadic Adjustment Scale (score = 105). He had told his partner that his erectile difficulties were due to the prostate surgery and would improve over time, which was the reason he was seeking treatment at this time point.

Assessment

Mr. V's sexual functioning was evaluated over the course of two, 1½-hour sessions, using a clinical interview that focused on the history of the presenting problem, current sexual functioning, psychosexual history, current relationship, and medical history. Mr. V also completed a questionnaire battery that included the International Index of Erectile Functioning (IIEF), Sexual Opinion Survey (SOS), Sexual Arousability Inventory (SAI), Dyadic Adjustment Scale (DAS), Depression Anxiety Stress Scales (DASS), SCL-90-R, and a medical history form. In addition, a copy of Mr. V's most recent urological evaluation was obtained. The IIEF was included in the questionnaire battery as a means of quantifying the severity of Mr. V's presenting problem and to serve as an outcomes measure. On the erectile functioning subscale, Mr. V scored in the range typically seen for men with erectile dysfunction (his score, 9; mean, 10.7; *SD,* 6.5 [Rosen et al., 1997]). However, Mr. V scored over 1 *SD* below the mean for men with erectile disorder on the desire (score, 4), intercourse satisfaction (score, 3), and overall satisfaction (score, 2) subscales. In addition, he rated his confidence at being able to achieve an erection as "very low." The SAI, SOS, and DAS were included in the questionnaire battery to complement information that was gathered in the interview. The SAI provided information about his subjective sexual arousal (score, 79), and the SOS provided information about his general emotional and attitudinal response to sexual situations (erotophilia–erotophobia). Mr. V scores on the SOS fell in the slightly erotophobic range (score, 52). The DAS was used to corroborate the information gathered in the interview about his current relationship. The DASS provided further information on Mr. V's level of overall anxiety, stress, and depression. Mr. V scored in the moderate range for anxiety (score, 12) and in the low range for both depression (score, 5) and stress (score, 9). The SCL-90 was utilized as a screen for other psychopathology (not used for basis of making the diagnoses) and was completed between the first and second assessment sessions. Based on his responses on the SCL-90 (area T score > 60 for interpersonal sensitivity and anxiety dimensions), a third assessment session was added. During this session (lasting about 2 hours), Mr. V's emotional functioning was formally evaluated using the Anxiety Disorders Interview Schedule for DSM-IV, non-lifetime version (ADIS-IV; Brown, Di Nardo, & Barlow, 1994). The ADIS-IV is a semistructured interview that focuses on anxiety, mood, and substance use disorders. Mr. V reported being highly anxious in a variety of social situations, including parties, small groups, public speaking, dating situations, interacting with authority figures, being assertive, and conversations.

Based on the information gathered during the assessment, Mr. V was assigned a principal diagnosis of social phobia, generalized (DSM-IV, 300.23), and an additional diagnosis of male erectile disorder, lifelong, situational, due to combined factors (DSM-IV, 302.72).

Case Formulation

Mr. V's case exemplifies how multiple factors contribute to and maintain sexual difficulties. In his case, erectile failures during his early sexual experiences developed into chronic difficulties due to performance worries, social anxiety, and avoidance of sexual activity. Organizing the information in terms of predisposing, precipitating, and maintaining factors can help clarify which contributing factors are most essential to address in the treatment plan. Lack of sexual information and experience, as well as significant social anxiety predisposed Mr. V to be uncomfortable in sexual situations and to worry about sexual performance and pleasing his partner. His inability to achieve an erection during his first attempt at intercourse and the negative reaction by the prostitute confirmed his fears and acted as a precipitating event. Intensified sexual performance worries, fears of embarrassment and rejection (social anxiety), and his pattern of avoiding sexual situations all interacted to maintain the sexual difficulties. In addition, organic or medical factors may also have contributed to his sexual dysfunction. Organic or medical contributing factors included advancing age, antihypertensive medications, and a history of prostate surgery. Unfortunately, his urologist did not formally evaluate his erectile capacity after the operation, which made it difficult to determine the unique variance accounted for by the medical factors. However, transurethral resection of the prostate is associated with only 11% to 17% postoperative erectile problems (Hammadeh et al., 1998; Perera & Hill, 1998). In addition, the type of antihypertensive medication (ACE inhibitor) used by Mr. V has been associated with a low incidence of erectile problems and in some instances may even facilitate vasodilation (Crenshaw & Goldberg, 1996). His ability to achieve at least a partial erection during masturbation indicates that the medical factors did not interfere completely with his erectile functioning.

Treatment Plan and Client Feedback

Since Mr. V's social phobia was causing greater distress and interference than his sexual problems and because the social anxiety was a contributing factor in his erectile problems, Mr. V was referred to cognitive-behavioral group therapy for social phobia (12 sessions). Although he was aware of the interference his social anxiety caused, Mr. V was initially reluctant to accept the referral for treatment. Providing Mr. V with an easily comprehended model that explained how all of the different factors, including his social anxiety, contributed to his sexual difficulties was an essential part of the feedback session. Specifically, it was explained that his performance worries, negative affect, and avoidance worked via a negative feedback-loop to maintain the sexual difficulties. Mr. V described being preoccupied during sexual activity with concerns about pleasing his partner and performing sexually. He feared that his inability to maintain erections and please his partner would eventually lead to her rejecting him. As a result of focusing on his past performance failures, worries about pleasing his partner, and possible partner rejection, Mr. V was unable to focus on the sexually pleasurable aspects of the situation. His generally low scores on the Sexual Arousability Inventory items supported this. Anxiety and negative affect produced by the focus on performance then functioned to motivate avoidance behavior. The avoidance of sexual situations, while reducing his anxiety in the short term, worked to increase his discomfort in sexual situations and failure predictions in the long term.

In addition, it was made clear to Mr. V how the skills he would learn during cognitive-behavioral treatment (e.g., cognitive restructuring and exposure to anxiety-provoking situations) would provide a springboard for addressing the erectile problems. Mr. V's treatment plan included individual sex therapy subsequent to completing anxiety treatment.

Perhaps motivated by his social anxiety, Mr. V was adamant that he did not want his partner to participate in the treatment. Based on his report and score on the DAS, it seemed that his reluctance to communicate with his partner about his sexual problems was not due to general relationship distress, thus not making it essential that the sexual problems be addressed via couples sexual therapy. His low SAI scores and low scores in the sexual satisfaction subscale of the IIEF indicated that increasing his ability to enjoy all forms of sexual activity, independent of whether he was able to achieve an erection, needed to be addressed in treatment. He agreed that the overall goal of treatment should be increasing his sexual satisfaction by developing a pleasure-focused approach to sex. In order to address the performance- and partner-related worries, the treatment plan emphasized building on the skills he would learn during the group by adapting cognitive restructuring skills to sexual performance-related thoughts and encouraging him not to avoid sexual activity. The treatment plan further included providing him with accurate sexual information to reduce misconceptions and sexual myths. In addition, direct discussions emphasizing the importance of focusing on pleasure in conjunction with sensate focus exercises were planned. In order to boast his sexual self-confidence and help overcome the potential negative effects of the surgery and antihypertensive medication, treatment with sildenafil citrate (Viagra) was included in Mr. V's treatment plan. Due to financial concerns, he was somewhat reluctant about the use of medication. Again, providing the client with a clear rationale was crucial in gaining his compliance with the treatment plan. It was explained how using Viagra on a temporary basis might increase his sexual confidence and provide a worry-free sexual environment that would allow him to focus on enjoying sexual activity.

CONCLUSION

Few disorders require the breadth and depth of assessment, and the careful attention to appropriate treatment planning than do sexual dysfunctions. And yet, few clinicians are aware of the wide variety of physical, psychological, and interpersonal factors that can contribute in a substantial way to sexual dysfunctions and which must be adequately assessed and conceptualized to produce fruitful and clinically useful treatment. Even in the area of erectile dysfunction where promising new drug treatments have appeared, most notably Viagra, it has become increasingly clear that this approach does not produce sexual satisfaction in the majority of cases (Virag, 1999). Additional attention to psychological and interpersonal factors is essential. In this chapter we have reviewed the fact that the sexual dysfunctions, particularly if defined liberally, seem to be the most prevalent of the "mental" disorders. And yet, clinics with the requisite medical and psychological expertise in the treatment of the sexual dysfunctions are few and far between. This means that only a few of even the most severe cases are able to avail themselves of a comprehensive multifaceted approach to their problem, and only if they happen to be appropriately referred to an existing clinic that specializes in sexual dysfunctions. For the time being, the vast majority of individuals who suffer from sexual dysfunctions, if they are predisposed to discuss the problem, receive interventions, such as they are, from primary care physicians. An existing challenge for clinicians who are highly trained in the assessment and treatment of sexual dysfunctions will be to devise efficient and effective methods for disseminating information on appropriate diagnosis, assessment, and treatment planning to these settings. At the very least, detailed information on the medical, psychological, and interpersonal factors that contribute to the variety of sexual dysfunctions should be disseminated so as to provide sufficient educational resources to reverse the problems in at least some patients. For the sexual dysfunctions, this is a particular challenge in view of the wide variety of dysfunctions that involve problems with either arousal, desire, performance, or pain across both sexes and the fact that several sexual dysfunctions often coexist in one individual. Nevertheless, and as alluded to earlier (Virag, 1999), comprehensive assessment and treatment planning is essential if any one of our treatments, either psychological or pharmacological, is to succeed to the extent that our patients desire. We hope that this chapter will assist current and future clinicians in achieving that goal.

REFERENCES

Althof, S. A., Corty, E. W., Levine, S. B., Levine, F., Burnett, A. L., McVary, K., Stecher, V., & Seftel, A. D. (1999). EDITS: Development of questionnaires for evaluating satisfaction with treatments for erectile dysfunction. *Urology, 53,* 793–799.

Aluja, A., & Torrubia, R. (1994). Sexual Arousability Inventory—Expanded (SAI-E): Subscales from factor analysis. *Revista de Psiquiatria de la Facultad de Medicina de Barcelona, 21,* 42–46.

Aluja, A., Torrubia, R., & Gallart, S. (1990). Spanish validation of the Sexual Arousability Inventory—Expanded (SAI-E). *Revista de Psiquiatria de la Facultad de Medicina de Barcelona, 17,* 252–268.

American Psychiatric Association. (1987). *Diagnostic and statistical manual of mental disorders* (3rd ed., rev.). Washington, DC: Author.

American Psychiatric Association. (1994). *Diagnostic and statistical manual of mental disorders* (4th ed.). Washington, DC: Author.

Andersen, B. L. (1981). A comparison of systematic desensitization and directed masturbation in the treatment of primary orgasmic dysfunction in females. *Journal of Consulting and Clinical Psychology, 49,* 568–570.

Andersen, B. L., & Cyranowski, J. M. (1995). Women's sexuality: Behaviors, responses, and individual differences. *Journal of Consulting and Clinical Psychology, 63,* 891–906.

Apfelbaum, B. (1989). Retarded ejaculation: A much-misunderstood syndrome. In S. R. Leiblum & R. C. Rosen (Eds.), *Principles and practice of sex therapy: Update for the 1990s* (2nd ed., pp. 168–206). New York: Guilford Press.

Bach, A. K., Brown, T. A., & Barlow, D. H. (1999). The effects of false negative feedback on efficacy expectancies and sexual arousal in sexually functional males. *Behavior Therapy, 30,* 79–95.

Bancroft, J. (1988). Sexual desire and the brain. *Sexual and Marital Therapy, 3,* 11–27.

Bancroft, J. (1992). Foreword. In R. C. Rosen & S. R. Leiblum (Eds.), *Erectile disorders: Assessment and treatment* (pp. vii–xv). New York: Guilford Press.

Barlow, D. H., (1986). Causes of sexual dysfunction: The role of anxiety and cognitive interference. *Journal of Consulting and Clinical Psychology, 54,* 140–148.

Beck, J. G. (1995). Hypoactive sexual desire disorder: An overview. *Journal of Consulting and Clinical Psychology, 63,* 919–927.

Beck, J. G., & Bozman, A. W. (1995). Gender differences in sexual desire: The effects of anger and anxiety. *Archives of Sexual Behavior, 24,* 595–612.

Beck, J. G., Bozman, A. W., & Qualtrough, T. (1991). The experience of sexual desire: Psychological correlates in a college sample. *Journal of Sex Research, 28,* 443–456.

Becker, J. V., Skinner, L. J., Abel, G. G., Axelrod, R., & Cichon, J. (1984). Sexual problems of sexual assault survivors. *Women and Health, 9,* 5–20.

Becker, J. V., Skinner, L. J., Abel, G. G., & Cichon, J. (1986). Level of postassault sexual functioning in rape and incest victims. *Archives of Sexual Behavior, 15,* 37–49.

Bergeron, S., Binik, Y. M., Khalife, S., Meana, M., Berkley, K. J., & Pagidas, K. (1997). The treatment of vulvar vestibulitis syndrome: Towards a multimodal approach. *Sexual and Marital Therapy, 12,* 305–311.

Bogaert, A. E., & Fisher, W. A. (1995). Predictors of university men's number of sexual partners. *Journal of Sex Research, 32,* 119–130.

Bradley, W. E., Timm, G. W., Gallagher, J. M., & Johnson, B. K. (1985). New method for continuous measurement of nocturnal penile tumescence and rigidity. *Urology, 26,* 4–9.

Brown, T. A., Di Nardo, P. A., & Barlow, D. H. (1994). *Anxiety Disorders Interview Schedule for DSM-IV (ADIS-IV).* San Antonio, TX: Psychological Corporation.

Campbell, B. C., & Udry, J. R. (1994). Implications of hormonal influences on sexual behavior for demographic models of reproduction. *Annals of the New York Academy of Sciences, 709,* 117–127.

Chambless, D. L., & Lifshitz, J. L. (1984). Self-reported sexual anxiety and arousal: The Expanded Sexual Arousability Inventory. *Journal of Sex Research, 20,* 241–254.

Chiechi, L. M., Granieri, M., Lobascio, A., Ferreri, R., & Loizzi, P. (1997). Sexuality in the climacterium. *Clinical and Experimental Obstetrics and Gynecology, 24,* 158–159.

Colpi, G. M., Fanciullacci, F., Beretta, G., Negri, L., & Zanolla, A. (1986). Evoked sacral potentials in subjects with true premature ejaculation. *Andrologia, 18,* 583–586.

Conte, H. R. (1986). Multivariate assessment of sexual dysfunction. *Journal of Consulting and Clinical Psychology, 54,* 149–157.

Cooper, A. J., & Magnus, R. V. (1984). A clinical trial of the beta blocker propranolol in premature ejaculation. *Journal of Psychosomatic Research, 28,* 331–336.

Cranston-Cuebas, M. A., & Barlow, D. H. (1990). Cognitive and affective contributions to sexual functioning. *Annual Review of Sex Research, 1,* 119–161.

Crenshaw, T. L. (1985). The sexual aversion syndrome. *Journal of Sex and Marital Therapy, 11,* 285–292.

Crenshaw, T. L., & Goldberg, J. P. (1996). *Sexual pharmacology: Drugs that affect sexual functioning.* New York: Norton.

Davies, S., Katz, J., & Jackson, J. L. (1999). Sexual desire discrepancies: Effects on sexual and relationship satisfaction in heterosexual dating couples. *Archives of Sexual Behavior, 28,* 553–567.

Davis, C. M., Yarber, W. L., Bauserman, R., Schreer, G., & Davis, S. L. (Eds.) (1998). *Handbook of sexuality-related measures.* Thousand Oaks, CA: Sage.

Davis, C, M., Yarber, W. L., & Davis, S. L. (Eds.). (1988). *Sexuality-related measures: A compendium.* Lake Mills, IA: Author.

Delehanty, R. (1982). Changes in assertiveness and changes in orgasmic response occurring with sexual therapy for preorgasmic women. *Journal of Sex and Marital Therapy, 8,* 198–208.

Delizonna, L. L., Wincze, J. P., Litz, B. T., Brown, T. A., and Barlow, D. H. (2001). A comparison of subjective and physiological measures of mechanically produced and erotically produced erections: Or, is an erection an erection? *Journal of Sex and Marital Therapy, 27,* 21–31.

Derflinger, J. R. (1998). Sex guilt among evangelical Christians in the 1990s: An examination of gender differences and salient correlates of sex guilt among married couples. *Dissertation Abstracts International, 58:* 5111. Abstract from PsychINFO Item: 1998–95006–439.

Derogatis, L. R. (1997). The Derogatis Interview for Sexual Functioning (DISF/DISF-SR): An introductory report. *Journal of Sex and Marital Therapy, 23,* 291–304.

Derogatis, L. R. (1998). The Derogatis Interview for Sexual Functioning. In C. M. Davis, W. L. Yarber, R. Bauserman, G. Schreer, & S. L. Davis (Eds.), *Handbook of sexuality-related measures* (pp. 267–269). Thousand Oaks, CA: Sage.

Derogatis, L. R., Fagan, P. J., Schmidt, C. W., Wise, T. N., & Gildem, K. S. (1986). Psychological subtypes of anorgasmia: A marker variable approach. *Journal of Sex and Marital Therapy, 12,* 197–210.

Derogatis, L. R., & Melisaratos, N. (1979). The DSFI: A multidimensional measure of sexual functioning. *Journal of Sex and Marital Therapy, 5,* 244–281.

Derogatis, L. R., Meyer, J. K., & Dupkin, C. (1976). Discrimination of organic versus psychogenic impotence with the DSFI. *Journal of Sex and Marital Therapy, 2,* 229–240.

Derogatis, L. R., & Rutigliano, P. J. (1996). Derogatis Affects Balance Scale. In B. Spiker (Ed.), *Quality of life and pharmacoeconomics in clinical trials* (2nd ed., pp. 160–177). Philadelphia: Lippincott-Raven.

Derogatis, L. R., & Savitz, K. L. (1999). The SCL-90-R, Brief Symptom Inventory, and matching clinical rating scales. In M. Maruish (Ed.), *The use of psychological testing for treatment planning and outcomes assessment* (2nd ed., pp. 679–724). Mahwah, NJ: Erlbaum.

Derogatis, L. R., Schmidt, C. W., Fagan, P. J., & Wise, T. N. (1989). Subtypes of anorgasmia via mathematical taxonomy. *Psychosomatics, 30,* 166–173.

Feldman, H. A., Goldstein, I., Hatzichristou, D. G., Krane, R. J., & McKinlay, J. B. (1994). Impotence and its medical and psychosocial correlates: Results of the Massachusetts Male Aging Study. *Journal of Urology, 151,* 54–61.

Feliciano, R., & Alfonso, C. A. (1997). Sexual side effects of psychotropic medications: Diagnosis, neurobiology, and treatment strategies. *International Journal of Mental Health, 26,* 79–89.

Finger, W. W., Lund, M., & Slagle, M. A. (1997). Medications that may contribute to sexual disorders: A guide to assessment and treatment in family practice. *Journal of Family Practice, 44,* 33–43.

Fisher, S. (1973). *The female orgasm: Psychology, physiology, fantasy.* New York: Basic Books.

Fisher, W. A. (1998). The Sexual Opinion Survey. In C. M. Davis, W. L. Yarber, R. Bauserman, G. Schreer, & S. L. Davis (Eds.), *Handbook of sexuality-related measures* (pp. 218–223). Thousand Oaks, CA: Sage.

Fisher, W. A., Byrne, D., White, L. A., & Kelley, K. (1988). Erotophobia–erotophilia as a dimension of personality. *Journal of Sex Research, 25,* 123–151.

Fugl-Meyer, A. R., & Sjogren Fugl-Meyer, K. (1999). Sexual disabilities, problems, and satisfaction in 18–74-year-old Swedes. *Scandinavian Journal of Sexology, 3,* 79–105.

Galindo, D., & Kaiser, F. E. (1995). Sexual health after 60. *Patient Care, 29,* 25–35.

Gebhard, P. (1966). Factors in marital orgasm. *Journal of Social Issues, 22,* 88–95.

Ghezzi, A., Malvestiti, G. M., Baldini, S., Zaffaroni, M., & Zibetti, A. (1995). Erectile impotence in multiple sclerosis: A neurophysiological study. *Journal of Neurology, 242,* 123–126.

Gilbert, F. S., & Gamache, M. P. (1984). The Sexual Opinion Survey: Structure and use. *Journal of Sex Research, 20,* 293–309.

Gordon, C. M., & Carey, M. P. (1995). Penile tumescence monitoring during morning naps to assess male erectile functioning: An initial study of healthy men of varied ages. *Archives of Sexual Behavior, 24,* 291–307.

Haavio-Mannila, E., & Kontula, O. (1997). Correlates of increased sexual satisfaction. *Archives of Sexual Behavior, 26,* 399–419.

Hammadeh, M. Y., Madaan, S., Singh, M., & Philp, T. (1998). Two-year follow-up of a prospective randomized trial of electrovaporization versus resection of prostate. *European Urology, 34,* 188–192.

Heiman, J. R., & Grafton-Becker, V. (1989). Orgasmic disorders in women. In S. R. Leiblum & R. C. Rosen (Eds.), *Principles and practice of sex therapy: Update for the 1990s* (2nd ed., pp. 51–88). New York: Guilford Press.

Heiman, J. R., & Meston C. M. (1997). Empirically validated treatment for sexual dysfunction. *Annual Review of Sex Research, 8,* 148–195.

Hillman, J. L. (2000). *Clinical perspectives in elderly sexuality.* New York: Kluwer Academic/Plenum.

Hite, S. (1976). *The Hite report: A nationwide study on female sexuality.* New York: Macmillan.

Hoon, E. F., & Chambless, D. (1998). Sexual Arousability Inventory and Sexual Arousability Inventory—Expanded. In C. M. Davis, W. L. Yarber, R. Bauserman, G. Schreer, & S. L. Davis (Eds.), *Handbook of sexuality-related measures* (pp. 71–74). Thousand Oaks, CA: Sage.

Hoon, E. F., & Hoon, P. W. (1978). Styles of sexual expression in women: Clinical implications of multivariate analyses. *Archives of Sexual Behavior, 7,* 105–116.

Hoon, E. F., Hoon, P. W., & Wincze, J. P. (1976). An inventory for the measurement of female sexual arousability: The SAI. *Archives of Sexual Behavior, 5,* 291–300.

Hudson, W. W. (1998). Index of Sexual Satisfaction. In C. M. Davis, W. L. Yarber, R. Bauserman, G. Schreer, & S. L. Davis (Eds.), *Handbook of sexuality-related measures* (p. 512). Thousand Oaks, CA: Sage.

Hudson, W. W., Harrison, D. F., & Crosscup, P. C. (1981). A short-form scale to measure sexual discord in dyadic relationships. *Journal of Sex Research, 17,* 157–174.

Huey, C. J., Kline-Graber, G., & Graber, B. (1981). Time factors in orgasmic response. *Archives of Sexual Behavior, 10,* 111–118.

Hulter, B. (1999). Sexual function in women with neurological disorders. *Comprehensive summaries of Uppsala dissertations from the faculty of medicine, 873.* Uppsala, Sweden: Acta Universitatis Upsaliensis.

Hunt, M. (1974). *Sexual behavior in the 1970s.* New York: Playboy Press.

Hurlbert, D. F., Apt, C., & Rabehl, S. M. (1993). Key variables to understanding female sexual satisfaction: An examination of women in nondistressed marriages. *Journal of Sex and Marital Therapy, 19,* 154–165.

Kameya, Y., Deguchi, A., & Yokota, Y. (1997). Analysis of measured values of ejaculation time in healthy males. *Journal of Sex and Marital Therapy, 23,* 25–28.

Kaplan, H. S. (1974). Group treatment for premature ejaculation. *Archives of Sexual Behavior, 3,* 443–452.

Kaplan, H. S. (1979). *Disorders of sexual desire.* New York: Brunner/Mazel.

Kaplan, H. S. (1989). *How to overcome premature ejaculation.* New York: Brunner/Mazel.

Kaplan, H. S., & Klein, D. F. (1987). *Sexual aversion, sexual phobias, and panic disorder.* Philadelphia: Brunner/Mazel.

Katz, R. C., Gipson, M., & Turner, S. (1992). Brief report: Recent findings on the Sexual Aversion Scale. *Journal of Sex and Marital Therapy, 18,* 141–146.

Kelly, M. P., Strassberg, D. S., & Kircher, J. R. (1990). Attitudinal and experiential correlates of anorgasmia. *Archives of Sexual Behavior, 19,* 165–177.

Kinsey, A. C., Pomeroy, W. B., & Martin, C. E. (1948). *Sexual behavior in the human male.* Philadelphia: Saunders.

Kinsey, A. C., Pomeroy, W. B., Martin, C. E., & Gebhard, P. (1953). *Sexual behavior in the human female.* Philadelphia: Saunders.

Laan, E., & Everaerd, W. (1995). Determinants of female sexual arousal: Psychophysiological theory and data. *Annual Review of Sex Research, 6,* 32–76.

Laumann, E. O., Paik, A., & Rosen, R. C. (1999). Sexual dysfunction in the United States: Prevalence and predictors. *Journal of the American Medical Association, 281,* 537–544.

Lazarus, A. A. (1989). Dyspareunia: A multimodal psychotherapeutic perspective. In S. R. Leiblum & R. C. Rosen (Eds.), *Principles and practice of sex therapy: Update for the 1990s* (2nd ed., pp. 89–112). New York: Guilford Press.

Lechtenberg, R., & Ohl, D. A. (1994). *Sexual dysfunction: Neurologic, urologic, and gynecologic aspects.* Malvern, PA: Lea & Febiger.

Leiblum, S. R. (1999, October). *Critical overview of the new consensus-based definitions and classification of female sexual dysfunction.* Paper presented at New Perspectives In the Management of Female Sexual Dysfunction, Boston.

Leiblum, S. R., & Rosen, R. C. (1989). Introduction: Sex therapy in the age of AIDS. In S. R. Leiblum & R. C. Rosen (Eds.), *Principles and practice of sex therapy: Update for the 1990s* (2nd ed., pp. 1–16). New York: Guilford Press.

Leiblum, S. R., & Rosen, R. C. (Eds.). (2000). *Principles and practice of sex therapy* (3rd ed.). New York: Guilford Press.

Leiblum, S. R., & Segraves, R. T. (1995). Sex and aging. *American Psychiatric Press Review of Psychiatry, 14,* 677–695.

Lindal, E., & Stefansson, J. G. (1993). The lifetime prevalence of psychosexual dysfunction among 55- to 57-year-olds in Iceland. *Social Psychiatry and Psychiatric Epidemiology, 28,* 91–95.

Locke, H. J., & Wallace, K. M. (1959). Short marital-adjustment and prediction tests: Their reliability and validity. *Marriage and Family Living, 21,* 251–255.

Masters, W. H., & Johnson, V. E. (1966). *Human sexual response.* Boston: Little, Brown.

Masters, W. H., & Johnson, V. E. (1970). *Human sexual inadequacy.* Boston: Little, Brown.

McCabe, M. P. (1994). Childhood, adolescent, and current psychological factors associated with sexual dysfunction. *Sexual and Marital Therapy, 9,* 267–276.

McCabe, M. P. (1998). Sexual Dysfunction Scale. In C. M. Davis, W. L. Yarber, R. Bauserman, G. Schreer, & S. L. Davis (Eds.), *Handbook of sexuality-related measures* (pp. 191–192). Thousand Oaks, CA: Sage.

McCabe, M. P., & Cobain, M. J. (1998). The impact of individual and relationship factors on sexual dysfunction among males and females. *Sexual and Marital Therapy, 13,* 131–143.

McCarthy, B. W. (1989). Cognitive-behavioral strategies and techniques in the treatment of early ejaculation. In S. R. Leiblum & R. C. Rosen (Eds.), *Principles and practice of sex therapy: Update for the 1990s* (2nd ed., pp. 141–167). New York: Guilford Press.

McGovern, K. B., Stewart, R. C., & LoPiccolo, J. (1975). Secondary orgasmic dysfunction: I. Analysis and strategies for treatment. *Archives of Sexual Behavior, 4,* 265–275.

Meana, M., & Binik, Y. M. (1994). Painful coitus: A review of female dyspareunia. *Journal of Nervous and Mental Disease, 182,* 264–272.

Meana, M., Binik, Y. M., Khalife, S., & Cohen, D. R. (1997a). Biopsychosocial profile of women with dyspareunia. *Obstetrics and Gynecology, 90,* 583–589.

Meana, M., Binik, Y. M., Khalife, S., & Cohen, D. R. (1997b). Dyspareunia: Sexual dysfunction or pain syndrome? *Journal of Nervous and Mental Disease, 185,* 561–569.

Metz, M. E., Pryor, J. L., Nesvacil, L. J., Abuzzahab, F., & Koznar, J. (1997). Premature ejaculation: A psychophysiological review. *Journal of Sex and Marital Therapy, 23,* 3–23.

Miller, R. S., & Johnson, J. A. (1998). Early Sexual Experiences Checklist. In C. M. Davis, W. L. Yarber, R. Bauserman, G. Schreer, & S. L. Davis (Eds.), *Handbook of sexuality-related measures* (pp. 23–25). Thousand Oaks, CA: Sage.

Miller, R. S., Johnson, J. A., & Johnson, J. K. (1991). Assessing the prevalence of unwanted childhood sexual experiences. *Journal of Psychology and Human Sexuality, 4,* 43–54.

Montejo-Gonzalez, A. L., Llorca, G., Izquierdo, J. A., Ledesma, A., Bousono, M., Calcedo, A., Carrasco, J. L., Ciudad, J., Daniel, E., de la Gandara, J., Derecho, J., Franco, M., Gomez, M. J., Macias, J. A., Martin, T., Perez, V., Sanchez, J. M., Sanchez, S., & Vicens, E. (1997). SSRR-induced sexual dysfunction: Fluoxetine, paroxetine, sertraline, and fluvoxamine in a prospective, multi-center, and descriptive clinical study of 344 patients. *Journal of Sex and Marital Therapy, 23,* 176–194.

Moody, G. A., & Mayberry, J. F. (1993). Perceived sexual dysfunction amongst patients with inflammatory bowel disease. *Digestion, 54,* 256–260.

Morokoff, P. (1978). Determinants of female orgasm. In J. LoPiccolo & L. LoPiccolo (Eds.), *Handbook of sex therapy* (pp. 147–165). New York: Plenum.

Morokoff, P. (1985). Effects of sex guilt, repression, sexual "arousability," and sexual experience on female sexual arousal during erotica and fantasy. *Journal of Personality and Social Psychology, 49,* 177–187.

Newcomb, M. D. (1984). Sexual behavior, responsiveness, and attitudes among women: A test of two theories. *Journal of Sex and Marital Therapy, 10,* 272–286.

Newman, F. L., Ciarlo, J. A., & Carpenter, D. (1999). Guidelines for selecting psychological instruments for treatment planning and outcome assessment. In M. Maruish (Ed.), *The use of psychological testing for treatment planning and outcomes assessment* (2nd ed., pp. 153–170). Mahwah, NJ: Erlbaum.

Newman, H. F., Reiss, H., & Northrup, J. D. (1982). Physical basis of emission, ejaculation, and orgasm in the male. *Urology, 19,* 341–350.

Perera, N. D., & Hill, J. T. (1998). Erectile and ejaculatory failure after transurethral prostatectomy. *Ceylon Medical Journal, 43,* 74–77.

Regan, P. C. (1999). Hormonal correlates and causes of sexual desire: A review. *Canadian Journal of Human Sexuality, 8,* 1–16.

Reissing, E. D., Binik, Y. M., & Khalife, S. (1999). Does vaginismus exist?: A critical review of the literature. *Journal of Nervous and Mental Disease, 187,* 261–274.

Reissing, E. D., Flory, N., & Binik, Y. M. (2000). Überlegungen zur Diagnose "Vaginismus" [Critical evaluation of the diagnostic concept of Vaginismus]. *Zeitschrift für Sexualforschung, 13,* 181–276.

Rise, J., Traeen, B., & Kraft, P. (1993). The Sexual Opinion Survey scale: A study on dimensionality in Norwegian adolescents. *Health Education Research, 8,* 485–494.

Rosen, R. C. (1996). Erectile dysfunction: The medicalization of male sexuality. *Clinical Psychological Review, 16,* 497–519.

Rosen, R. C. (1998). Quality of life assessment in sexual dysfunction trials. *International Journal of Impotence Research, 10,* S21–S23.

Rosen, R. C., Brown, C., Heiman, J., Leiblum, S., Meston, C., Shabsigh, R., Ferguson, D., & D'Agostino, R. (2000). The Female Sexual Function Index (FSFI): A multidimensional self-report instrument for the assessment of female sexual function. *Journal of Sex and Marital Therapy, 26,* 191–208.

Rosen, R. C., Kostis, J. B., Jekelis, A., & Taska, L. S. (1994). Sexual sequelae of antihypertensive drugs: Treatment effects on self-report and physiological measures in middle-aged male hypertensives. *Archives of Sexual Behavior, 23,* 135–152.

Rosen, R. C., Leiblum, S. R., & Spector, I. P. (1994). Psychologically based treatment for male erectile disorder: A cognitive-interpersonal model. *Journal of Sex and Marital Therapy, 20,* 67–85.

Rosen, R. C., Riley, A., Wagner, G., Osterloh, I. H., Kirkpatrick, J., & Mishra, A. (1997). The International Index of Erectile Function (IIEF): A multidimensional scale for assessment of erectile dysfunction. *Urology, 49,* 822–830.

Rosen, R. C., Taylor J. F., Leiblum, S. R., & Bachmann, G. A. (1993). Prevalence of sexual dysfunction in women: Results of a survey study of 329 women in an outpatient gynecological clinic. *Journal of Sex and Marital Therapy, 19,* 171–188.

Rosser, B. R., Metz, M. E., Bockting, W. O., & Buroker, T. (1997). Sexual difficulties, concerns, and satisfaction in homosexual men: An empirical study with implications for HIV prevention. *Journal of Sex and Marital Therapy, 23,* 61–73.

Roughan, P. A., & Kunst, L. (1981). Do pelvic floor exercises really improve orgasmic potential? *Journal of Sex and Marital Therapy, 7,* 223–229.

Rust, J., & Golombok, S. (1986). The GRISS: A psychometric instrument for the assessment of sexual dysfunction. *Archives of Sexual Behavior, 15,* 157–165.

Rust, J., & Golombok, S. (1998). The GRISS: A psychometric scale and profile of sexual dysfunction. In C. M. Davis, W. L. Yarber, R. Bauserman, G. Schreer, & S. L. Davis (Eds.), *Handbook of sexuality-related measures* (pp. 192–194). Thousand Oaks, CA: Sage.

Sakheim, D. K., Barlow, D. H., Abrahamson, D. J., & Beck, J. G. (1987). Distinguishing between organogenic and psychogenic erectile dysfunction. *Behaviour Research and Therapy, 25,* 379–390.

Schiavi, R. C., Derogatis, L. R., Kuriansky, J., O'Connor, D., & Sharpe, L. (1979). The assessment of sexual function and marital satisfaction. *Journal of Sex and Marital Therapy, 5,* 169–224.

Schover, L. R., & LoPiccolo, J. (1982). Treatment effectiveness for dysfunctions of sexual desire. *Journal of Sex and Marital Therapy, 8,* 179–197.

Segraves, K. B., & Segraves, R. T. (1991). Hypoactive sexual desire disorder: Prevalence and comorbidity in 906 subjects. *Journal of Sex and Marital Therapy, 17,* 55–58.

Segraves, K. B., Segraves, R. T., & Schoenberg, H. W. (1987). Use of sexual history to differentiate organic from psychogenic impotence. *Archives of Sexual Behavior, 16,* 125–137.

Segraves, R. T., & Althof, S. (1998). Psychotherapy and pharmacotherapy of sexual dysfunction. In P. E. Nathan & J. M. Gorman (Eds.), *A guide to treatments that work* (pp. 447–471). New York: Oxford University Press.

Segraves, R. T., & Segraves, K. B. (1991). Diagnosis of female arousal disorder. *Sexual and Marital Therapy, 6,* 9–13.

Sherwin, B. B. (1988). A comparative analysis of the role of androgen in human male and female sexual behavior: Behavioral specificity, critical thresholds, and sensitivity. *Psychobiology, 16,* 416–425.

Sim, M. J. (1861). On vaginismus. *Clinical Obstetrics and Gynecology, 3,* 356–367.

Simons, J. S., & Carey, M. P. (2001). Prevalence of the sexual dysfunctions: Results from a decade of research. *Archives of Sexual Behavior, 30,* 177–219.

Smith, E. R., Becker, M. A., Byrne, D., & Przybyla, D. P. J. (1993). Sexual attitudes of males and females as predictors of interpersonal attraction and marital compatibility. *Journal of Applied Social Psychology, 23,* 1011–1034.

Spector, I. P., & Carey, M. P. (1990). Incidence and prevalence of the sexual dysfunctions: A critical review of the empirical literature. *Archives of Sexual Behavior, 19,* 389–408.

Spector, I. P., Carey, M. P., & Steinberg, L. (1996). The Sexual Desire Inventory: Development, factor structure, and evidence of reliability. *Journal of Sex and Marital Therapy, 22,* 175–190.

Spector, I. P., Carey, M. P., & Steinberg, L. (1998). Sexual Desire Inventory. In C. M. Davis, W. L. Yarber, R. Bauserman, G. Schreer, & S. L. Davis (Eds.), *Handbook of sexuality-related measures* (pp. 174–175). Thousand Oaks, CA: Sage.

Spiess, W. F., Geer, J. H., & O'Donohue, W. T. (1984). Premature ejaculation: Investigation of factors in ejaculatory latency. *Journal of Abnormal Psychology, 93,* 242–245.

Strassberg, D. S., Mahoney, J. M., Schaugaard, M., & Hale, V. E. (1990). The role of anxiety in premature ejaculation: A psychophysiological model. *Archives of Sexual Behavior, 19,* 251–257.

Talmadge, L. D., & Talmadge, W. C. (1990). Sexuality assessment measures for clinical use: A review. *American Journal of Family Therapy, 18,* 80–105.

Tiefer, L. (1994). The medicalization of impotence: Normalizing phallocentrism. *Gender and Society, 8,* 363–377.

Tiefer, L., & Melman, A. (1989). Comprehensive evaluation of erectile dysfunction and medical treatments. In S. R. Leiblum & R. C. Rosen (Eds.), *Principles and practice of sex therapy: Update for the 1990s* (2nd ed., pp. 207–236). New York: Guilford Press.

van der Velde, J., & Everaerd, W. (1999). Voluntary control over pelvic floor muscles in women with and without vaginistic reactions. *International Urogynecology Journal and Pelvic Floor Dysfunction, 10,* 230–236.

van der Velde, J., Laan, E., & Everaerd, W. (in press). *Vaginismus, a component of a general defensive reaction: An investigation of pelvic floor muscle activity during exposure to emotion inducing films excerpts in women with and without vaginismus.*

Ventegodt, S. (1998). Sex and the quality of life in Denmark. *Archives of Sexual Behavior, 27,* 295–307.

Virag, R. (1999). Indications and early results of sildenafil (Viagra) in erectile dysfunction. *Urology, 54,* 1073–1077.

Wagner, T. H., Patrick, D. L., McKenna, P., & Proese, P. S. (1996). Cross-cultural development of a quality of life measure for men with erectile difficulties. *Quality of Life Research, 5,* 443–449.

Waldinger, M. D., Hengeveld, M. W., Zwinderman, A. H., & Olivier, B. (1998). An empirical operationalization study of DSM-IV diagnostic criteria for premature ejaculation. *International Journal of Psychiatry in Clinical Practice, 2,* 287–293.

Watters, W. W., Askwith, J., Cohen. M., & Lamont, J. A. (1985). An assessment approach to couples with sexual problems. *Canadian Journal of Psychiatry, 30,* 2–11.

Werlinger, K., King, T. K., Clark, M. M., Pera, V., & Wincze, J. P. (1997). Perceived changes in sexual functioning and body image following weight loss in an obese female population: A pilot study. *Journal of Sex and Marital Therapy, 23,* 74–78.

Wiederman, M. W. (2000). Women's body image self-consciousness during physical intimacy with a partner. *Journal of Sex Research, 37,* 60–68.

Wincze, J. P., & Barlow, D. H. (1996). *Enhancing sexuality (client workbook).* San Antonio, TX: Psychological Corporation.

Wincze, J. P., & Carey, M. P. (2001). *Sexual dysfunction: A guide for assessment and treatment* (2nd ed.). New York: Guilford Press.

Zilbergeld, B. (1992). *The new male sexuality.* New York: Bantam Books.

Zilbergeld, B. (1999). *The new male sexuality* (rev. ed.). New York: Bantam.

15

Insomnia

Josée Savard
Charles M. Morin

Insomnia is a problem that is frequently reported by patients in various clinical settings. Insomnia complaints are often associated with emotional distress, as well as impaired social and occupational functioning. Despite its prevalence and clinical significance, insomnia is frequently underdiagnosed and, consequently, undertreated. The general goal of this chapter is to emphasize the importance of conducting a thorough evaluation of insomnia to select an effective treatment course. Specifically, this chapter aims to (1) review the diagnostic classification, clinical characteristics, and natural course of insomnia; (2) present the range of available sleep assessment modalities with their respective strengths and weaknesses; (3) provide practical recommendations for insomnia assessment (including differential diagnosis) and its integration with treatment planning; and (4) suggest how insomnia assessment can be integrated in managed care and primary care settings.

OVERVIEW OF INSOMNIA

Nature of Insomnia Complaints

Insomnia is a heterogeneous complaint that typically reflects an unsatisfactory duration, efficiency, or quality of sleep. Presenting complaints vary, according to the part of the night when sleep is most disturbed. They include difficulties falling asleep at bedtime (i.e., initial or sleep onset insomnia), trouble staying asleep with prolonged nocturnal awakenings (i.e., middle or maintenance insomnia), early morning awakening with inability to resume sleep (i.e., terminal or late insomnia), and nonrestorative sleep. These difficulties are not mutually exclusive, as a person may present with mixed difficulties in initiating and in maintaining sleep. Age is an important factor for determining the type of insomnia an individual suffers. Young adults usually complain of difficulties initiating sleep, whereas older adults tend to complain more of waking up in the middle of the night (with incapacity to resume sleep) and awakening too early in the morning (Bixler, Kales, & Soldatos, 1979; Mellinger, Balter, & Uhlenhuth, 1985).

The Continuum of Insomnia Symptoms

Insomnia varies greatly in terms of frequency, severity, duration, and daytime sequelae. Almost everyone has occasional sleep difficulties at some point in life, but not all are clinical insomniacs or in need of treatment. Severity levels for sleep difficulties can be viewed on a continuum that ranges from no sleep difficulties to chronic insomnia. Although the presence of an insomnia disorder is a clear indication for treatment, it is not the only one. Individuals with moderate and persistent insomnia symptoms can also benefit significantly from treatment.

When combining criteria of the International Classification of Sleep Disorders (ICSD; American Sleep Disorders Association, 1997), the *Diagnostic and Statistical Manual of Mental Disorders,* fourth edition (DSM-IV; American Psychiatric Association, 1994), and those typically used in clinical research, the insomnia disorder (or insomnia syndrome) can be defined as (1) difficulty initiating (i.e., 30 minutes or more to fall asleep) or maintaining sleep (i.e., 30 minutes or more of nocturnal awakenings), with a corresponding sleep efficiency (i.e., ratio of total sleep time to time spent in bed) lower than 85%; (2) the sleep problem occurs at least three nights per week; and (3) the sleep disturbance causes significant daytime impairment (e.g., fatigue, mood disturbances) or marked distress. The insomnia disorder is considered chronic when its duration is more than 6 months, subacute when its duration is less than 6 months but more than 1 month, and transient when its duration is 1 month or less.

Prevalence, Risk Factors, Longitudinal Course, and Potential Consequences of Insomnia

Prevalence

Insomnia is the most common of all sleep disorders (Bixler et al., 1979). Prevalence rates for insomnia vary considerably across surveys, ranging from as low as 2% (Liljenberg, Almqvist, Hetta, Roos, & Agren, 1989) to as high as 48% (Karacan, Thornby, & William, 1983), with an average of approximately 20% (Ohayon, Caulet, & Lemoine, 1998). This extensive variability is mainly attributable to differences in data collection techniques (e.g., questionnaires vs. interviews) and the failure to distinguish between insomnia symptoms and insomnia disorder. Based on the most cited epidemiological surveys, insomnia affects one-third of the adult population, including between 9% and 12% on a chronic basis (Ford & Kamerow, 1989; Gallup Organization, 1991; Mellinger et al., 1985).

Risk Factors

Studies conducted in the general population suggest that some demographic variables are associated with an increased risk to develop insomnia, including gender, age, and marital and employment status. Specifically, the risk to develop insomnia increases with aging and is higher in women; in unemployed, separated, and widowed individuals; and in people living alone (Bixler et al., 1979; Ford & Kamerow, 1989; Mellinger et al., 1985; Ohayon, Caulet, Priest, & Guilleminault, 1997).

Insomnia is also more prevalent in patients with psychiatric symptomatology, particularly those with depression and anxiety disorders (Morin & Ware, 1996). In one study, Ford and Kamerow (1989) found that 40% of patients with insomnia displayed other psychiatric symptoms, compared to only 16.4% of normal sleepers. Mellinger et al. (1985) also found higher levels of psychological distress and symptoms of major depression in insomnia sufferers.

The prevalence of insomnia is also higher in individuals with medical disorders. In an elderly sample, physical health was found to be the strongest risk factor for insomnia, even though mental health factors (e.g., depressed mood) were also related to insomnia (Morgan & Clarke, 1997). In another recent study, chronic medical conditions including cardiovascular disease (e.g., angina), chronic pain (e.g., arthritis), gastric problems (e.g., peptic ulcer), and prostate problems were associated with insomnia, even after controlling for depression (Katz & McHorney, 1998). There is also accumulating evidence to suggest that insomnia is highly prevalent in individuals with medical illnesses such as cancer, end-stage renal disease, cerebrovascular diseases, and multiple sclerosis (Pressman, Gollomp, Benz, & Peterson, 1997; Savard & Morin, 2001).

Some studies suggest that a past history of insomnia is another factor that increases the risk of future insomnia episodes (Vollrath, Wicki, & Angst, 1989) and that family history is also a potential risk factor (Bastien & Morin, 2000). Finally, stressful life events such as personal losses (e.g., death of a loved one), family stressors (e.g., marital difficulties), health-related difficulties (e.g., hospitalization), and work and financial problems (e.g., job overload) are other potential risk factors for insomnia (Cernovsky, 1984). Although a more recent study could not replicate these results (Friedman, Brooks III, Bliwise, Yesavage, & Wicks, 1995), an early study found that poor sleepers reported experiencing a greater number of stressful life events during the year of insomnia onset than did good sleepers (Healy et al., 1981). Because most of the studies conducted on risk factors for insomnia have been cross-sectional in design, at this point few conclusions can be made regarding the causal role of these factors.

Longitudinal Course

Insomnia can begin at any time during the course of the life span, but onset of the first episode is most common in young adulthood (Kales & Kales, 1984). In a small subset of cases, insomnia begins in childhood, in the absence of psychological or medical problems, and persists throughout adulthood (Hauri & Olmstead, 1980). Insomnia is a frequent problem among women during menopause and often persists even after associated symptoms (e.g., hot flashes) have resolved (Krystal, Edinger, Wohlgemuth, & Marsh, 1998). The first episode of insomnia can also occur late in life, although it must be distinguished from normal age-related changes in sleep patterns and from sleep disturbances due to medical problems or prescribed medications.

For the large majority of insomnia sufferers, sleep difficulties are transient in nature, lasting a few days, and resolving themselves once the initial precipitating event (e.g., stressful life event) has subsided or the individual has adapted to it. Its course may also be intermittent, with repeated brief episodes of sleep difficulties following a close association with the occurrence of stressful events (Vollrath et al., 1989). Even when insomnia has developed a chronic course, typically there is extensive night-to-night variability in sleep patterns, with an occasional restful night's sleep intertwined with several nights of poor sleep. The subtype of insomnia (i.e., sleep onset, maintenance, or mixed insomnia) may also change over time (Hohagen et al., 1994).

Potential Consequences

Fatigue is one of the most common complaints of patients with insomnia. In a study conducted in individuals with a variety of sleep disorders, fatigue was elevated in all sleep disordered patients but was significantly higher in patients with insomnia (Lichstein, Means, Noe, & Aguillard, 1997). Individuals with insomnia also frequently report daytime impairments such as poor concentration and memory, difficulties accomplishing simple tasks, and more drowsiness (Gallup Organization, 1991). These cognitive impairments have been corroborated by objective measurement in some (Hart, Morin, & Best, 1995; Hauri, 1997), but not all, studies. Recent findings also validate the widespread assumption that insomnia is associated with an overall decrease in quality of life (Chevalier et al., 1999; Zammit, Weiner, Damato, Sillup, & McMillan, 1999). Since most studies have been cross-sectional, more research is needed to determine whether these impairments are really caused by insomnia.

Psychological disturbances are other potential consequences of insomnia. For example, in the long run, individuals with insomnia can worry about the consequences of their sleep disorder and feel helpless and dysphoric about their inability to overcome this problem. There is also increasing evidence that insomnia can lead to psychiatric disorders. Indeed, longitudinal studies showed that individuals with persistent insomnia are at higher risk for developing subsequent depressive, anxiety, and substance use disorders up to 30 years later (Breslau, Roth, Rosenthal, & Andreski, 1996; Chang, Ford, Mead, Cooper-Patrick, & Klag, 1997; Ford & Kamerow, 1989; Gillin, 1998; Livingston, Blizard, & Mann, 1993; Weissman, Greenwald, Nino-Murcia, & Dement, 1997).

Finally, there is some evidence to suggest that sleep disturbance negatively affects health. In cross-sectional studies, individuals with insomnia report a higher frequency of health problems, medical consultations, and hospitalizations relative to good sleepers (Gislason & Almqvist, 1987; Kales et al., 1984; Mellinger et al., 1985; Simon & Von Korff, 1997). Further evidence for a link between insomnia and health is provided by data from prospective epidemiological surveys, which indicate that short sleep duration is associated with increased mortality (Kripke, Simons, Garfinkel, & Hammond, 1979; Wingard & Berkman, 1983). However, since insomnia is a clinical syndrome that is characterized by several symptoms other than a shorter sleep duration, these findings may not be generalizable to insomnia. Finally, some psychoneuroimmunological research suggests that insomnia can alter immunocompetence, although these findings are based on cross-sectional studies and the clinical impact of this effect on health is unknown (Cover & Irwin, 1994; Irwin, Smith, & Gillin, 1992; Savard et al., 1999).

REVIEW OF SLEEP/INSOMNIA ASSESSMENT MODALITIES

It is a common mistake to view insomnia as a simple symptomatic problem that can be treated with all-purpose interventions. In reality, a thorough evaluation of all aspects associated with the sleep problem is extremely helpful—if not necessary—to select an appropriate and effective treatment plan. Ideally, the evaluation should include the use of various and complementary assessment methods such as clinical interview, sleep diary, and self-report measures. The use of mechanical devices and laboratory sleep assessments can also be useful to corroborate the subjective complaint with objective data (see Table 15.1 for a list of insomnia measures with their respective advantages and limitations).

Semistructured Clinical Interviews

The clinical interview is certainly the most important component of the insomnia assessment. Besides evaluating the nature of the complaint (e.g., insomnia type), the clinical interview collects a detailed history of the sleep problem (i.e., longitudinal course) and allows a functional analysis. A complete functional analysis should include the identification of sleep habits, insomnia severity, consequences of insomnia, symptoms of other sleep disorders,

TABLE 15.1. Summary of Advantages and Limitations of Different Sleep Assessment Modalities

Assessment modality	Instruments	Advantages	Limitations
Semistructured interviews	Insomnia Interview Schedule (IIS; Morin, 1993) Structured Interview for Sleep Disorders (SIS-D; Schramm et al., 1993)	Assess thoroughly the nature, course, and severity of the sleep disturbance and associated aspects; allow a functional analysis and differential diagnosis with other forms of pathology	Require good knowledge of the sleep disorders spectrum and interviewers need to receive training (except for computerized interviews); because data are mainly subjective, not a good outcome measure
Sleep diary		Assess nightly variations in the nature, frequency, and severity of sleep difficulties, and some maladaptive behaviors; flexible; ecological validity (assessment undergone in the patient's natural environment); allow prospective evaluation over extensive periods of time; excellent outcome measure; economical	Moderate convergent validity with polysomnographic (objective) data; reactivity to the measure is possible; adherence problems in some patients
Self-report measures	Insomnia Severity Index (ISI; Morin, 1993) Pittsburgh Sleep Quality Index (PSQI; Buysse et al., 1989) Dysfunctional Beliefs and Attitudes about Sleep (DBAS; Morin, 1994) Arousal Predisposition Scale (APS; Coren, 1988) Sleep Hygiene Awareness and Practice Scale (SHAPS; Lacks & Rotert, 1986) Pre-Sleep Arousal Scale (PSAS; Nicassio et al., 1985)	Practical and economical; no need for trained staff; can be administered repeatedly and used as an outcome measure	Retrospective and global assessment; risk of overestimation of sleep difficulties; most of the existing scales are not fully validated
Mechanical devices	Wrist actigraphy Sleep assessment device Switch-activated clock	Self-administered; no need for a trained technician; economical; unobtrusive; ecological validity	Do not measure sleep stages; convergent validity with polysomnography needs to be further studied
Laboratory polysomnography		The "gold standard" for the evaluation and diagnosis of all sleep disorders; provides objective measures for the entire range of sleep parameters, including sleep stages; excellent outcome measure	Expensive; trained technician needed throughout the night and to score data; relatively invasive; low ecological validity; need for repeated measures to reliability assess insomnia; "first-night effect"
Ambulatory polysomnography		All advantages of laboratory polysomnography; ecological validity; reduction of the "first-night effect"	Higher risk of artifacts and invalidation; lack of behavioral observations

and self-help strategies used, including medication (Bootzin & Engle-Friedman, 1981; Spielman & Glovinsky, 1997). The functional analysis should also include an assessment of causal factors that have been involved in the development of insomnia including (1) predisposing factors, or enduring traits that increase the individual's general vulnerability to develop insomnia (e.g., trait hyperarousalability, family or personal history of insomnia); (2) precipitating factors, or situational conditions that trigger the onset of insomnia (e.g., divorce, work difficulties, illness); and (3) perpetuating factors, or variables that contribute to the maintenance of insomnia over time. Of particular importance for determining the treatment plan is the identification of perpetuating factors—that is maladaptive sleep habits (e.g., spending too much time in bed) and dysfunctional cognitions (e.g., worrying excessively about the consequences of insomnia)—that the person develops and entertains in reaction to sleep disturbance.

Insomnia Interview Schedule (IIS)

The IIS (Morin, 1993) is a semistructured interview that gathers a wide range of information about the nature (i.e., problems falling asleep, staying asleep, waking up too early in the morning, problem staying awake during the day) and severity or the sleep problem, along with the current sleep/wake schedule, which includes information such as typical bedtime and arising times, time of the last awakening in the morning, frequency and duration of daytime naps, frequency of difficulties sleeping, time to fall asleep, number and duration of awakenings per night, and total duration of sleep. The IIS also assesses the onset (e.g., gradual or sudden, precipitating events), course (e.g., persistent, episodic, seasonal), and duration of insomnia; past and current use of sleeping aids (i.e., prescribed and over-the-counter medications, alcohol); and health habits that might influence sleep (i.e., exercise, caffeine intake, smoking, alcohol use). Information is also gathered about environmental factors (e.g., bed partner, mattress, noise level, temperature), as well as on sleep habits (e.g., watching TV in the bedroom, staying in bed when awake) and other factors (e.g., stress, vacation) that impair/facilitate sleep. In addition, the IIS assesses the effect of insomnia on daytime functioning and quality of life. Finally, symptoms of other sleep disorders and psychiatric disorders are evaluated for differential diagnosis. Although the IIS provides all relevant clinical information for the assessment of insomnia and a diagnosis based on ICSD or DSM-IV classifications, its psychometric properties remain to be demonstrated. For instance, its reliability (e.g., interrater reliability) and concurrent validity with other insomnia assessment methods (both subjective and objective) have yet to be verified.

Structured Interview for Sleep Disorders (SIS-D)

The SIS-D (Schramm et al., 1993) uses the format of the Structured Clinical Interview for DSM to assess sleep–wake disorders according to the DSM-III-R criteria. The SIS-D first provides a brief semistructured overview of physical health, drug and alcohol use, and history of mental illness, as well as a screening of sleep apnea and narcolepsy. It is followed by structured questions inquiring about specific symptoms of sleep disorders. Similar to the ISS, the SIS-D was designed to be used by trained and experienced interviewers who are capable of making clinical judgments. Overall, the SIS-D interrater reliability has been found to be adequate for the assessment of sleep disorders, with higher agreement rates obtained for the insomnia diagnosis. Moreover, a concordance rate of 90% between the SIS-D and a polysomnographic assessment has been obtained (Schramm et al., 1993).

Computerized Assessments

The Sleep-EVAL is designed to assist interviewers in diagnosing sleep disorders according to DSM-IV and ICSD criteria (Ohayon, Guilleminault, et al., 1997). This expert system contains 1,543 possible questions that are automatically selected based on the individual's previous answers. The interviewer asks the question as selected by the system and enters the answer according to several formats. During the course of the interview, the system poses a series of diagnostic hypotheses that are later confirmed or rejected with further questioning or deductions. All diagnostic trees are consecutively explored and eliminated until a final diagnosis is reached. The interview takes between 20 to 30 minutes to conduct in individuals with no sleep disorder and 60 to 120 minutes in those with sleep difficulties. Validation studies have revealed high levels of agreement between diagnoses obtained from the Sleep-EVAL and those made by clinician psychiatrists and psychologists, including agreement for the diagnosis of insomnia (Hoch et al., 1994; Ohayon, Guilleminault, et al., 1997). The major advantages of computerized assessments over standard clinical interviews are their uniformity of administration and the minimal training required for interviewers. By contrast, computerized assessments are less flexible and are unable to take into account temporal relationships among different symptoms (Ohayon, Guilleminault, et al., 1997).

Sleep Diary

Description

Sleep diary monitoring is the most widely used method for assessing insomnia (Bootzin & Engle-Friedman, 1981). This method is extremely helpful for both clinical and research purposes. Sleep diary monitoring gives a general overview of patient's sleep patterns for an entire week. At a glance, the clinician can quickly gain an understanding of the nature, frequency, and intensity of insomnia, as well as nightly variations of sleep difficulties and the presence of certain perpetuating factors (e.g., naps, spending too much time in bed).

A typical daily sleep diary form collects information about bedtime, arising time, time to fall asleep, number and duration of awakenings, time of last awakening, sleep duration, naps, medication intake, and indices of sleep quality and daytime functioning (Lacks, 1987). Figure 15.1 is an example of diary that can be used. The diary can be simplified or adapted to a patient's specific needs. Sleep variables that are derived from this information are as follows: sleep-onset latency, waking after sleep onset, early morning awakening, time in bed, total time awake, total time asleep, and sleep efficiency. Usually, the sleep diary is completed for a period of at least 2 weeks before treatment is begun, and throughout treatment thereafter. This procedure allows the clinician to establish baseline insomnia severity and to monitor progress over the course of treatment. It is very useful to provide patients with clear instructions on how to complete the diary, along with an example. Training may be necessary for some patients.

Validation Data

Early research conducted on the validity of sleep diaries has revealed modest concurrent validity with polysomnographic assessments, which are often considered the "gold standard." Specifically, insomnia patients tend to overestimate sleep-onset latency and to underestimate sleep duration, in comparison to what is found by polysomnographic measurement (Bixler, Kales, Leo, & Slye, 1973; Carskadon et al., 1976; Frankel, Coursey, Buchbinder, & Snyder, 1976; Monroe, 1967). Using a different analysis method (i.e., averaging all possible

	Today's date	3/25					
1.	Yesterday, I napped from ___ to ___. (Note the times of all naps.)	*1:50 to 2:30 P.M.*					
2.	Yesterday, I took ___ mg of medication and/or ___ oz of alcohol as a sleep aid.	*Halcion 0.125 mg*					
3.	Last night, I went to bed at ___ o'clock and turned the lights off at ___ o'clock.	*10:45 P.M. 11:15 P.M.*					
4.	After turning the lights out, I fell asleep in ___ minutes.	*40 min.*					
5.	My sleep was interrupted ___ times. (Specify number of nighttime awakenings.)	*2*					
6.	Each time, my sleep was interrupted ___ minutes. (Specify duration of each awakening.)	*10 45*					
7.	This morning, I woke up at ___ o'clock. (Note time of last awakening.)	*6:20*					
8.	This morning, I got out of bed at ___ o'clock. (Specify the time.)	*6:40*					
9.	Last night, my sleep was ___ % recuperative. (Specify a percentage.)	*30%*					
10.	Overall, I am ___ % satisfied with my quality of sleep last night. (Specify a percentage.)	*54%*					

FIGURE 15.1. Example of a sleep diary form. Adapted from Morin (1993). Copyright 1993 by The Guilford Press. Adapted by permission.

combinations of internight correlations), Coates et al. (1982) concluded that daily estimates of sleep-onset latency and waking after sleep onset that were obtained by diary yield a reliable and valid relative index of insomnia, even though they do not reflect the absolute values that are obtained from polysomnography.

Advantages and Limitations

Sleep diary monitoring is a practical and economical method to assess sleep in patients' natural environments. In addition, sleep diary monitoring allows for the prospective evaluation of sleep over extensive periods of time, thereby yielding a more representative sample of a person's sleep. This is a major advantage over polysomnography, which is usually only used for a few nights (e.g., at pre- and posttreatment) because of the costs involved. Also, sleep diary data can reflect how sleep patterns change over time, which can help pinpoint the situational and temporal factors that contribute to these variations. It can also have a therapeutic effect by making patients realize that their sleep is not as disturbed as they thought it was. Hence, sleep diary monitoring is less subject to exaggeration of sleep difficulties than is a single, global, and retrospective measure. The main limitations of sleep diary monitoring have to do with convergent validity (as discussed here), reactivity, and compliance. Reactivity can be attenuated by extending baseline monitoring for at least 2 weeks, which is the standard in current outcome research (Lacks & Morin, 1992). Compliance can be a problem in some patients, and this issue is discussed later in this chapter.

Self-Report Measures

Insomnia Severity Index (ISI)

The ISI (Morin, 1993) yields a quantitative index of insomnia severity. The ISI is composed of seven items assessing, on a 5-point scale, the perceived severity of problems with sleep onset, sleep maintenance, and early morning awakenings; the dissatisfaction with the current sleep pattern; the degree of interference with daily functioning; the noticeability of impairment due to the sleep disturbance; and the degree of worry or concern caused by the sleep problem (see Figure 15.2). The total ISI score, which is obtained by summing the seven ratings, ranges from 0 to 28. A higher score indicates more severe insomnia. The ISI takes less than 5 minutes to complete and score. A cutoff score of 8 has been suggested to detect clinical insomnia (Bastien, Vallières, & Morin, 2001), although additional research is needed to determine whether it yields the optimal sensitivity and specificity rates. Two parallel versions—clinician and significant other (e.g., spouse, roommate) versions—are available to provide collateral validation of patients' perception of their sleep difficulties. Psychometric studies have revealed acceptable internal consistency (Cronbach's alpha = .77), good concurrent validity when compared with a sleep diary, and adequate concurrent validity when compared with polysomnographic data. Finally, the ISI has been found to be sensitive to clinical change following treatment with pharmacotherapy, cognitive-behavioral therapy, and a combination of both, which supports its use as an outcome measure in clinical research (Bastien et al., 2001).

Pittsburgh Sleep Quality Index (PSQI)

The PSQI (Buysse, Reynolds, Monk, Berman, & Kupfer, 1989) is a self-rating scale that is frequently used to assess general sleep disturbances. The PSQI is composed of 19 self-rated items assessing sleep quality and disturbances over a 1-month interval. Aspects of sleep cov-

Please answer the following questions by using this scale and circling the appropriate number.

Not at all	Mild	Moderate	Severe	Very severe
0	1	2	3	4

1. Please rate the current SEVERITY of your insomnia problem(s):
   a. Difficulty falling asleep:

0	1	2	3	4

   b. Difficulty staying asleep:

0	1	2	3	4

   c. Problem waking up too early:

0	1	2	3	4

2. How satisfied/dissatisfied are you with your current sleep pattern?

Very satisfied		Moderately satisfied		Very dissatisfied
0	1	2	3	4

3. To what extent do you consider your sleep problem to INTERFERE with your daily functioning (e.g., daytime fatigue, ability to function at work/daily chores, concentration, memory, mood, etc.)?

Not at all	A little	Somewhat	Much	Very much
0	1	2	3	4

4. How NOTICEABLE to others do you think your sleeping problem is in terms of impairing the quality of your life?

Not at all	A little	Somewhat	Much	Very much
0	1	2	3	4

5. How CONCERNED are you about your current sleep problem?

Not at all	A little	Somewhat	Much	Very much
0	1	2	3	4

FIGURE 15.2. The Insomnia Severity Index. Adapted from Morin (1993). Copyright 1993 by The Guilford Press. Adapted by permission.

ered include subjective sleep quality, sleep latency, sleep duration, sleep efficiency, sleep disturbances, use of sleeping medication, and daytime dysfunction. A summation of these seven component scores yields a global score, ranging from 0 to 21, of sleep quality. The first four items are open-ended questions, while the remaining items are rated on a 4-point Likert scale, ranging from 0 to 3. Available psychometric data indicate high internal consistency (Cronbach's alpha = .83) and test–retest reliability ($r = .85$). It also discriminates well between poor and good sleepers (Buysse et al., 1989). The convergent validity with the ISI studied in a French Canadian sample has been found to be fair ($r = .44$) (Blais, Gendron, Mimeault, & Morin, 1997). A total PSQI score higher than 5 provides an effective screening tool for psychophysiological insomnia, with a sensitivity of 89.6% and a specificity of 86.5% (Buysse et al., 1989).

Dysfunctional Beliefs and Attitudes about Sleep Scale (DBAS)

The DBAS (Morin, 1994) is a 30-item self-report scale that is designed to assess sleep-related beliefs and attitudes that are believed to be instrumental in maintaining sleep difficulties (Morin, 1993; Morin, Savard, & Blais, 2000). The patient indicates the extent to which he or she agrees or disagrees with each statement on a visual analogue scale that ranges from 0 (strongly disagree) to 100 (strongly agree). Ratings are summed to yield a total score; a higher score suggests more dysfunctional beliefs and attitudes about sleep. The content of the items reflects several themes, such as faulty causal attributions (e.g., "I feel that insomnia is basically the result of aging"), misattribution or amplification of the perceived consequences of insomnia (e.g., "I am concerned that chronic insomnia may have serious consequences for my physical health"), unrealistic sleep requirement expectations (e.g., "I need 8 hours of sleep to feel refreshed and function well during the day"), diminished perception of control and predictability of sleep (e.g., "I am worried that I may lose control over my abilities to sleep"), and faulty beliefs about sleep-promoting practices (e.g., "When I have trouble getting to sleep, I should stay in bed and try harder"). Although initially designed as an assessment device to evaluate the severity of dysfunctional sleep cognitions, the DBAS is also a useful tool for clinicians to select relevant targets for cognitive therapy sessions. Initial psychometric data indicate that the DBAS has good internal consistency (Cronbach's alpha = .80) and an average item–total correlation of .37 (Morin, 1994; Morin, Stone, Trinkle, Mercer, & Remsberg, 1993). The DBAS discriminates well between good and poor sleepers (Morin et al., 1993) and is sensitive to clinical change following cognitive-behavioral therapy (Morin, Blais, & Savard, in press).

Arousal Predisposition Scale (APS)

The APS (Coren, 1988) is a 12-item self-report instrument that was designed to assess arousability as a relatively stable predisposition rather than as strictly limited to sleep time. It is a good predictor of sleep disturbance, but it has not been validated in a clinical population.

Sleep Hygiene Awareness and Practice Scale (SHAPS)

The SHAPS (Lacks & Rotert, 1986) is a 33-item scale that is useful for examining the role played by poor sleep hygiene in perpetuating insomnia. It measures whether an individual believes that various activities are beneficial, disruptive, or have no effect on sleep, and whether several foods, beverages, and nonprescription drugs contain caffeine. It also assesses the extent to which sleep is disturbed by environmental factors and the frequency with which individuals engage in poor sleep hygiene practices. To our knowledge, the psychometric properties of this scale have not been studied.

Pre-Sleep Arousal Scale (PSAS)

The PSAS is a 16-item self-report scale that was designed to assess cognitive (e.g., racing thoughts, worries) and somatic (e.g., heart racing, muscle tension) arousal states at bedtime. It yields two scores, measuring the relative contributions of intrusive cognitions and physiological factors to sleep-onset difficulties (Nicassio, Mendlowitz, Fussell, & Petras, 1985). Internal consistency of this scale is adequate for both subscales (Cronbach's alphas from .67 to .88), as is the temporal stability of the subscales (cognitive: $r = .72$; somatic: $r = .76$). The PSAS also successfully discriminates individuals with insomnia from normal sleepers. The

PSAS is correlated with a wide range of sleep variables, but most importantly with sleep-onset latency.

Advantages and Limitations

Self-report measures offer several practical and economical advantages for assessing sleep. They can easily be used in a variety of contexts to provide a global assessment of sleep difficulties and can be administered by untrained staff. They can also be administered repeatedly to measure the clinical changes that are associated with treatment. The most important limitation of self-report scales is their retrospective nature and their risk of recall biases. Typically, insomnia is present only some nights in a given week, even in individuals with chronic insomnia. Also, the nature and severity of sleep difficulties can vary considerably from night to night, which makes it difficult for the individual to retrospectively give precise information on these variables. Because individuals with insomnia are distressed by their sleep difficulties, they may tend to recall mostly those nights that were difficult, resulting in an overestimation of insomnia. Another limitation is that many of the paper-and-pencil instruments presented here have not been submitted to complete validation studies, so it remains uncertain whether they provide valid measures of insomnia and its associate features.

Mechanical Devices

Wrist Actigraphy

Wrist actigraphy devices provide measures of body movements. Essentially, a small sensing device that looks like a wristwatch is worn throughout the day and the night on the wrist (Hauri & Wisbey, 1992; Mullaney, Kripke, & Messin, 1980). This ambulatory monitoring system uses a microprocessor to record and store data along with actual clock time. Data are transferred and processed through microcomputer software, and an algorithm is used for estimating several sleep parameters. In good sleepers, estimates of sleep duration and total wake time are highly correlated with data from polysomnography. However, mixed results have been obtained in individuals with insomnia, with some studies showing a strong association (e.g., Kripke, Mullaney, Messin, & Wyborney, 1978) and others showing no association (e.g., Kupfer, Detre, Foster, Tucker, & Delgado, 1972) between wrist actigraphy and polysomnographic recordings. These discrepancies are particularly pronounced in insomniacs with low levels of activity while awake (e.g., depressed insomniacs).

Sleep Assessment Device

The Sleep Assessment Device (Lichstein, Nickel, Hoelscher, & Kelley, 1982) works by generating a brief, soft tone at fixed intervals (usually every 10 minutes) throughout the night. After each tone, a tape recorder is activated for 10 seconds and records the patient's verbal response. Absence of a verbal response ("I'm awake") is interpreted as evidence of sleep. This device yields measures of sleep-onset latency, number of awakenings, duration of awakenings, total wake time, and sleep efficiency. Studies comparing these estimates against polysomnographic evaluations have yielded excellent support for the validity of this device (Espie, Lindsay, & Espie, 1989; Lichstein, Hoelscher, Eakin, & Nickel, 1983; Lichstein & Johnson, 1991; Lichstein et al., 1982), although it tends to slightly underestimate wakefulness.

Switch-Activated Clock

The switch-activated clock consists of a remote hand-held switch that is connected to an electric or battery-operated clock (Franklin, 1981). A momentary switch connection is designed so that the clock runs only when pressure is applied to the switch level. On retiring to bed, the patient activates the clock by holding the switch in his or her hand and depressing the lever with the thumb. Relaxation of thumb pressure upon falling asleep releases the switch lever and automatically stops the clock, yielding a measure of sleep-onset latency. Validation of this device against polysomnographic measurement showed that the switch is released within 5 to 10 minutes of polysomnography-defined sleep onset, with the correspondence being closer to stage 2 than stage 1 sleep (Morin & Schoen, 1986; Viens, De Koninck, Van Den Bergen, Audet, & Christ, 1988).

Advantages and Limitations

These behavioral assessment devices offer several advantages. Because they are self-administered and do not require scoring by trained technicians, they are much less expensive than is polysomnography. Moreover, these measures are relatively unobtrusive and minimally affect the sleep process being measured. Finally, they have the marked advantage of measuring sleep in the natural environment, which is particularly important for assessing an environmentally conditioned problem such as insomnia. However, these mechanical devices do not provide measure of sleep stages and cannot detect more subtle changes in sleep such as microarousals. As is the case with polysomnography, these measures are not always readily available for clinical use. In addition, the convergent validity with polysomnography needs to be further investigated in the context of insomnia assessment (Sateia, Doghramji, Hauri, & Morin, 2000). Therefore, these devices should probably be viewed as a supplement to other measures.

Nocturnal Polysomnography

Laboratory Polysomnography

A polysomnographic evaluation involves all-night electrophysiological monitoring of sleep, as measured by electroencephalography (EEG), electrooculography (EOG), and electromyography (EMG). These three parameters provide the necessary information to distinguish sleep from wake and to determine the specific sleep stages. These three types of recording are generally sufficient for monitoring and scoring sleep patterns, but respiration, electrocardiogram, oxygen desaturation, and leg movements are also often assessed, at least during the first night, to detect the presence and severity of sleep pathologies other than insomnia (e.g., sleep apnea, periodic limb movement). For insomnia sufferers, a laboratory evaluation is helpful for assessing the nature and severity of the sleep problem and to provide data on the full range of sleep variables from sleep-onset latency to proportion of time spent in various sleep stages. It is also useful for determining the level of discrepancy between the subjective complaint and actual sleep disturbances, and it can have a therapeutic role in some cases by showing a patient that he or she is getting more sleep than actually perceived. In addition, EEG monitoring provides information about atypical polysomnographic features (e.g., alpha–delta sleep) that are otherwise undetectable. Finally, a laboratory setting provides an ideal opportunity for observing behaviors (e.g., body movements) and for monitoring physiological variables (e.g., frontalis EMG) that can yield important clues on the role played by physiological arousal in sleep disturbances. Although polysomnography has several utilities in the assessment of insomnia, its necessity has been questioned (Edinger et al., 1989; Jacobs, Reynolds, Kupfer, Lovin, & Ehrenpreis, 1988; Kales & Kales, 1984).

Ambulatory Polysomnography

Several ambulatory devices have been commercialized for conducting polysomnographic evaluations in the patient's natural environment. The typical portable recorder is self-contained and allows data storage throughout the night. Data are then transferred to a computer for analysis. Although a high concordance has been found between laboratory and home-based polysomnographic data (Ancoli-Israel, 1997), most validation studies have focused on the diagnosis of sleep-related respiratory disorders. Hence, the validity of home-based polysomnography in the assessment of insomnia remains to be demonstrated (Chesson et al., 2000).

Advantages and Limitations

Polysomnography is clearly the method that provides the most comprehensive assessment of sleep. It is the only sleep measure that allows quantification of sleep stages and can confirm or rule out the presence of another form of sleep pathology. However, although laboratory polysomnography is recognized as the "gold standard," it is not without limitations. Because it requires a sophisticated equipment and the presence of a trained technician throughout the night, nocturnal polysomnograpy is quite expensive, precluding its routine use. In addition, laboratory polysomnography is a fairly invasive assessment method that may cause reactivity. Because the individual is not in his or her natural environment, he or she may sleep differently in the laboratory, especially the first night (often called the "first-night effect"). The reactivity can be minimized by discarding the data from the first night of recording and using only the data from subsequent nights. Although outcome research on insomnia has mostly used two or three nights of polysomnography recordings, a recent study concluded that an entire week of recording was necessary to achieve adequate temporal stability of polysomnographic data (Wohlgemuth, Edinger, Fins, & Sullivan, 1999). Unfortunately, such a lengthy assessment is very costly, largely unpractical, and unacceptable to many patients.

Some of these disadvantages are circumvented by the use of ambulatory polysomnographic assessment in the patient's home, which facilitates repeated measurement, improves patients' acceptance, reduces the "first-night effect," and increases ecological validity. But, again, this does not represent the perfect alternative. The risk of artifacts and invalidation in some ambulatory studies is higher (e.g., there is no technician to correct problems that may arise during the night), and the lack of behavioral observations from technicians can make some records more difficult to interpret.

Summary

In this section, several methods of sleep assessment were presented, each with a description of the relative strengths and weaknesses. The choice of assessment strategies depends on the goal of the evaluation. A multifaceted assessment that combines a clinical interview to obtain a sleep history and the use of objective (e.g., polysomnography) and subjective (e.g., sleep diary, self-report scales) measures is ideal. However, polysomnography is not always necessary, especially when the clinician has no suspicion about the presence of an underlying sleep disorder such as sleep apnea.

PRACTICAL RECOMMENDATIONS FOR THE ASSESSMENT OF SLEEP DISORDERS

Distinguishing Insomnia from Other Sleep Disorders

When a patient presents in clinic with a chief complaint of insomnia, it is crucial to make a differential diagnosis with other sleep pathologies. No fewer than 88 distinct sleep–wake disorders, including 12 insomnia subtypes, are described in the most recent version of the ICSD (American Sleep Disorders Association, 1997). Several of these disorders can produce a subjective complaint of insomnia, including sleep apnea, periodic limb movements, restless legs syndrome, circadian rhythm disorders, parasomnias, and narcolepsy. Although a thorough clinical interview can help the clinician suspect the presence of such disorders, polysomnography is almost always necessary to confirm the diagnosis.

Sleep Apnea

Sleep apnea is a physical condition that is characterized by episodes of impaired breathing during sleep, although respiration is normal during wakefulness (Guilleminault, 1989). Sleep apnea is most frequently found in obese men between the ages of 30 and 60 years (Partinen, 1994; Young et al., 1993). Although sleep apnea is rare in young women, its prevalence increases in the postmenopausal years. Patients are often unaware of the main symptoms of apnea, which include loud snoring, pauses in breathing during sleep, and restless and fragmented sleep. These manifestations frequently lead to excessive daytime sleepiness, which is the typical complaint of patients with apnea. In some cases, prolonged respiratory pauses lead to nocturnal awakenings, another common complaint of these patients, and may be misdiagnosed as insomnia.

Restless Legs Syndrome

Insomnia should also be distinguished from the restless legs syndrome, which is described as an uncomfortable aching sensation in the legs. This sensation can occur during the day but is usually worse at bedtime and is accompanied by an irresistible urge to move the legs. It may also involve the thighs, feet, knees, and even the arms. Walking or stretching of the legs can alleviate this unpleasant sensation. Prolonged sleep-onset latency is a frequent consequence of restless legs syndrome, which may be confounded with insomnia. Most individuals with restless legs syndrome also present with periodic limb movements during sleep.

Periodic Limb Movements

Periodic limb movements (or nocturnal myoclonus) consist of repetitive, highly stereotyped movements of the limbs (legs and arms) that occurs during sleep, most commonly during the first third of the night. These movements are often associated with episodes of arousal, but not necessarily with full awakenings. Since the patient is often unaware of these movements, the bed partner is habitually the best source of information for assessing this disorder. Periodic limb movements must be distinguished from "hypnic jerk," which occurs at sleep onset (i.e., muscle contraction associated with a feeling of falling down a cliff) and from phasic limb twitches of rapid eye movement (REM) sleep, both of which are normal phenomena. The prevalence of this disorder increases with age and is higher in patients with chronic pain and renal diseases, as well as in patients with medical conditions that cause poor blood circulation (e.g., diabetes). The subjective complaints associated with periodic limb movements that may be confounded with insomnia manifestations include night-time awakenings and daytime sleepiness.

Circadian Rhythm Sleep Disorders

Circadian rhythm sleep disorders (CRSDs) comprise a variety of disorders that have in common a misalignment between the individual's endogenous sleep–wake rhythm and the sleep–wake schedule imposed on the individual by occupational and social demands. The resulting complaint is that the individual can neither sleep nor stay awake when he or she wishes or needs to do so. Estimates from clinical cases series suggest that CRSDs account for approximately 2% of all patients seen at sleep disorders centers (Coleman et al., 1982). These conditions are to be distinguished from insomnia because they may require different interventions (e.g., light therapy, chronotherapy). In the phase-delay syndrome, particularly frequent in college students and people working at night or on rotating shifts, sleep onset is delayed until late in the night (e.g., 3:00 A.M.). However, it is usually uninterrupted for the remainder of the night (Weitzman et al., 1981). In the phase-advanced syndrome, most commonly found in the elderly, the patient is unable to stay awake until the desired time in the evening, goes to bed early, and wakes early in the morning. However, total sleep duration is not shortened as it is in maintenance insomnia, which can sometimes be confounded with this syndrome.

Narcolepsy

Insomnia must also be distinguished from narcolepsy, which is characterized by excessive sleepiness, daytime napping, cataplexy, sleep paralysis, and hypnagogic hallucinations. Excessive daytime sleepiness is typically the first symptom to appear and usually develops during adolescence or young adulthood. Other symptoms of the disorder may develop several years after the onset of excessive daytime sleepiness, or not at all. Narcolepsy is a relatively rare hereditary condition, with about 1 case per 10,000 to 20,000 individuals, and a slightly higher prevalence among men than women (Guilleminault, 1994; Karacan & Howell, 1988).

Parasomnias

Finally, insomnia must be differentiated from parasomnia. Parasomnias are characterized by abnormal behaviors during sleep that are readily detectable and include sleepwalking, sleep talking, sleep terrors, nightmares, and sleep paralysis. Parasomnias do not necessarily lead to a complaint of insomnia, though in the most severe forms insomnia may be present.

Distinguishing between Primary and Secondary Insomnia

The distinction between primary and secondary insomnia is often a difficult task for the clinician. Primary insomnia is defined as a sleep problem with a predominant psychophysiological etiology, whereas secondary insomnia is established when the trouble sleeping is due to another psychiatric disorder (e.g., mood disorder), a medical illness, substance use, or another sleep disorder. Hence, the distinction between primary and secondary insomnia implies that the clinician is able to determine the underlying cause, a process that is often based more on clinical judgment than on objective findings. This task is rather straightforward when insomnia has a clear physical or environmental etiology but can become quite challenging when psychological disturbances are present. In the latter case, the clinician must determine whether these psychological disturbances represent causes or consequences of insomnia. It is also complex to determine whether insomnia is a pure physiological consequence of a medical illness or a psychological reaction to it. These difficulties probably explain in large part that only a moderate degree of concordance has been found between insomnia subgroups identified via an empirical cluster analysis and diagnostic subgroups as defined on the basis of either DSM or ICSD criteria (Edinger et al., 1996).

Primary Insomnia

Primary insomnia may co-occur with psychiatric or medical disorders, but it is viewed as an independent disorder that is etiologically unrelated to any other coexisting condition, including mood disturbances. Primary insomnia is fairly prevalent, inasmuch as approximately one in five patients who present to specialty sleep disorders centers seemingly meet criteria for this diagnosis (Buysse et al., 1994; Coleman et al., 1982).

According to the ICSD classification, there are three distinct types of primary insomnia: psychophysiological insomnia, subjective insomnia (or sleep state misperception), and idiopathic insomnia. Psychophysiological insomnia is the most common form; it affects about half of patients requiring treatment for insomnia (Morin, Stone, McDonald, & Jones, 1994). This disorder is believed to develop as the result of learned sleep-preventing associations—that is, conditioning between stimuli that are normally conducive to sleep (e.g., bed, bedroom) and sleeplessness. Another factor believed to be an important contributor is somatic tension, which leads to hyperarousal as bedtime approaches. A vicious cycle emerges in which repetitive unsuccessful sleep attempts reinforce the patient's anticipatory anxiety, which, in turn, leads to more insomnia. Through their repetitive association with unsuccessful sleep efforts, the bedroom environment and pre-sleep rituals often become cues or stimuli for poor sleep. In this type of primary insomnia, the complaint is corroborated by polysomnographic recording.

Conversely, in the sleep-state misperception disorder, the insomnia complaint, although genuine, is not corroborated by objective polysomnographic data. To some degree, all insomniacs tend to overestimate the time it takes them to fall asleep and to underestimate the time they actually sleep. However, in sleep-state misperception, the subjective complaint of poor sleep is clearly out of proportion with any objective finding. This disorder, also called subjective, pseudoinsomnia, or experiential insomnia, is often associated with more severe daytime sequelae compared to patients with psychophysiological insomnia. This disorder constitutes about 5% to 10% of all patients with insomnia (Coleman et al., 1982; Trinder, 1988; Zorick, Roth, Hartze, Piccione, & Stepanski, 1981). This condition is poorly understood, and there is controversy as to whether it should even be a separate diagnostic entity (McCall & Edinger, 1992; Trinder, 1988). First, most clinicians do not have access to polysomnography equipment to confirm or refute the patient's subjective complaint. Second, the mismatch between subjective and objective data may simply be due to the limits of current EEG technology, which is not sensitive enough to detect subtle brain wave patterns that are erroneously coded as sleep rather than wakefulness.

By definition, idiopathic insomnia is of unknown origin. It presents an insidious onset in childhood, is unrelated to psychological trauma or medical disorders, and has a chronic course throughout the adult life. It is one of the most persistent forms of insomnia and does not present the nightly variability observed with other forms of primary insomnia. A mild defect in basic neurological sleep–wake mechanisms may be a predisposing factor (Hauri & Olmstead, 1980). Idiopathic insomniacs tend to minimize the impact of disturbed sleep on their lives and display less psychological distress than patients with psychophysiological insomnia, even though their sleep is objectively more impaired (Hauri, 1983).

Secondary Insomnia

Insomnia can occur secondary to a variety of problems, including the other sleep disorders discussed here. Other conditions that may cause secondary insomnia are psychiatric disorders, medical conditions, and alcohol or drug use. Sleep disturbances are common clinical features of several psychiatric disorders. To diagnose insomnia secondary to another mental disorder, the sleep disturbance must be temporally and causally related to the underlying psychopathology and should be of sufficient concern to the patient to warrant a specific treatment. Estimates from clinical case series suggest that between 35% and 44% of patients presenting to sleep disorders centers with a complaint of insomnia meet diagnostic criteria for this disorder (Buysse et al., 1994; Coleman et al., 1982; Edinger et al., 1989). The most common diagnoses associated with insomnia are mood disorders (e.g., major depressive disorder, dysthymic disorder) and anxiety disorders (e.g., generalized anxiety disorder). Major depression and dysthymia are characterized by difficulty falling asleep, frequent or prolonged nocturnal awakenings, and premature awakening in the morning with an inability to resume sleep. Difficulties falling asleep and increased awakenings are also common in patients with anxiety disorders, including generalized anxiety disorder and obsessive–compulsive disorder. In panic disorder, panic attacks can arise from sleep and lead to insomnia symptoms, particularly sudden awakenings. Difficulties initiating sleep may also develop secondarily because of the anticipatory anxiety about having nocturnal panic attacks. Patients with posttraumatic stress disorder often experience various forms of sleep disturbances, including insomnia, nightmares, and sleep terrors.

A diagnosis of insomnia due to a general medical condition is established when the sleep disturbance is thought to be induced by a medical condition and when sleep difficulties are of such severity that they warrant separate clinical attention. Physical illnesses that may be etiologically responsible for insomnia include, but are not restricted to, cerebrovascular disease, congestive heart failures and chronic pulmonary diseases, degenerative neurological conditions, hyperthyroidism, gastrointestinal diseases, chronic bronchitis, and degenerative neurological conditions. Also, almost any condition that produces pain or physical discomfort is likely to cause insomnia. These conditions include low back pain, arthritis, osteoporosis, headaches, and cancer (Atkinson, Ancoli-Israel, Slater, Garfin, & Gillin, 1988; Pilowsky, Crettenden, & Townley, 1985; Savard & Morin, 2001; Wittig, Zorick, Blumer, Heilbroon, & Roth, 1982). Whenever possible, the insomnia treatment should first directly address the contributing medical condition in order to improve sleep (e.g., decrease pain by opioid use). However, a specific intervention is often necessary to treat residual insomnia symptoms.

Insomnia can also develop secondary to substance use or withdrawal. Substances that are likely to cause insomnia are alcohol, prescribed and over-the-counter medications, and illicit drugs. Substance-induced insomnia is often diagnosed concurrently with a DSM-IV substance use disorder diagnosis and is most frequently related to excessive use or abrupt discontinuation following regular use (i.e., rebound effect) of alcohol, sedative-hypnotic medications (e.g., benzodiazepines), and stimulants (e.g., amphetamines, cocaine, caffeine, nicotine). Between 4% (Buysse et al., 1994) and 12% (Zorick et al., 1981) of patients presenting to sleep disorders centers are diagnosed with a substance-induced sleep disorder.

Multistep Assessment Battery

The optimal insomnia assessment strategy combines the use of a clinical interview, sleep diary, self-report questionnaires, and polysomnography. Each of these methods is complementary to the others and provides information with some level of specificity and relevance for the selection of an appropriate treatment.

Usually, the assessment of insomnia begins with a clinical interview; the extent of this evaluation largely depends on the assessment context. For example, the interview is often more extensive when conducted in sleep disorders clinics than in primary care settings. A detailed clinical history is the most important component of the evaluation of insomnia. It should include information and questions about the nature of the sleep complaint; its duration, onset, and course; the presence of exacerbating and alleviating factors; the use of sleep aids; and prior treatment and outcomes. Ideally, at the end of interview, the clinician should have all information in his or her hands to determine whether the symptoms reported by the patient are more consistent with a diagnosis of insomnia than another sleep problem and whether the insomnia symptoms are primary or secondary to another disorder. To attain that goal, the clinical interview should include a specific assessment of medical and psychiatric comorbidity. The most valid and reliable strategy is to incorporate in the clinical interview some sections of a semistructured interview such as the Structured Clinical Interview for DSM-IV (SCID; First, Spitzer, Gibbon, & Williams, 1996). Another possibility, though not as effective, is to administer self-report questionnaires that were designed to screen for psychological disturbances. Instruments such as the Brief Symptom Inventory (BSI; Derogatis & Melisaratos, 1983), the Beck Depression Inventory–II (Beck, Steer, & Brown, 1996), and the State–Trait Anxiety Inventory (STAI; Spielberger, 1983) can yield valuable information about the presence of psychological symptomatology, although none of those instruments should be used alone to make a diagnosis.

A laboratory evaluation (i.e., polysomnogram) can provide very valuable information to determine the nature and severity of the sleep disturbances, but it is generally not indicated for the routine evaluation of insomnia (Sateia et al., 2000). However, a polysomnogram is essential to diagnose several other sleep disorders. Although insomnia may be the presenting complaint, the underlying problem may be another sleep disorder, unknown to the patient, that can only be detected by an overnight sleep laboratory evaluation.

Because diaries can provide valuable information across assessment and treatment settings, collection of daily data on a sleep diary should be initiated in all patients following the clinical interview, for a minimum of 2 weeks. In fact, sleep diaries can be completed throughout treatment as well to monitor sleep improvements and to guide the clinician in the application of treatment strategies. Finally, self-report questionnaires that assess the severity of insomnia or cognitive and behavioral aspects of insomnia can be added to the initial assessment battery to collect complementary information that is useful for tailoring insomnia interventions.

Procedural Problems and Potential Solutions

A potential problem encountered in the evaluation of insomnia is poor adherence to assessment procedures. This problem is particularly common when patients are asked to complete sleep diaries, which require some time and effort on a daily basis. One of the most common reasons reported by patients for not completing their diaries is forgetfulness. Other reasons frequently reported by patients include the fact that sleep diaries are too cumbersome or make them feel overly self-conscious. Consequently, patients may feel more anxious about their sleep difficulties, as a result of attempting to complete sleep diaries. Completing a daily sleep diary may produce anxiety, especially in patients with obsessive–compulsive personality traits who are excessively concerned about giving precise information about their sleep (e.g., estimating duration of nocturnal awakenings).

Various strategies can be applied to circumvent these barriers. Initially, the rationale for completing the sleep diary should be explained to the patient; it is also important to continue emphasizing the utility of this assessment method throughout the assessment and the treatment phase. This may be done by explaining the importance of quantifying the patient's sleep complaints, measuring day-to-day variations of his or her sleep difficulties, and evaluating the progress achieved with treatment. Otherwise, because the therapeutic gains generally occur gradually, patients may minimize the gains obtained from treatment. It is also essential to systematically review the sleep diary with the patient and to provide corrective feedback at each visit to ensure it is completed correctly and to maximize adherence to the monitoring procedure. Clinicians should remain alert to the possibility of retrospective assessment (e.g., completion of all the weekly diaries at the same time, just before the therapy session). The therapist should inspect the data carefully to detect any stereotyped pattern (i.e., no variations from night to night), and address any problems with the patient by emphasizing the importance of completing the diary each day. Another strategy is to require patients to mail, fax, or call in their diary data on a daily basis (Friedman, Bliwise, Yesavage, & Salom, 1991; Lacks, Bertelson, Gans, & Kunkel, 1983; Spielman, Saskin, & Thorpy, 1987), but this may not always be practical or readily accepted by patients. The perception of burden and anxiety can also be alleviated by explaining to the patients that rough estimations are sufficient. This suggestion is particularly important since, during the course of behavioral treatment, patients are discouraged to compulsively watch their bedroom clock during the night. Finally, patients should also be instructed to leave the sleep diary form in a place that will remind them to complete it upon waking each morning (e.g., near the bed, on the kitchen table). Reminders can also be placed elsewhere in the house (e.g., on the refrigerator).

Summary

The assessment of insomnia is much more challenging than it may appear at first. Because sleep difficulties can result from other sleep pathologies, psychiatric disorders, and medical conditions, a thorough evaluation is usually necessary. The differential diagnosis is more effectively achieved in the context of a clinical interview. Another essential part of the assessment battery is the use of daily sleep diaries, which allows quantification of the sleep complaint, the assessment of temporal fluctuations, and the monitoring of therapeutic gains throughout the treatment. The most common problem encountered in the assessment of insomnia is adherence to the evaluation protocol. However, this problem is usually easily circumvented by the implementation of several simple strategies.

INTEGRATING ASSESSMENT WITH TREATMENT PLANNING AND OUTCOME MEASUREMENT

Overview of Empirically Supported Treatments for Insomnia

Pharmacological Treatment

Hypnotic medication is by far the most commonly used treatment for insomnia. It includes benzodiazepines that are specifically marketed as hypnotics (e.g., flurazepam, temazepam, triazolam), several other benzodiazepines that are marketed as anxiolytics (e.g., lorazepam, clonazepam, oxazepam), and newer nonbenzodiazepine hypnotics (e.g., zolpidem, zopiclone, zaleplon). These latest medications have more selective or specific hypnotic effects and fewer residual effects the next day. Some antidepressant medications (those with sedating properties such as trazodone, amitriptyline, doxepin) can be of some utility in the treatment of insomnia in depressed patients, but more specific hypnotic agents or psychological interventions are often needed, especially when activating antidepressants are used such as selective serotonin reuptake inhibitors (e.g., fluoxetine [Rush et al., 1998]).

Placebo-controlled studies show that benzodiazepines are an efficacious treatment for the short-term management of insomnia, as indicated by reduced sleep latency, fewer awakenings, and increased total sleep duration and efficiency (Kupfer & Reynolds, 1997; Nowell et al., 1997; Parrino & Terzano, 1996; Roth & Roehrs, 1991). However, because placebo-controlled studies have typically not included follow-ups (median duration of treatment: 7 days), the long-term efficacy of hypnotic medications is unknown (Morin, 2001; Nowell et al., 1997). Furthermore, a recent meta-analysis of benzodiazepine efficacy suggests that benzodiazepines only improve sleep duration and that patients overestimate the efficacy of these medications (Holbrook, Crowther, Lotter, Cheng, & King, 2000). Specifically, results based on polysomnographic data showed that sleep latency was reduced by only 4 minutes, whereas total sleep duration was increased by 62 minutes. Subjective sleep latency was reduced by 14 minutes.

Moreover, the use of hypnotic medications is associated with a number of risks and limitations. Long-acting agents (e.g., flurazepam, quazepam) can produce residual effects the next day, including daytime drowsiness, dizziness or lightheadedness, and cognitive and psychomotor impairments (Hall, 1998; Holbrook et al., 2000). Because of their slower metabolism of medications, elderly people are more vulnerable to experience these effects. Elderly patients are also at greatest risk for falls and hip fractures when using long-acting hypnotics, compared to using short-acting medications or no medication at all (Ray, Griffin, & Downey, 1989). Benzodiazepines are also likely to cause or aggravate cognitive impairments in the elderly (Foy et al., 1995; Gray, Lai, & Larson, 1999; Tune & Bylsma, 1991). Other important limitations of hypnotic medications are their risks of tolerance (i.e., reduction of efficacy with prolonged usage and need to increase the dosage to maintain therapeutic effects) and dependence (particularly psychological dependence), which are associated with prolonged usage (Hall, 1998; Morin, 1993; Morin, 2001).

These limitations have led sleep experts to recommend using hypnotic medications primarily for situational insomnia and to use the lowest effective dosage of hypnotics for the shortest period of time. Treatment should start with a small dosage, with a subsequent gradual increase only if necessary. Generally, it is recommended that the treatment duration not exceed 4 weeks in order to avoid the development of tolerance and to minimize the risk of dependency. Then, if the problem persists or is recurrent, the main intervention should be non pharmacological, with hypnotic medication used only as adjunctive therapy (Morin, 2001; National Institutes of Health, 1996).

Psychological Therapies

Several nonpharmacological interventions have been used for the treatment of insomnia. Research efforts have been mainly devoted to evaluating the efficacy of behavioral and, more recently, cognitive-behavioral treatments. Two recent meta-analyses (based on approximately 60 studies) revealed that these interventions are efficacious for treating insomnia (Morin, Culbert, & Schwartz, 1994; Murtagh & Greenwood, 1995). The effect sizes fell in the moderate to large range, with larger therapeutic effects obtained for sleep-onset latency (0.87 and 0.88), ratings of sleep quality (0.94), and duration of awakenings (0.65), and medium-size effects obtained on total sleep time (0.42 and 0.49) and number of awakenings (0.53 and 0.63). Interestingly, the magnitude of these changes is comparable to those obtained with hypnotic medications (Nowell et al., 1997), and, overall, between 70% and 80% of patients benefit from psychological treatment. Sleep improvement derived from psychological management of insomnia is well maintained up to 24 months after the initial treatment.

Stimulus control, sleep restriction, and multimodal treatments (i.e., combining several approaches) have generally been found to be the most effective nondrug interventions, whereas education in sleep hygiene produces only modest gains when it is used alone (Morin, Culbert, & Schwartz, 1994). Other commonly used strategies include relaxation training and cognitive therapy. Relaxation procedures have been shown efficacious to treat insomnia (Lichstein, 2000); however, this procedure can sometimes have a paradoxical effect and exacerbate performance anxiety and insomnia. The efficacy of cognitive therapy as a single treatment for insomnia has never been evaluated, but studies that have incorporated this intervention into a multicomponent treatment have reported clinically meaningful therapeutic benefits (Morin et al., 2000). The goals and procedures of each of these interventions are described briefly in Table 15.2.

TABLE 15.2. Goals and Procedures of Commonly Used Psychological Treatments for Insomnia

Intervention	Goals	Procedures
Stimulus control therapy	Reassociate temporal (bedtime) and environmental (bed and bedroom) stimuli with rapid sleep onset; establish a regular circadian sleep–wake rhythm	Leave at least an hour to relax before going to bed; develop a ritual to do before going to bed; go to bed only when sleepy; when unable to fall asleep or go back to sleep within 15 to 20 minutes, get out of bed and leave the bedroom, and return to bed only when sleepy; maintain a regular time to get out of bed in the morning; use the bed/bedroom for sleep and sex only (do not watch TV, listen to the radio, eat, or read in the bed); do not nap during the day
Sleep restriction procedures	Curtail time in bed to the actual sleep time, thereby creating mild sleep deprivation, which results in more consolidated and more efficient sleep	Restrict the amount of time spent in bed to the actual amount of time asleep; time in bed is progressively increased as sleep efficiency improves
Relaxation training	Reduce somatic and cognitive arousal that interferes with sleep	Progressive muscle relaxation, autogenic training, biofeedback, imagery training, hypnosis, thought stopping
Cognitive therapy	Change dysfunctional beliefs and attitudes about sleep and insomnia that exacerbate emotional arousal, performance anxiety, and learned helplessness related to sleep (e.g., unrealistic expectations regarding sleep requirements, faulty appraisals of sleep difficulties, misattributions of daytime impairments, misconceptions about the causes of insomnia)	Identify sleep cognitive distortions (mainly by self-monitoring), challenge the validity of sleep cognitions (by using probing questions such as "What is the evidence that supports this idea? Is there an alternative explanation?"); reframe dysfunctional cognitions into more adaptive thoughts by using cognitive restructuring techniques (e.g., decatastrophizing, reattribution, reappraisal, and attention shifting)
Sleep hygiene education	Change health practices and environmental factors that interfere with sleep	Avoid stimulants (e.g., caffeine and nicotine) and alcohol around bedtime; do not eat heavy or spicy meals too close to bedtime; exercise regularly, but not too late in the evening; maintain a dark, quiet, and comfortable sleep environment

Summary

Medication is the most frequently used treatment for insomnia. Although it is a simple and often efficacious strategy, pharmacotherapy is associated with several limitations including potential residual effects the next day and the associated risks of tolerance and dependence. Cognitive-behavioral therapy has produced outcomes equivalent to those obtained with hypnotic medications, without their side effects. Moreover, there is evidence to suggest that the therapeutic gains derived from cognitive-behavioral therapy are well maintained over time, an effect that has not been documented yet with pharmacotherapy. The major limitation of cognitive-behavioral therapy is the need for the clinician to obtain specific training and the degree of commitment that is required from the patient during treatment, which may lead to adherence problems. The selection of a treatment for a given patient should take into account the advantages and limitations of both approaches and the patient's preferences. In addition, the clinician can attempt to match the intervention with the patient's characteristics, as will be discussed in the following section. Finally, cognitive-behavioral and pharmacological treatments are not mutually exclusive, and their combined use may represent an effective strategy (Morin, Colecchi, Stone, Sood, & Brink, 1999).

The Role of Assessment in Treatment Planning

Developing a Case Formulation

As mentioned earlier, a thorough evaluation of a sleep complaint is essential for accurate diagnosis and effective treatment planning. Ideally, treatment planning should be based on a well-defined case formulation that takes into account several factors, such as the nature and duration of the sleep complaint, as well as the types of precipitating, perpetuating, and exacerbating factors. The initial case formulation often needs to be modified, as additional information becomes available during the course of treatment.

Matching the Case Formulation with the Intervention

There is limited evidence regarding the direct link between assessment and treatment planning for insomnia. Most clinical studies of psychological interventions for insomnia have compared the relative efficacy of single or combined interventions. Only two studies have attempted to tailor treatment to patients' characteristics (i.e., relaxation with tensed patients and stimulus control for those with sleep incompatible activities), and the results have been equivocal. For example, Espie, Brooks, and Lindsay (1989) found that randomized treatment produced greater improvements in sleep than did treatment that was tailored to patients' characteristics. Sanavio (1988) found no differential improvements when patients with high tension level at baseline were assigned to EMG biofeedback treatment and patients with a high rate of intrusive thoughts were assigned to cognitive therapy, compared to mismatched conditions. Despite the equivocal evidence regarding tailored treatment approaches, it is unlikely that any single treatment will be effective with all patients and all insomnia subtypes. Effective clinical management of insomnia will often require the clinician's flexibility and a combination of different procedures. As most interventions are not incompatible with one another, treatments may need to be combined to optimize outcome.

Several general principles can guide practitioners as they select optimal treatment strategies. These guidelines are functions of several factors, including the nature (primary vs. secondary), duration (acute vs. chronic), and course of insomnia; the presence of comorbid psychological or medical conditions; the prior use of hypnotic medications; and the patient's treatment preference.

For acute and situational insomnia, treatment should focus first on alleviating the precipitating factors when possible (i.e., stress, medical illness). In some instances (e.g., bereavement, divorce, jet lag), a hypnotic medication may be necessary and very useful to alleviate sleep difficulties. For chronic and primary insomnia, cognitive-behavioral treatment should be the main intervention, with hypnotic medications serving as an adjunct.

The presence of comorbid medical or psychological disorders is another factor to consider when selecting the most appropriate treatment for insomnia. For instance, hypnotic medications are contraindicated during pregnancy, when there is a history of alcohol or substance abuse, and with patients who present with renal or hepatic diseases. When insomnia is associated with another form of psychopathology or with another medical condition, the general principle is to treat the underlying condition first. However, this is not always possible. Nor does this approach always resolve the concurrent sleep difficulties. For example, treatment of chronic pain or major depression does not always alleviate an associated sleep disturbance. In such instances, it may be necessary to add treatment (cognitive-behavioral or pharmacological) that focuses directly on the sleep disturbance.

Prior use of hypnotic drugs is another important consideration for selecting the most appropriate treatment for insomnia. Two different scenarios are likely to arise in clinical practice. The first one, most commonly encountered by psychologists, involves a patient who has already been using sleep medications for a prolonged period and is unable to discontinue their use. The most appropriate intervention for this type of hypnotic-dependent insomnia would involve a gradual tapering of the sleep medication, accompanied by cognitive-behavioral therapy. Another possible scenario is that of a patient who may have used hypnotic medications only infrequently or not at all in the past. In this case, a short-term trial on hypnotic medications could be useful during the initial course of treatment in order to provide some immediate relief and reduce performance anxiety. Cognitive-behavioral therapy would be initiated simultaneously and continued upon drug withdrawal.

The patient's preference is another important, although often neglected, factor for selecting among psychological and pharmacological therapies. Regardless of how effective a treatment is, if a patient fails to comply with the treatment regimen (because of side effects or for other reasons), this treatment will be of little benefit. Thus, if a patient is unwilling to use a sleep medication, behavioral interventions may be the only alternative available. Likewise, if a patient is unwilling to invest time and effort in a cognitive-behavioral approach, medication may be a better choice of treatment. Although cognitive-behavioral approaches are often more acceptable than medication to patients, this issue of treatment preference needs to be addressed systematically when discussing the various treatment options with a patient.

Assessing Progress throughout Treatment

It is essential to monitor progress throughout treatment. Although regular monitoring is most frequently used in the context of cognitive-behavioral interventions, it should also be standard procedure to adjust the hypnotic medication regimen. Relying exclusively on the patient's global and subjective report is inadequate because it is nonspecific and does not identify the particular sleep parameters that have improved, deteriorated, or remained unchanged. Also, in addition to a tendency to overestimate their sleep difficulties, patients with insomnia tend to underestimate their progress during treatment.

The best method to monitor progress throughout treatment is the daily sleep diary because of its flexibility (i.e., various variables can be evaluated) and its capacity to assess day-to-day symptom fluctuations. A daily sleep log is also very useful for monitoring adherence to behavioral treatment recommendations, such as sleep restriction procedures, stimulus-control instructions, and sleep hygiene education. Hence, it is possible to correlate treatment adherence with therapeutic outcome. For example, the sleep diary can reveal that a lack of improvement is due to noncompliance with treatment. Daily recording is also essential when using sleep restriction procedures to determine the patient's allowable time in bed. Self-report questionnaires such as the ISI and the PSQI are valuable complements to the daily sleep diary for periodic reevaluation of insomnia severity.

Evaluating Treatment Outcome

There is currently no consensus regarding how we should measure treatment effectiveness and what should be the optimal outcome when treating insomnia. Traditionally, investigators have focused exclusively on symptom reductions (e.g., reduction of the time required to fall asleep, frequency and duration of nocturnal awakenings, increase in the amount of total sleep time). The primary treatment goals are typically to reduce the time to fall asleep and the time awake after sleep onset below 30 minutes per night, to increase total sleep time to above 6½ hours, and to increase sleep efficiency to above 85%. Although these sleep indices are important for evaluating outcome, insomnia is more than just a complaint about poor sleep. It is often the emotional distress about sleep loss and its perceived consequences (e.g., fatigue, impaired daytime functioning), rather than insomnia per se, that prompts individuals to seek treatment. Thus, an important marker of progress should be the patient's degree of concern about sleep and his or her perception of control over sleep. Likewise, measures of functional impairment (fatigue, impaired concentration), mood disturbances, psychological well-being and quality of life, and even utilization of health-care services and hypnotic medications provide additional, clinically meaningful indices for measuring the impact of treatment.

ASSESSMENT OF INSOMNIA IN MANAGED CARE AND PRIMARY CARE SETTINGS

There is a significant gap between our current knowledge about assessment and treatment of insomnia and what is actually done in clinical practice. In this last section, we review several barriers to the assessment of insomnia in primary care settings, outline a brief assessment protocol, and discuss the main indications for referring patients to specialized sleep disorders centers.

Barriers to Insomnia Assessment

Potential barriers to insomnia assessment and treatment are related to the patient, to the clinician, or to the economic context (National Institutes of Health, 1996). First, there is often a stigma associated with acknowledging a sleep problem because it implies a loss of self-control over an important function. Some individuals are also reluctant to discuss sleep difficulties with their physician because they are concerned that the only recommendation will involve a prescription for sleeping pills. Likewise, some health care practitioners tend to ignore or minimize the effect of insomnia complaints, either because of lack of time or lack of training in sleep medicine. A comprehensive assessment of insomnia can be time-consuming, and some clinicians may be reluctant to ask questions about sleep. Also, because the effect of insomnia is not life threatening and is often less visible than is the effect of other health conditions (e.g., chronic pain), some practitioners may not see this problem as a priority, especially when it is part of a more complex medical problem. Another important barrier to assessment is reimbursement. Some insurance carriers still do not recognize insomnia as a condition that requires medical treatment, and, therefore, they do not reimburse for the assessment and treatment of this condition. Finally, very few health care practitioners, either in medicine or in clinical psychology, have received any formal training or even minimal exposure to the assessment and management of sleep disorders.

Streamlining the Assessment Procedure

Despite these barriers to assessing and treating insomnia, the evidence is increasingly clear that untreated insomnia may be a much more costly problem than that associated with treating this condition (Chilcott & Shapiro, 1996). For this reason, some inquiries about sleep should be an integral component of the assessment of any new patient evaluated for psychological or medical problems. Sleep is a basic need, similar to eating and drinking, and both its quality and duration can be affected by numerous psychological and medical problems. A complete sleep evaluation can be fairly time-consuming and should be reserved for those whose primary complaint is about sleep. For the majority of patients seen in primary care settings, insomnia is often part of a larger problem and it may not be always necessary to provide a thorough evaluation. A few key screening questions may be sufficient to gather critical information and make a preliminary decision about the need for further evaluation or treatment. Here are some of the key questions to ask as part of the initial clinical interview:

1. Have you had difficulties sleeping at night or staying awake in the day during the last month? If no, stop the sleep assessment.
2. What is the nature of the sleep complaint (i.e., problems sleeping at night, excessive sleepiness during the day, or abnormal behaviors during sleep)?
3. How long have these difficulties been present? If less than one month, keep monitoring.
4. What is the clinical significance of this problem (frequency, severity, and effect)?
5. Do the onset and course of this problem coincide with another medical or psychological problem? If yes, treat the underlying problem first, if possible.
6. Are there symptoms of other sleep disorders (e.g., sleep apnea, narcolepsy, restless legs syndrome)? If yes, refer to a sleep disorders center.

Completion of this screening assessment will usually take less than 10 minutes and is often sufficient to make a preliminary decision about the need for further evaluation, the need for insomnia-specific treatment, or referral to a sleep disorders center. In addition to this screening assessment, asking the patient to keep a sleep diary will provide valuable information about the nature, severity, and impact of the sleep problem.

Guidelines for Referral

In most cases, insomnia is a condition that can be effectively evaluated and treated in primary care settings (Walsh & Schweitzer, 1999). The main indications for referral to a sleep disorders center include the presence of symptoms suggesting sleep apnea (e.g., loud snoring, pauses in breathing during sleep, excessive daytime sleepiness), restless legs syndrome or periodic limb movements (e.g., restless legs, twitches or cramps in the legs at night), and narcolepsy (e.g., recurrent and unpredictable/uncontrollable sleep attacks). When the presenting complaint is excessive daytime sleepiness, referral to a sleep disorders center is also essential. In addition to a nocturnal polysomnogram, patients with excessive daytime sleepiness should undergo a multiple sleep latency test during the day. This test involves five 20-minute nap opportunities scheduled at 2-hour intervals throughout the day. The patient is asked to lie down in bed and simply try to go to sleep. The test is terminated at the end of 20 minutes, and the speed with which an individual falls asleep provides an objective measure of physiological sleepiness.

It may also be indicated to refer to a sleep clinic for a more thorough evaluation when the initial diagnosis is uncertain or when the initial treatment trial is unsuccessful. This evaluation might detect symptoms of another condition that were not captured during the initial clinical evaluation.

When referring to a sleep disorders center, it is important to inquire about the availability of a behavioral sleep medicine consultant to implement insomnia treatment. Because most sleep clinics are part of tertiary care centers, they may only have resources available to evaluate the sleep problem and treat some conditions such as sleep apnea and narcolepsy. Only a few centers have a behavioral sleep consultant specifically trained in treating insomnia. It is important to inquire about the availability of such resources if the referral is not only for evaluation but also for treatment of insomnia.

CONCLUSION

Insomnia is a prevalent complaint in primary care settings, and it is associated with significant psychosocial and health care costs (Ford & Kamerow, 1989; Simon & Von Korff, 1997). Paradoxically, insomnia complaints are often ignored or trivialized by practitioners and, consequently, this condition often remains untreated (Katz & McHorney, 1998). When treatment is indeed initiated, it is often based more on idiosyncratic factors such as the resources available in a clinical setting and the practitioner's training, rather than on evidence-based guidelines. Although significant advances have been made in the assessment and treatment of insomnia in the past decade, there is still a major gap between the knowledge available and its integration into current clinical practices. This chapter was designed to present empirically valid and clinically useful information to help clinicians use that knowledge more effectively in their daily practice to evaluate and treat patients with insomnia.

ACKNOWLEDGMENT

Preparation of this chapter was supported in part by grants from the Medical Research Council of Canada (No. MT-14039) and the National Institute of Mental Health (No. MH55469).

REFERENCES

American Psychiatric Association. (1994). *Diagnostic and statistical manual of mental disorders* (4th ed.). Washington, DC: Author.

American Sleep Disorders Association. (1997). *International classification of sleep disorders: Diagnostic and coding manual.* Rochester, MN: Author.

Ancoli-Israel, S. (1997). The polysomnogram. In M. R. Pressman & W. Orr (Eds.), *Understanding sleep: The evaluation and treatment of sleep disorders* (Vol. 1, pp. 177–191). Washington, DC: American Psychological Association.

Atkinson, J. H., Ancoli-Israel, S., Slater, M. A., Garfin, S. R., & Gillin, J. C. (1988). Subjective sleep disturbance in chronic back pain. *Clinical Journal of Pain, 4,* 225–232.

Bastien, C. H., & Morin, C. M. (2000). Familial incidence of insomnia. *Journal of Sleep Research, 9,* 1–6.

Bastien, C. H., Vallières, A., & Morin, C. M. (2001). Validation of the Insomnia Severity Index as an outcome measure for insomnia research. *Sleep Medicine, 2,* 297–307.

Beck, A. T., Steer, R. A., & Brown, G. K. (1996). *Beck Depression Inventory Manual* (2nd ed.). San Antonio, TX: Psychological Corporation.

Bixler, E. O., Kales, A., Leo, L. A., & Slye, T. (1973). A comparison of subjective estimates and objective sleep laboratory findings in insomniac patients. *Sleep Research, 2,* 143.

Bixler, E. O., Kales, A., & Soldatos, C. R. (1979). Sleep disorders encountered in medical practice: A national survey of physicians. *Behavioral Medicine, 6,* 1–6.

Blais, F. C., Gendron, L., Mimeault, V., & Morin, C. M. (1997). évaluation de l'insomnie: Validation de trois questionnaires. *L'Encéphale, 23,* 447–453.

Bootzin, R. R., & Engle-Friedman, M. (1981). The assessment of insomnia. *Behavioral Assessment, 3,* 107–126.

Breslau, N., Roth, T., Rosenthal, L., & Andreski, P. (1996). Sleep disturbance and psychiatric disorders: A longitudinal epidemiological study of young adults. *Biological Psychiatry, 39,* 411–418.

Buysse, D. J., Reynolds, C. F., Kupfer, D. J., Thorpy, M. J., Bixler, E., Manfredi, R., Kales, A., Vgontzas, A., Stepanski, E., Roth, T., Hauri, P., & Mesiano, D. (1994). Clinical diagnoses in 216 insomnia patients using the International Classification of Sleep Disorders (ICSD), DSM-IV and ICD-10 categories: A report from the APA/ NIMH DSM-IV field trial. *Sleep, 17,* 630–637.

Buysse, D. J., Reynolds, C. F., Monk, T. H., Berman, S. R., & Kupfer, D. J. (1989). The Pittsburgh Sleep Quality Index: A new instrument for psychiatric practice and research. *Psychiatry Research, 28,* 193–213.

Carskadon, M. A., Dement, W. C., Mitler, M. M., Guilleminault, C., Zarcone, V., & Spiegel, R. (1976). Self-report versus sleep laboratory findings in 122 drug-free subjects with complaints of insomnia. *American Journal of Psychiatry, 133,* 1382–1388.

Cernovsky, Z. Z. (1984). Life stress measures and reported frequency of sleep disorders. *Perceptual and Motor Skills, 58,* 39–49.

Chang, P. P., Ford, D. E., Mead, L. A., Cooper-Patrick, L., & Klag, M. J. (1997). Insomnia in young men and subsequent depression. *American Journal of Epidemiology, 146,* 105–114.

Chesson, A., Hartse, K., Anderson, W. M., Davila, D., Johnson, S., Littner, M., Wise, M., & Rafecas, J. (2000). Practice parameters for the evaluation of chronic insomnia. *Sleep, 23,* 237–241.

Chevalier, H., Los, F., Boichut, D., Bianchi, M., Nutt, D. J., Hajak, G., Hetta, J., Hoffmann, G., & Crowe, C. (1999). Evaluation of severe insomnia in the general population: Results of a European multinational survey. *Journal of Psychopharmacology, 13*(4, Suppl. 1), S21–S24.

Chilcott, L. A., & Shapiro, C. M. (1996). The socioeconomic impact of insomnia. *PharmacoEconomics, 10*(Suppl. 1), 1–14.

Coates, T. J., Killen, J. D., George, J., Marchini, E., Silverman, S., & Thoresen, C. (1982). Estimating sleep parameters: A multitrait–multimethod analysis. *Journal of Consulting and Clinical Psychology, 50,* 345–352.

Coleman, R. M., Roffwarg, H. P., Kennedy, S. J., Guilleminault, C., Cinque, J., Cohn, M. A., Karacan, I., Kupfer, D. J., Lemmi, H., Miles, L. E., Orr, W. C., Phillips, E. R., Roth, T., Sassin, J. F., Schmidt, H. S., Weitzman, E. D., & Dement, W. C. (1982). Sleep-wake disorders based on a polysomnographic diagnosis: A national cooperative study. *Journal of the American Medical Association, 247,* 997–1003.

Coren, S. (1988). Prediction of insomnia from arousability predisposition scores: Scale development and cross-validation. *Behaviour Research and Therapy, 26,* 415–420.

Cover, H., & Irwin, M. (1994). Immunity and depression: Insomnia, retardation, and reduction of natural killer cell activity. *Journal of Behavioral Medicine, 17,* 217–223.

Derogatis, L. R., & Melisaratos, N. (1983). The Brief Symptom Inventory: An introductory report. *Psychological Medicine, 13,* 595–605.

Edinger, J. D., Fins, A. I., Goeke, J. M., McMillan, D. K., Gersh, T. L., Krystal, A. D., & McCall, W. V. (1996). The empirical identification of insomnia subtypes: A cluster analytic approach. *Sleep, 19,* 398–411.

Edinger, J. D., Hoelscher, T. J., Webb, M. D., Marsh, G. R., Radtke, R. A., & Erwin, C. W. (1989). Polysomnographic assessment of DIMS: Empirical evaluation of its diagnostic value. *Sleep, 12,* 315–322.

Espie, C. A., Brooks, D. N., & Lindsay, W. R. (1989). An evaluation of tailored psychological treatment of insomnia. *Journal of Behavior Therapy and Experimental Psychiatry, 20,* 143–153.

Espie, C. A., Lindsay, W. R., & Espie, L. C. (1989). Use of the Sleep Assessment Device to validate insomniacs' self-report of sleep pattern. *Journal of Psychopathology and Behavioral Assessment, 11,* 71–79.

First, M., Spitzer, R. L., Gibbon, M., & Williams, J. B. W. (1996). *Structured Clinical Interview for DSM-IV Axis I Disorders—Patient Edition (SCID-I/P, Version 2.0).* New York: Biometrics Research Department, New York State Psychiatric Institute.

Ford, D. E., & Kamerow, D. B. (1989). Epidemiologic study of sleep disturbances and psychiatric disorders: An opportunity for prevention? *Journal of the American Medical Association, 262,* 1479–1484.

Foy, A., O'Connell, D., Henry, D., Kelly, J., Cocking, S., & Halliday, J. (1995). Benzodiazepine use as a cause of cognitive impairment in elderly hospital inpatients. *Journal of Gerontology, Series A, Biological Sciences and Medical Sciences, 50,* M99–M106.

Frankel, B. L., Coursey, R., Buchbinder, R., & Snyder, F. (1976). Recorded and reported sleep in primary chronic insomnia. *Archives of General Psychiatry, 33,* 615–623.

Franklin, J. (1981). The measurement of sleep onset latency in insomnia. *Behaviour Research and Therapy, 19,* 547–549.

Friedman, L., Bliwise, D. L., Yesavage, J. A., & Salom, S. R. (1991). A preliminary study comparing sleep restriction and relaxation treatments for insomnia in older adults. *Journal of Gerontology, 46,* 1–8.

Friedman, L., Brooks III, J. O., Bliwise, D. L., Yesavage, J. A., & Wicks, D. S. (1995). Perceptions of life stress and chronic insomnia in older adults. *Psychology and Aging, 10,* 352–357.

Gallup Organization. (1991). *Sleep in America.* Princeton, NJ: Author.

Gillin, J. C. (1998). Are sleep disturbances risk factors for anxiety, depressive and addictive disorders? *Acta Psychiatrica Scandinavica, 98*(Suppl. 393), 39–43.

Gislason, T., & Almqvist, M. (1987). Somatic diseases and sleep complaints: An epidemiological study of 3201 Swedish men. *Acta Medica Scandinavica, 221,* 475–481.

Gray, S. L., Lai, K. V., & Larson, E. B. (1999). Drug-induced cognition disorders in the elderly: Incidence prevention and management. *Drug Safety, 21,* 101–122.

Guilleminault, C. (1989). Clinical features and evaluation of obstructive sleep apnea. In M. H. Kryger, T. Roth, & W. C. Dement (Eds.), *Principles and practice of sleep medicine* (pp. 552–558). Philadelphia: Saunders.

Guilleminault, C. (1994). Narcolepsy syndrome. In M. H. Kryger, T. Roth, & W. C. Dement (Eds.), *Principles and practice of sleep medicine* (2nd ed., pp. 549–561). Philadelphia: Saunders.

Hall, N. (1998). Taking policy action to reduce benzodiazepine use and promote self-care among seniors. *Journal of Applied Gerontology, 17,* 318–351.

Hart, R. P., Morin, C. M., & Best, A. M. (1995). Neuropsychological performance in elderly insomnia patients. *Aging and Cognition, 2,* 268–278.

Hauri, P. J. (1983). A cluster analysis of insomnia. *Sleep, 6,* 326–338.

Hauri, P. J. (1997). Cognitive deficits in insomnia patients. *Acta Neurologica Belgica, 97,* 113–117.

Hauri, P. J., & Olmstead, E. M. (1980). Childhood-onset insomnia. *Sleep, 3,* 59–65.

Hauri, P. J., & Wisbey, J. (1992). Wrist actigraphy in insomnia. *Sleep, 15,* 293–301.

Healy, E. S., Kales, A., Monroe, L. J., Bixler, E. O., Chamberlin, K., & Soldatos, C. R. (1981). Onset of insomnia: Role of life-stress events. *Psychosomatic Medicine, 43,* 439–451.

Hoch, C. C., Dew, M. A., Reynolds III, C. F., Monk, T. H., Buysse, D. J., Houck, P. R., Machen, M., & Kupfer, D. J. (1994). A longitudinal study of laboratory- and diary-based sleep measures in healthy "Old Old" and "Young Old" volunteers. *Sleep, 17,* 489–496.

Hohagen, F., Kappler, C., Schramm, E., Riemann, D., Weyerer, S., & Berger, M. (1994). Sleep onset insomnia, sleep maintaining insomnia and insomnia with early morning awakening: Temporal stability of subtypes in a longitudinal study on general practice attenders. *Sleep, 17,* 551–554.

Holbrook, A. M., Crowther, R., Lotter, A., Cheng, C., & King, D. (2000). Meta-analysis of benzodi-azepine use in the treatment of insomnia. *Canadian Medical Association Journal, 162*, 225–233.

Irwin, M., Smith, T. L., & Gillin, J. C. (1992). Electroencephalographic sleep and natural killer activity in depressed patients and control subjects. *Psychosomatic Medicine, 54*, 10–21.

Jacobs, E. A., Reynolds, C. F., Kupfer, D. J., Lovin, P. A., & Ehrenpreis, A. B. (1988). The role of polysomnography in the differential diagnosis of chronic insomnia. *American Journal of Psychiatry, 145*, 346–349.

Kales, A., & Kales, J. D. (1984). *Evaluation and treatment of insomnia.* New York: Oxford University Press.

Kales, J. D., Kales, A., Bixler, E. O., Soldatos, C. R., Cadieux, R. J., Kashurba, G. J., & Vela-Bueno, A. (1984). Biopsychobehavioral correlates of insomnia: V. Clinical characteristics and behavioral correlates. *American Journal of Psychiatry, 141*, 1371–1376.

Karacan, I., & Howell, J. W. (1988). Narcolepsy. In R. L. Williams, I. Karacan, & C. A. Moore (Eds.), *Sleep disorders: Diagnosis and treatment* (pp. 87–108). New York: Wiley.

Karacan, I., Thornby, J., & William, R. (1983). Sleep disturbance: A community survey. In C. Guilleminault & E. Lugaresi (Eds.), *Sleep/wake disorders: Natural history, epidemiology, and long-term evolution* (pp. 37–60). New York: Raven.

Katz, D. A., & McHorney, C. A. (1998). Clinical correlates of insomnia in patients with chronic illness. *Archives of Internal Medicine, 158*, 1099–1107.

Kripke, D. F., Mullaney, D. J., Messin, S., & Wyborney, V. G. (1978). Wrist actigraphic measures of sleep and rhythms. *Electroencephalography and Clinical Neurophysiology, 44*, 674–676.

Kripke, D. F., Simons, R. N., Garfinkel, L., & Hammond, E. C. (1979). Short and long sleep and sleeping pills: Is increased mortality associated? *Archives of General Psychiatry, 36*, 102–116.

Krystal, A. D., Edinger, J., Wohlgemuth, W., & Marsh, G. R. (1998). Sleep in peri-menopausal and post-menopausal women. *Sleep Medicine Reviews, 2*, 243–253.

Kupfer, D. J., Detre, T. P., Foster, G., Tucker, G. J., & Delgado, J. (1972). The application of Delgado's telemetric mobility recorder for human studies. *Behavioral Biology, 7*, 585–590.

Kupfer, D. J., & Reynolds, C. R. (1997). Management of insomnia. *New England Journal of Medicine, 336*, 341–346.

Lacks, P. (1987). *Behavioral treatment of persistent insomnia.* New York: Pergamon.

Lacks, P., Bertelson, A. D., Gans, L., & Kunkel, J. (1983). The effectiveness of three behavioral treatments for different degrees of sleep onset insomnia. *Behavior Therapy, 14*, 593–605.

Lacks, P., & Morin, C. M. (1992). Recent advances in the assessement and treatment of insomnia. *Journal of Consulting and Clinical Psychology, 60*, 586–594.

Lacks, P., & Rotert, M. (1986). Knowledge and practice of sleep hygiene techniques in insomniacs and poor sleepers. *Behaviour Research and Therapy, 24*, 365–368.

Lichstein, K. L. (2000). Relaxation. In K. L. Lichstein & C. M. Morin (Eds.), *Treatment of late-life insomnia* (pp. 185–206). Thousand Oaks, CA: Sage.

Lichstein, K. L., Hoelscher, T. J., Eakin, T. L., & Nickel, R. (1983). Empirical sleep assessment in the home: A convenient, inexpensive approach. *Journal of Behavioral Assessment, 5*(2), 111–118.

Lichstein, K. L., & Johnson, R. S. (1991). Older adults' objective self-recording of sleep in the home. *Behavior Therapy, 22*, 531–548.

Lichstein, K. L., Means, M. K., Noe, S. L., & Aguillard, N. (1997). Fatigue and sleep disorders. *Behaviour Research and Therapy, 35*, 733–740.

Lichstein, K. L., Nickel, R., Hoelscher, T. J., & Kelley, J. E. (1982). Clinical validation of a sleep assessment device. *Behaviour Research and Therapy, 20*, 292–297.

Liljenberg, B., Almqvist, M., Hetta, J., Roos, B. E., & Agren, H. (1989). Age and the prevalence of insomnia in adulthood. *European Journal of Psychiatry, 3*, 5–12.

Livingston, G., Blizard, B., & Mann, A. (1993). Does sleep disturbance predict depression in elderly people? A study in inner London. *British Journal of General Practice, 43*, 445–448.

McCall, W. V., & Edinger, J. E. (1992). Subjective total insomnia: An example of sleep state misperception. *Sleep, 15*, 71–73.

Mellinger, G. D., Balter, M. B., & Uhlenhuth, E. H. (1985). Insomnia and its treatment: Prevalence and correlates. *Archives of General Psychiatry, 42*, 225–232.

Monroe, L. J. (1967). Psychological and physiological differences between good and poor sleepers. *Journal of Abnormal Psychology, 72,* 255–264.

Morgan, K., & Clarke, D. (1997). Risk factors for late-life insomnia in a representative general practice sample. *British Journal of General Practice, 47,* 166–169.

Morin, C. M. (1993). *Insomnia: Psychological assessment and management.* New York: Guilford Press.

Morin, C. M. (1994). Dysfunctional beliefs and attitudes about sleep: Preliminary scale development and description. *Behavior Therapist, 17,* 163–164.

Morin, C. M. (2001). Combined treatment of insomnia. In M. T. Sammons & N. B. Schmidt (Eds.), *Combined treatments for mental disorders: A guide to psychological and pharmacological interventions* (pp. 111–129). Washington, DC: American Psychological Association.

Morin, C. M., Blais, F. C., & Savard, J. (in press). Are changes in beliefs and attitudes about sleep related to sleep improvements in the treatment of insomnia? *Behavior Research and Therapy.*

Morin, C. M., Colecchi, C., Stone, J., Sood, R., & Brink, D. (1999). Behavioral and pharmacological therapies for late-life insomnia: A randomized controlled trial. *Journal of the American Medical Association, 281,* 991–999.

Morin, C. M., Culbert, J. P., & Schwartz, S. M. (1994). Nonpharmacological interventions for insomnia: A meta-analysis of treatment efficacy. *American Journal of Psychiatry, 151*(8), 1172–1180.

Morin, C. M., Savard, J., & Blais, F. C. (2000). Cognitive therapy for late-life insomnia. In K. L. Lichstein & C. M. Morin (Eds.), *Treatment of late-life insomnia* (pp. 207–230). Newbury Park, CA: Sage.

Morin, C. M., & Schoen, L. (1986, November). *Validation of an electromechanical timer to measure sleep/wake parameters.* Paper presented at the Association for Advancement of Behavior Therapy, Chicago, IL.

Morin, C. M., Stone, J., McDonald, K., & Jones, S. (1994). Psychological management of insomnia: A clinical replication series with 100 patients. *Behavior Therapy, 25,* 291–309.

Morin, C. M., Stone, J., Trinkle, D., Mercer, J., & Remsberg, S. (1993). Dysfunctional beliefs and attitudes about sleep among older adults with and without insomnia complaints. *Psychology and Aging, 8*(3), 463–467.

Morin, C. M., & Ware, J. C. (1996). Sleep and psychopathology. *Applied and Preventive Psychology, 5,* 211–224.

Mullaney, D. J., Kripke, D. F., & Messin, S. (1980). Wrist-actigraphic estimation of sleep time. *Sleep, 3,* 83–92.

Murtagh, D. R. R., & Greenwood, K. M. (1995). Identifying effective psychological treatments for insomnia: A meta-analysis. *Journal of Consulting and Clinical Psychology, 63,* 79–89.

National Institutes of Health. (1996). NIH releases statement on behavioral and relaxation approaches for chronic pain and insomnia. *American Family Physician, 53,* 1877–1880.

Nicassio, P. M., Mendlowitz, D. R., Fussell, J. J., & Petras, L. (1985). The phenomenology of the pre-sleep state: The development of the pre-sleep arousal scale. *Behaviour Research and Therapy, 23,* 263–271.

Nowell, P. D., Mazumdar, S., Buysse, D. J., Dew, M. A., Reynolds, C. F., & Kupfer, D. J. (1997). Benzodiazepines and zolpidem for chronic insomnia: A meta-analysis of treatment efficacy. *Journal of the American Medical Association, 278,* 2170–2177.

Ohayon, M. M., Caulet, M., & Lemoine, P. (1998). Comorbidity of mental and insomnia disorders in the general population. *Comprehensive Psychiatry, 39,* 185–197.

Ohayon, M. M., Caulet, M., Priest, R. G., & Guilleminault, C. (1997). DSM-IV and ICSD–90 insomnia symptoms and sleep dissatisfaction. *British Journal of Psychiatry, 171,* 382–388.

Ohayon, M. M., Guilleminault, C., Paiva, T., Priest, R. G., Rapoport, D. M., Sagales, T., Smirne, S., & Zulley, J. (1997). An international study on sleep disorders in the general population: Methodological aspects of the use of the Sleep-EVAL system. *Sleep, 20,* 1086–1092.

Parrino, L., & Terzano, M. G. (1996). Polysomnographic effects of hypnotic drugs: A review. *Psychopharmacology, 126,* 1–16.

Partinen, M. (1994). Epidemiology of sleep disorders. In M. H. Kryger, T. Roth, & W. C. Dement (Eds.), *Principles and practice of sleep medicine* (2nd ed., pp. 437–452). Philadelphia: Saunders.

Pilowsky, I., Crettenden, I., & Townley, M. (1985). Sleep disturbance in pain clinic patients. *Pain, 23,* 27–33.

Pressman, M. R., Gollomp, S., Benz, R. L., & Peterson, D. D. (1997). Sleep and sleep disorders in noncardiopulmonary medical disorders. In M. R. Pressman & W. C. Orr (Eds.), *Understanding sleep: The evaluation and treatment of sleep disorders* (pp. 371–384). Washington, DC: American Psychological Association.

Ray, W. A., Griffin, M. R., & Downey, W. (1989). Benzodiazepines of long and short elimination half-life and the risk of hip fracture. *Journal of the American Medical Association, 262,* 3303–3306.

Roth, T., & Roehrs, T. A. (1991). A review of the safety profiles of benzodiazepine hypnotics. *Journal of Clinical Psychiatry, 52,* 38–41.

Rush, A. J., Armitage, R., Gillin, J. C., Yonkers, K. A., Winokur, A., Moldofsky, H., Vogel, G. W., Kaplita, S. B., Fleming, J. B., Montplaisir, J., Erman, M. K., Albala, B. J., & McQuade, R. D. (1998). Comparative effects of nefazodone and fluoxetine on sleep in outpatients with major depressive disorder. *Biological Psychiatry, 44,* 3–14.

Sanavio, E. (1988). Pre-sleep cognitive intrusions and treatment of onset-insomnia. *Behaviour Research and Therapy, 26,* 451–459.

Sateia, M. J., Doghramji, K., Hauri, P. J., & Morin, C. M. (2000). Evaluation of chronic insomnia. *Sleep, 23,* 243–308.

Savard, J., Miller, S. M., Mills, M., O'Leary, A., Harding, H., Douglas, S. D., Mangan, C. E., Belch, R., & Winokur, A. (1999). Association between subjective sleep quality and depression on immunocompetence in low-income women at risk for cervical cancer. *Psychosomatic Medicine, 61,* 496–507.

Savard, J., & Morin, C. M. (2001). Insomnia in the context of cancer: A review of a neglected problem. *Journal of Clinical Oncology, 19,* 895–908.

Schramm, E., Hohagen, F., Grasshoff, U., Riemann, D., Hajak, G., Weeb, H.-G., & Berger, M. (1993). Test–retest reliability and validity of the structured interview for sleep disorders according to DSM-III-R. *American Journal of Psychiatry, 150,* 867–872.

Simon, G. E., & Von Korff, M. (1997). Prevalence, burden, and treatment of insomnia in primary care. *American Journal of Psychiatry, 154,* 1417–1423.

Spielberger, C. D. (1983). *Manual for the State–Trait Anxiety Inventory (Form Y).* Palo Alto, CA: Mind Garden.

Spielman, A. J., & Glovinsky, P. B. (1997). The diagnostic interview and differential diagnosis for complaints of insomnia. In M. R. Pressman & W. C. Orr (Eds.), *Understanding sleep: The evaluation and treatment of sleep disorders* (pp. 125–160). Washington, DC: American Psychological Association.

Spielman, A. J., Saskin, P., & Thorpy, M. J. (1987). Treatment of chronic insomnia by restriction of time in bed. *Sleep, 10,* 45–56.

Trinder, J. (1988). Subjective insomnia without objective findings: A pseudo diagnostic classification? *Psychological Bulletin, 103,* 87–94.

Tune, L. E., & Bylsma, F. W. (1991). Benzodiazepine-induced and anticholinergic-induced delirium in the elderly. *International Psychogeriatrics, 3,* 397–408.

Viens, M., De Koninck, J., Van Den Bergen, H., Audet, R., & Christ, G. (1988). A refined switch-activated time monitor for the measurement of sleep-onset latency. *Behaviour Research and Therapy, 26(3),* 271–273.

Vollrath, M., Wicki, W., & Angst, J. (1989). The Zurich study: VIII. Insomnia—Association with depression, anxiety, somatic syndromes, and course of insomnia. *European Archives of Psychiatry and Neurological Sciences, 239,* 113–124.

Walsh, J. K., & Schweitzer, P. K. (1999). Ten-year trends in the pharmacological treatment of insomnia. *Sleep, 22,* 371–375.

Weissman, M. M., Greenwald, S., Nino-Murcia, G., & Dement, W. C. (1997). The morbidity of insomnia uncomplicated by psychiatric disorders. *General Hospital Psychiatry, 19,* 245–250.

Weitzman, E. D., Czeisler, C. A., Coleman, R. M., Spielman, A. J., Zimmerman, J. C., Dement,

W. C., Richardson, G. S., & Pollack, C. P. (1981). Delayed sleep phase syndrome: A chronobiologic disorder with sleep onset insomnia. *Archives of General Psychiatry, 38,* 737–746.

Wingard, D. L., & Berkman, L. F. (1983). Mortality risk associated with sleeping patterns among adults. *Sleep, 6,* 102–107.

Wittig, R. M., Zorick, F. J., Blumer, D., Heilbroon, M., & Roth, R. (1982). Disturbed sleep in patients complaining of chronic pain. *Journal of Nervous and Mental Disease, 170,* 429–431.

Wohlgemuth, W. K., Edinger, J. D., Fins, A. I., & Sullivan, R. J. (1999). How many nights are enough? The short-term stability of sleep parameters in elderly insomniacs and normal sleepers. *Psychophysiology, 36,* 233–244.

Young, T., Palta, M., Dempsey, M., Skatrud, J., Weber, S., & Badr, S. (1993). Occurrence of sleep disordered breathing among middle-aged adults. *New England Journal of Medicine, 328,* 1230–1235.

Zammit, G. K., Weiner, J., Damato, N., Sillup, G. P., & McMillan, C. A. (1999). Quality of life in people with insomnia. *Sleep, 22*(Suppl. 2), S379–S385.

Zorick, F. J., Roth, T., Hartze, K. M., Piccione, P. M., & Stepanski, E. J. (1981). Evaluation and diagnosis of persistent insomnia. *American Journal of Psychiatry, 138,* 769–773.

Author Index

Subject Index